THE ROUTLEDGE COMPANION TO DIGITAL MEDIA AND CHILDREN

This companion presents the newest research in this important area, showcasing the huge diversity in children's relationships with digital media around the globe, and exploring the benefits, challenges, history, and emerging developments in the field.

Children are finding novel ways to express their passions and priorities through innovative uses of digital communication tools. This collection investigates and critiques the dynamism of children's lives online with contributions fielding both global and hyper-local issues, and bridging the wide spectrum of connected media created for and by children. From education to children's rights to cyberbullying and youth in challenging circumstances, the interdisciplinary approach ensures a careful, nuanced, multi-dimensional exploration of children's relationships with digital media.

Featuring a highly international range of case studies, perspectives, and socio-cultural contexts, *The Routledge Companion to Digital Media and Children* is the perfect reference tool for students and researchers of media and communication, family and technology studies, psychology, education, anthropology, and sociology, as well as interested teachers, policy makers, and parents.

Lelia Green is Professor of Communications at Edith Cowan University, Perth, Australia.

Donell Holloway is a Senior Research Fellow at Edith Cowan University, Perth, Australia.

Kylie Stevenson is a Research Associate and HDR Communication Adviser in the Centre for Learning and Teaching at Edith Cowan University, Perth, Australia.

Tama Leaver is an Associate Professor in Internet Studies at Curtin University, Perth, Australia.

Leslie Haddon is a Senior Researcher and Lecturer in the Department of Media and Communications at the London School of Economics and Political Science, London, UK.

THE ROUTLEDGE COMPANION TO DIGITAL MEDIA AND CHILDREN

Edited by Lelia Green, Donell Holloway, Kylie Stevenson, Tama Leaver, and Leslie Haddon

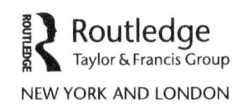

Routledge
Taylor & Francis Group
NEW YORK AND LONDON

First published 2021
by Routledge
52 Vanderbilt Avenue, New York, NY 10017

and by Routledge
2 Park Square, Milton Park, Abingdon, Oxon, OX14 4RN

Routledge is an imprint of the Taylor & Francis Group, an informa business

© 2021 Taylor & Francis

The right of Lelia Green, Donell Holloway, Kylie Stevenson, Tama Leaver, and Leslie Haddon to be identified as the authors of the editorial material, and of the authors for their individual chapters, has been asserted in accordance with sections 77 and 78 of the Copyright, Designs and Patents Act 1988.

All rights reserved. No part of this book may be reprinted or reproduced or utilised in any form or by any electronic, mechanical, or other means, now known or hereafter invented, including photocopying and recording, or in any information storage or retrieval system, without permission in writing from the publishers.

Trademark notice: Product or corporate names may be trademarks or registered trademarks, and are used only for identification and explanation without intent to infringe.

Library of Congress Cataloging-in-Publication Data
A catalog record for this title has been requested

ISBN: 978-1-138-54434-5 (hbk)
ISBN: 978-0-367-55906-9 (pbk)
ISBN: 978-1-351-00410-7 (ebk)

Typeset in Bembo
by River Editorial Ltd, Devon, UK

CONTENTS

List of Tables   x
List of Figures   xii
List of Contributors   xiii

Introduction: Children and Digital Media   1
Lelia Green, Donell Holloway, Kylie Stevenson, Tama Leaver, and Leslie Haddon

Acknowledgements   15

PART I
Creation of Knowledge   17

1. Child Studies Meets Digital Media: Rethinking the Paradigms   19
   Natalie Coulter

2. Engaging in Ethical Research Partnerships with Children and Families   28
   Madeleine Dobson

3. Platforms, Participation, and Place: Understanding Young People's Changing Digital Media Worlds   38
   Heather A. Horst and luke gaspard

4. Methodological Issues in Researching Children and Digital Media   48
   Rebekah Willett and Chris Richards

5. Young Learners in the Digital Age   57
   Christine Stephen

6. Children Who Code   67
   Jamie C. Macbeth, Michael J. Lee, Jung Soo Kim, and Tony Boming Zhang

7 Young Children's Creativity in Digital Possibility Spaces: What Might Posthumanism Reveal?   75
   Kylie J. Stevenson

8 The Domestication of Touchscreen Technologies in Families with Young Children   87
   Leslie Haddon

9 Grandparental Mediation of Children's Digital Media Use   96
   Nelly Elias, Dafna Lemish, and Galit Nimrod

PART II
Digital Media Lives   **109**

10 Young Children's Haptic Media Habitus   111
    Bjørn Nansen

11 Early Encounters with Narrative: Two-Year-Olds and Moving-Image Media   120
    Cary Bazalgette

12 Siblings Accomplishing Tasks Together: Solicited and Unsolicited Assistance When Using Digital Technology   130
    Sandy Houen, Susan Danby, and Pernilla Miller

13 Children as Architects of Their Digital Worlds   144
    Joanne O'Mara, Linda Laidlaw, and Suzanna So Har Wong

14 Teens' Online and Offline Lives: How They Are Experiencing Their Sociability   152
    Sara Pereira, Joana Fillol, and Pedro Moura

15 Teens' Fandom Communities: Making Friends and Countering Unwanted Contacts   161
    Julián de la Fuente and Pilar Lacasa

16 Identity Exploration in Anonymous Online Spaces   173
    Mary Anne Lauri and Lorleen Farrugia

17 Supervised Play: Intimate Surveillance and Children's Mobile Media Usage   185
    William Balmford, Larissa Hjorth, and Ingrid Richardson

18 Challenging Adolescents' Autonomy: An Affordances Perspective on Parental Tools   195
    Bieke Zaman, Marije Nouwen, and Karla Van Leeuwen

PART III
Complexities of Commodification   205

19 Children's Enrolment in Online Consumer Culture   207
    Ylva Ågren

20 The Emergence and Ethics of Child-Created Content as Media Industries   217
    Benjamin Burroughs and Gavin Feller

21 Pre-School Stars on YouTube: Child Microcelebrities, Commercially
    Viable Biographies, and Interactions with Technology   226
    Crystal Abidin

22 Balancing Privacy: Sharenting, Intimate Surveillance, and the Right to
    Be Forgotten   235
    Tama Leaver

23 Parenting Pedagogies in the Marketing of Children's Apps   245
    Donell Holloway, Giovanna Mascheroni, and Ashley Donkin

24 Digital Literacy/'Dynamic Literacies': Formal and Informal Learning Now
    and in the Emergent Future   256
    John Potter

25 Being and Not Being: 'Digital Tweens' in a Hybrid Culture   265
    Inês Vitorino Sampaio, Thinayna Máximo, and Cristina Ponte

26 "Technically They're Your Creations, but . . .": Children Making, Playing,
    and Negotiating User-Generated Content Games   275
    Sara M. Grimes and Vinca Merriman

27 Marketing to Children through Digital Media: Trends and Issues   285
    Wonsun Shin

PART IV
Children's Rights   295

28 Child-Centred Policy: Enfranchising Children as Digital Policy-Makers   297
    Brian O'Neill

29 Law, Digital Media, and the Discomfort of Children's Rights   308
    Brian Simpson

30 No Fixed Limits? The Uncomfortable Application of Inconsistent Law to
    the Lives of Children Dealing with Digital Media   318
    Brian Simpson

31	Children's Agency in the Media Socialisation Process *Claudia Riesmeyer*	327
32	Digital Citizenship in Domestic Contexts *Lelia Green*	337
33	Digital Socialising in Children on the Autism Spectrum *Meryl Alper and Madison Irons*	348
34	Disability, Children, and the Invention of Digital Media *Katie Ellis, Gerard Goggin, and Mike Kent*	358
35	Children's Moral Agency in the Digital Environment *Joke Bauwens and Lien Mostmans*	368
36	Children's Rights in the Digital Environment: A Challenging Terrain for Evidence-Based Policy *Sonia Livingstone, Amanda Third, and Gerison Lansdown*	378

PART V
Changing and Challenging Circumstances — 391

37	Caring Dataveillance: Women's Use of Apps to Monitor Pregnancy and Children *Deborah Lupton*	393
38	Digital Media and Sleep in Children *Alicia Allan and Simon Smith*	403
39	Sick Children and Social Media *Ana Jorge, Lidia Marôpo, and Raiana de Carvalho*	414
40	Children's Sexuality in the Context of Digital Media: Sexualisation, Sexting, and Experiences with Sexual Content in a Research Perspective *Liza Tsaliki and Despina Chronaki*	424
41	Digital Inequalities Amongst Digital Natives *Ellen J. Helsper*	435
42	Street Children and Social Media: Identity Construction in the Digital Age *Marcela Losantos Velasco, Lien Mostmans, and Guadalupe Peres-Cajías*	449
43	Perspectives on Cyberbullying and Traditional Bullying: Same or Different? *Robin M. Kowalski and Annie McCord*	460

44	Digital Storytelling: Opportunities for Identity Investment for Youth from Refugee Backgrounds *Lauren Johnson and Maureen Kendrick*	469
45	Children, Death, and Digital Media *Kathleen M. Cumiskey*	480

PART VI
Local Complexities in a Global Context — 489

46	Very Young Children's Digital Literacy: Engagement, Practices, Learning, and Home–School–Community Knowledge Exchange in Lisbon, Portugal *Vítor Tomé and Maria José Brites*	491
47	The Voices of African Children *Chika Anyanwu*	500
48	Limiting the Digital in Brazilian Schools: Structural Difficulties and School Culture *Daniela Costa and Juliana Doretto*	508
49	Australia and Consensual Sexting: The Creation of Child Pornography or Exploitation Materials? *Amy Shields Dobson*	518
50	Revisiting Children's Participation in Television: Implications for Digital Media Rights in Bangladesh *S M Shameem Reza and Ashfara Haque*	527
51	Chinese Teen Digital Entertainment: Rethinking Censorship and Commercialisation in Short Video and Online Fiction *Xiang Ren*	539
52	Sexual Images, Risk, and Perception among Youth: A Nordic Example *Elisabeth Staksrud*	549
53	US-Based Toy Unboxing Production in Children's Culture *Jarrod Walczer*	562
54	The Role of Digital Media in the Lives of Some American Muslim Children, 2010–2019 *Nahid Afrose Kabir*	572
	Index	*584*

TABLES

9.1	Grandparental mediation	102
9.2	Pearson's correlations between past and current involvement in mediation	104
12.1	Key transcription conventions employed in this chapter	133
14.1	Number and gender of the youngsters by school and class	154
16.1	Participants in interviews and focus groups	176
16.2	Motivations for using Ask.fm	177
16.3	Demographics of respondents	179
16.4	Estimated class shares	179
16.5	The four latent classes emerging from the model	180
16.6	poLCA logistic regression model with USE as a predictor of class membership	180
16.7	For each respective class, the probability that respondents are in that class if they are users/non-users of anonymous platforms	181
18.1	Conceptual comparison between parental mediation practices and parenting dimensions	196
23.1	Case study analysis of download pages (example)	249
41.1	Inequalities in potential and actual access (Europe)	438
41.2	Actualised access (UK)	439
41.3	Internet and smartphone skills (Europe)	439
41.4	Internet and smartphone skills (UK)	440
41.5	Online opportunities and risks (Europe)	441
41.6	Number of different activities undertaken monthly (UK)	441
41.7	Negative outcomes of internet and smartphone use (Europe)	442
41.8	Negative and positive outcomes of Internet use (UK)	443
50.1	Children's shows for analysis	533
52.1	EU Kids Online classification of online risks	550
52.2	Norwegian youth (15–17) definition of sexual content, in percentage (2018)	553
52.3	Where Norwegian children (9–17) have seen sexual content past 12 months (2018), by percentage	554
52.4	How Norwegian children felt after being exposed to sexual content online, by age and gender (2018)	555
52.5	Stated feelings of Norwegian children after seeing sexual images (on- or offline), by gender 2018	556

Tables

52.6	Intentionality of seeing sexual images online among Norwegian children, by gender (2018)	556
52.7	Parental awareness of children's experience with sexual images versus child's answer (Norwegian sample, 2018)	557
52.8	Risks Norwegian parents worry about a lot, as a percentage, according to child's gender and age (2018)	558
54.1	Participants, with pseudonyms, from Massachusetts, Michigan, New York, and Virginia, USA, aged 15–18 years. Interviews conducted in 2010* and 2016–2019^	574

FIGURES

9.1	Familiarity with children's media: mean scores	99
9.2	Attitudes toward children's media: mean scores	100
9.3	Involvement in mediation in the past (as parents): mean scores	103
12.1	Tina and Trae lying side by side playing with their own devices	133
12.2	Siblings playing a motion-sensor-based virtual tennis game	135
12.3	Siblings navigating YouTube Junior	139
12.4	Revisiting *Fragment 2*: the management and negotiation of assistance	141
16.1	Survey instrument investigating users' responses to platforms and apps that allow anonymous communication	178
38.1	Possible mechanisms for disruption to sleep onset from digital media	404
42.1	Joanna's Facebook post, 14 August 2018	453
42.2	Leonor's Facebook post, 21 March 2018	453
42.3	Natalia's Facebook post, 23 December 2018	454
42.4	A call for help. Facebook post, 9 December 2017	455
42.5	Street adolescent Facebook profile photo	456
42.6	Street adolescent Facebook profile photo	456
44.1	Somali refugee camp run by UNHCR. Young boy attending Koranic school holding a piece of wood inscribed with Koranic script. Moslem United Nations High Commissioner for Refugees	475
44.2	Mechanic in Hargeisa, Somaliland	475
44.3	The long hall and the clock tower of the UCC quadrangle	476
52.1	Logistic regression of probability for being bothered by seeing sexual images by age and gender (Norwegian Children, 2018)	555

CONTRIBUTORS

Crystal Abidin is Senior Research Fellow and ARC DECRA Fellow in Internet Studies at Curtin University, Australia. She is a socio-cultural anthropologist of vernacular internet cultures, particularly young people's relationships with internet celebrity, self-curation, and vulnerability. Her books include *Internet Celebrity: Understanding Fame Online* by Emerald Publishing and the co-authored *Instagram: Visual Social Media Cultures* by Polity Press. Her most recent publication is the co-edited *Mediated Interfaces: The Body on Social Media* by Bloomsbury Academic.

Ylva Ågren is Senior Lecturer in Child and Youth Studies in the Department of Education, Communication, and Learning at the University of Gothenburg, Sweden. Her research focusses on childhood in social media and children's interactions with electronic media in their everyday lives.

Alicia Allan is Research Fellow at the Institute for Social Science Research at The University of Queensland, Australia, and has multidisciplinary expertise in psychology, health, and design. Having received her PhD from Queensland University of Technology in 2016, her current research addresses how sleep occurs in context, particularly the environmental influences on sleep and wellbeing, sleep in the home setting, and the role of light environments in regulating sleep and wake.

Meryl Alper is Assistant Professor in the Department of Communication Studies at Northeastern University, Boston, Massachusetts, USA. She has extensive professional experience as a researcher, strategist, and consultant with Sesame Workshop, PBS Kids, Nickelodeon, and Disney, and her current research interests include the social and cultural implications of communication technologies, focussing on children and families' technology use. Alper has authored *Giving Voice: Mobile Communication, Disability, and Inequality* and *Digital Youth with Disabilities*, both published by MIT Press.

Chika Anyanwu is Associate Professor of Media and Research Associate at Hugo Centre for Migration and Population Research at the University of Adelaide, Australia. He is the Founding Partner of C3N2 Educational Empowerment, a social enterprise designed to empower people and institutions from emerging communities. He has received many awards, including the Leslie Humanities Cyberdisciplinarity Fellowship at Dartmouth, as well as holding a myriad of academic leadership positions across Australia and internationally.

Contributors

William Balmford is a sessional Lecturer in the Bachelor of Design (Games) program, member of the Digital Ethnographic Research Centre, and is part of the Design & Creative Practice Engaging Capabilities Platform at RMIT University, Australia. His research uses innovative ethnographic methods and an interdisciplinary approach to collaboration, and explores the impacts of domestic videogame and new media usage, with a keen interest in digital play, social exchange, and the relationship between device and person.

Joke Bauwens is Professor of Media and Communication Studies at Vrije Universiteit Brussel, Belgium, where she heads the research centre for Culture, Emancipation, Media and Society. Drawing upon sociological and philosophical approaches, her research interests and expertise include the social, cultural, and moral consequences of media. She has published on children's and young people's engagement with media, the relationship between digital media and morality, and the digitisation of media, culture, and social life.

Cary Bazalgette taught English in London schools in the 1960s and 1970s before joining the British Film Institute in 1979. As Head of BFI Education from 1999–2006 she led the development of new approaches to education about moving-image media for the 3–14 age group. In 2018 she completed her PhD at UCL Institute of Education, investigating how two-year-olds learn to understand moving-image media. She continues to research and write on this subject.

Maria José Brites is Associate Professor at the Lusófona University, Portugal, and researcher at CICANT. Her research interests include participatory methodologies, youth, journalism and participation, and civic literacy. She has coordinated and participated within a number of international projects and COST Actions, previously being the Portuguese coordinator of the Media In Action project and the RadioActive project. She is currently the Coordinator of the co-funded project Delinquency Centres with Digital and Civic Competencies.

Benjamin Burroughs is Assistant Professor of Emerging Media in the Hank Greenspun School of Journalism and Media Studies at the University of Nevada, Las Vegas (UNLV), USA. His research interests include streaming culture, media industries, and social media. His work has been published in journals including *New Media and Society*, *Journal of Broadcasting and Electronic Media*, and *Critical Studies in Media and Communication*.

Despina Chronaki is Adjunct Lecturer at the National and Kapodistrian University of Athens and the Hellenic Open University, Greece. Her research focusses on audiences of popular culture, media ethics, porn studies, sexuality, and children's experiences with media. For the past decade she has been collaborating with media scholars from around the world on a number of EU-funded Greek, European, and International projects and has presented her findings to international audiences.

Daniela Costa is Coordinator of a national Brazilian-based research project conducted by the Regional Centre for Studies on the Development of the Information Society, investigating the role of ICT in education. She has a PhD in Education from the Pontifical Catholic University of São Paulo and her research interests include education, children, technologies, and social participation.

Natalie Coulter is Associate Professor and Director of the Institute for Digital Literacies (IRDL) at York University, Toronto, Canada. Her research explores the promotional ecologies of children's media and entertainment. She is co-editor of *Youth Mediations and Affective Relations*, published by Palgrave Macmillan, and is author of *Tweening the Girl*, published by Peter Lang. She has been published in the *Journal of Consumer Culture*, *Girlhood Studies* and the *Journal of Children and Media*.

Kathleen M. Cumiskey is Professor of Psychology at the College of Staten Island, part of the City University of New York, USA. Her research examines mobile media, affect, intimacy and loss. Currently serving on the editorial board of *Mobile Media and Communication*, published by Sage, she has also authored numerous publications and companions, her most recent being *Mobile Media Practices, Presence and Politics: The Challenges of Being Seamlessly Mobile* published by Routledge.

Susan Danby is Professor in the Faculty of Education at Queensland University of Technology, Australia, and is Director of the Australian Research Council Centre of Excellence for the Digital Child (2020–2026). She has received an Honorary Doctorate in Education from Uppsala University, Sweden, recognising her leadership in child studies and young children's digital technologies. Her research areas include children's lives across home and school contexts, and in clinical and helpline settings.

Raiana de Carvalho is a PhD student in Mass Communications in the S.I. Newhouse School of Public Communications at Syracuse University, New York, USA. Her most recent research explores how social media and mass media impact the way people experience health and illness. She has been interested in studies on digital media, media and identity, children and media, health communication, and narrative studies.

Julián de la Fuente is Assistant Professor of Audiovisual Communication at the University of Alcalá, Spain. His research is multidisciplinary, sharing perspectives and approaches from psychology, anthropology, history, and sociology. Often collaborating with architects, engineers, and artists, he uses qualitative and ethnographic methodologies and the analysis of multimodal discourse. He has authored and co-authored numerous publications examining social media, technology, and young people's digital engagement. He has also conducted several outreach projects for film heritage.

Amy Shields Dobson is Lecturer in Internet Studies at Curtin University, Perth, Australia. Their work focusses on youth, gender politics, social media, and feminine subjectivities. They are the author of *Postfeminist Digital Cultures* and co-editor of *Digital Intimate Publics and Social Media*, both published by Palgrave Macmillan. Their most recent projects include research into cybersafety and sexting education, female genital cosmetic surgery, and girls' and young women's social media cultures.

Madeleine Dobson is Senior Lecturer and the Director of Student Experience and Community Engagement in the School of Education at Curtin University, Perth, Australia. Her research interests include media, digital technologies, social justice, children's rights, and resilience and wellbeing within educational contexts. As an advocate for participatory, ethically literate research that empowers participants to collaborate in the research process, she is particularly passionate about experiential research where participants' experiences and perspectives are elicited and honoured.

Ashley Donkin is a PhD candidate in the School of Arts and Humanities at Edith Cowan University, Perth, Australia. Her PhD is investigating the benefits and risks to 5–12-year-old

Australians whilst playing and socialising within online games that have social networking capabilities. She is also a trained high school teacher.

Juliana Doretto is Assistant Professor at the Postgraduate Program in Languages, Media and Arts at the Pontifical Catholic University of Campinas, Brazil. She has published her research on the relationship between journalism and children, specifically within a digital context, while her PhD in Communications from the Universidade NOVA de Lisboa focussed on the contact and engagement Brazilian and Portuguese youth had with the news and the participatory channels that journalist media can offer them.

Nelly Elias is Associate Professor in the Department of Communication Studies at Ben-Gurion University of the Negev, Israel. Her research focusses on psychological, sociological, and cultural aspects of media use in early childhood, including the media effects on parent–child relations and overall child development.

Katie Ellis is Professor and Director of the Centre for Culture and Technology at Curtin University, Australia. She has authored *Disability and Digital Television Cultures* published by Taylor & Francis, as well as having recently co-edited a number of publications including *The Routledge Companion to Disability and Media*, *Manifestos for the Future of Critical Disability Studies*, and *Interdisciplinary Approaches to Disability: Looking Towards the Future*, all published by Routledge.

Lorleen Farrugia is a PhD candidate, Visiting Lecturer, and Dissertation Supervisor within the Faculty for Social Wellbeing at the University of Malta. A member of the EU Kids Online research network, as well as a member of the Maltese Safer Internet Centre Advisory Board, BeSmartOnline!, her research interests include children, youth, risk, and new media. Her PhD is researching children's social representations of online risks.

Gavin Feller is a Postdoctoral Research Fellow in Digital Humanities at Umeå University, Sweden. His research uses the relationship between technology and culture to explore theoretical questions surrounding power, identity, and community.

Joana Fillol is a journalist and a PhD candidate in Communication Sciences in the Communication and Society Research Centre at the University of Minho, Portugal. Her PhD examines children, teenagers, and news, aiming to create a news outlet for and with this specific audience. As a journalist she has worked in various media and as a researcher she has been a part of the team of the European Project Transmedia Literacy.

luke gaspard is a post-doctoral researcher in the Department of Media and Communications at The University of Sydney, Australia. His research explores a range of digital youth practices centred around sociality and informal learning. Recent publications include "Australian high school students and their Internet use: perceptions of opportunities vs 'problematic situations'" in *Children Australia*, and the co-authored paper "Media practices of young Australians: tangible and measurable reflections on a digital divide" in the journal *Kome*.

Gerard Goggin is Wee Kim Wee Chair in Communication Studies at Nanyang Technological University, Singapore, and Professor of Media and Communications at the University of Sydney, Australia. He has a longstanding research interest in disability, media, technology, and culture. His publications include *Digital Disability* published by Rowman & Littlefield, *Disability and the*

Media published by Palgrave Macmillan, and the *Routledge Companion to Disability and Media* published by Routledge.

Lelia Green is Professor of Communications at Edith Cowan University, Perth, Australia, and ECU node leader and Chief Investigator with the Australian Research Council's (ARC) Centre of Excellence for the Digital Child. Researching children's lives in digital contexts for 20 years, Lelia has published more than 180 papers, written two books, and co-edited three more. Many of her publications have been grounded in work funded by the ARC and/or associated with the EU Kids Online project.

Sara M. Grimes is Director of the Knowledge Media Design Institute and Associate Professor in the Faculty of Information at the University of Toronto, Canada. Her research focusses on the intersection of children's media, culture, technology, and play. She has published widely on the commercialisation of children's digital play and creativity online, and the impact of intellectual property regimes on children's cultural rights. She was Principal Investigator of the Kids DIY Media Partnership.

Leslie Haddon is Senior Researcher and Lecturer in the Department of Media and Communications at the London School of Economics and Political Science, UK. Recently, his research has focussed on children's digital experiences, helping to co-ordinate the EU Kids Online project, and being on the team for the ARC Toddlers and Tablets project, which looked at smartphone and tablet use of 0–5 year olds. He has published numerous journal publications, book chapters, encyclopaedia entries, and books.

Ashfara Haque is a researcher and educator in media and communication. She has degrees in Communications from Edith Cowan University, Australia, and training in Media and Journalism from Scripps College of Communication, Ohio University, Ohio, USA. She specialises in children and media, media law and ethics, environmental communication, and broadcast journalism. She has published several articles in academic journals including *Media Asia*. She was a Fellow Broadcast Journalist at Deutsche Welle, Germany, and SUSI academic scholar in the USA.

Ellen J. Helsper is Professor in the Media and Communications Department at the London School of Economics and Political Science, UK. She is a Visiting Scholar at universities around the world, consults for intergovernmental organisations and NGOs on issues of participation and engagement in increasingly digital societies, and works in commercial audience research. Her research considers the links between social and digital inequalities and methodological innovation in quantitative and qualitative media and communications research.

Larissa Hjorth is Distinguished Professor at RMIT University, Australia, an artist, and digital ethnographer. She has two decades of experience working in cross-cultural, interdisciplinary, collaborative creative practice and socially innovative digital media research that explores intergenerational literacies around play and sociality. She is currently the Design & Creative Practice ECP Platform Director at RMIT. The Platform focusses on interdisciplinary collaboration and creative solutions to real-world problems, especially in relation to ageing well, through careful and multisensorial methods.

Donell Holloway is Senior Research Fellow at Edith Cowan University, Australia. She is currently Chief Investigator on three Australian Research Council grants: the ARC Centre of Excellence for the Digital Child; The Internet of Toys: benefits and risks of connected toys for children; and Toddlers and Tablets: exploring the risks and benefits 0–5s face online. Her research centres on the domestic context of children's media use for children and their families.

Heather A. Horst is Director of the Institute for Culture and Society at Western Sydney University, Australia. A sociocultural anthropologist by training, she researches material culture, mobility, and the mediation of social relations, through digital media and technology. Her most recent publication is *Location Technologies in International Context* published by Routledge, and she is co-editor of *The Moral Economy of Mobile Phones: Pacific Island Perspectives* published by ANU Press.

Sandy Houen is Senior Research Associate in the Faculty of Education at Queensland University of Technology, Australia. Her research interests include children's social interactions in home and classroom contexts, and early childhood education. Her PhD work has contributed fine-grained understandings of teacher–child interactions in prior-to-school settings and she has published numerous co-authored journal articles and conference papers.

Madison Irons is a 2018 graduate of Northeastern University, Boston, Massachusetts, USA, where she received a Bachelor in Communication Studies and a minor in English and Psychology. During her time at Northeastern she worked as a Special Events Assistant Manager for the Asperger/Autism Network.

Lauren Johnson works as an English language instructor in Manchester, UK, and develops arts-based community literacy programmes for newcomer youth. Completing a Master of Arts in Literacy Education at the University of British Columbia, Canada, her research focussed on multimodal approaches to literacy engagement with youth from refugee and immigrant backgrounds.

Ana Jorge is Research Coordinator at the Centre for Research in Applied Communication, Culture, and New Technologies at Lusófona University, Portugal. She has researched children and youth as media audiences, as objects of media representation, and as content producers, specifically in regards to the topic of celebrity and microcelebrity. She has co-edited *Digital Parenting* published by Nordicom, as well as a number of journal articles in *Celebrity Studies* and *Communications*, among others.

Nahid Afrose Kabir is Professor of History in the Department of English and Humanities, BRAC University, Bangladesh, a Visiting Researcher at Georgetown University, USA, and Adjunct Professor at Edith Cowan University and the University of South Australia, both in Australia. With publications in numerous peer-reviewed journals and edited collections, her recent books include *Muslim Americans: Debating the Notions of American and Un-American* published by Routledge, and *Young American Muslims: Dynamics of Identity* published by Edinburgh University Press.

Maureen Kendrick is Professor in the Department of Language and Literacy Education at the University of British Columbia, Canada. Having a keen interest in visual communication, her research examines literacy and multimodality as integrated communicative practices, specifically in marginalised populations in East Africa and Canada. She has authored and co-authored numerous journal articles and book chapters and has also co-edited volumes on youth literacies, and family and community literacies.

Mike Kent is Professor in the Centre for Culture and Technology at Curtin University, Australia. His research is centred on the intersections of disability, social media, and eLearning. He has authored, co-authored, and co-edited numerous publications, with his most recent being the co-edited *Manifestos for the Future of Critical Disability Studies* and *Interdisciplinary Approaches to Disability: Looking Towards the Future*, both published by Routledge.

Jung Soo Kim is a product owner with FactSet Research Systems, having received a Master of Science in Software Engineering and Computer Science from Fairfield University, Fairfield, Connecticut, USA. A two-time recipient of the Porter Academic Scholarship Award, she wrote her Master's thesis on the self-teaching experience of Gidget users in a CS101 course.

Robin M. Kowalski is Centennial Professor of Psychology at Clemson University, Clemson, South Carolina, USA. Her research addresses aversive interpersonal behaviours, notably complaining, teasing, and bullying, with a particular focus on cyberbullying. Named by *The Princeton Review* as one of the best 300 professors in the nation, she has received several awards including the Phil Prince Award for Excellence and Innovation in the Classroom, and Clemson Women's Commission Outstanding Female Faculty Member.

Pilar Lacasa is Emeritus Professor of Audiovisual Communication and Researcher in the Faculty of Humanities at the University of Alcalá, Spain. She has coordinated the Images, Word and Ideas Research Group since 1998 and has been a visiting researcher at universities across the globe. Pilar is the author of *Learning in Virtual and Real Worlds* published by Palgrave Macmillan and *Adolescent Fans: Practices, Discourses, Communities* published by Peter Lang.

Linda Laidlaw is Professor in Language and Literacy Education at the University of Alberta, Canada. Her research considers digital and mobile technologies in primary education, and she is particularly interested in the relationship between children's digital practices at home and their experiences at school. Her current projects, funded by the Social Sciences and Humanities Research Council of Canada, investigate new pedagogical frames and strategies for literacy education in a changing world.

Gerison Lansdown is an international consultant, having published and lectured widely on children's rights. Founder Director of the Children's Rights Alliance for England and former Vice Chair of UNICEF-UK, she currently chairs a number of advisory boards including Child to Child and the ODI Gender and Adolescence: Global Evidence Advisory Board. She is an Adjunct Professor at Carleton University, Ottawa, Canada, and is on the editorial advisory board of the *Canadian Journal of Children's Rights*.

Mary Anne Lauri is Professor in Psychology at the Faculty for Social Wellbeing at the University of Malta and is an active member of many voluntary, media, and political organisations. She has authored several works published in both Maltese and international journals. Her co-authored book *Exploring the Maltese Media Landscape*, published by Allied Publications, won a prize awarded by the National Book Council in Malta. She is a current member and researcher of the EU Kids Online network.

Tama Leaver is Associate Professor in Internet Studies at Curtin University in Perth, Australia. He is a Chief Investigator in the Australian Research Council Centre of Excellence for the Digital Child. His books include *Artificial Culture: Identity, Technology and Bodies* published by Routledge, the co-edited *Social, Casual and Mobile Games* published by Bloomsbury, and the co-authored *Instagram: Visual Social Media Cultures* published by Polity.

Contributors

Michael J. Lee is the Dorman-Bloom Assistant Professor of Informatics at the New Jersey Institute of Technology, Newark, New Jersey, USA, where he directs the Gidget Lab, which focusses on designing, creating, and testing technology-focussed educational tools. His research in computing education is funded by the National Science Foundation and Oculus Research, and has received numerous best paper awards. He holds a PhD in Information Science from the University of Washington, and a Master's from UC Berkeley.

Dafna Lemish is Distinguished Professor and Associate Dean of Programs at the School of Communication and Information at Rutgers University, New Jersey, USA. Founding editor of the *Journal of Children and Media*, and Fellow of the International Communication Association, her research specifically addresses children, media, and gender representations. One of her most recent publications is the co-authored *KakaoTalk and Facebook: Korean American Youth Constructing Hybrid Identities*, published by Peter Lang.

Sonia Livingstone (OBE) is Professor in the Department of Media and Communications at the London School of Economics and Political Science, UK. She researches young people's risks and opportunities, media literacy, and rights in the digital environment, and is the author of 20 books. Founder of the 33-country EU Kids Online research network, she currently directs the projects Children's Data and Privacy Online, Parenting for a Digital Future and Global Kids Online (with UNICEF).

Marcela Losantos Velasco is the Coordinator of the Research Institute of Behavioural Sciences at Universidad Católica Boliviana 'San Pablo', Bolivia, and has been Coordinator of the Alalay Foundation, which designs care intervention models for at-risk children and adolescents in Bolivia. Her PhD examined the permanence of children on the streets of La Paz in Bolivia and, in 2018, she received the Marie Curie Award from the National Science Academy for her work researching street children.

Deborah Lupton is SHARP Professor in the Faculty of Arts & Social Sciences at the University of NSW, Australia. Working in two research centres and leading the Vitalities Lab, she is author and co-author of 17 books. These include *Fat* (2nd edition), published by Routledge, and *Data Selves*, published by Polity. She is Fellow of the Academy of the Social Sciences in Australia, and Honorary Doctor of Social Science awarded by the University of Copenhagen.

Jamie C. Macbeth is Assistant Professor in the Department of Computer Science at Smith College, Northampton, Massachusetts, USA, and a Martin Luther King Jr. Visiting Scholar at the Massachusetts Institute of Technology. His research is focussed on building computing systems that demonstrate a human-like capability for in-depth understanding and production of natural language, and that thus can achieve richer interactions with human users.

Annie McCord is a Doctoral candidate in Industrial-Organizational Psychology at Clemson University, Clemson, South Carolina, USA. Her research addresses online communications and social psychology, and how these principles can apply to workplace incivility and counterproductive workplace behaviours. Annie has extensive knowledge of the literature pertaining to cyberbullying and workplace cyberincivility. She was awarded Master in General Experimental Psychology at Western Carolina University.

Lidia Marôpo is Assistant Professor at the Polytechnic Institute of Setubal, Portugal, and researcher at the Interdisciplinary Centre of Social Sciences at Nova University of Lisbon,

Portugal. Undertaking cross-national studies between Portugal and Brazil, her research addresses the relationship between young people and the news media, their reception of news content, and more broadly media and identity, audience studies, digital media, and digital media activism. She has published her findings both nationally and internationally.

Giovanna Mascheroni, PhD, is Associate Professor of Sociology of Media and Communication in the Department of Communication and Performing Arts, Università Cattolica of Milan, Italy. She is part of the EU Kids Online management team and WP6 leader in the H2020 project ySKILLS. Her work focusses on the social shaping and the social consequences of the internet, mobile media, and IoTs for children and young people, especially on datafication and its implications for digital citizenship.

Thinayna Máximo holds a Master's in Communication from the Federal University of Ceará, Brazil. Member of the Research Lab on Children, Youth and Media (LabGRIM), she researches the relationship that children have with the internet, especially social networking sites.

Vinca Merriman was primary research assistant on Children Making Games, a sub-project of the Kids DIY Media Partnership, providing game-related and child-centred insight into the 'do-it-yourself' media-making phenomenon. She also contributed to a global study of children's rights in the digital age led by Western Sydney University and the London School of Economics and Political Science. A Master of Information at the University of Toronto, Canada, she's currently an account manager at Ipsos Canada.

Pernilla Miller is a Research Associate in the Faculty of Education at Queensland University of Technology, Australia. She is a qualified primary school teacher who undertook the research pathway. Her research interests include pre-service teachers' global imagination, children's peer and sibling relationships, and children's digital lives.

Lien Mostmans is Research Advisor for Erasmus University College Brussels, Belgium, where she coordinates international research projects in the fields of children, education, and healthcare. Holding a PhD in Media and Communication Studies from Vrije Universiteit Brussels, she has extensive research experience in the field of children and media cultures, using a wide range of qualitative, such as ethnographic and visual, methodologies.

Pedro Moura is a PhD student in Communication Sciences at the University of Minho, Portugal, and a Researcher at the Communication and Society Research Centre. Part of the Portuguese team that participated in the European research project Transmedia Literacy, his research interests relate to media reception, transmedia storytelling, and media education and literacy. His PhD research project is focussed on the reception of transmedia narratives by young people.

Bjørn Nansen is a Senior Lecturer in Media and Communications at the University of Melbourne, Australia. He has published widely across studies of technology innovation and adoption, digital media industries, and cultural practices of media use in everyday and family life. His work often focusses on emerging and marginal digital practices, and is based in interdisciplinary approaches to research. His current projects investigate children's YouTube, digital memorialising, and sleep management technologies.

Galit Nimrod is Professor at the Department of Communication Studies and Research Fellow at the Center for Multidisciplinary Research in Aging at Ben-Gurion University of the Negev,

Israel. Aiming to contribute to the understanding of wellbeing in later life, she studies psychological and sociological aspects of leisure, media, and technology use among older adults. She has published extensively on this topic in leading scientific journals and has presented her studies at numerous international conferences.

Marije Nouwen is a researcher at the Meaningful Interactions Lab in the Institute for Media Studies at the KU Leuven, Belgium. She is pursuing a PhD degree in Social Sciences on the topic of playful tangible interactions between dislocated grandparents and grandchildren. She has worked previously on several research projects, primarily focussed on children and digital media.

Joanne O'Mara is Associate Professor in Language and Literature Education in the Faculty of Arts and Education at Deakin University, Australia. An experienced English and Drama teacher, she continues to work with young people through her university research, focussing on emergent literacies and new textual practices, digital games, and the spatial and social dimensions of teachers' work. Her research is dedicated to working in collaboration with students, teachers, schools, professional associations, and key education authorities.

Brian O'Neill is Director of Research at Technological University Dublin, Ireland. His research addresses youth and digital technologies, specifically online safety and policy for the digital environment. He has conducted research for the European Commission and UNICEF. He chairs the Steering Group of Media Literacy Ireland and is a member of Ireland's National Advisory Council for Online Safety. He co-authored *Towards a Better Internet for Children? Policy Pillars, Players and Paradoxes*, published by Nordicom.

Sara Pereira is Associate Professor at the Department of Communication Sciences and researcher at the Communication and Society Research Centre at the University of Minho, Portugal. Co-coordinator of the Observatory on Media and Information Literacy (MILObs), her research interests are children, young people and media, media literacy and education, and media audiences. She coordinated the Portuguese team of the European research project Transmedia Literacy.

Guadalupe Peres-Cajías is Head of the Communication Research Center at Cibescom-Universidad Católica Boliviana San Pablo, La Paz, Bolivia, and main editor of its journal. She is a PhD student of Communication Studies in the Vrije Universiteit Brussel, Belgium. Her research focusses on social and cultural processes, based on communication analysis and innovative methodologies. She published a book about festivities and youth identities in La Paz and Bogotá (PIEB-UCB) and writes regularly for two national newspapers, *Página-Siete* and *El-Deber*.

Cristina Ponte is Full Professor of Media and Journalism Studies and member of ICNOVA, at Universidade NOVA de Lisboa, Portugal. Her research examines children, youth and media, and media and generations, with a focus on the family, digital inclusion, media, journalism, and society.

John Potter is Associate Professor (Reader) in Media in Education at the University College London Institute of Education, UK. His research and publications focus on media education, new literacies, creative activity, and learner agency; teaching and learning responses to media technologies in formal and informal settings.

Xiang Ren is Research Fellow in Chinese Media and Culture at Western Sydney University, Australia, and a member of the Institute for Culture and Society and the Australia-China Institute for Arts and Culture. He has published widely on digital publishing, creative industries, and open knowledge. Working for over a decade in Chinese media industries, his current research focusses on the globalisation of Chinese digital popular culture in the fields of webnovel, short video, and live streaming.

S M Shameem Reza teaches Development Communication, Media Policy, and Public Communication at the University of Dhaka, Bangladesh, and was Ford Asia Fellow at IKMAS, Malaysia. His research and academic publications examine issues in young people and media, community broadcasting, media policy and regulations, NGO and media development, right to information, and environmental advocacy. As a communication consultant, he has worked for, among others, the World Bank, UNICEF, IFAD, BRAC, and Save the Children.

Chris Richards retired from the Institute of Education at the University of London in November 2013, having begun teaching in 1974 with Waltham Forest's West Indian Supplementary Service. He has authored three books, the most recent being *Young People, Popular Culture and Education* published by Bloomsbury. He has also co-edited *Children's Games in the New Media Age* published by Routledge and co-authored *Children, Media and Playground Cultures* published by Springer.

Ingrid Richardson is Professor of Digital Media in the School of Media and Communication at RMIT University, Melbourne, Australia. Interested in the 'human–technology relation', she has published widely on topics such as scientific technovision, virtual and augmented reality, games, mobile media and small-screen practices, and web-based content creation and distribution. She is co-author of both *Gaming in Social, Locative and Mobile Media* published by Palgrave Macmillan and *Ambient Play* published by MIT Press.

Claudia Riesmeyer is Research Associate in the Department of Media and Communication at the Ludwig-Maximilians-University Munich, Germany. Her research interests address the media socialisation process as an intergenerational project, media literacy, and qualitative research methods. She deals with the effects of media literacy, such as political participation, the recognition of dangerous content, or health communication, as well as the self-representation of children and adolescents on social networks.

Wonsun Shin is Senior Lecturer in Media and Communications at the University of Melbourne, Australia. Areas of research include youth and digital media, marketing communications, consumer socialisation, and parental mediation. Her work has been published in the *Journal of Children and Media* and *New Media and Society*, among others. She serves on the Editorial Review Boards of the *Journal of Advertising* and the *International Journal of Advertising*.

Brian Simpson was formerly Professor of Law in the School of Law, University of New England, Australia. Before retiring he taught child and family law for more than 30 years in both Australia and the UK. His research has been interdisciplinary, focussing on children's rights, law and new technologies, and urban justice. He continues to co-convene the IT Law and Cyberspace stream at the UK Socio-Legal Studies Association Annual Conference.

Simon Smith is Professor of Sleep and Health in the Institute for Social Science Research at the University of Queensland, Australia. He is a clinical neuropsychologist and has published widely on sleep, circadian rhythms, health, and social context across the lifespan.

Elisabeth Staksrud is Professor at the Department of Media and Communication, University of Oslo, Norway. She is part of the management team of the EU Kids Online project, and chair of the ECREA Children, Youth and Media section. Her research interests examine children and online risk and opportunities, including rights-based issues and transgressive online behaviour, freedom of expression and media censorship, and research ethics.

Christine Stephen was a research fellow at the University of Stirling, Scotland, and has recently retired. Her research concerns young children's learning and the ways in which this is supported at home and in educational settings, and the influence of culture and children's everyday experiences. She has co-directed a series of studies of young children's engagement with digital technologies, has published many journal articles, and co-authored two books about growing up with new technologies.

Kylie J. Stevenson, PhD, is an interdisciplinary researcher and HDR Communications Adviser in the Centre for Learning and Teaching at Edith Cowan University, Perth, Australia. Her research spans children and technology, creativity and reflective practice, arts education, higher degree by research pedagogy, and experiences of welfare dependency. Previously a Research Associate on several Australian Research Council grants, she has authored over 20 articles and book chapters. An accomplished poet, Kylie has two collections published in anthologies.

Amanda Third is Professorial Research Fellow in the Institute for Culture and Society and Co-Director of the Young and Resilient Research Centre at Western Sydney University, Australia. Researching technology practices of marginalised youth through rights-based and intergenerational approaches, she also co-directs the Intergener8 Living Lab, and is a Program Co-Leader in the Centre for Resilient Communities and Inclusive Societies. She recently led the authorship of *Young People in Digital Society: Control/Shift* published by Palgrave Macmillan.

Vítor Tomé is Assistant Professor at the Autonoma University of Lisbon, Portugal, Researcher at the University Institute of Lisbon, and a professional journalist. He is involved in numerous international projects, including as International Expert for Digital Citizenship Education (DCE) for the Council of Europe, International Advisor for DCE in General Education (Shota Rustaveli National Science Foundation of Georgia), Scientific Coordinator for the Portuguese Ministry of Education, and Coordinator of the Digital Citizenship Academy (Lisbon area).

Liza Tsaliki is Associate Professor in the Department of Communication and Media Studies at the National and Kapodistrian University of Athens, Greece. Investigating teens' access to sexual content across four countries, her research spans political engagement and participation, celebrity culture and activism, gender and technology, porn studies, children, youth and sexualisation. She is commentaries editor for *The International Journal of Media and Cultural Politics* and editorial board member of *Convergence* and *Information, Communication and Society*.

Karla Van Leeuwen is Professor in Family Studies at the Faculty of Psychology and Educational Sciences at KU Leuven, Belgium. Affiliated with the Parenting and Special Education Research Unit, she conducts research on child/adolescent characteristics such as temperament, personality, and genes, as well as environment (parenting) interactions in the prediction of child/adolescent outcome, assessment of parenting, differential parenting, co-parenting, parenting of children with special needs, and evaluation of parenting support programmes.

Inês Vitorino Sampaio is Associate Professor of Communication Sciences and a member of the Research Lab on Children, Youth and Media (LabGRIM) at the Institute of Culture and Art, Federal University of Ceará, Brazil. Her research focusses on children, youth and media, digital cultures and advertising with a background in sociology and communication. Her research has been published in numerous international journals, including *Communication Studies* and the *Journal of Communication Studies*.

Jarrod Walczer is pursuing his PhD in Media and Communications at the Queensland University of Technology's Digital Media Research Centre, Australia. Fusing cultural studies with digital methods, he explores the impact that toy unboxing creator culture on YouTube has had on the children's media industry in the US. He received his Master of Arts from the University of Southern California and his Master of Science from the London School of Economics and Political Science.

Rebekah Willett is Associate Professor in the Information School at the University of Wisconsin-Madison, USA. She has conducted research on children's media cultures, focussing on issues of play, literacy, identity, and learning. Her publications investigate makerspaces, playground games, amateur camcorder cultures, families' screen media practices, and children's story writing. She has numerous publications in journals of education and childhood studies, among others, and has co-authored and edited five books.

Suzanna So Har Wong is Adjunct Professor and Lecturer in Elementary Education, Language and Literacy at the University of Alberta, Canada. Her research focusses on young children's home digital literacy practices and the connections between literacy learning and makerspaces in elementary classrooms. She worked with researchers across the world during her Postdoctoral Fellowship. She is currently a Research Collaborator in a 'maker literacies' project funded by the Social Sciences and Humanities Research Council of Canada.

Bieke Zaman is Associate Professor and Head of the Meaningful Interactions Lab at KU Leuven, Belgium. Her research addresses the intersection of Communication Sciences and Human–Computer Interaction research. She conducts research on children and technologies, player–computer interaction, and progressive research and dissemination methods.

Tony Boming Zhang is a Bay State Master Student at the University of Massachusetts, Boston, USA, majoring in computer science. His current research is about science learning and educational games. He was previously a summer camp instructor with iD Tech Camps in Amherst, where he taught coding and machine learning to children aged 13 to 17.

INTRODUCTION
Children and Digital Media

Lelia Green, Donell Holloway, Kylie Stevenson, Tama Leaver, and Leslie Haddon

Children continuously reinvent digital technologies in ways that serve their purposes and passions. From cheap text messages that innovated with a language of their own, to today's child-led political activism using digital connectivity, under-18s have challenged the status quo and claimed new spaces of agency and authority. In doing this, children have encountered risks, and sometimes harm; and taken opportunities and experienced benefits while resetting adults' priorities in their families, their localities, and across the world. This book explores these dynamics and the multi-faceted nature of children's complex and evolving relationships with digital media.

Divided into six parts, *The Routledge Companion to Digital Media and Children* provides insights into the digital lives of under-18s around the globe, in good circumstances and in challenging situations. It also considers the many ways in which adults construct and understand children's lives; and the activities and wellbeing of the young people they care for, create policy about, and seek to support. Drawing upon children's voices and perspectives, the 54 chapters include content from six of the seven continents, and from a wide variety of disciplinary perspectives.

Part I, the Creation of Knowledge, introduces the collection by examining the ways in which researchers work with and alongside children to construct the data which informs understandings of children's interactions with digital media. It also begins the exploration of how children learn through their uses of information and communication technologies. Digital Media Lives, Part II, interrogates children's use of digital media in the active embrace of opportunities for agency. It also considers how young people teach each other about technology use and connected sociability, and parents' engagement with children through mediation and via caring, intimate surveillance. Part III, Complexities of Commodification, centrally addresses the challenges posed by patterns of profit-making that construct children as consumers and as target markets; and which monetise young people's activities and data.

The second half of the book turns from the objectification of children by industry and markets to the acknowledgement of children as global citizens, as young people with rights. Part IV, Children's Rights, acknowledges a conversation which reached a crucial turning point in 1989 with the promulgations of the United Nations Convention on the Rights of the Child, currently being revisited with specific reference to the digital environment. Changing and Challenging Circumstances, Part V, examines children's digital media use across a range of contexts, some of which highlight gross inequalities in children's access. The final section, Part VI, addresses Local Complexities in a Global Context, highlighting the diversity of the ways in which children's digital culture is manifest around the globe. Each of these parts will be briefly introduced and discussed in the remainder of this Introduction, which concludes with observations about digital media and the children who use it, alongside those children who can't or don't have access.

PART I: Creation of Knowledge

Natalie Coulter starts the collection (Chapter 1) by considering a range of ways in which social and cultural discourse constructs the notion of the child, children, and childhood. Her contribution, Child Studies Meets Digital Media: Rethinking the Paradigms, provides the *Companion* with a starting point which is subsequently developed through and across other chapters. Coulter highlights the ways in which (mainly) adults construct the idea of the child, and notes that these constructions reflect the specifics of a social, technological, political, and cultural moment in time. Within that discursive space, the notions of the child circulating in and through culture nonetheless have implications for the opportunities enjoyed by actual children in their everyday uses of digital media, while influencing the future opportunities available to young people in connected space. In addition to recognising the importance of the everyday construction of the child, conversations about children and digital media are often replete with hopes, fears, and judgements. Further, such discussions frequently include ethical dimensions. It is to this aspect of digital media and children that Madeleine Dobson turns in Chapter 2, Engaging in Ethical Research Partnerships with Children and Families. Using the United Nations Convention on the Rights of the Child (UNCRC) as a litmus test for researchers' approaches to children and their data, Dobson argues that children are citizens from birth and deserving of engaged research practices that are democratic, inclusive, and empowering. Eschewing one-dimensional and one-way research, where the power is almost entirely in the hands of the researcher, the chapter demonstrates that not only is it possible to build reciprocal inclusive research partnerships with children and their families, but it leads to better research and more reliable outcomes.

In Platforms, Participation, and Place: Understanding Young People's Changing Digital Media Worlds (Chapter 3), Heather Horst and luke gaspard identify three critical aspects of young people's digital media activities that enable and support participatory culture. The authors argue that the challenges and opportunities provided by these lenses for viewing digital culture are not mutually exclusive but mutually constitutive, building upon one another while delineating how young people understand and engage in dynamic media landscapes. This chapter critically engages with any assumption that digital media is available to young people for them to mould as they wish, according to their choices. The intersections of platforms, participation, and place highlight how commercial interests and technical infrastructure remain determining factors of much of the inequality that characterises children's digital media experiences around the globe. Continuing the focus on contemporary childhood in Chapter 4, Rebekah Willett and Chris Richards address Methodological Issues in Researching Children and Digital Media. They argue for the importance of researching children's media engagement in terms of the digital culture created and experienced by young people themselves. Willett and Richards's chapter explores the value of combining reflective observation and interviews with children on the one hand and working with children as participant researchers on the other. Drawing attention to the inherent interpolations and intertextual references relating to digital media in online and offline contexts (and the essential permeability of the apparent boundaries between these), the authors note that children are both 'beings' and 'becomings', negotiating socio-cultural structuring forces through agency, and their own agency through such structures. They argue that engagement with the agentic child, alongside careful reflection by researchers, will help create meaningful understandings of children's digital cultures.

Christine Stephen's focus (Chapter 5) on Young Learners in the Digital Age invites consideration of the emergence of the digital child through nuanced, situated interactions with digital media in the age group from birth to eight years old. At the same time, Stephen's chapter continues the emphasis on relationships, values, and choices that inform and constitute children's engagement with digital media, especially within the home. A cultural-historical perspective illuminates empirical evidence to highlight children's agency in relation to digital media use, alongside the activities of parents, peers, and educators. Stephen reveals that, even at very young ages, children's interests and preferences can be gleaned from their personalised digital media experiences.

The ways in which people learn about children and digital media are complemented by research into the ways in which children learn about people, and themselves, through their use of digital media. This shift in focus constitutes the second element of the Part 1 theme, Creation of Knowledge, and is introduced in Chapter 6: Children Who Code. Here, Jamie C. Macbeth, Michael J. Lee, Jung Soo Kim and Tony Boming Zhang turn their attention to the potentially life-changing impact of a child's understanding of the ways in which coding can deliver control over media devices and experiences. Drawing upon research into children's responses to a ten-week coding project that aimed to redress structured disadvantage, and harnessing young people's memories of their first experiences of coding, the authors argue that coding skills equip young people to become power users of digital media, aware of the risks, benefits, and affordances of digital media that children who are less aware might simply take for granted. Kylie J. Stevenson's work (Chapter 7) similarly explores children's creativity in digital contexts, although her focus is on a younger age group. Interrogating the notions of Craft's *little c* creativity, and Vygotsky's construction of play as creativity, Stevenson examines the means and technologies through which children entangle themselves in digital play. Applying posthuman perspectives and possibility thinking to children's everyday technological experiences with the Internet of Toys, makerspaces, and apps, Stevenson delivers on her chapter's title: Young Children's Creativity in Digital Possibility Spaces: What Might Posthumanism Reveal? She argues that the conceptual tools and literature around creativity, digital media, and posthumanism enable careful consideration of the emergent assemblages of the human child and the digital non-human.

Children's informal learning around digital media often takes place within the home. In Chapter 8, The Domestication of Touchscreen Technologies in Families with Young Children, Leslie Haddon applies a domestication framework to explore the diverse reasons – in addition to 'education' – underlying parents' decisions to introduce their very young children to touchscreen media. Drawing upon material collected as part of an Australian/UK project, *Toddlers and Tablets*, which examined children's digital media use between birth and five years old, Haddon examines parents' nuanced support for their children's digital media experiences while also noting that, in talking about media content with children, parents often engage with non-digital and philosophical topics. Haddon's discussion also highlights unanticipated aspects of children's digital engagement, the guilt that parents sometime feel about this area of their parenting practice, and the frequent requirement for adult intervention and support in this younger age group. Although the value of digital media in connecting children to absent grandparents has been a long-standing focus of research, less attention has been paid to the ways in which grandparents mediate their grandchildren's digital activities when they are acting in a caregiving role of children aged two to seven. Differentiating between the mediation of interactive media and non-interactive media, the research presented by Nelly Elias, Dafna Lemish, and Galit Nimrod in Grandparental Mediation of Children's Digital Media Use (Chapter 9) underlines that the management of children's digital media use is an area of concern for many grandparents. Although grandparents' attitudes, behaviour, and knowledge about digital media is variable, the mediation role they commonly play is an integral and important component of contemporary grandparenting duties. Part of the complexity of these activities lies in the fact that grandparents find themselves negotiating their grandchildren's expectations around digital media use alongside the expectations of their own children, their grandchildren's parents.

PART II: Digital Media Lives

This section of the *Companion* transitions from a consideration of how researchers gain knowledge about digital media and children, and how they come to understand children's growing engagement with digital media, to an appreciation of the ways in which children and young people come to integrate digital media into their lives. Part II begins with the youngest children, whose natural gestures are particularly suited to touchscreen technology – or so it might appear. In Chapter 10, Young Children's Haptic Media Habitus, Bjørn Nansen identifies that there is limited research on children's engagement with haptic interfaces and few studies of how designers take account of very young children's gestural repertoires when developing these haptic interfaces. Phenomenological writings and the concept of habitus are suggested as constituting a useful framework for understanding body-technology relations in children's experiences of haptic technologies. Nansen demonstrates the value of this approach using material from an ethnographic study where children do not just interact 'naturally' with the interface but need to discipline their gestures in order to learn the grammar of interaction that designers have mapped into devices, partly based on videos of young children's gestures.

Continuing the focus on younger media users, Cary Bazalgette uses Chapter 11, Early Encounters with Narrative: Two-Year-Olds and Moving-Image Media, to examine how young children learn to make sense of moving images. Based on observations and videos of her grandchildren, the author considers the conventions children need to learn to engage with and become immersed in visual media. Drawing attention to the overlooked specificities of children's consumption of audio-visual material, she argues that children are doing far more than 'just looking' at a screen and proposes that moving-image media are not facsimiles of what is observed by children in the everyday, but constructed artefacts that employ complex protocols and codes to support meaning-making. Bazalgette sensitises the reader to what two-year-olds might observe; what may be motivating young children in, for example, their repeated viewing of the same moving images; and the cognitive and emotional processes that can come into play. In addition to learning audio-visual conventions from repeated engagement with media content, young children also learn from each other's experiences as Sandy Houen, Susan Danby, and Pernilla Miller show in Chapter 12, Siblings Accomplishing Tasks Together: Solicited and Unsolicited Assistance when Using Digital Technology. These researchers use a linguistic analysis of Australian sibling conversational interactions to demonstrate how young children collaborate to achieve digital goals, and how they learn in this process. Houen, Danby, and Miller first indicate different ways in which children might try to recruit assistance, and then they use fragments from case studies to show how children manage both solicited and unsolicited assistance from their siblings. Such management of help may involve negotiation of goals, resisting assistance, and modifying strategies in the light of resistance; for example, providing verbal instructions rather than demonstrating how to solve a problem. Relevantly, sibling learning is a multi-directional process with younger siblings supporting older sibling learning, and vice versa.

Conceptualising Children as Architects of Their Digital Worlds, Joanne O'Mara, Linda Laidlaw, and Suzanna So Har Wong's Chapter 13 uses case studies from Canada and Australia to explore how children aged five to ten can engage creatively with digital materials, working as designers. Providing examples from controlling robots, creating digital worlds with Minecraft, and developing games, O'Mara, Laidlaw, and Wong demonstrate that some children are motivated to learn programming skills and develop their digital literacy. These processes require open-ended applications that provide some freedom for children to set specific goals and include social elements. Informed by the Maker movement, the authors also indicate how adults, especially teachers, can encourage and support the process of learning for children to become their own digital architects. Sara Pereira, Joana Fillol, and Pedro Moura use Chapter 14, Teens' Online and

Introduction

Offline Lives: How They Are Experiencing Their Sociability, to note debates about whether online options to communicate are displacing or stimulating sociability among young people. Putting this discussion into a media-embedded perspective, they draw on Floridi and other researchers, highlighting how the online/offline distinction is itself fading. Based on multi-method data from a Portuguese study, Pereira, Fillol, and Moura demonstrate the profound role played by digital media in teenagers' performance of sociability. Such practices blur old boundaries between online and offline, even as teens' social engagements highlight the various ways in which online sociability is embedded in offline life, mostly with known friends, complementing other forms of interaction. At the same time, the authors note that these teen sociability practices mainly exclude adults and are differently experienced by rural and urban students.

Although many teens use social media as a means of maintaining and deepening their friendship networks, some take part in fan-based affinity networks and make new friends through shared interests. This is an area of interest for Julián de la Fuente and Pilar Lacasa in Chapter 15, Teens' Fandom Communities: Making Friends and Countering Unwanted Contacts. The authors use a three-year Spanish ethnographic study of online fandom relating to celebrities such as Harry Styles and One Direction to explore girls' contact management practices. Outlining various processes at work in this online community of interest, especially concerning the fans' diverse relationships with each other, de la Fuente and Lacasa analyse the behaviour of tweens and early adolescents, typically girls aged between eight and fourteen. As they decide whether or not to engage with other unknown online fans, community members also negotiate the nature of fanfiction production, the commitment implied in writing for other fans, the multiple profiles of individual fans, and the different places they can hang out online. At the same time as learning how to manage relationships with people they are yet to meet in real life, the children use digital media in a way often characterised by an exploration of personal identity. In Chapter 16, Identity Exploration in Anonymous Online Spaces, Mary Anne Lauri and Lorleen Farrugia focus on the use by adolescents of social networking sites supporting anonymous communication. Although these sites have attracted criticism for being risky spaces, especially where they might appear to support cyberbullying practices, the authors review the literature to show that such online spaces can have a value for identity exploration and production. Lauri and Farrugia subsequently draw on qualitative and quantitative Maltese data from the *EU Kids Online* project to examine the various attractions of such sites, the role of peer pressure, and adolescent users' awareness of the risks involved, even if, in some young people's judgements, those risks are outweighed by benefits.

Parents and educators are implicated as key resources in supporting children's negotiation of risky digital encounters. But when does support become intrusive? In Supervised Play: Intimate Surveillance and Children's Mobile Media Usage (Chapter 17), William Balmford, Larissa Hjorth, and Ingrid Richardson review the growing literature on different and subtle forms of surveillance in everyday life that have been enabled by mobile technologies, focussing on parental monitoring of their children. Noting that not all forms of surveillance should be considered negative, and that judgements around intrusiveness tend to reflect the age of the children being monitored, the authors use examples from the Australian *Games of Being Mobile* project to explore parents' friendly, intimate, and caring surveillance practices. Adults' favoured strategies include unobtrusively communicating parental availability via mobile games, following children on social media, only allowing the use of digital devices where children can be observed, and co-playing games with children as a means of knowing more about children's activities. Parents' management of anxiety over their children's digital activities also informs Bieke Zaman, Marije Nouwen, and Karla Van Leeuwen's chapter (18), Challenging Adolescents' Autonomy: An Affordances Perspective on Parental Tools. Exploring the different types of parenting implied by parental choice of different tools for monitoring or controlling their children's digital experiences, these researchers critique the standard nomenclature of parental mediation practices, arguing that parents' active engagement with children's activities can in one context be a form of control, and in another parental support, allowing privacy and encouraging autonomy. Zaman, Nouwen, and Van Leeuwen show how the concept of affordances is complex, covering features of design but also the meaning that parents assign to design; for example, an affordance not correlating with the type of parent they want to be. Finally, the researchers examine parenting tools and the ways in which these are marketed to show how these strategies address different groups of parents and styles of parenting.

PART III: Complexities of Commodification

The culmination of Part II acknowledges that many affordances of digital culture reflect the marketing strategies of technology companies towards children and their families. In Part III, Complexities of Commodification, Ylva Ågren begins discussion of children as consumers by arguing against simplistic understandings of children's relationship to consumer culture. In her chapter (19), Children's Enrolment in Online Consumer Culture, Ågren suggests that young people are often positioned as either naïve or fully competent in terms of comprehending and negotiating the commercial underpinnings of consumption, especially in digital contexts. Challenging this polarisation through two case studies of Swedish children, she highlights the multifaceted engagement by children of different ages in virtual worlds while playing the mobile game *Pokémon Go*. The case studies demonstrate how the practices exhibited by children in responding to the game's commercialism are inevitably intertwined in their everyday lives, including their play spaces and digitally infused imaginative activities. Indeed, Ågren's chapter underlines that children's understanding of consumption and their roles as consumers is a crucial part of their emerging appreciation of how contemporary society works.

Benjamin Burroughs and Gavin Feller in Chapter 20, The Emergence and Ethics of Child-Created Content as Media Industries, take a deep dive into the world of child YouTube stars, asking some hard questions about child labour and aspiration. While they argue that each new medium comes with new questions about children's labour and participation, to date the children featured in YouTube videos, even those featured almost every day, are not specifically covered by many legal systems, including in the US which is not, as it happens, a signatory to the 1989 UN Convention on the Rights of the Child. While children view, enjoy, mimic and idealise child YouTubers, their attention and activity are both incentivised and completely monitored by commercial platforms such as Google, the owners of YouTube. Questions of transparency and ethics are also central to Crystal Abidin's chapter (21), Pre-School Stars on YouTube: Child Microcelebrities, Commercially Viable Biographies, and Interactions with Technology. Abidin utilises three pre-school YouTubers as case studies – one from South Korea, one from the US, and the last from Singapore – and examines their presence on screen, and the explicit and implicit parental practices framing the online presence and profitability of these children. While each of the three offers a different window into the life of a pre-school YouTuber, the commonalities provoke significant questions. Indeed, Abidin concludes with a call for greater transparency in terms of the contracts, labour expectations, parental management, and general terms of work that govern the lives of these pre-school YouTube stars.

Adopting a broader perspective on the rights of all children in their everyday digital lives, Tama Leaver uses Chapter 22, Balancing Privacy: Sharenting, Intimate Surveillance, and the Right to be Forgotten, to argue that in the era of sharenting, apps, platforms, and infant wearables, protecting children's right to privacy is a thankless task that all too often falls on the shoulders of new parents. At an incredibly busy time of their lives, when they are learning as they go, parents frequently find themselves ill-equipped to manage their child's initial online presence and navigate the many challenges that come with protecting a young child's data. Leaver examines the function served by popular parent and child influencers as privacy role models, explores new questions provoked by (over)sharenting, and weighs the digital traces young people leave against any right they might have to one day have their childhoods forgotten, at least by big data giants and social media platforms. In Chapter 23, Parenting Pedagogies in the Marketing of Children's Apps, Donell Holloway, Giovanna Mascheroni, and Ashley Donkin maintain the focus on parents as the digital decision-makers for their children, examining apps specifically aimed at preschoolers. Extrapolating from the app store listings for a range of popular education apps, these researchers argue that such digital tools situate parents and carers as online educators from the beginning of children's lives. Indeed, promotional discourses not only build the notion of parental responsibility for using education apps from a very young age but also implicitly criticise parents who are not participating in the data economy relating to shifting educational aspirations, metrics, and norms. Holloway, Mascheroni, and Donkin raise issues that continue to resonate in the wake of, for example, the spread of the Coronavirus pandemic and the resulting requirement upon parents to educate millions of school children in their homes, often adopting apps and online platforms at very short notice.

In Chapter 24, Digital Literacy/'Dynamic Literacies': Formal and Informal Learning Now and in the Emergent Future, John Potter warns against existing, relatively static notions of digital literacy and media literacy. Instead of stasis, argues Potter, the broadly conceptualised fields in which literacies and digital technologies interact are deeply contingent on lived everyday experiences which constantly shift. To capture the changing nature of lived experiences, approaches to learning, and the many emergent areas of digital technology in contemporary culture, Potter uses young people's digital media production experiences to offer the concept of 'dynamic literacies' which inherently remind everyone that the literacies needed to navigate the current, evolving digital and material world are fluid, changing, and responsive. Reflecting Potter's insights, it is the very complexity and contingency of children's digital lives that is exemplified in Chapter 25, Inês Vitorino Sampaio, Thinayna Máximo, and Cristina Ponte's work on Being and Not Being: 'Digital Tweens' in a Hybrid Culture. These researchers highlight major differences between Brazilian experiences of digital culture, relating these to inequalities across experiences of childhood, while also highlighting many points of continuity. A country characterised by inequality, Brazil celebrates affluent child stars who produce YouTube videos about product consumption while simultaneously accommodating almost five million children without regular internet access. Focusing on tweens, aged 11 to 12 years old, Sampaio, Máximo, and Ponte highlight different forms of online interactivity, often characterised by the fact that tweens tend to access the internet using mobile phones. Some of the most popular content for this cohort is the aspirational child YouTubers who review consumer products while also suggesting that fame is within the reach of every child.

In "Technically They're Your Creations, but ...": Children Making, Playing, and Negotiating User-Generated Content Games (Chapter 26), Sara M. Grimes and Vinca Merriman explore children's understanding of copyright, ownership, and intellectual property in user-generated content (UGC) games such as *Minecraft*. While there is a significant body of work exploring the educational and pedagogical uses of UGC games, Grimes and Merriman address a relatively under-researched gap by asking how children aged between six and twelve understand intellectual property. Their game-jam group interview sessions reveal complex ideas about ownership and copyright, some close to existing legal realities, others based on the notion that the owners of games would do the right thing by players. Dishearteningly, while the children interviewed had emergent ideas about copyright, all of them indicated that it was something corporations owned, and they did not. Grimes and Merriman end their chapter with a call to include children in public discussions about digital authorship rights.

In Chapter 27, Marketing to Children through Digital Media: Trends and Issues, Wonsun Shin offers a big picture overview of the approaches and concerns raised when advertisers target children. Shin notes that, while older children are directly targeted since they themselves hold increasing purchasing power, this is also true of younger children. The marketing strategies to the latter, however, revolve around prompting younger children to actively and repeatedly ask parents to make specific purchases. Formal advertising on various platforms and channels, branded experiences in games, and even influencer marketing on Instagram and YouTube, are all arenas where children must learn to negotiate marketing and commercialism in various forms. Children are far from passive, often pushing back against marketing intrusions, but the sheer scale of advertising and marketing in children's digital worlds can become insidious. Shin concludes by arguing that an era of social media demands more nuanced studies of children's understanding of marketing in order to encompass a comprehensive model of persuasion that acknowledges the diversity of media and platforms through which children participate and consume.

PART IV: Children's Rights

Discussions of marketing, commodification, and privacy inevitably raise the issue of children's rights, and particularly their rights in the context of digital environments. The 1989 adoption of the United Nations Convention on the Rights of the Child (UNCRC) was reprised 25 years later when the UN Committee on the Rights of the Child met to discuss 'Digital Media and Children's Rights'. The resulting Digital Rights Framework reconfigured approaches to children's needs, agency, and vulnerability to harm in today's digital world. That framework implies and assigns roles and responsibilities to a variety of social actors, including the state, families, schools, commercial entities, researchers, and children themselves. Part IV of the *Companion*, Children's Rights, centrally addresses children's rights in the digital world. It gathers together research from around the globe that focusses on these children's rights as agential citizens to provision and participation regarding digital devices and content, as well as their right to protection from harm. Interwoven throughout this part is an acknowledgement that children of various ages, abilities, socioeconomic and geographic backgrounds should have equal access to digital media. This part also highlights children's right to have a voice when decisions regarding their rights are being made.

Brian O'Neill's chapter (28) on Child-Centred Policy: Enfranchising Children as Digital Policy Makers, discusses children's right to be consulted by policymakers. Referencing the UNCRC, O'Neill emphasises the importance of children having an active role in the making of decisions that affect their lives. The contribution addresses ways in which children's participation in policymaking can be enhanced and heightened, arguing that doing so will also improve policymaking decisions. As O'Neill suggests, the digital environment both demands and offers new approaches to meaningful processes for engaging children and young people in policymaking.

In the first of two related chapters, Law, Digital Media, and the Discomfort of Children's Rights (Chapter 29), Brian Simpson argues that many conventional rights approaches to children's use of digital media are centred on the negative goal of protecting children from potential harm. This perspective reflects political, ideological, economic, and romantic conceptions of the child that result in a legal narrative inclined towards child protection. Simpson challenges this dominant paradigm by identifying a variety of flaws in relation to 'avoid harm' approaches to children's rights. He argues that more focus needs to be placed on supporting children's rights to autonomy and active engagement in the digital world. Chapter 30, No Fixed Limits? The Uncomfortable Application of Inconsistent Law to the Lives of Children Dealing with Digital Media, explores the notion of the best interest of the child, investigating how the concept of best interest may be re-articulated to focus on children's rights to agency. Simpson discusses legal cases from the US within which notions of the immature or wicked child obfuscate, or impede, more nuanced understandings of children's rights to digital speech and discourses that address the broader rights of children in a digital world.

In Children's Agency in the Media Socialisation Process (Chapter 31), Claudia Riesmeyer focusses on children's agency and media socialisation. She argues that research into media socialisation often concentrates on how children and young people are socialised through interactions with their elders, parents, teachers, and their peers. The role of the individual within this socialisation process is largely ignored, however. Riesmeyer provides a systematic literature review to highlight the importance of the concepts of self-socialisation and agency within the media socialisation process. She concludes her work by formulating four theses aimed at guiding future research in this area. Lelia Green, in Digital Citizenship in Domestic Contexts (Chapter 32), notes how the notion of digital citizenship has become an important topic in policy circles where the rights of the child are addressed. In this context, digital citizenship rights tend to function as a way of highlighting what policymakers might deem to be appropriate media use, as well as supporting children's fundamental right to online participation. Green draws on ethnographic work with a group of male teen gamers and their parents to demonstrate that many children negotiate their digital rights in the domestic realm. She argues that parents have an important role in helping develop their children's understanding of digital citizenship.

The rights of vulnerable or disadvantaged children form the focus of the next three chapters. In Chapter 33, Meryl Alper and Madison Irons discuss Digital Socialising in Children on the Autism Spectrum. Drawing upon theoretical and conceptual frameworks relevant to disability, autism, and youth, the authors investigate autistic youth and their use of digital technologies. Three areas are foregrounded in this analysis of autistic youth and media: technologies for socialisation, materials for socialising, and media that supposedly promote anti-social behaviour. Alper and Irons echo previous authors' views that disproportionate attention is paid to harm (avoidance) rather than benefit, noting that neurodivergent children's digital socialising has received much less notice than their digital socialisation and anti-social uses of digital media. They conclude that there are tensions and contradictions in how social norms are shaped, transformed, and communicated through media at both the interpersonal and institutional level. Chapter 34, Disability, Children, and the Invention of Digital Media, investigates this topic area more broadly. Authors Katie Ellis, Gerard Goggin, and Mike Kent note that discourses and research about children's media use tend to omit or overlook children with disabilities. They argue that more research in this area is urgently needed because, without it, a full and comprehensive understanding of children's media use will remain partial and incomplete. In addition, the chapter argues that important theoretical, policy, and practice insights may be gained through the lens of critical disabilities studies, and that those insights will benefit research into digital media and children in general.

Joke Bauwens and Lien Mostmans use Chapter 35 to address Children's Moral Agency in the Digital Environment. They argue that digital engagement provides a practice ground in which children learn about ethical and moral responsibilities to themselves, each other, and society at large. It is through digital conversations with others that children learn what it is to have and express moral agency. Although the literature tends to focus on the moral crises thrown up by such topics as sexting and cyberbullying, Bauwens and Mostmans suggest that active agency lies in the negotiation of moral and social dimensions of peer culture and risk management. Noting that an everyday understanding of moral agency mandates that more attention be paid to the role of digital media in supporting children to lead meaningful and fulfilling lives, these authors call for a greater emphasis upon the experiences of children outside Anglophone cultures. In the final chapter in Part IV (36), Sonia Livingstone, Amanda Third, and Gerison Lansdown discuss Children's Rights in the Digital Environment: A Challenging Terrain for Evidence-Based Policy. They highlight that the UNCRC has many policy implications for children's digital lives, but that its 1990 ratification means that it easily predates the widespread adoption of the internet. Critically evaluating the challenges facing policymakers who seek to recognise and support children's rights in a rapidly evolving digital world, Livingstone, Third, and Lansdown note that the UN Committee on the Rights of the Child has recently committed to developing a UN General Comment on Children's Rights in Relation to the Digital Environment. In this, the authors call for global consultation with children as part of a positive framework that recognises children as agential actors and rights holders.

PART V: Changing and Challenging Circumstances

From pregnancy apps which instil habits that support parents through their children's early years to questions about how children understand death and express grief, digital media accompany many of life's changes and challenges: the focus of Part V of the *Companion*. This part starts at the beginning of a young child's life with Deborah Lupton's chapter (37) on Caring Dataveillance: Women's Use of Apps to Monitor Pregnancy and Children. Highlighting that dataveillance can be caring as well as, or instead of, intrusive, Lupton draws upon two qualitative research projects with young mothers to explore their use of apps in relation to conception, pregnancy, and the care of babies. Examining the data with a feminist new materialism lens, which considers human-nonhuman assemblages that generate 'thing-power', Lupton argues that people learn both how to become and how to live with data. In the case of new mothers, this is complicated by social expectations of what it is to be a good mother and a rejection of the old personal apps that women had previously used to monitor their own fitness, but which they now felt guilty about as their mothering role increasingly requires them to attend to the baby's wellbeing rather than their own.

Health apps often monitor the quality and quantity of sleep, and this is the focus of Alicia Allan and Simon Smith's chapter (38) relating to Digital Media and Sleep in Children. Highlighting that device use can be linked to poorer sleep and a range of adverse health outcomes, Allan and Smith explore a range of reasons why this might be the case. While arguing that more nuanced research is required, these authors also offer evidence-based recommendations for the management of children's digital media use prior to bedtime.

While social media use, particularly at bedtime, may not be an optimally healthy choice, Ana Jorge, Lidia Marôpo, and Raiana de Carvalho use their chapter (39) to consider possible interactions between positive and negative aspects of the relationship between Sick Children and Social Media. Their central case study examines Lorena Reginato and *CarecaTV*, the YouTube channel started by Lorena when she was 12 years old and fighting brain cancer. Arguing that social media use can allow sick children and their families agency in constructing a network that connects health professionals, friends, family members, supporters, and other children in similar challenging circumstances, Jorge, Marôpo, and de Carvalho suggest that such activist-based activities can raise awareness of the experiences of children living with, and sometimes recovering from, serious illness. Children's use of digital media to explore and communicate their sexuality is a more closely regulated, contested, and censored space than their use of social media in circumstances of illness. In Chapter 40, Children's Sexuality in the Context of Digital Media: Sexualisation, Sexting, and Experiences with Sexual Content in a Research Perspective, Liza Tsaliki and Despina Chronaki note that the growth of digital media use has been associated with increasing fears about the sexualisation of children and teens. Rejecting a simplistic effects and risk narrative, Tsaliki and Chronaki highlight the benefits of adopting cultural studies-based approaches that offer nuanced understandings of self-presentations and representations of children's sexuality in their social and historical context. These researchers advocate the application of a children's rights framework in this area that recognises and respects young people's claims to sexual rights and citizenship.

Introduction

Ellen J. Helsper uses Chapter 41, Digital Inequalities Amongst Digital Natives, to provoke consideration of the many inequities that persist in terms of children's access to, understandings, and uses of digital media. Critiquing the notion of the digital native, she argues that it is the socio-technical ecology, rather than the generation that a child is born into, that has the greatest impact upon their future digital lives. Such ecologies comprise more than the family of the child and extend to neighbourhoods, peer groups, and values systems. Using internationally comparative datasets, Helsper demonstrates that inequalities are directly related to variable positive and negative outcomes which reflect the specific circumstances of children. Considering socio-economic disadvantage, age, and gender differences, and young people with emotional vulnerabilities, she proposes that inequalities need to be addressed via changes to young people's socio-digital environments. Helsper calls for more research on disadvantaged children in the Global South, and one aspect of this is considered in Chapter 42, Street Children and Social Media: Identity Construction in the Digital Age, by Marcela Losantos Velasco, Lien Mostmans, and Guadalupe Peres-Cajías. Researching the digital lives of street children in Bolivia, these authors argue that many street children are on Facebook, with most participants accessing the app daily. Indeed, mobile phones are readily converted to money, so digital media technologies operate as a desirable exchange commodity. Noting that street children use social media to build and maintain links with each other, with aid organisations, and with volunteers and professionals, Losantos Velasco, Mostmans, and Peres-Cajías analyse a selection of children's posts to explore their constructed identities and the strategies used to manage relationships with imagined online and offline audiences.

Robin M. Kowalski and Annie McCord turn to the thorny issue of adolescent experiences of bullying and being bullied in Chapter 43, Perspectives on Cyberbullying and Traditional Bullying: Same or Different? The researchers consider different aspects of social aggression both online and off, drawing upon the experiences of adolescents who have encountered bullying in a range of different circumstances. Noting the conceptual importance of distinguishing the two types of behaviour, given that there are concomitant risk and protective factors and outcomes, Kowalski and McCord conclude by highlighting the importance of intervention strategies, including young people's suggestions for parents who may be worried about how to support a child who is dealing with victimisation.

In Digital Storytelling: Opportunities for Identity Investment for Youth from Refugee Backgrounds (Chapter 44), Lauren Johnson and Maureen Kendrick examine the pedagogical benefits of using personal storytelling to provide opportunities for young people from refugee backgrounds. As well as practising digital literacies, such stories allow young people to explore different aspects of their identities. Adolescents from refugee backgrounds often struggle to reach the language and literacy proficiency of their peers while also dealing with the added burden of living with trauma, and thus this pedagogical approach offers notable benefits. Johnson and Kendrick use a case study, Abdullahi's story, to indicate how creating his digital record offered Abdullahi a specific learning experience and helped him communicate his knowledge and identity to peers and the wider community. The authors argue that communicating his past experiences in an agentic manner enabled Abdullahi to build his identity within a new social context, allowing him to develop hope and plan for his future.

The final chapter in Part V of the *Companion* continues the focus on children's experiences of trauma. Children, Death, and Digital Media, by Kathleen M. Cumiskey (Chapter 45), records how children and adolescents may turn to digital media as a means of navigating experiences of grief and bereavement. In circumstances of grief, loss, and longing, the storage, retrieval, and sharing of digital content around people who are loved, but now gone, can help young people continue to feel connected with those who have died. The chapter uses two case studies to explore nuanced complexities around children's use of digital media as a means of trying to manage traumatic experiences and the processes of grieving. Cumiskey suggests that people in the child's circle can help the child reconnect, build support networks, and take part in collective activities while the young bereaved person engages in meaning-making around death.

PART VI: Local Complexities in a Global Context

The final part of this volume, Local Complexities in a Global Context, foregrounds the fact that nuanced understandings of children's digital media use need to be located within specific contexts. This introduces huge complexity, but also recognises the creative capacity of young people to use the social, communicative, and technological tools at their disposal to express themselves, their identities, and their hopes for the future. Although the preceding parts have drawn their content from around the globe, each of the chapters in this part is specifically associated with one country or continent.

In Chapter 46, Very Young Children's Digital Literacy: Engagement, Practices, Learning, and Home–School–Community Knowledge Exchange in Lisbon, Portugal, researchers Vítor Tomé and Maria José Brites provide an account of an innovative fieldwork project entitled *Digital Citizenship Education for Democratic Participation*, in which they worked with young Portuguese children aged three to eight, their parents and teachers, and the local neighbourhood of the Caneças district in inner-city Lisbon. The aim was to use digital media to foster social participation. Tomé and Brites demonstrate how this community-based action research project developed very young children's digital literacy competencies through the application of an intervention model. They argue that adaptive in-service teacher training around digital media use can assist to rapidly overcome the gap between high digital use at home and low digital use at school.

Chika Anyanwu uses Chapter 47 to shift the geographical focus by addressing the under-considered topic of The Voices of African Children. Drawing on data collected from *Young and Online: Children's Perspectives on Life in the Digital Age* (The State of the World's Children 2017 companion report), the *South African Kids Online* report, and selected UNICEF reports, while freely acknowledging that the data analysed comprises mere snapshots of a complex continent of 54 countries, Anyanwu argues that the global nature of digital platforms that cross geo-cultural and political landscapes give impetus to a collective analysis of the experiences of African children. This contribution gives voice to the challenges these children face in engaging with digital media and notes that promising young African entrepreneurs have used their experiences of childhood challenges to craft creative solutions that increase African children's participation in the online world.

Limiting the Digital in Brazilian Schools: Structural Difficulties and School Culture (Chapter 48) showcases Daniela Costa and Juliana Doretto's presentation of data from two research surveys conducted in Brazil involving 1,106 participating schools, alongside interviews with more than 14,000 students and 1,854 teachers. They highlight contradictions between the data gathered and the existing public policies on the educational use of digital technologies. Noting a range of issues for schools including inadequate internet connections and digital technology, and how teachers often needed to use their own mobiles to access the internet for tasks within the curriculum, Costa and Doretto call for government policies that make a difference in paying real heed to the social discourses that position Brazilian children's digital technology skills as vital to addressing education dilemmas and disadvantage.

Amy Shields Dobson's chapter (49), Australia and Consensual Sexting: The Creation of Child Pornography or Exploitation Materials?, presents her argument that the framing of youth sexting practices as 'child pornography' or sexual exploitation materials, both legally and culturally, has significant unintended negative impacts on young people and those who care for and about them. Dobson's research demonstrates that current laws pathologise and potentially criminalise

Introduction

children's and teens' sexuality as expressed and experienced through digital media, arguing that the debate requires reframing to address youth sexting as an issue of young people's sexual rights. She explains why young people remain vulnerable under child pornography laws but acknowledges that the prohibitions around the making and circulating of child sexual abuse materials are crucial in the historical and cultural context of digital media and potential adult exploitation.

S M Shameem Reza and Ashfara Haque use Chapter 50, Revisiting Children's Participation in Television: Implications for Digital Media Rights in Bangladesh, to present field research conducted with Bangladeshi children who participated in child-led TV shows or attended TV shows with children mostly as presenters or performers. They identify a range of changes associated with the deregulation and the liberalisation of communications coinciding with economic growth in South Asia, the result of which has been a sudden expansion of conventional broadcast and digital media. Reza and Haque argue that such significant disruption makes it imperative for signatories to the UN Convention on the Rights of the Child, like Bangladesh, to have a charter to support children's rights and participation in both digital and legacy media contexts. The authors explain that the parallel developments of a digital media space and legacy media highlight the importance of acknowledging and protecting children's rights, fostering their participation in the digital age.

Xiang Ren's contribution, Chinese Teen Digital Entertainment: Rethinking Censorship and Commercialisation in Short Video and Online Fiction (Chapter 51), examines problems in Chinese teenagers' online cultural engagement and civic participation. He argues that, while internet regulations and censorship in China effectively control political agendas, they are less successful in protecting children's safety and rights, particularly when children view unsuitable content. Xiang Ren further posits that Chinese teenagers are being engaged in 'playbour', or the rapid commodification of informal creative labour, and he calls for China's teen digital entertainment sphere to be subject to greater scrutiny by academics and policymakers, along with increased action via platform governance and regulation, to attend to teenagers' rights as participatory creators.

In Sexual Images, Risk, and Perception among Youth: A Nordic Example (Chapter 52), Elisabeth Staksrud provides insights from a Norwegian study of children aged nine to sixteen (and their parents) about young people's exposure to sexual images on the internet. Staksrud details how Norwegian parents find sexual risk in general, and sexual content specifically, worrisome. This is especially the case for parents of younger children and parents of daughters. The results from Staksrud's study demonstrate that younger children and girls are most upset, and most likely to experience negative feelings, after seeing sexual images online, while older boys appear to be the least affected by such content. Such results, she argues, identify a need for more research on the gendered nature of sexual risk assessment and experience among young people.

Jarrod Walczer's chapter (53), US-Based Toy Unboxing Production in Children's Culture, addresses a younger age group but also deals with challenges posed by adults' perceptions of the impact of content upon children. Critically examining YouTube creators in the US who make toy unboxing videos for children, Walczer draws upon 25 interviews with top-ranking toy unboxers to argue that, as children's culture changes to encompass digital media, longstanding anxieties and new concerns have arisen in response to toy unboxing content. Using a circuit of culture approach, Walczer declares that children's digital practices should not be seen as separate from those in the 'real world'. He further suggests that before governments, regulators, and industry rush to constrain such materials, close attention should be paid to the circuit of culture theory as it relates to toy unboxing media, and the agency implicit in children's engagement with these programmes on YouTube. Doing this may result in new perspectives that help shape more nuanced understandings of toy unboxing videos.

The final chapter in the *Companion* remains in the US and considers older teens' negotiations of their religious-cultural identity as Muslims within the context of a sometimes Islamophobic socio-political environment. In Chapter 54, The Role of Digital Media in the Lives of Some American Muslim Children, 2010–2019, Nahid Afrose Kabir synthesises some nine years of field interviews to demonstrate how young American Muslim children use digital media to negotiate community relations, develop friendships, and explore personal, cultural, and religious differences. Kabir gives an account of the challenges faced by some of these children, such as negotiating the cultural dilemmas of family expectations and peer group pressures. She suggests that digital media assists Muslim children in their identity formation, identity negotiation, and their communication skills, while also helping to keep them globally connected. In this final chapter on digital media and children, Kabir reflects on the sophisticated ways in which some Muslim American children use digital media to negotiate complex aspects of their identity, moving between being an American child and a Muslim child, while belonging to a local peer group and also remaining a member of a cultural/ethnic diaspora.

Taken together these 54 chapters provide a broad but deep interrogation of the many issues raised and challenges addressed by children's digital media use. Even as this volume was being developed and curated, the impacts of digital media continue to transform and disrupt what children and their families deem to be everyday life. As this Introduction goes to press, the world is in the grip of the COVID-19 pandemic with unprecedented numbers of children and parents locked down in their homes, reliant on their digital media skills, technology, and infrastructure to work, learn, and play. While that is a subject for many other volumes, this *Companion* has set out to capture and interrogate the rich diversity of young people's imaginings for and interactions with the digital materials that help constitute their lives. It provides a firm foundation upon which others will continue to build.

ACKNOWLEDGEMENTS

This volume had its beginnings in a modest proposal to address the digital lives of under-6s. Erica Wetter at Taylor & Francis suggested the outline could be expanded into a more ambitious work, while Emma Sherriff acquired the project in 2018 as a newly minted Taylor & Francis editorial assistant. We are grateful to them both for their vision and support.

A volume of this length and breadth requires a prolonged period of work, across organisational areas, institutions, and geographical boundaries, with the five editors equally sharing the demands of producing this *Companion*. In this case a tireless editors' assistant kept the team on track and moved the project forward. The existence of the published outcome is a testament to the support provided by Linda Jaunzems. We are immeasurably grateful to Linda for her tenacity, sticking power, good humour, and eye for detail. Thank you, Linda.

Given its beginnings in work associated with the Australian Research Council (ARC) Discovery Project, DP150104734: Toddlers and Tablets: Exploring the Risks and Benefits 0-5s Face Online (led by Lelia Green), we are indebted to the ARC for their support for that project, and consequently some of the support for Linda's work on this book, since she supplied administrative assistance on that grant. The *Companion* is partly an output of that Discovery Project, especially selected chapters in Parts I and II.

At the point when it was accepted, the volume was expanded to include children and teenagers. This broader vision has also allowed the inclusion of outputs from a more recent ARC Discovery Project, DP190102435: Adolescents' Perceptions of Harm From Accessing Online Sexual Content (led by Lelia Green). As DP150104734 admin support ended, so DP190102435 support began, and the book similarly owes the ARC a debt of gratitude for that assistance, with related outputs in Parts VI, V, and VI.

More recently, the project has also been supported by Edith Cowan University's (ECU) research focus on Digital Citizenship and Human Behaviour. We're grateful to Tony Marceddo, the university-wide research theme leader for his vision around building impact, and for ECU's commitment to supporting this publication.

Other people also helped along the way. We are especially grateful to Ashley Donkin and Claire Hanlon for their assistance, which allowed us (and Linda) to progress other aspects of the volume when there was a lot to do and not much time in which to do it. Ashley's work occurred in the context of her Research Assistant appointment on the ARC Discovery Project DP180103922, The Internet of Toys: Benefits and Risks of Connected Toys for Children (led by Donell Holloway). This book is thus partly an output of that funding stream.

Acknowledgements

In the interests of chasing quality and creating a collection of value, we complicated our lives a little more than is usual with an edited volume. For example, every chapter in this collection has been double-blind peer-reviewed by two reviewers. This means that the scholars reviewing the chapter didn't know who wrote it or who else was reviewing and the authors didn't know who their reviewers were. Every reviewer added value and every chapter benefited from the feedback offered. It is with great pleasure and the sincerest appreciation that we thank our community of reviewers, some of whom were kind enough to review more than one chapter. We acknowledge their contribution here:

Kath Albury, Beth Almeida, Chika Anyanwu, Tom Apperley, Catherine Archer, Veronica Barassi, Jamal Barnes, Carla Barros, Jo Bird, Mindy Blaise, Anna Bunn, Patricio Cabello, Daniel Cardosa, Charlotte Chalklen, Bertha Chin, Despina Chronaki, Natalie Coulter, Sky Croeser, Leen D'Haenes, Lorenzo Dalvit, Julie Dare, Christina Davidson, Melissa Davis, Jos De Haan, Lenka Dědková, Madeleine Dobson, Veronica Donoso, Juliana Doretto, Elza Dukels, Katie Ellis, Toby Emert, Liese Exelmans, Lorleen Farrugia, Neil Ferguson, Kim Flintoff, Carmelo Garitaonandia, luke gaspard, Laura Glitsos, Abigail Hackett, John Hartley, Geoffrey Hawker, Patrik Hernvall, Larissa Hjorth, Jonathon Hutchinson, Estefania Jimenez, Nicola Johnson, Nahid Kabir, Daniel Kardefelt-Winther, Louise Kay, Michael Keane, Brendan Keogh, Robin Kowalski, Dafna Lemish, Catharine Lumby, Deborah Lupton, Lidia Marôpo, Giovanna Mascheroni, Anneleen Masschelein, Jane Mavoa, Jill McLachlan, Cori More, Karen Murcia, Maria Fransesca Murru, Bjørn Nansen, Linda Nesby, Michelle Neumann, Raphael Nowak, Kjartan Ólafsson, Joanne O'Mara, Kate Orton-Johnson, Cristina Ponte, Pille Pruulmann-Vengerfeldt, Claudia Riesmeyer, Ana Rivoir, Eleanor Sandry, Fiona Scott, Julian Sefton-Green, Andra Siibak, Gavin Sim, Suzanne Smythe, Barbara Spears, Elisabeth Staksrud, Daniel Süss, Amanda Third, Christine Trueltzsch-Wijnen, Liza Tsaliki, Panayiota Tsatsou, Anca Valecu, Sofie Vandoninck, Jane Vincent, Jarrod Walczer, Lynn Whitaker, Pamela Wisniewski, Dylan Yamada-Rice, Bieke Zaman, Elaine Zhao.

This book exists in its current form as a result of the dedication of all the people named above. We are extremely grateful to you all.

Lelia Green,
Donell Holloway,
Kylie Stevenson,
Tama Leaver,
and Leslie Haddon

PART I
Creation of Knowledge

1
CHILD STUDIES MEETS DIGITAL MEDIA
Rethinking the Paradigms

Natalie Coulter

Introduction

Children are often the focus of much public concern regarding the impacts of digital culture. A quick google search on digital media and children lists links to websites that make such claims as children are: addicted to screens, bullied online, obsessed with social media, corrupted by online pornography, and in danger of ruining their reputations. Stories abound of the perils of the digital for children, as if children are unwitting victims of this new technology. These refrains echo the sentiments of technological determinism as if, somehow, this technology is colonising and controlling children.

These statements reveal as much about societal anxieties of digital culture as they do about definitions of contemporary childhood, and by extension adulthood. Each of these same refrains could easily be made with regards to adults, but it is most often children that are deemed to be susceptible to the internet's dangers. While there are many ways that these arguments can be unpacked and critiqued, they do reveal some of the ways in which society defines, frames, and knows young people. Understanding why these debates often become centred on children begins with basic ontological questions, including what is a child and what is childhood? Who gets to be defined as children, and who are not defined as children? And, as Jenks has suggested, "how is the child possible as such?" (Jenks, 2005, p. 4): a question that explores why children are defined in these ways, and what this reveals about society. How society defines and frames the child and childhood has major implications for how it understands the digital child, what voices they are given, how their relationships with technology are understood, and which children are framed in these debates and which are not.

The child that is held up in these fearful refrains of technology is not an actual child, but an image of a child that fits the ideological logics of the rhetoric of the arguments. There is a distinction between the imagined child that is framed as an 'unwitting victim' of this technology and the lived experiences of the estimated 2.2 billion children in the world (UNICEF, 2017).

Research on children and digital culture needs to take into account what the term child actually means. Of course, the embodied child always becomes the constructed child, once it is positioned within discourse. But what does the term 'child' actually mean in the context of digital media and children? The purpose of this chapter is to begin to unpack the cultural, social discursiveness of the terms child, children, and childhood, and think critically about how these terms are employed.

History of Children as a Construction

Perhaps one of the best starting points in unpacking the concept of the child is the work of Phillipe Ariès. Emerging in the 1960s, Ariès' scholarship incited a debate on the 'invention of the child'. Phillipe Ariès' work *Centuries of Childhood: A Social History of Family Life* (1965) suggests that childhood, as a meaningful concept, is an invention of the emerging modern society. Prior to this, Ariès contends, childhood was not recognised or valued as a distinct phase of life. Despite the fact that scholars such as Lawrence Stone and Natalie Zemon Davis have suggested that Ariès' work is methodologically flawed (see Wilson, 1980), his research opened up the possibility of thinking about children and childhood as a social construct and not a natural, universal category of being. While Ariès is largely credited with initiating this debate, earlier scholars have also pushed against the reification of childhood. Consider, for example, Margaret Mead's *Coming of Age in Samoa* (2017), originally published in 1943, which suggested that adolescence is shaped by social and cultural conditions. But it was Airès' work in the 1960s that was foundational in establishing that child, children, and childhood are not universal concepts; instead they are constituted discursively within the social, cultural, political, and economic institutions and structures of a historical moment.

At the heart of these lines of thinking is the debate around the role of culture in shaping categories of being. The child is a social and cultural construction constituted through discourse. It is not a natural category of being, determined solely by biological stages of development. Nor is it a universal category that is fixed and remains unchanging across historical and cultural boundaries. Instead, childhood, as Henry Jenkins suggests:

> is not timeless but rather subject to the same historical shifts and institutional factors that shape all human experience. Children's culture is not the result of purely top-down forces of ideological and institutional control, nor is it a free space of individual expression. Children's culture is a site of conflicting values, goals and expectations.
>
> *(1998, p. 14)*

Jenkins highlights the complex tensions at play. The child is a discursive and social construction, and the meanings of childhood are in constant processes of struggle and negotiation, in both public discourse and in interpersonal relationships.

This is not to deny that there are biological realities of the stages of childhood, nor that biology plays a role in the framing of young people. But it is to assert, instead, that the biological realities of this stage of life are named, given meaning, and understood discursively. To quote Jenks, the child is "a status of person which is comprised through a series of, often heterogeneous, images, representations, codes and constructs" (Jenks, 2005, p. 29). The notion of a child is not merely illusionary, however. The definition of the child has real-life consequences that are felt deeply by those who are defined as children. Nor is the definition of the child fixed, stable, or even an objective definition, but is, instead, in a perpetual process of change, mutating alongside other social and cultural shifts, often according to the needs and logics of adult institutions such as the church, the government, the schools, and even the media.

Vivian Zelizer's work *Pricing the Priceless Child* (1994) provides a poignant example of Jenks' quote as it reveals the changing relationships between the economic value of children and their sociocultural worth. Zelizer traces a complex social trajectory of how childhood changed in meaning around the end of the 19th century and early 20th century when the sacred/sentimental child displaced the worker/labourer child. Zelizer shows how childhood as a social construct is tied to an array of social, political, economic, and cultural factors, which are all implicated in framing and defining childhood in very particular ways, with dramatic results for the lives of actual children. For example, as Zelizer highlights, shifts in constructions of children as paid labourers, and the types of children desired for adoption (from work-ready boys to sentimentalised baby girls), have real consequences for those children. The discursive ties between childhood and labour is again a shifting ground in digital culture. Scholarship by Crystal Abidin (2015) on babies as microcelebrities (famous within small niche networks) and Alicia Blum-Ross's work on 'sharenting' (share-parenting) (2015) opens up new questions about how the curation of children's digital images are leveraged as digital capital for an intimate public in the digital economy.

The child that is framed in the opening refrains of this chapter, the one who is 'addicted', 'coerced', etc., fits an assumption of children as not having developed the tools to successfully negotiate digital culture: the corresponding assumption is that adults have these skills. The child is often "locked within binary reasoning", in which the child is being conditioned or socialised to become an adult (Jenks, 2005, p. 3). Childhood is a processional stage of becoming, towards an ambiguously defined notion of adult as the full completion of the processes. Such framings assume that childhood is presocial, in a teleological process of becoming adult, and not in a liminal stage of being.

The children in these narratives are deemed as being influenced or 'effected' – both brought into being and impacted, or not (Gauntlett, 1998), by digital technology. Children are not considered social actors who engage in meaning-making practices themselves (Cook, 2011; James, Jenks, & Prout, 1998; Jenks, 2005). Nor do these narratives address the diverse and complex ways in which different children engage with digital media. Instead, in these narratives, childhood is conceptualised as a period of mostly powerlessness. The child, presumed innocent and devoid of social agency, is considered to be 'immature', 'irrational' (Jenkins, 1998, p. 2), and vulnerable to exploitation and manipulation.

These framings position childhood as inherently separate from the media, where the media is seen as somehow external to childhood and children's everyday lives (Buckingham, 2018, p. iii). This slips quickly into assumptions of media effects, where the media is conceptualised as having a direct impact on children's consciousness and behaviour. Such understandings are too simplistic; not only do they position the child as having very little agency, they also assume that childhood is experienced separately or externally from digital media (Buckingham, 2018, p. iii), as opposed to appreciating how children's lives are deeply engaged with digital media. The media are not separate from children's lives, but are instead embedded within the practices of children's everyday experiences. Children are actively engaged with digital media, as they consume, use, respond to, resist, are influenced by, negotiate, and produce digital media as part of their daily activities. Digital media is not something external to childhood but is integrated within children's lives.

The scholarship in the rest of this book builds upon the theoretical framings of critical childhood studies that conceptualise the child as a social and historical construct, born out of a multidimensional network of social forces, institutional regimes, economic demands, and historical developments. While these constitutions often serve the needs of adult-centred social, cultural, political, and economic systems, young people are not completely passive; they are "active in the construction and determination of their own social lives, the lives of those around them and of the societies in which they live" (James & Prout, 2003, p. 8). Young people are active agents of change. They do not simply respond to narratives provided by media culture but instead actively participate in the construction of their own subjectivities and practices.

Paradigms of Scholarship

As a starting point in the scholarship on digital media and children, it is helpful to turn to the work of Allison James and Alan Prout (2003, 2015) whose foundational texts offer deep insight into research on the child. In the mid-1990s Prout and James established a new paradigm for the sociology of childhood. The authors outline six key features of this paradigm, which will all be individually explored in the following section. Each of these six features provide useful starting points for thinking about children and digital media.

The first feature of the paradigm is that "childhood is understood as a social construction". It is an "interpretive frame for contextualising the early years of human life". While this chapter has already started to address this idea, there is more to add in specific relation to children and digital media. With digital media there are multiple perspectives, structures, and institutions that discursively construct the child. Digital media is embedded in capitalism, which is perhaps one of the key institutions to define childhood in the past century and which is largely dominated by multinational organisations. Daniel Cook's work on the child in the marketplace provides a useful starting point to reflect upon the social constructions of childhood. Cook argues that the child is defined, articulated, and framed according to the logics and needs of the marketplace. The child is a "figment of the commercial imagination" produced to meet the needs of the cultural industries of children (advertising, marketing, media, retail, and technology) as these industries research, target, and trade their knowledge of children and youth and vie for children's attention in the marketplace (Cook, 2004, p. 7). In his later work, Cook calls these the "commercial epistemologies", the ways of 'knowing' about children and youth that serve the interests and needs of the 'knower' (2011, p. 258). Alluding to the ideological constructions of childhood, Cook's work provides a useful insight into understanding the discursive forces of capitalism. In digital capitalism, much of the 'knowing' about young people depends upon data mining and surveillance of young people online in order to harness young people as potential customers, users, creators, and audiences of digital media.

Social media platforms, digital games, and internet-connected toys produce endless reams of data that can be instantaneously harvested or mined by corporations. This data is often then curated, commodified, and sold to third-party advertisers and becomes the means by which audiences are understood, defined, and framed. This process is a commercial epistemology, in which the digital child is known only through and according to the logics of data mining, which functions as a means to create profit. The process of data mining of children's digital spaces was noticed in the early stages of digital media. In 2005, before the development of most social media platforms, Sara Grimes and Leslie Regan Shade (2005) called out how seemingly benign children's digital games, such as Neopets, were in reality data-mining platforms gathering data on their players to sell to market research companies. A year earlier in 2004, Ellen Seiter observed that Neopets wasn't selling a media product, instead it was "selling information about the children and young adults who are its fans" (p. 98). These scholars, along with the early work of Sonia Livingstone (2003) and Juliet Schor (2004), raised awareness of how digital media was in the business of harvesting data well before scholars such as Mark Andrejevic (2007) and Christian Fuchs (2010) took notice and began to explore how users/followers perform unpaid labour in the workings of digital capitalism (although Tatiana Terranova had begun to write about free labour in 2000 and Greg Elmer wrote about data profiling in 2004).

It is important to note this trajectory of scholarship. Scholars of children's digital media were recognising early on the exploitive nature of digital media, and yet most of their work has been left out of current scholarship on digital labour. Take Trebor Scholz's foundational edited collection, *Digital Labour: The Internet as Playground and Factory* (2012), which completely ignores children. The absence of children from wider debates on digital media, privacy, and free labour continues today, although hopefully this edited collection will begin to address the marginalisation of children's digital cultures from the wider field.

A more recent example of children's digital media raising the flag on wider issues with regards to digital culture, in that it addresses worries about internet-connected smart toys (see Holloway & Green, 2016), has drawn attention to concerns surrounding data surveillance by corporations, privacy issues, geolocation and tracking, and the digital hacking of other technologies included in the internet of things.

Returning to the original paradigm discussed in this section, that childhood is a social construction, recent scholarship in children's studies suggests that it is not just the discursive that frames the child, but the material (James & Prout, 2015). Drawing upon the theoretical frames of posthumanism and new materialism as a way to move beyond the limitations of social construction, and the subject/object and agency/structure binaries (see Prout, 2011), this newer work acknowledges the affective entanglements of young people with material objects and assemblages. Instead of setting the subject apart from the material, posthumanism insists upon the importance of material encounters, as the child is relational, in process, and constituted by conceptual and material forces (Murris, 2017).

The second paradigmatic feature considers childhood as a "variable of social analysis that cannot be divorced from such variables as class, gender or ethnicity" (Prout & James, 2003, p. 8). Prout and James call for research that is intersectional, comparative, and cross-cultural to reveal a diverse childhood instead of a singular universal phenomenon (2003). The child is never solely an aged subjectivity, childhood is lived as an intersectional subjectivity.

The child that is often understood within digital culture and media is an imagined global child who is often Western, due largely to the discursive impact of the dominance of multinational corporations in the digital mediascape. As Dafna Lemish has argued, in regards to the production of content (both digital and analog) for the international marketplace, there is a tendency to erase the cultural symbols and signs that mark a children's text as foreign or national, to produce the "neutral grounds of global culture" (in Chan, Lemish, McMillin, & Parameswaran, 2013, p. 213). This perceived neutrality is based on an imagined global child and a universalising notion of childhood (Hogan & Sienkiewicz, 2013) that emerges from corporations' need to sell content globally. The universal child (who is predominately constructed as a Western middle-class boy) allows global corporations to justify the sale of one program to dozens of nations. As Havens (2007) notes, this "myth of a global child" essentialises childhood, implying that there are unified tastes and desires of children that make it feasible to sell across a multitude of local markets. Such discourse homogenises young people as gendered and aged consuming subjects to the exclusion of collective and regional subjective experiences (Buckingham, 2011; Wise, 2008).

A similar discursive bias can be seen in children's rights. Boyden asks, in the context of the United Nations Convention on the Rights of the Child (UNCRC), whose rights are being addressed? And, in whose interests are the best interests of the child being addressed? Boyden suggests that the view of childhood is Western and it is a European conception of childhood that is exported to the Global South. Its values are white, urban, and middle class (Boyden, 2003). To rectify these types of biases, Prout and James call on scholarship to be intersectional, to see the child as more than a gendered and aged subject. This child, and the lived experiences of children, are intersectionally intertwined with a child's race, sexuality, socio-economic status, and geographic locale. James and Prout call for us to think of childhoods, not childhood, by pushing for a world view of childhood that is a comparative, historical, cross-cultural analysis of a variety of childhoods, and not just a simple, single phenomenon (2003, p. 4).

The third feature of the paradigm for a new sociology of childhood argues that "children's social relationships and cultures are worthy of study in their own right, independent of the perspectives and concerns of adults" (Prout & James, 2003, p. 8). This is particularly relevant in regards to children and digital media as children's content is often evaluated from the perspective of adults. A common concern about children's digital media is that the content is 'bad' and of poor quality. Terms like vacuous, silly, and ridiculous are often bandied about when adults comment on children watching the latest YouTube videos from Ryan's Toys (over 1.1 billion views at the time of writing) or Sophia Grace (583 million views). Deeming children's content to be 'bad' suggests that children need to be protected from themselves – from the consequences of their own dubious tastes and uncultured desires. The assumption seems to be that, left to their own desires, children would naturally consume vulgar, sensational content with simplistic stereotypes (Davies, Buckingham, & Kelley, 2000). Adult assumptions about children's content often reveal more about adult culture than children's culture. Disparaging children's cultural consumption is an act of power that works to perpetuate and reinforce distinctions between the child and the adult, often reinscribing adult culture as the 'valued' culture.

Allison James' work on children's candy argues that children's attraction to content that is deemed as poor by adult culture can be a small act of resistance. Consuming and enjoying that which is judged as not having value is a means for children to forge alternative systems of meaning, reinterpret social models, and semantically reorder adult signs (James, 1998, p. 394). James' work here reminds us of the need for scholarship on the child and digital media that recognises "children's agency in constructing and defining their own tastes and identities" (Davies et al., 2000, p. 8). Digital content is often more complex than it might appear to be on the surface. Patricia Lange's (2014) work on YouTube, for example, reveals the collaborative social networks that young people use to negotiate identity and develop digital literacies, even in content that is disparaged. Digital media is a space for young people to make and remake meaning, often in contention with the adult world. Scholarship on young people and digital media needs to reveal these creative processes of interdependence between child and adult cultures.

The fourth feature of the paradigm states that children are "active in the construction and determination of their own lives, the lives of those around them and of the societies in which they live" (Prout & James, 2003, p. 8). This feature reminds us that children are not "passive subjects of social structures and processes" and, it could be added, "materialities", but are active participants. Children are social actors and are part of culture, not a precursor to culture (James & Prout, 2003, p. vii). The opening refrains of this chapter that position children as 'obsessed with', 'bullied on', and 'corrupted by' digital media do not consider the child as agentive. The child in such framing is passive and manipulated by technological forces. Nor do these frames recognise that children and children's culture actually help shape and direct the way digital media is organised and functions.

Children are creators of digital content, from producing videos on YouTube to building online games. They often create content in ways that challenge and contest the limited and limiting options provided by corporate entities. Young people also find ways to "appropriate digital media to find spaces of personal autonomy while their parents and teachers try to deploy digital media normatively to shape young people's present achievements and future prospects" (Livingstone & Sefton-Green, 2016, p. 56). Children can demonstrably shape the way content is circulated online and the means through which it is monetised, effectively impacting the political and economic structures of digital platforms. But more work needs to be done on how young people's participation in digital media influences the workings of digital capitalism.

On the flip side of recognising children as agentive within the political economic structures of digital media, there is a danger of romanticising children's agency, or celebrating them as 'digital natives', a narrative that has been highly critiqued. Work on young people needs to balance the notion that children have agency but also recognise the deep constraints on children's participation as they are beholden to structures that are often designed, created, and policed without their input. As Livingstone and Haddon note, children's activities can be highly constrained both online, through the design of platforms and websites for example, and offline through the constraining role of families, communities, and schools (2012).

Feature five of the paradigm calls for methodological approaches that give children a direct voice and active participation in the production of data (Prout & James, 2003). Allison James suggests that the true nature of the culture of childhood is often hidden from adults (1998).

Scholarship on and with young people must take a 'child-centred approach' which identifies children's experiences, voices, and actions, and then contextualises these within the concentric circles of structuring social influences, such as the family, community, and culture (Livingstone & Haddon, 2012). For Prout and James, this requires ethnographic research methods as opposed to "experimental or survey styles of research" (2003, p. 8). A recent example of an excellent ethnography in scholarship on children and digital media is Sonia Livingstone and Julian Sefton-Green's work *The Class* (2016), which tracked a group of students over three semesters as a way of challenging existing assumptions by the adult world of policymakers, parents, and educators, about young people's digital worlds.

Currently, innovative strategies are being explored to 'decolonise' childhood research by positioning children as co-researchers or collaborators in the research process, and understand children as aware of their own worlds. Drawing from postcolonial research (see Tuhiwai Smith, 1999), these strategies acknowledge the power dynamics of positioning the child as a data subject of an adult researcher, and offer alternative methodological practices based on collaboration. Digital technologies allow for new forms of creative methods, such as photo voice techniques, that utilise the digital competencies of children as active researchers in their own digital lives (see Thomson, Berriman, & Bragg, 2018).

Another methodological possibility is to use a phenomenological approach to understand how young people are living contemporary lives in digital spaces. Poyntz and Kennelly suggest that phenomenology "permits the focus of meaning-making to rest with the experiences of youth themselves within the context of a much larger historical frame" (2015, p. 3). Using a methodological approach that incorporates children's voices, perspectives, opinions, and experiences about digital media is an important methodological tool in counteracting the narrow and limiting arguments of digital media as a corrupting force on children, as outlined in the opening paragraphs of this chapter.

For the sixth and last feature of this paradigm, Prout and James acknowledge that the new sociology of childhood is complicit in its own reproduction. It is a double hermeneutic, they suggest. To proclaim a new paradigm of childhood is to discursively reconstruct the child. Extending this to digital media means that to begin research on children and digital media from the position that childhood is a social construction, separate from the realities of the living child, discursively frames the child. This is a reminder that the social sciences are not "neutral commentaries on children [and childhood] but active factors in its construction and reconstruction" (Prout & James, 2003, p. 29). Such research encourages scholars to reflect upon tensions in their work between the child as a social institution and the lived experiences of the embodied child within the social institution. It acknowledges that the act of research is always a political act. And it exhorts those that are interested in understanding the child, childhood, and the experiences of children to be aware of ethical responsibilities to produce nuanced narratives of digital engagement that are reflective of a wide range of experiences and perspectives.

Conclusion

The meaning of the child is always fluid and in process of development, reflecting the ebb and flows of social, technological, political, and cultural change. As the digital intensifies and shifts, the definitions and framings of what it means to be a child also shift. And the reverse is also true, as cultural understandings of childhood and the experiences of children shift, so too does thinking about the digital. For example, current shifts that locate the child and the digital within a rights-based perspective and which advocate for children's rights to both participate in and be protected in digital environments, forces a rethinking of the figure of the child and the meaning of the digital (see Livingstone & Third, 2017). As another example, children's roles as influencers, and as online microcelebrities, open up new questions around children's creative labour in digital capitalism, which require both a rethinking of the child as labourer and also the meaning of work in digital capitalism.

While it is over 20 years old, James and Prout's paradigm of the sociology of childhood still provides a useful starting point for scholarship on the child and digital media. Its six features offer avenues to think through the child in digital environments, in ways that position the child as an agentive subject. The basic premise that "children should be regarded as part of society and culture, not precursor to it; and that children should be seen as already social actors not being in the process of becoming such" (James & Prout, 2003, p. vii), is critical for scholarship on the child and digital media. For the child, the digital is not a neutral or benign space, created by adults, where the child enters into it as a preformed environment. Instead, the digital is a space where young people have been and continue to be productively engaged in forming and shaping the contours of their experiences.

References

Abidin, C. (2015). Micromicrocelebrity: Branding babies on the internet. *M/C Journal, 18*(5). Retrieved from: http://journal.media-culture.org.au/index.php/mcjournal/article/view/1022.

Andrejevic, M. (2007). *iSpy: Surveillance and power in the interactive era*. Lawrence, KS: University Press of Kansas.

Ariès, P. (1965). *Centuries of childhood: A social history of family life*. New York, NY: Vintage Books.

Blum-Ross, A. (2015, June 17). 'Sharenting': Parent bloggers and managing children's digital footprints. Retrieved from: http://eprints.lse.ac.uk/76347.

Boyden, J. (2003). Childhood and the policy makers: A comparative perspective on the globalization of childhood. In A. James & A. Prout (Eds.), *Constructing and reconstructing childhood: Contemporary issues in the sociological study of childhood* (2nd ed., pp. 190–216). London, UK: Falmer Press.

Buckingham, D. (2011). *The material child: Growing up in consumer culture*. Cambridge, UK: Polity Press.

Buckingham, D. (2018). Foreword. In R. Thomson, L. Berriman, & S. Bragg (Eds.), *Researching everyday childhoods: Time technology and documentation in a digital age* (pp. vii–xi). London, UK: Bloomsbury.

Chan, K., Lemish, D., McMillin, D., & Parameswaran, R. (2013). Beyond 'the West to the Rest': A roundtable on global children's media flows. *Interactions: Studies in Communication and Culture, 4*(3), 211–220.

Cook, D. (2004). *The commodification of childhood: The children's clothing industry and the rise of the child consumer*. Durham, NC: Duke University Press.

Cook, D. (2011). Commercial epistemologies of childhood: "Fun" and the leveraging of children's subjectivities and desires. In D. Zwick & J. Cayla (Eds.), *Inside marketing: Practices, ideologies and devices* (pp. 257–268). Oxford, UK: Oxford University Press.

Davies, H., Buckingham, D., & Kelley, P. (2000). In the worst possible taste: Children, television and cultural value. *European Journal of Cultural Studies, 3*(1), 5–25.

Elmer, G. (2003). *Profiling machines: Mapping the personal information economy*. Cambridge, MA, USA: MIT Press.

Fuchs, C. (2010). Labor in informational capitalism and on the Internet. *The Information Society, 26*(3), 179–196.

Gauntlett, D. (1998). Ten things wrong with the 'effects' model. In R. Dickinson, R. Harindranath, & O. Linne (Eds.), *Approaches to audiences: A reader* (pp. 120–130). London, UK: Arnold.

Grimes, S. M., & Shade, L. R. (2005). Neopian economics of play: Children's cyberpets and online communities as immersive advertising in NeoPets.com. *International Journal of Media & Cultural Politics, 1*(2), 181–198.

Havens, T. (2007). Universal childhood: The Global trade in children's television and changing ideals of childhood. *Global Media Journal, 6*(10), 1–8.

Hogan, L., & Sienkiewicz, M. (2013). 1001 markets: Independent production, 'Universal childhood' and the global kids' television industry. *Interactions: Studies in Communication & Culture, 4*(3), 221–238.

Holloway, D., & Green, L. (2016). The internet of toys. *Communication Research and Practice, 2*(4), 506–519.

James, A. (1998). Confections, concoctions, and conceptions. In H. Jenkins (Ed.), *The children's culture reader* (pp. 394–405). New York, NY: NYU Press.

James, A., Jenks, C., & Prout, A. (1998). *Theorizing childhood*. Williston, VT: Teachers College Press.

James, A., & Prout, A. (2003). Preface to second edition. In A. James & A. Prout (Eds.), *Constructing and reconstructing childhood: Contemporary issues in the sociological study of childhood* (2nd ed., pp. ix–xvii). London, UK: Falmer Press.

James, A., & Prout, A. (2015). Introduction. In A. James & A. Prout (Eds.), *Constructing and reconstructing childhood* (3rd ed., pp. 1–5). New York, NY: Routledge.

Jenkins, H. (Ed.). (1998). Introduction: Childhood innocence and other modern myths. In H. Jenkins (Ed.), *The children's culture reader* (pp. 1–37). New York, NY: NYU Press.

Jenks, C. (2005). *Childhood*. New York, NY: Routledge.

Lange, P. (2014). *Kids on YouTube: Technical identities and digital literacies*. Walnut Creek, CA: Left Coast Press.

Livingstone, S. (2003). Children's use of the internet: Reflections on the emerging research agenda. *New Media & Society, 5*(2), 147–166.

Livingstone, S., & Haddon, L. (2012). *Children, risk and safety on the internet: Research and policy challenges in comparative perspective*. Bristol, UK: Policy Press.

Livingstone, S., & Sefton-Green, J. (2016). *The class: Living and learning in the digital age*. New York, NY: NYU Press.

Livingstone, S., & Third, A. (2017). Children and young people's rights in the digital age: An emerging agenda. *New Media & Society, 19*(5), 657–670.

Mead, M. (2017). *Coming of age in Samoa: A study of adolescence and sex in primitive societies*. Penguin Books Limited (original work published 1943).

Murris, K. (2017). The post-human child: III. In D. Kennedy & B. Bahler (Eds.), *Philosophy of childhood today: Exploring the boundaries* (pp. 185–197). Lanham, MD: Lexington Books.

Poyntz, S. R., & Kennelly, J. (2015). Introduction. In S. Poyntz & J. Kennelly (Eds.), *Phenomenology of youth cultures and globalization: Lifeworlds and surplus meaning in changing times* (pp. 1–22). Abingdon, UK: Routledge.

Prout, A. (2011). Taking a step away from modernity: Reconsidering the new sociology of childhood. *Global Studies of Childhood, 1*(1), 4–14.

Prout, A., & James, A. (2003). A new paradigm for the sociology of childhood? In A. James & A. Prout (Eds.), *Constructing and reconstructing childhood: Contemporary issues in the sociological study of childhood* (2nd ed., pp. 7–33). London, UK: Falmer Press.

Scholz, T. (Ed.). (2012). *Digital labor: The internet as playground and factory*. Abingdon, UK: Routledge.

Schor, J. (2004). *Born to buy: The commercialized child and the new consumer culture*. New York, NY: Simon and Schuster.

Seiter, E. (2004). The internet playground. In J. Goldstein, D. Buckingham, & G. Brougére (Eds.), *Toys, games, and media* (pp. 93–108). Mahwah, NJ: Lawrence Erlbaum Associates.

Terranova, T. (2000). Free labor: Producing culture for the digital economy. *Social Text, 18*(2), 33–58.

Thomson, R., Berriman, L., & Bragg, S. (2018). *Researching everyday childhoods: Time technology and documentation in a digital age*. London, UK: Bloomsbury.

Tuhiwai Smith, L. (1999). *Decolonizing methodologies: Research and Indigenous peoples*. London, UK: Zed Books.

UNICEF. (2017). *The state of the world's children 2017 statistical tables*. Retrieved from: https://data.unicef.org/resources/state-worlds-children-2017-statistical-tables.

Wilson, A. (1980). The infancy of the history of childhood: An appraisal of Philippe Ariès. *History and Theory, 19*(2), 132–153.

Wise, M. (2008). *Cultural globalization: A user's guide*. Carlton: Blackwell.

Zelizer, V. A. (1994). *Pricing the priceless child: The changing social value of children*. Princeton, NJ: Princeton University Press.

2

ENGAGING IN ETHICAL RESEARCH PARTNERSHIPS WITH CHILDREN AND FAMILIES

Madeleine Dobson

Introduction

Research with children and families presents exciting and significant opportunities. Through working with children and families, researchers can obtain important insight into their ways of being, their perspectives, and their lived experiences. In the space of digital media, this kind of insight is crucial. Examining the ways in which children and families live with and engage with digital media has the potential to further researchers' understandings around the nature of digital media, its present place and purpose, and possible future directions. Nonetheless, there are conceptual and ethical complexities of which researchers must be aware and which require prioritisation and careful navigation.

This chapter encompasses a range of conceptual and ethical issues related to research with children and families in the space of digital media. Influenced by a strong image of children, the chapter begins by examining researchers' conceptualisations of children, digital media, and their nexus, which has great relevance to research ethics. Thus, the chapter next raises ethical issues that researchers in this space may face and frameworks they may benefit from utilising. Finally, the chapter focusses on ethical considerations for exploring digital media in the lives of children and families, with a mind towards serving, supporting, and honouring children and families.

Conceptualising Children, Digital Media, and Their Nexus

Beliefs about children shape adults' interactions with and observations of them. Thus, clarifying what conceptions of children, childhood, and digital media researchers bring to the process is essential if research is to proceed in an ethically literate manner. This influences the lens through which the researcher looks, and how they make sense of what is being explored (Rallis, 2018), and consequently impacts on ethical matters. When researching children, families, and digital media, two key conceptual questions arise: how do researchers conceptualise children? And, how do researchers conceptualise the nexus of children and digital media?

Conceptualising Children

The ways in which researchers conceptualise children has incredible influence over a research project, from its inception and preparation, through the generation and analysis of data, and into the finalisation and dissemination of the project. Unpacking the conceptualisation of children involves critical reflection about who a researcher believes children to be and how children are situated in the adults' world, and, thus, in research.

Traditionally, children have been viewed and positioned as voiceless (Smith & Taylor, 2000), passive (Mittal, 2005), lacking in knowledge and capacity (Freeman & Mathison, 2009), and existing in binary opposition to adults (Robinson & Jones-Diaz, 2016). The consequence of this conceptualisation of children tends to be that they become objects of research, rather than subjects, and their expertise regarding their own lives is disregarded. Conversely, children can be conceptualised as important, active, and agentic individuals with their own views, voices, and values. This shift towards new and stronger conceptualisations of the child is seen in the work of poststructuralist and feminist theories (Robinson & Jones-Diaz, 2016), in the discourse of socioculturalism (Dunn, 2015), and through the lens of the educational project of Reggio Emilia (as explored by Britt & McLachlan, 2015). By viewing children through this respectful and appreciative lens, an imperative emerges: for researchers to partner with children and to empower them as collaborators and co-creators in research. Analogously, there is powerful potential in creating similar partnerships with children's families, and empowering parents/guardians/carers to share in the research journey alongside their children.

Therefore, a central question for researchers working with children is: what image of the child is mobilised in the research? This question stems from the work of Malaguzzi and is embraced by educators and researchers working in the tradition of Reggio Emilia (Irving, 2018). Britt and McLachlan (2015, p. xv) identify this question as a challenging one, and elaborate: "the question's significance becomes clear when we consider that what we see, expect, and believe about children powerfully shapes our response to them". Further questions that will help researchers in navigating their image of the child include:

- What capacities are children believed to possess?
- What kind of citizenship do children hold?
- How are children viewed in relation to adults?
- How does the research project position child participants?

Like the central question, these questions are challenging and significant. They encompass themes of power and potential, and merit close and careful attention. By engaging in this critically reflective conceptual work, a researcher can reach a more nuanced understanding of their role and responsibilities. And while there are many ways to conceptualise children, and certainly many images of children that have emerged historically, culturally, and politically, there is immense potential in embracing a strong and nuanced image of the child. By seeing children as capable and competent (Rinaldi, 2013), as thinkers and theorists (Duncan, 2018), as meaning-makers (Clark & Moss, 2017), and as active citizens (Britt & McLachlan, 2015) who are entitled to rights, respect, and recognition (Freeman, 2011), researchers can move in responsive, creative, and promising directions.

Conceptualising the Nexus of Children and Digital Media

The nexus of children and digital media – that is, the relationship that exists between children and digital media and how the researcher conceptualises these intersections – is a key locus for research contemplation. It is well-acknowledged that digital media have a pivotal presence in children's lives (Reid Chassiakos, Radesky, Christakis, Moreno, & Cross, 2016; Rideout, Foehr, & Roberts, 2010; Selwyn, 2011; Stephen & Edwards, 2017) – but how is this presence conceptualised? Key questions for reflection include:

- How is the power dynamic between children and digital media conceptualised?
- Does the research position children as 'digital natives'? Why/why not?

These questions encourage researchers to further examine their image of children with specific regard to digital media. Issues of power arise – for example, it is often observed that children are immersed in the world of digital media (Reid Chassiakos et al., 2016; Stephen & Edwards, 2017). The framing of this immersion is key, particularly in terms of the power dynamic between children and digital media. Children who have grown up amidst digital technologies have been referred to as 'digital natives' (Prensky, 2001) – a conceptualisation which this chapter explores and critiques. There is sometimes a tendency towards polarised views where the dynamic is framed as positive/negative or beneficial/harmful, which ignores the inherent complexities of children and media (Qvarsell, 2000). In particular, to construct children as wholly vulnerable in this equation is to deny them their full humanity. Conversely, constructing children as active and agentic in this equation reinforces a strong image of the child and has the potential to empower children.

The question of whether or not to embrace a view of children as digital natives is one worthy of consideration for researchers working in this space. While the term 'digital natives' is relatively commonplace, this way of conceptualising children's relationships with digital media is divisive and contested. It is argued that the characterisation of children as digital natives is lacking in evidence (Bennett, Maton, & Kervin, 2008) and presents a homogeneous view of a generation of children and young people (Palfrey & Gasser, 2011). There is potential for presumptions to be made about children's readiness to engage with digital media and their levels of interest and investment, rather than recognising diversity and difference in children. As part of their conceptual framing, researchers are encouraged to critically consider whether or not they buy into the idea of children as digital natives, and to contemplate the variety of ways in which children live, in terms of their upbringing and education, and the range of perspectives and passions that children may possess.

Ultimately, establishing a clear and informed conceptualisation of how children and digital media intersect informs and supports a researcher's next steps, especially with regards to the ethical and methodological aspects of their project.

Ethical Research Partnerships with Children and Families

Engaging in Ethically Literate Research

The importance of research ethics cannot be overstated. Research ethics have significant bearing upon the researcher, their practice, the project at hand, and the participants and their context. A researcher's engagement with ethics should not be singular or cursory – rather, it is imperative that researchers engage in ethically literate practice. This involves considering ethics in a holistic, critical, and comprehensive manner, and placing it at the very heart of the research endeavour. Engagement in ethically literate research ensures that children and families are protected and supported during projects in which they are involved, and, ultimately, honoured. This section deals with the centrality of research ethics and key considerations for researchers working with children and families. Rather than exacting prescriptive standards, the intention is to raise provocations that illuminate the rich potential of a holistic approach to ethics.

Research ethics are sometimes viewed as a 'tick and flick' exercise, where priority is placed on satisfying the protocols of the researcher's institution and the context in which they seek to undertake research. This view fails to recognise the pervasive presence and complexity of ethics and the necessity of considering the ethics of research before, during, and after any given study. The centrality of ethics is well recognised, particularly with regards to working with children (Abebe & Bessell, 2014; Barblett, Hydon, & Kennedy, 2017), which is an inherently ethical endeavour (Clark & Moss, 2017). Ethics also extend beyond matters of access and assent or consent, and encompass respect, rights, and equality (Alderson & Morrow, 2011). Furthermore, engaging in ethical research practice on an ongoing basis is advocated for by Flick (2007, p. 70), who writes:

> Reflection of ethics is not only relevant while you are in the field and it is not only something to work on while you prepare a proposal – for the ethics committee or the institutional review board of your institution. Ethics should play a role in your considerations of how to plan a study, of who you want to work with, and how you (or your fieldworkers) should act in the field.

While research ethics hinge on the context and circumstances of each project (Rose, 2012), there are overarching issues related to researching digital media with children and families. The ways in which a researcher relates to children and families, which is inextricably linked to their conceptual understandings, is a definitive component of the research process and a major aspect of research ethics. Strong and respectful conceptualisations of children invite researchers to engage in their work in ways that honour children's rights and capacities. Namely, a rights-based approach can be of immense value (Beazley, Bessell, Ennew, & Waterson, 2011). Human rights have immense ethical significance and are grounded in recognition of worth and dignity (Monteiro, 2014). A rights-based approach involves aligning research ethics to the United Nations Convention on the Rights of the Child (UNCRC), which advocates for and articulates children's citizenship and rights. While the UNCRC is not specifically focussed on research, it provides valuable guidance and groundwork for engaging ethically with children (Abebe & Bessell, 2014). Here, the following articles come into play:

- Article 3.3: Children have the right to expect the highest possible standards of services from professionals who work with them;
- Article 12: Children have the right to express their opinions in matters concerning them;
- Article 13: Children have the right to express themselves in any way they wish – not limited to the verbal expressions used by adults; and
- Article 36: Children have the right to be protected from all forms of exploitation, including being exploited through research processes and through the dissemination of information.

In aligning research ethics to these articles, researchers can afford children agency and voice, and ensure that their needs and rights are met. Potential implications of a rights-based research approach are explored later in this chapter.

As well as considering the UNCRC, researchers engaged in work with children and families can draw on a range of relevant ethical codes such as the European Early Childhood Education Research Association (EECERA) Ethical Code (EECERA, 2014) and the Early Childhood Australia (ECA) Code of Ethics (ECA, 2016). The EECERA Ethical Code is guided by an ethic of respect around the following principles:

1   The child, family, community, and society;
2   Democratic values;

3   Justice and equity;
4   Knowing from multiple perspectives;
5   Integrity, transparency, and respectful interactions;
6   Quality and rigour;
7   Academic scholarship; and
8   Social contribution.

Similarly, the ECA Code of Ethics – though developed with a pedagogical focus – has relevance for researchers. There is distinct advocacy for a strong image of children and an appreciation of children's rights. Key principles for consideration include:

- Each child has unique interests and strengths and the capacity to contribute to their communities;
- Children are citizens from birth with civil, cultural, linguistic, social, and economic rights;
- Partnerships with families and communities support shared responsibility for children's learning, development, and wellbeing; and
- Democratic, fair, and inclusive practices promote equity and a strong sense of belonging.

The principles articulated by EECERA and ECA align to the UNCRC and reinforce the notion of children as competent individuals. While these codes are intended to apply to children in the early years (i.e., birth to eight years of age), the principles have applicability for all children and young people, and their families as well. Researchers are invited to consider a multitude of ethical issues with regards to participants and their contexts. Key questions for critical reflection include:

- How can the project support children's rights and citizenship?
- How can the researcher plan for inclusivity? For example – are multiple modes of expression supported? What strategies can be put in place to honour and accommodate diversity and difference in children and families?
- What is the potential impact of the project in the short, medium, and long term?
- Are the participants thoroughly versed in the foreseeable outcomes of the project?

These questions can guide and support planning for ethics in the initial stages. Critical reflection should continue throughout the entirety of the project, both in terms of the bigger picture and the minutiae. Researchers should engage with the aforementioned questions with careful consideration towards their participants' identities. One aspect of identity which is key here is the age and stage of the participants, particularly with regards to how they may or may not understand the project's foreseeable outcomes. For instance, when working with younger children, the process of inviting participation may require adjustments. Such adjustments may include amending the format and/or language of the documentation, involving parents to a greater extent, and ensuring there are comprehensive checks for understanding employed. With regards to children's assent to engage in research, there are a range of options available to researchers that may enhance the process. For example, it is recommended that researchers individualise assent processes with consideration towards children's personal factors and family dynamics, as well as the complexity of the project design and any researcher and organisational factors (Oulton et al., 2016). There are also creative options in obtaining informed consent, such as making use of picture books that depict participation in the research process (Pyle & Danniels, 2016) or utilising technology such as video clips explaining the methods and context of the research (Parsons, Sherwood, & Abbott, 2016).

As research unfolds, the ways in which researchers relate to children is of critical consequence. Ethical interactions with children are characterised by active and respectful listening, a commitment to empowering children and eliciting their voices, staying attuned to children's needs, and working adaptively in recognition of diversity and difference in terms of – for example – language, culture, and socio-economic status. This requires a sensitive and adaptive disposition from the researcher, and can present challenges when working across different cohorts of children and families. Recognising the diversity of children's abilities and preferences is also key (Merewether & Fleet, 2014), the implications of which are discussed in the next section of this chapter.

While ethical issues will vary from project to project, and while different complexities, questions, and quandaries may emerge, researchers can remain ethically attuned by engaging in ongoing reflection informed by the principles from EECERA and ECA and the relevant articles from the UNCRC, and by remaining focussed on the ways in which they relate to their participants. By embracing an ethical code that encompasses relevant articles and principles from the aforementioned documents, researchers can enter into child-centric practices that aim to give children choice and voice. There are many possibilities in centring children in research, including positioning them as storytellers of their own experiences (Bloch & Bailey, 2016), as philosophers (Britt & McLachlan, 2015), and as experts and co-researchers (McGladrey, 2015). This type of practice ensures a socially just approach (Freeman & Mathison, 2009) and supports the growth of children's citizenship (Noddings & Brooks, 2017). It leads researchers towards responsive, reciprocal, and respectful methodologies that honour children and families.

Key Considerations for Ethical Research Partnerships

If researchers embrace the view that their work should be underpinned by a strong image of children and infused with ethical literacy, then an imperative emerges to engage in responsive, reciprocal, and respectful partnerships. There are extensive possibilities in terms of methodological approaches and research methods, including – but not limited to – surveys (e.g., Nikken & Opree, 2018; Rideout et al., 2010), questionnaires (e.g., Johnson, 2012; Mourgela & Pacurar, 2018), case studies (e.g., Heydon, McKee, & Daly, 2017; Teichert & Anderson, 2014), and ethnographies (e.g., Dahya, 2017; Dezuanni, 2018). This section details considerations that have relevance across designs and methods, and which support a strong image of children and a holistic and continuous approach to ethics.

Stemming from a strong image of children is the prospect of partnering with children in research. This is a complex endeavour. It requires a commitment to taking the time to build a positive rapport (Clark & Moss, 2017) characterised by active, careful, and ethical listening (Pascal & Bertram, 2009), and then working continually to sustain an authentic, collaborative, and reciprocal working relationship (Freeman & Mathison, 2009). Working in an adaptive and responsive manner is also key (Merriam & Tisdell, 2016). McLachlan (2012, p. 27), offering pedagogical insight into centring children and following their interests:

> Following the interests of children is not a predictable process, no matter what the context. Children see differently, walk differently, care differently and talk differently from adults and from each other. Walking beside children, rather than leading them, requires constant and committed reflection with every step. It means getting down low, adjusting your pace regularly, and following through to completion. It requires negotiation, questioning and risk, recognising and respecting the differences that exist among a group of thinkers.

The provocations here – to commit to reflection, to adapt to children's ways of being and seeing, and to work in a cooperative and responsive manner – have great relevance for researchers. This connects to the ethics of the project and, in terms of the generation of data, can contribute depth and richness. While these provocations are of distinct significance to research with children, they can also apply to working with children's families. There are implications for:

- The allocation of time (e.g., at what pace do the research activities occur? Can the pace be adjusted to accommodate greater opportunity for voice and choice for the participants? Do context- or individual-specific adjustments need to be made?).
- The nature of communication (e.g., is accessible language used and is it aligned to the participants' needs? Are multiple modes of expression supported for participants? How might language be adjusted when working with multi-age cohorts or with children and families who are linguistically diverse?).
- The researcher/participant dynamic (e.g., when is it time for the researcher to lead? When is it time to follow the participant?).

Adjusting the pace of the research conveys a respect for participants and their contributions. For many children and families, research can seem intimidating – slowing the pace can contribute to building a sense of trust and supports positive working relationships. It also creates space for deeper engagement in research activities and potentially opens up the project beyond the researcher's lens and framework, to include the participants' ways of being and seeing. This is particularly important when working with very young children, who often require more time to ease into research activities and who may benefit from a slower and more patient style of interaction. In terms of research activities, there is a broad range of options that have the potential to invite children's engagement and inspire their contributions. For instance, Teichert and Anderson's (2014) case study of digital media in the life of a five-year-old involved three interviews which involved elicitation devices and activities. These included relevant picture books, a digital camera and related software, and iPhone apps. The use of these elicitation devices and activities were targeted at engaging the child, gaining insight into their perspectives and interests, and working responsively with their interests. Furthermore, permitting children to have agency over the pacing of the research can be helpful. In research involving interviews and focus groups with children aged between four and thirteen, Leeson's (2014) participants were able to use age-appropriate strategies to signal when they did not want to answer a question or when they preferred the interview to end. While the older participants were able to vocalise their preferences, the younger participants used strategies including pre-determined code words, tokens, or pictures. These types of considerations are illustrative of an ethical approach which responds to and respects the children in question.

The use of accessible and flexible language is critical. This hinges on the cohort – for example, are there participants with English as an additional language? At what level are the children in terms of their listening, speaking, reading, and writing? Do some of the terms relevant to the project require clarification, elaboration, or re-wording to ensure accessibility? When working with children of many different ages, what strategies are in place for adjusting the language used in documentation (e.g., assent letters, surveys, and/or questionnaires) and face-to-face communication? A variety of strategies were employed in the EU Kids Online project to ensure children's readiness to engage in the research, including cognitive testing to ensure questions were comprehendible, checking for understanding during face-to-face interviews, carefully defining terminology, and translating to include a wide range of languages (Livingstone, Haddon, Görzig, & Ólafsson, 2011). Researchers can also consider multiple modes of expression, including non-verbal modes of communication that children and families may utilise in the research process.

The integration of visual resources may also support participation, both in terms of including visual aspects in documentation (e.g., colour coding or illustrative imagery in assent letters for children) or including opportunities for participants to express themselves visually (e.g., photography, drawing, painting, mind-mapping) as part of the research method.

The question of who leads, and how, and when, is also imperative. This requires a commitment to ethical and respectful practice. Researchers working with children and families may benefit from maintaining a critical consciousness towards when it is the researcher's time to speak and act, and when it is time to 'open the floor' to the participants and, perhaps, follow their lead. Such an approach requires a commitment to listening to participants in an authentic and meaningful way. Good guidance in this regard is offered by Rinaldi (2012), who characterises listening as a sensitive, curious, patient, and inclusive experience which gives people and their perspectives visibility and legitimacy. By embracing this critical consciousness, researchers can balance the scales, empower participants, and create space for participants to make meaningful contributions to the project. There are many ways that this ethic of listening can be pursued. For example, in the author's own study focussing on young girls' relationships with different types of media across their home, school, and community contexts, an emphasis was placed on empowering the girls to share their perspectives and experiences (Dobson & Beltman, 2019). The girls were positioned as storytellers and the researcher sought their perspectives and experiences through curious and compassionate listening and questioning which was personalised to each girl engaged in the research. Through this type of listening, strong researcher–participant relationships emerged, which contributed to the generation of rich experiential data about the girls' ways of relating to the variety of media in their lives. The approach was also highly regarded by the girls, who reflected that they appreciated the opportunity to have their voices and views heard (Dobson & Beltman, 2019).

While these ethical approaches have merit, however, they can also present challenges and tensions. For instance, slowing the pace of research is difficult given the realities of time constraints for researchers, children, and families – so striking a balance is key. While permitting children to influence the pace and parameters of research activities is important in respecting and supporting their agency, it may present perceived difficulties or obstacles at times. Accounting for linguistic diversity may – depending on the cohort and their context – prove demanding for researchers and their resources. Supporting multiple modes of expression is complex and requires attention to detail and investment of time, effort, and expertise. Distributing power between the researcher and participants can also prove a navigational challenge. With regards to all of these potential issues, persistence and sensitivity are essential. Persistence is important in committing to this type of practice in a meaningful way, while sensitivity on the part of the researcher elicits an awareness of challenges, tensions, and possible resolutions. Here, ethics return to the fore, as the researcher can refer to their ethical framework to determine a respectful and constructive response to any issues.

There is distinct potential and worth in pursuing approaches that encompass a strong image of children and a deep commitment to ethical literacy. These approaches can be adapted to ensure alignment to the purpose, context, and complexities of the project. In the realm of researching digital media with children and families, such approaches open up possibilities for understanding digital media use through multiple lenses with a deserved emphasis on lived experience.

Conclusion

This chapter has examined conceptual and ethical issues related to researching digital media with children and their families. It is grounded in a strong and nuanced image of children and a research ethic that encompasses respect, care, and rights. Provocations are raised for researchers intending to engage in work with children and families around weaving ethics throughout the entirety of the project and engaging in partnerships which are supportive and inclusive. By pursuing research of this nature, researchers can create collaborative, equitable, and productive projects which have the potential to progress people's understandings of digital media in the lives of children and families.

References

Abebe, T., & Bessell, S. (2014). Advancing ethical research with children: Critical reflections on ethical guidelines. *Children's Geographies, 12*(1), 126–133. doi:10.1080/14733285.2013.856077.

Alderson, P., & Morrow, V. (2011). *The ethics of research with children and young people: A practical handbook* (2nd ed.). London, UK: SAGE.

Barblett, L., Hydon, C., & Kennedy, A. (2017). *Ethics in action: A practical guide to implementing the Early Childhood Australia Code of Ethics*. Deakin West, ACT: Early Childhood Australia.

Beazley, H., Bessell, S., Ennew, J., & Waterson, R. (2011). How are the human rights of children related to research methodology? In A. Invernizzi & J. Williams (Eds.), *The human rights of children: From visions to implementation* (pp. 159–178). Surrey, UK: Ashgate.

Bennett, S., Maton, K. A., & Kervin, L. (2008). The 'digital natives' debate: A critical review of the evidence. *British Journal of Educational Technology, 39*(5), 775–786. doi:10.1111/j.1467-8535.2007.00793.x.

Bloch, M., & Bailey, C. (2016). The matter of lives: Towards an everyday politics of action. In R. R. Scarlet (Ed.), *The anti-bias approach in early childhood* (3rd ed., pp. 343–349). Sydney, NSW: Multiverse.

Britt, C., & McLachlan, J. (2015). *Unearthing why: Stories of thinking and learning with children*. Mt Victoria, NSW: Pademelon Press.

Clark, A., & Moss, P. (2017). *Listening to young children: The mosaic approach* (3rd ed.). London, UK: Jessica Kingsley Publishers.

Dahya, N. (2017). Critical perspectives on youth digital media production: 'Voice' and representation in educational contexts. *Learning, Media, and Technology, 42*(1), 100–111. doi:10.1080/17439884.2016.1141785.

Dezuanni, M. (2018). Minecraft and children's digital making: Implications for media literacy education. *Learning, Media, and Technology, 43*(3), 236–249. doi:10.1080/17439884.2018.1472607.

Dobson, M., & Beltman, S. (2019). Powerful and pervasive, or personal and positive? Views of young girls, parents and educators about media. *Issues in Educational Research, 29*(1), 38–54.

Duncan, R. (2018). *Journeys of inquiry*. Osborne Park, WA: Association of Independent Schools Western Australia.

Dunn, J. (2015). Insiders' perspectives: A children's rights approach to involving children in advising on adult-initiated research. *International Journal of Early Years Education, 23*(4), 394–408. doi:10.1080/09669760.2015.1074558.

Early Childhood Australia. (2016). *ECA Code of Ethics – Core principles*. Retrieved from: www.earlychildhoodaustralia.org.au/our-publications/eca-code-ethics/code-of-ethics-core-principles.

European Early Childhood Education Research Association. (2014). *Ethical code for early childhood researchers*. Retrieved from: www.eecera.org/custom/uploads/2016/07/EECERA-Ethical-Code.pdf.

Flick, U. (2007). *Designing qualitative research*. London, UK: SAGE.

Freeman, M. (2011). *Children's rights: Progress and perspectives*. Leiden and Boston, MA: Martinus Nijhoff Publishers.

Freeman, M., & Mathison, S. (2009). *Researching children's experiences*. New York, NY: The Guilford Press.

Heydon, R., McKee, L., & Daly, B. (2017). iPads and paintbrushes: Integrating digital media into an intergenerational art class. *Language and Education, 31*(4), 351–373. doi:10.1080/09500782.2016.1276585.

Irving, E. (2018). What is a child? Conceptions and images of childhood. In E. Irving & C. Carter (Eds.), *The child in focus: Learning and teaching in early childhood education* (pp. 3–29). South Melbourne, Victoria: Oxford University Press.

Johnson, G. (2012). Learning, development, and home digital media use among 6 to 8 year old children. *Problems of Psychology in the 21st Century, 1*, 6–16.

Leeson, C. (2014). Asking difficult questions: Exploring research methods with children on painful issues. *International Journal of Research & Method in Education, 37*(2), 206–222. doi:10.1080/1743727X.2013.820643.

Livingstone, S., Haddon, L., Görzig, A., & Ólafsson, K. (2011). *EU Kids Online: Final report*. Retrieved from: http://eprints.lse.ac.uk/39351.

McGladrey, M. (2015). Lolita is in the eye of the beholder: Amplifying preadolescent girls' voices in conversations about sexualization, objectification, and performativity. *Feminist Formations, 27*(2), 165–190. doi:10.1353/ff.2015.0012.

McLachlan, J. (2012). No, it's not okay: Drawing a line in the sand. In A. Fleet., C. Patterson, & J. Robertson (Eds.), *Insights: Behind early childhood pedagogical documentation* (pp. 25–36). Mt Victoria, NSW: Pademelon Press.

Merewether, J., & Fleet, A. (2014). Seeking children's perspectives: A respectful layered research approach. *Early Child Development and Care, 184*(6), 897–914. doi:10.1080/03004430.2013.829821.

Merriam, S. B., & Tisdell, E. J. (2016). *Qualitative research: A guide to design and implementation* (4th ed.). San Francisco, CA: Jossey-Bass.

Mittal, S. (2005). *Children and media* (Vol. 3). Adarsh Nagar, Delhi: Isha Books.

Monteiro, A. R. (2014). *Ethics of human rights*. Switzerland: Springer International.

Mourgela, V., & Pacurar, E. (2018). Children, extracurricular activities, and digital media: The process of displacement and school performance. *Journal of Educational Computing Research, 56*(2), 202–225. doi:10.1177/0735633117707792.

Nikken, P., & Opree, S. (2018). Guiding young children's digital media use: SES-differences in mediation concerns and competence. *Journal of Child and Family Studies, 27*(6), 1844–1857. doi:10.1007/s10826-018-1018-3.

Noddings, N., & Brooks, L. (2017). *Teaching controversial issues: The case for critical thinking and moral commitment in the classroom*. New York, NY: Teachers College Press.

Oulton, K., Gibson, F., Sell, D., Williams, A., Pratt, L., & Wray, J. (2016). Assent for children's participation in research: Why it matters and making it meaningful. *Child: Care, Health and Development, 42*(4), 588–597. doi:10.1111/cch.12344.

Palfrey, J., & Gasser, U. (2011). Reclaiming an awkward term: What we might learn from 'digital natives'. In M. Thomas (Ed.), *Deconstructing digital natives: Young people, technology, and new literacies* (pp. 186–204). New York, NY: Routledge.

Parsons, S., Sherwood, G., & Abbott, C. (2016). Informed consent with children and young people in social research: Is there scope for innovation? *Children & Society, 30*(2), 132–145. doi:10.1111/chso.12117.

Pascal, C., & Bertram, T. (2009). Listening to young citizens: The struggle to make real a participatory paradigm in research with young children. *European Early Childhood Education Research Journal, 17*(2), 249–262. doi:10.1080/13502930902951486.

Prensky, M. (2001). Digital natives, digital immigrants – Part 1. *On the Horizon, 9*(5), 2–6.

Pyle, A., & Danniels, E. (2016). Using a picture book to gain assent in research with young children. *Early Child Development and Care, 186*(9), 1438–1452. doi:10.1080/03004430.2015.1100175.

Qvarsell, B. (2000). Children's use of media as transformed experience: Educological and psychological dimensions. In B. Van den Bergh & J. Van den Bergh (Eds.), *Children & media: Multidisciplinary approaches* (pp. 33–47). Leuven-Apeldoorn: Garant.

Rallis, S. F. (2018). Conceptual framework. In B. B. Frey (Ed.), *The SAGE encyclopaedia of educational research, measurement, and evaluation* (pp. 354–356). Thousand Oaks, CA: SAGE.

Reid Chassiakos, Y. L., Radesky, J., Christakis, D., Moreno, M. A., & Cross, C. (2016). Children and adolescents and digital media. *Pediatrics, 138*(5), 1–18. doi:10.1542/peds.2016-2593.

Rideout, V. J., Foehr, U. G., & Roberts, D. F. (2010). *Generation M^2: Media in the lives of 8- to 18-year-olds*. Menlo Park, CA: Kaiser Family Foundation.

Rinaldi, C. (2012). The pedagogy of listening: The listening perspective from Reggio Emilia. In C. Edwards, L. Gandini, & G. Forman (Eds.), *The hundred languages of children: The Reggio Emilia experience in transformation* (3rd ed., pp. 233–246). Santa Barbara, CA: Praeger.

Rinaldi, C. (2013). *Re-imagining childhood: The inspiration of Reggio Emilia education principles in South Australia*. Adelaide, SA: Government of South Australia.

Robinson, K., & Jones-Diaz, C. (2016). *Diversity and difference in childhood* (2nd ed.). Berkshire, UK: Open University Press.

Rose, G. (2012). *Visual methodologies: An introduction to researching with visual materials* (3rd ed.). London, UK: SAGE.

Selwyn, N. (2011). *Schools and schooling in the digital age: A critical analysis*. Abingdon, Oxon: Routledge.

Smith, A., & Taylor, N. (2000). Introduction. In A. Smith, N. Taylor, & M. Gollop (Eds.), *Children's voices: Research, policy and practice* (pp. ix–xiii). Auckland: Pearson Education New Zealand.

Stephen, C., & Edwards, S. (2017). *Young children playing and learning in a digital age: A cultural and critical perspective*. Abingdon, Oxon: Routledge.

Teichert, L., & Anderson, A. (2014). "I don't even know what blogging is": The role of digital media in a five-year-old girl's life. *Early Child Development and Care, 184*(11), 1677–1691. doi:10.1080/03004430.2013.875540.

3

PLATFORMS, PARTICIPATION, AND PLACE

Understanding Young People's Changing Digital Media Worlds

Heather A. Horst and luke gaspard

Introduction

Over the past few decades, the media worlds available to young people have changed dramatically. The generation of adults who began their computing lives with home-based Commodore 16s or 64s or the Sinclair Spectrum ranges of computers are now the parents of young people who have in their possession a handheld computing device in the form of a smartphone with about 1,500 times the Commodore's processing power. Gaming in the form of non-networked gaming consoles has given way to the option of playing on the move via iPods, smartphones, and tablets; downloaded or streamed games via a variety of platforms using a desktop or laptop computer and an ever-expanding range of consoles and dedicated hand-held devices offer the possibility of 3D, haptic, and virtual-reality gaming. During this time, huge shifts have also taken place in the way young people interact and their ability to create media content. Communication between friends has shifted from lengthy (and often pre-arranged) phone conversations and conference calls to a wide variety of computer-mediated communication services that enable the sharing of a range of multi-media and linkable content within large and small personally known and unknown groups on a smartphone, tablet, and via computer apps. The ability to create music, photographs, films, and other creative content has been enhanced through cheaper and more accessible digital cameras and smartphones, often equipped with a variety of basic editing software and the means to share these creations easily and widely. These and many other changes have transformed how young people communicate.

This chapter focusses upon three developments that have fundamentally shaped young people's media worlds. The first development revolves around the proliferation of cross-media *platforms* and the capacity for these new platforms to be used across a range of technology tools and contexts. The second development involves how platforms and associated technologies such as public wi-fi can now support greater *participation*, sometimes thought of as participatory culture, which facilitates young people's ability to communicate, learn, play, and share in ways unforeseeable even a generation ago. The third development, *place*, highlights the spread and uneven mainstreaming of practices using social media and gaming in the different local and national contexts in which young people live. Whilst the issues that underpin place are not necessarily caused by media and technology, the chapter highlights the importance of attending to place's persistence in shaping the varied practices among youth from different backgrounds, and acknowledge the ways in which place shapes young people's different – and differentiated – media worlds in contrasting and dynamic ways. In order to highlight these important historical shifts, examples of practices among youth in Melbourne, Australia, are provided from recent research.[1] These examples show that platforms, participation, and place are not mutually exclusive or bounded entities; instead, they build upon each other to reconfigure young people's contemporary media landscapes.

Platforms

Rapid changes in technology and the possibilities this opens up have provided the grounds for some of the most optimistic accounts of changes in young people's lives. Within a generation, enormous shifts have occurred not only in the availability of digital computing platforms for young people but also in how technologies are utilised by youth. Established and dominant media forms have given way to new technologies and media uses that only a short while ago were unknown or only viable for a small minority of (adult) users. Television, for example, is no longer the dominant media form in a young person's media world; instead, the internet has become their go-to media platform for leisure, entertainment, homework, and a range of other activities. In the UK, for example, between 2008 and 2017, while television viewing in a typical week among eight- to fifteen-year-olds had declined by 15%, internet use had increased by 45% (OFCOM, 2008, 2017). The smartphone has grown to become the principal media tool for many young people with recent reports suggesting that US youth spend more time with this device than any other in an average day (Rideout, 2015, p. 21). Nearly all US teens (94%) aged 13 to 17 use social media (AP-NORC, 2017) and video gaming has emerged as the most favoured media activity among this group (Rideout, 2015, p. 21). Among Australian youth, social media is the most commonly mentioned of any offline or online media activity taking place 'every day' (gaspard, Horst, Pink, & Gomez Cruz, 2020).

These shifts in media focus among young people can broadly be understood via a dual lens of access and the multi-functionality of technology. In terms of access, many young people, particularly those of the developed West, are now able to access the internet in numbers and at speeds unimaginable only a short time ago. Taking the US as a case in point, at the turn of the millennium the majority of US teens did not possess internet access in the home (Roberts, Foehr, & Rideout, 2005, p. 77), and even five years later just as many youths were accessing the internet via a dial-up telephone modem as were using high-speed connections (ibid, p. 78). Today, combining reporting data from the EU, UK, and USA, current estimates suggest around 88% of five to sixteen-year-olds live in a household with a high-speed internet connection (Livingstone, Haddon, Görzig, & Ólafsson, 2011; OFCOM, 2017; Rideout, 2015).

At the same time, free public wi-fi access in shopping malls, cafes, transport, and other venues has helped provide internet opportunities a young person can enjoy beyond the traditionally fixed locations of the home, school, and public library. Between 2016 and 2017 alone, the number of public wi-fi hotspots worldwide was estimated to have nearly doubled to 179 million (Statista, 2017). Hardware platforms for accessing the internet have also become cheaper, smaller, and increasingly mobile. Following the commercial market introduction of laptops, tablets, and smartphones in the early 2000s, these devices now supersede the desktop computer in terms of prevalence within a young person's home (Rideout, 2015, p. 22). Alongside the shrinking size of computing technology, the costs associated with going online have also witnessed dramatic declines (BLS, 2015). These changes in the media profile of many youths have allowed the smartphone to become the most commonly used device by youth to access the internet (Byrne, Kardefelt-Winther, Livingstone, & Stoilova, 2016).

The pre-eminence of the mobile phone has also been aided by device convergence, which exponentially increases the range of functions that a single media appliance can perform (Jenkins, 2006). For example, as mobile phones have increased in technical sophistication, a typical smartphone can function as a telephone, camera, video-recorder, geo-locater, facilitate computer-mediated communication (e.g., via email, instant messaging, and social network sites), and act as a web browser, document reader, and an audio and video player. Smartphones also offer (online and offline) gaming opportunities. Moreover, with the roll-out of 5G networks in October of 2018, there is the possibility to eliminate network latency (the time data takes to travel between sender and receiver) and increase download speeds to 20 times faster than with 4G. Industry professionals promoting these changes, such as Ronan Dunne, Executive Vice President and Group President, Verizon Wireless, characterise the impact of the technology as akin to ushering in a "Fourth Industrial Revolution" (verizon.com).

Lastly, social media and social network sites (SNS) have emerged as key platforms for youth interaction and identity exploration. The use of social media tools has grown exponentially as they have fundamentally lowered "barriers to communication and sharing", and in doing so have reshaped "the kinds of networks that people are able to build and support" (Ellison & boyd, 2013, p. 9). As Ellison and boyd (2013) stress, this has also been aided by online users being prepared to shift their coming together within interest-driven virtual communities to build more intimate and social relationships via the sharing of highly personalised information and content. boyd (2008) has addressed how these sites offer for parents a safe space for their children to 'hang-out' with peers where issues of time pressure, transportation, and broader societal fears can be mitigated. Meanwhile, for youth, valuable space is provided to explore questions of identity and taste by presenting and managing aspects of a user's identity that can be viewed, discussed, and altered (boyd, 2008; Stern, 2008; Willett, 2008).

But, as will be even clearer in the later sections, the picture is always more complex than is captured by the focus on changes in technological possibilities outlined above. As a word of caution even at this stage, there are pressures associated with the kinds of perpetual engagement, being *always on*, which have now been enabled by smartphones and other platforms. For example, Sherry Turkle (2011) has argued that such heightened inter-connectedness breeds increased expectations to be constantly available for friends online. At the same time, she argues, the new technologies' possibilities for mediating young people's interactions offer the allure of companionship without the demands of building strong and intimate friendships, while arguably also reducing the ability to engage in quality of thought due to the over-stimulus demanded by engagement with multiple media applications (ibid.).

Participation

Digital access offers the potential for the creators of media content and those who use and consume media content to interact with each other in new ways. Traditional top-down broadcast models of communication emblematic of 'old' media systems have given way to opportunities for individuals to 'broadcast themselves', both through personal social networks but also more widely to unseen and unknown masses via video aggregation platforms such as YouTube, Vimeo, or the specialist video gaming platform Twitch. As such, the positions of the media producer and media consumer need no longer be separate and exclusive but instead give rise to participants that can amalgamate these once distinct roles into a 'prosumer' or 'producer' (Bruns, 2008; Jenkins, 2006; Lange, 2014). With the ability to circulate and create culture, share knowledge, build social networks, and connect and play with others in ways never previously envisaged, this 'participatory culture' can drive the acquisition of new media literacy skills. These can also be thought of as social skills whereby youth can learn from each other as exploration and ingenuity are valued in ways that traditional classrooms struggle to accommodate (Ito et al., 2010; Jenkins, Purushotma, Weigel, Clinton, & Robison, 2009).

A notable example of this process comes in a seminal study of 800 youth in the United States, the Digital Youth project, that identified the different 'genres of participation' – hanging out, messing around, and geeking out – that young people use in their everyday life; and the ways in which these practices reflect learning (Ito et al., 2010). For example, many young people in the US at the time participated in early social networking sites like MySpace and learned norms of interacting, or what might be thought of as socialisation with their peers, through 'Hanging Out' with their friends by posting pictures and comments online when they returned home from school. Others who were curious about where information came from or wanted to know how to do things such as changing their profiles on social media, engaged in what Ito's co-author Dan Perkel described as 'copy and paste literacy' by using bits of pre-written code to transform the look and feel of their social media profiles. This, the authors argued, could be conceived of as a form of exploration ('messing around') to learn how things work. The third genre of participation, geeking out, often emerged when young people became intensely interested in an activity such as gaming or making videos. In some instances this meant gaining expertise as to how to do a particular activity, joining a community of people who shared that interest, and enjoying the reputation associated with such expertise, including teaching others how to do activities. This was, for many young people, an expression of expertise not always acknowledged in adult-driven institutions such as schools or families.

An important location for youth participation was illustrated in a recent netnography of Steam, a platform downloaded to the computer that is situated at the centre of diverse networks ranging from economic, informational, and social (Gomez Cruz, Horst, gaspard, & Pink, forthcoming). The Steam study was part of a broader project on Transmedia Literacies designed to understand how young people are learning skills outside the school. The authors and their collaborators undertook research in Melbourne, Australia, and surveyed 860 students at four secondary schools and one primary, held two workshops focussed upon transmedia storytelling and gaming, and carried out 36 in-depth interviews. Teens celebrated the Steam platform on many levels as it provided a fully immersive participatory space for communicating, learning about games, sharing knowledge, and game-playing that offered an opportunity for community building and developing a shared identity. As one participant commented, "It's like the go-to for everything", while another described the platform as "social media for games ... it is a chat thing ... it's like the apps-store but with friends ... like the apps store and iMessage kind of mashed together ...".

The ability to socialise with like-minded gaming enthusiasts was especially prominent for many users. For example, War Owl, a 13-year-old boy, demonstrated the considerable number of people he had in his Friends List, 'half' of which he had known offline while the other 'half' he had met online within the platform. Many participants discussed the recommender systems for games within the platform wherein people post their recommendations and reviews of games, as well as let's play and walk-through videos. These aspects of metagaming, i.e., the emerging cultures around gaming beyond playing the game itself (Kow, Young, & Tekinbaş, 2014), are also able to be incorporated into the Steam platform via access to YouTube and other platforms, which further support the gaming ecology. The creation of such content proves valuable for gamers as it enables recognition of gaming expertise honed through many hours of gaming. War Owl, for example, developed and refined his presentation and video-making skills through three YouTube channels and more than 30 videos. In so doing, War Owl had identified a niche gaming activity where he was able to monetise his gaming exploits. Here, expertise converges with social networks and the tools to make, share, and circulate content associated with participatory culture.

However, there are difficulties and exposure to risks that can impact a youth's ability to participate allied to these possibilities of increased connection and learning. Issues of contact, content, and inappropriate behaviour plague youth participation in online spaces. Although popular media stories often overstate the occurrence of offline contact with strangers and the number of contacts young people possess in their social media networks, many young people continue to leave themselves vulnerable to identification by maintaining a public profile often with personal information including phone numbers or addresses (Livingstone et al., 2011, pp. 38–9). Moreover, inappropriate, nasty, or hateful content online are everyday experiences for many young people, while the incidence of cyber-bullying is on the rise (Livingstone, Mascheroni, Ólafsson, & Haddon, 2014; OFCOM, 2017). Alongside this, more than half of young people reported that they had blocked a message from a person they did not want to hear from (OFCOM, 2017, pp. 167–8). Meeting a person face to face having first met online is a practice undertaken by only one in four youth (Livingstone et al., 2011, pp. 38–9).

Apart from such risks, a 'ladder of opportunities' is in place that shapes how much or how little youth actually exploit the digital technologies at their disposal. Nearly two decades ago David Buckingham (in Seiter, 2005, p. 6) observed that in practice the majority of youth under-used technology and rarely engaged "in relatively more creative or technologically complex activities". More recent research indicates that the majority of youths' media uses remain clustered around a small number of activities. Principally these are communication, content consumption, gaming, and schoolwork, with few users engaging in more technically challenging activities such as file-sharing, content creation, and civic participation (EU Kids Online, 2014; Livingstone, 2012). It is also important to bear in mind how factors such as 'knowledge' and 'social context' impact a youth's technological inclusion or exclusion and ability to exploit technology (Buckingham & Willett, 2006; Seiter, 2005, 2008). How parents perceive the role of technology within the family home, e.g., as a tool of education or entertainment, how it is embedded within the routines and spaces of the household, parental skill and knowledge levels, and their ability to mediate youth access, have all been addressed as crucial factors that can cultivate or hinder young people's relationships and uses of digital technology (boyd & Hargittai, 2013; gaspard, 2015; Horst, 2012; Lally, 2002; Schofield Clark, 2013; Tripp, 2010).

Finally, further complicating youth participation is the issue of how young people often struggle to contextualise the environments in which their web browsing takes place, further driving calls for an increased focus on digital literacy (Buckingham, 2007). With youth tending to congregate on websites with explicit commercial motivations (see ebizmba.com), Patti Valkenburg (2004) argues that young surfers fail to understand the commercial imperatives underpinning the existence of their favourite sites. This positioning of the young body as an economic body is, however, not a recent development borne from the advent of online digital engagement. Instead, this exploitation has a long history, taking into account differing historical periods, including the use of free or cheap youth labour within pre-industrial and industrial eras (Aries, 1973; Qvortrup, 2005). Later, at the turn of the twentieth century, the department store industry marketed to the needs and desires of young people in previously unseen ways in order to attract mothers into these "palaces of consumption" (Cook, 2004); more recent marketing developments point to the deep entrenchment of boundary marking between youth age groups as a way of further encouraging differing consumption practices among young people (see Cody, 2012 for discussion). Indeed, even within the media industry, creators of culture have a long history of finding novel and not so novel ways of framing youth participation in their own culture as a commercial practice (Cook, 2004; Kinder, 1999; Kline, 1993). In the digital age, media corporations have expertly navigated the media worlds that youth inhabit in order to create spaces for participation, including those for entertainment, game-playing, citizenship, and community which are intrinsically tied to consumption (Banet-Weiser, 2007; Grimes, 2008a, 2008b; Hill, 2011).

Place

The ladder of opportunities discussion suggests that not all young people have access to the same opportunities and choices. This raises issues of access, equity, and digital disadvantage, which are often associated with place as well as other demographic factors. Despite government efforts in many countries to reduce the digital inequalities some groups encounter in comparison with others, there are essential divides that must be acknowledged concerning the quality of the digitally mediated life a young person can and does encounter. A young person's social-economic status (SES), their age, gender, household structure, but also region within their national context, all remain essential determinants of their digital experience. On the one hand, a young person's wealth is a likely indicator of the type of social media platform they use (Lenhart, 2015); older children, boys, and youth from middle-class families enjoy better quality home internet access than girls, as well as younger and lower-class children (Livingstone & Helsper, 2007). On the global stage, UNICEF reports that significant disparities exist worldwide between urban and rural home internet access for youth, with those from the lowest-income countries using the internet the least (UNICEF, 2017).

Globally, 12% fewer women are using the internet than men, and in some developing countries, where girls encounter severe restrictions on their rights in comparison with boys, substantial digital gender gaps are present. In India, for example, less than a third of online users are women (UNICEF, 2017). Even within OECD countries gender differences in digital use are present. More boys go online daily than girls, boys use the internet at an earlier age, and are much more likely to use a desktop computer to access the internet, whereas twice as many girls use a smartphone (Mascheroni & Ólafsson, 2014). Conversely, girls encounter more online risk than boys, experience higher levels of cyber-bullying and being bothered by others, encounter more upsetting content, while also experiencing higher levels of parental mediation of their internet use (Ito & Horst, 2019; Livingstone et al., 2014).

This high proportion of girls utilising mobile phone technology as a critical access route to the internet is significant as it raises issues of concern also found with low-income youth. More impoverished youth, especially if the young person belongs to an ethnic minority, have lower levels of home internet access (Child Trends, 2015), are more likely to rely on mobile-only access within the home, either via a tablet or smartphone, and have the smartphone as the most commonly found computing device in the home (Rideout & Katz, 2016). In these low- and moderate-income homes, despite internet access being near-universal, families experience severe impediments to the quality of their computing experience. Interruptions to service, slow service, use of out-dated technology, and youth unable to gain sufficient time on computing technology due to sharing device time with other members of the household, are all common challenges facing more impoverished digital youth (ibid.), impacting upon opportunity and digital creativity and skill development. While parents cite the high cost of a home computer and internet access as the principal reason for not investing in these, the report *Opportunity for All* points to many implications of mobile-centric internet access for youth (ibid.). Such youth are less likely to use their technology to complete homework when compared with those using a computer or laptop at home, as well as playing fewer educational games and looking up less information that interests them (ibid., pp. 34–5). The increased flexibility and privacy afforded by mobile devices for youth to access the internet also increases exposure to risk (O'Neill & Dinh, 2015), while reducing the parental opportunity for mediation and support of their children's media use. At the same time, Byrne and colleagues (2016, p. 36) argue that the use of a small screen negatively impacts the 'complexity' and scope of content that can be accessed.

It is also important to remember that inequalities also exist within developed and highly connected cities, such as Melbourne, Australia, voted annually since 2011 as the world's most liveable city by the Economist Intelligence Unit. In work carried out by gaspard and colleagues (2020) exploring transmedia and informal learning practices among teens aged 12–18, they found that, of 838 school students, a little under 2% of teens surveyed did not possess an internet connection at home. Tim, a 13-year-old boy who attended a school in a multicultural lower-class suburb in the east of the city, provides a case in point. Although born in Melbourne, Tim was from a South Pacific island background and he found school difficult. His teacher commented that he would often play-up in class and his dedication to completing work was a rarity rather than the norm. His principal carer, his grandmother, did not have an internet connection at her home, meaning Tim's opportunities for digital participation were severely limited. With a tablet device as the sole piece of digital household technology available to access the internet, school and the occasional visit to a friend's home offered his only sources of going online. The local library was not a consideration, which meant his game-playing was restricted to downloading free games from the App store while at school, which he could play later offline. However, because of the school policy to block many websites, including social media platforms such as Facebook, there was only so much he could achieve in his internet exploration.

Due to the curbs on his internet time, Tim was not able to participate to the same degree in online culture as many of his friends. He did not play web-based multiplayer games or examine game reviews or consume YouTube videos on game-play (the platform found by the research team to be the hegemonic learning tool in youths' media culture and in many cases their principal source of information). Despite having three social media accounts, Tim had only ever posted two photos to these and was generally a very infrequent user; he was also unable to utilise the internet for any of his school work. Whether embodying the limitations of his internet participation that his situation dictated or because he did not see value in the affordances of being online, when questioned as to how he felt about his degree of internet use, Tim claimed "I think I'm doing all right. I don't need to be on the internet more than I should be".

Platforms, Participation, and Place: Looking Ahead

Platforms, participation, and place represent three key developments that have altered how digital youth engage in and create their media worlds. While important individually, when overlaid together they provide a more balanced and more complex framework to account for the dynamism of the media worlds that underpin digital youth engagement. On the one hand, digital devices and evolution in software tools and platforms have led some to paint a landscape of abundant opportunity for young people that resonates with narratives of 'digital natives' advocated by Prensky (2001) and Barnes, Simun, Gasser, and Palfrey (2009). Yet the infrastructure and hardware that supports these practices, the software architecture facilitating the exploitation of online opportunities, and how these opportunities are made more or less available to particular young people, include many factors that remain outside their direct control.

If computing technology keeps to the experience curve it has so far produced, it will become even cheaper, smaller, and more powerful than the technology of today. This means that one possible future may be the offer of more complex software platforms with greater degrees of immersion and participation, possibly to degrees that, even from a current viewpoint, may seem unlikely or even absurd. Yet, important questions remain as to how youth are best positioned to exploit the advances of this brave new world. Are the increases in computing power and internet speeds likely to overcome the bottlenecks that appear in the way youth use technology? Moreover, if the above technological scenario is to occur, what measures or forms of digital literacy can help mitigate the increased risks that accompany the opportunities from further digital engagement? Manuel Castells has argued that the internet is being increasingly geared towards supporting the economic interests of a few commercial entities (Castells, 2002). Has the hope of an internet geared more toward achieving broader social good been all but extinguished as conglomerations increasingly determine the internet's evolving architecture rather than nation-states and its users?

Moreover, what of the digital inequalities that impact many different groups in society as youths' digital contexts typically continue to reflect the social disadvantages they experience offline? Even if smartphone penetration is likely to increase among the economically disadvantaged youth of the Global South (e.g., Kant, Horst, & Drugunalevu, 2019), will 5G roll-outs in the developed North further exacerbate the divides already present? Without critical intervention into the way media worlds are constrained and restricted by institutions and the structural dimensions of society, existing research suggests that there are already indicators of the answers to many of these questions.

Note

1 This refers to research funded by the European Union's Horizon 2020 research and innovation programme under grant agreement No. 645238. Further details about the Transmedia Literacies project are available online: https://transmedialiteracy.org.

References

(AP-NORC) The Associated Press-NORC Center for Public Affairs Research. (2017). *Instagram and snapchat are most popular social networks for teens; Black teens are most active on social media, messaging apps.* Retrieved from: www.apnorc.org/PDFs/Teen%20Social%20Media%20Messaging/APNORC_Teens_SocialMedia_Messaging_2017_FINAL.pdf.

Aries, P. (1973). *Centuries of childhood.* Harmondsworth: Penguin.

Banet-Weiser, S. (2007). *Kids rule: Nickelodeon and consumer citizenship.* Durham, NC and London: Duke University Press.

Barnes, R. F., Simun, M., Gasser, U., & Palfrey, J. (2009). Youth, reativity, and copyright in the digital age. *International Journal of Learning & Media, 1*(2), Spring, 79–97.

BLS (Bureau of Labor Statistics). (2015). *Long-term price trends for computers, TVs, and related items.* Retrieved from: www.bls.gov/opub/ted/2015/long-term-price-trends-for-computers-tvs-and-related-items.htm.

boyd, d. (2008). Why youth (heart) social network sites: The role of networked publics in teenage social life. *Youth, identity, and digital media* (pp. 119–142). Cambridge, MA, USA: MIT Press.

boyd, d., & Hargittai, E. (2013). Connected and concerned: Variations in parents' online safety concerns. *Policy & Internet, 5*(3), 245–269.

Bruns, A. (2008). *Blogs, Wikipedia, Second Life, and beyond: From production to produsage.* New York, NY: Peter Lang.

Buckingham, D. (2007). *Beyond technology: Children's learning in the age of digital culture.* Cambridge and Malden, MA: Polity.

Buckingham, D., & Willett, R. (Eds.). (2006). *Digital generations: Children, young people, and new media.* Manhwah, NJ: Lawrence Erlbaum Associates Inc.

Byrne, J., Kardefelt-Winther, D., Livingstone, S., & Stoilova, M. (2016). *Global Kids Online research synthesis, 2015–2016.* UNICEF Office of Research Innocenti and London School of Economics and Political Science. London: LSE. Retrieved from: http://eprints.lse.ac.uk/71299.

Castells, M. (2002). *The internet galaxy: Reflections on the internet, business, and society.* Oxford: Oxford University Press.

Child Trends. (2015). *Home computer access and internet use: Indicators of child and youth well-being.* Retrieved from: www.childtrends.org/wp-content/uploads/2015/12/69_Computer_Use.pdf.

Cody, K. (2012). "BeTween two worlds": Critically exploring marketing segmentation and liminal consumers. *Young Consumers, 13*(3), 284–302.

Cook, D. T. (2004). *The commodification of childhood: The children's clothing industry and the rise of the child consumer.* Durham, NC: Duke University Press.

ebizmba.com. (2018). *Top 15 most popular Kid websites.* Retrieved from: www.ebizmba.com/articles/kids-websites.

Ellison, N., & boyd, d. (2013). Sociality through social network sites. *The Oxford handbook of internet studies.* Oxford: Oxford University Press. doi:10.1093/oxfordhb/9780199589074.013.0008.

EU Kids Online. (2014). *EU Kids Online: Findings, methods, recommendations (deliverable D1.6)*. London: EU Kids Online, LSE.

gaspard, l. (2015). *Ecologies of the televisual: children's use of the televisual in Melbourne, Australia*. RMIT University.

gaspard, l., Horst, H., Gomez Cruz, E. & Pink, S. (2020). Media practices of young Australians: Tangible and measurable reflections on a digital divide. *KOME – An International Journal of Pure Communication Inquiry, 2020* 8(1), 80–96. doi: 10.17646/KOME.75672.42.

Gomez Cruz, E., Horst, H., gaspard, L., & Pink, S. (forthcoming). Navigating moral universes: Young people's strategies for managing digital media worlds. [Manuscript submitted for publication].

Grimes, S. M. (2008a). Saturday morning cartoons go MMOG. *Media International Australia Incorporating Culture & Policy, 126*, 120–131.

Grimes, S. M. (2008b). Kid's ad play: Regulating children's advergames in the converging media context. *International Journal of Communications Law & Policy, 12*, 161–178.

Hill, J. A. (2011). Endangered childhoods: How consumerism is impacting child and youth identity. *Media Culture Society, 33*(3), 347–362.

Horst, H. A. (2012). New media technologies in everyday life. In H. A. Horst & D. Miller (Eds.), *Digital anthropology* (pp. 61–79). New York, NY: Berg Publications.

Ito, M., Baumer, S., Bittanti, M., boyd, d., Cody, R., Herr-Stephenson, R., . . . Tripp, L. (2010). *Hanging out, messing around, and geeking out: Kids living and learning with new media*. Cambridge: MIT Press.

Ito, M., & Horst, H. (2019). Preface. In M. Ito, S. Baumer, M. Bittanti, d. boyd, R. Cody, R. Herr-Stephenson, . . . L. Tripp (Eds.), *Hanging out, messing around, and geeking out: Kids living and learning with new media* (10th anniversary ed.; pp. xiii–xxxvi). Cambridge: MIT Press.

Jenkins, H. (2006). *Convergence culture: Where old and new media collide*. New York, NY: NYU Press.

Jenkins, H., Purushotma, R., Weigel, M., Clinton, K., & Robison, A. J. (2009). *Confronting the challenges of participatory culture: Media education for the 21st century*. Cambridge, MA: MIT Press.

Kant, R., Horst, H., & Drugunalevu, E. (2019). *Parenting in the smart age: Fijian perspectives*. Documentary film, 27 min.

Kinder, M. (1999). *Kid's media culture*. Durham, NC: Duke University Press.

Kline, S. (1993). *Out of the garden: Toys and children's culture in the age of TV marketing*. London: Verso.

Kow, Y. M., Young, T., & Tekinbaş, K. S. (2014). *Crafting the metagame: Connected learning in the StarCraft II community*. Irvine, CA: Digital Media and Learning Research Hub.

Lally, E. (2002). *At home with computers*. Oxford and New York, NY: Berg.

Lange, P. G. (2014). *Kids on YouTube: Technical identities and digital literacies*. Walnut Creek, CA: Routledge.

Lenhart, A. (2015). *Teen, social media and technology overview 2015*. Washington, DC: Pew Research Center.

Livingstone, S. (2012). Understanding the relation between risk and harm: Theory, evidence and policy regarding children's internet use. Keynote lecture to the 62nd Annual Conference of the International Communication Association, Phoenix, May 2012.

Livingstone, S., Haddon, L., Görzig, A., & Ólafsson, K. (2011). *Risks and safety on the internet: The perspective of European children: Full findings and policy implications from the EU Kids Online survey of 9-16-year-olds and their parents in 25 countries*. EU Kids Online, Deliverable D4. London: EU Kids Online Network.

Livingstone, S., & Helsper, E. (2007). Gradations in digital inclusion: Children, young people and the digital divide. *New Media & Society, 9*(4), 671–696.

Livingstone, S., Mascheroni, G., Ólafsson, K., & Haddon, L. (2014). *Children's online risks and opportunities: Comparative findings from EU Kids Online and Net Children Go Mobile*. London: London School of Economics and Political Science.

Mascheroni, G., & Ólafsson, K. (2014). *Net Children Go Mobile: Risks and opportunities* (Second ed.). Milano: Educatt.

OFCOM. (2008). *Media literacy audit: Report on UK children's media literacy*. Retrieved from: www.stakeholders.ofcom.org.uk/binaries/research/media-literacy/media-lit-2010/ml_childrens08.pdf.

OFCOM. (2017). *Children and parents: Media use and attitudes report*. Retrieved from: www.ofcom.org.uk/__data/assets/pdf_file/0020/108182/children-parents-media-use-attitudes-2017.pdf.

O'Neill, B., & Dinh, T. (2015). Mobile technologies and the incidence of cyberbullying in seven European countries: Findings from Net Children Go Mobile. *Societies, 5*(2), 384–398.

Prensky, M. (2001). Digital natives, digital immigrants part 1. *On the Horizon, 9*(5), 1–6.

Qvortrup, J. (2005). Introduction. In J. Qvortrup (Ed.), *Studies in modern childhood: Society, agency, culture* (pp. 1–20). Hampshire: Palgrave Macmillan.

Rideout, V. (2015). *The common sense census: Media use by tweens and teens*. Retrieved from: www.commonsensemedia.org/sites/default/files/uploads/research/census_researchreport.pdf.

Rideout, V. J., & Katz, V. S. (2016). *Opportunity for all? Technology and learning in lower-income families*. A report of the Families and Media Project. New York, NY: The Joan Ganz Cooney Center at Sesame Workshop.

Roberts, D. F., Foehr, U. G., & Rideout, V. (2005). *Generation M: Media in the lives of 8-18 year-olds*. Kaiser Family Foundation. Retrieved from: https://kaiserfamilyfoundation.files.wordpress.com/2013/01/generation-m-media-in-the-lives-of-8-18-year-olds-report.pdf.

Schofield Clark, L. S. (2013). *The parent app: Understanding families in the digital age*. New York, NY: Oxford University Press.

Seiter, E. (2005). *The internet playground: Children's access, entertainment and mis-education*. New York, NY and Oxford: Peter Lang.

Seiter, E. (2008). Practicing at home: Computers, pianos, and cultural capital. In T. McPherson (Ed.), *Digital youth, innovation, and the unexpected (The John D. and Catherine T. Macarthur Foundation series on digital media and learning)* (pp. 27–52). Cambridge, MA: MIT Press. doi:10.1162/dmal.9780262633598.027.

Statista.com. (2017). *Number of public Wi-Fi hotspots worldwide from 2016 to 2021* (in millions). Retrieved from: www.statista.com/statistics/677108/global-public-wi-fi-hotspots.

Stern, S. (2008). Producing sites, exploring identities: Youth online authorship. In D. Buckingham (Ed.), *Youth, identity, and digital media* (pp. 95–118). Cambridge, MA: MIT Press.

Tripp, L. M. (2010). "The computer is not for looking around, it is for school work": Challenges for digital inclusion as Latino immigrant families negotiate children's access to the internet. *New Media & Society, 13*(4), 552–567.

Turkle, S. (2011). *Alone together: Why we expect more from technology and less from each other*. New York, NY: Basic Books.

UNICEF. (2017). *The State of the world's children 2017: Children in a digital world*. New York, NY: Author.

Valkenburg, P. M. (2004). *Children's responses to the screen: A media psychological approach*. Mahwah, NJ and London: Lawrence Erlbaum Associates Inc.

Verizon.com. (n.d.). What is 5G? Retrieved from: www.verizon.com/about/our-company/5g/what-5g.

Willett, R. (2008). Consumer citizens online: Structure, agency, and gender in online participation. In D. Buckingham (Ed.), *Youth, identity, and digital media* (pp. 49–70). Cambridge, MA: MIT Press.

4
METHODOLOGICAL ISSUES IN RESEARCHING CHILDREN AND DIGITAL MEDIA

Rebekah Willett and Chris Richards

Introduction

Researching children's digital mediascapes presents exciting challenges for scholars attempting to understand modern childhood (Appadurai, 1996). Statistics from various sources indicate that many children's lives, at least in the Global North, are permeated with media. For example, a study by the technology education non-profit group Common Sense Media found that children in the United States aged 8 to 12 years consume on average six hours of media daily, not including for school or homework (Rideout, 2015). Although there are questions about the meanings of these measurements, such as what constitutes consuming media, few would deny that media are an important presence in children's lives. Not only are media embedded in the everyday activities of children, media appear as various iterations across the landscape of their daily lives, as in Appadurai's concept of mediascapes. A globally popular children's television show might appear in a family living room on a shared television screen and as a game on a family's mobile device; children's bedrooms might feature toys, posters, books, and drawings referencing the show; characters from the show might feature on lunchboxes and backpacks in school corridors; key phrases, actions, and plotlines from the show might appear in children's play; and the list could go on. Even spaces that seem discreetly different, such as online and offline, have permeable boundaries (Leander & McKim, 2003). It seems essential, then, to include media in any study of modern childhood.

In addition to viewing media as important parts of the landscape of modern childhood, the way childhood and the individual child are theorised also plays a key role in how researchers approach the study of children's media. Researchers studying the sociology of childhood theorise the child as a social actor and aim to reveal the multiple childhoods experienced by children in different socio-cultural contexts (see, for example, James, Jenks, & Prout, 1998; Qvortrup, Corsaro, & Honig, 2009). Questioning developmental approaches to childhood, these theorists analyse childhood as a social construct and emphasise children's agency in relation to the structures that create the conditions of modern childhood. In this context, various authors have argued for an understanding of children as both 'becomings' and 'beings', drawing on developmental and socio-cultural aspects of children's experiences (e.g., Johansson, 2010; Uprichard, 2008). Researchers across disciplinary fields are investigating both how children negotiate agency through structures, and how structures figure in individual agency. Writing in the field of social semiotics, Gunther Kress describes children's interactions with cultural texts in this way:

As children are drawn into culture, 'what is to hand', becomes more and more that which the culture values and therefore makes readily available. The child's active, transformative practice remains, but it is more and more applied to materials which are already culturally formed. In this way children become the agents of their own cultural and social making.

(Kress, 1997, p. 13)

Applying Kress's theories to the study of children's digital media implies that research must focus on the social nature of sign making, the transformative work that children undertake, and the cultural meanings of the signs through which children communicate. Given the embedded nature of media in children's lives, these theoretical approaches create challenges when trying to distinguish media from other texts or semiotic resources available to children.

In addition to challenges raised by these theoretical positions are methodological considerations about how to access children's media cultures and how to interpret data. Viewing children's media consumption and production as cultural practice aligns with anthropological approaches, and particularly those ethnographic methods of study originating in social and cultural anthropology. Among the questions raised in this field are those focussing on the ethics of studying an 'other' culture. Further, arguably, children's media culture is 'other' to those adults who render it an object of study. Various researchers apply a children's rights agenda to research connected with children and discuss the nuanced ethical dilemmas and considerations they face (e.g., Alderson & Morrow, 2011; see also Dobson, this volume). In addition to questions about the ethics of accessing children's digital media culture, there are related problems in the interpretation of such 'other' data. Ethnography requires researchers to immerse themselves in a culture to create thick descriptions, yet as adults, there are limitations on how much a researcher can be immersed in children's cultural spaces. Both areas of study connected with children and media – ethics and interpretation – have a well-developed body of literature and theory. Rather than attempting to distil these bodies of literature in this chapter, in the sections that follow, examples of methods of studying children's media culture are provided with a discussion of some methodological questions and dilemmas raised by these research practices. The examples start with a premise, as indicated in this introduction, that children's media cultures are complex sites of interaction that require nuanced interpretive research methodologies.

The Interrelationship between Observation and Interviewing

Given that children's experience of the media is often substantial, research has tended to focus on how 'saturated' their leisure and play might be, in the past by television and now by digital media. There has also been a growing body of research, however, giving attention to how children engage productively with the media they enjoy. In seeking to explore how children interpret and remake media texts, considerable attention has been paid to their play activities. Though play takes place in the home and in public playgrounds, school playgrounds are key sites for extended fantasy play between peers. In this section, the discussion draws on research conducted in school playgrounds in London in 2009–2011 and outlines methodological issues both particular to that research and of broader relevance to qualitative research with children. The research in question was specifically framed as an enquiry into the relationship between children's playground games and the old and new digital media.

The study described in this section involved multiple data collection methods which took place over a two-year period, including (but not limited to) written observations, video recordings, and interviews with children (see Willett, Richards, Marsh, Burn, & Bishop, 2013). Broadly construed as ethnographic, these methods, the resulting data, and subsequent analytical approaches invoke different sets of debates and bodies of literature concerning research methods and methodologies. Fundamentally, the project recognises the advantages of adopting an outsider perspective (and indeed, out of necessity, maintaining an etic perspective on children's cultural spaces) whilst also employing methods to gain more of an insider perspective, including engaging children as participant researchers as described in the following section (see Headland, Pike, & Harris, 1990 for an introduction to the insider/outsider debate). Similar to the 'Day in the Life' methodology, the project also involved iterative discussions and reflexive work, moving between insider and outsider perspectives to gain an understanding of children's media cultures (Gillen & Cameron, 2010). Collecting video footage creates challenges in terms of ethics, data collection decisions, and analysis, with the project drawing from a body of literature on using visual methods with children (see, for example, Thomson, 2009) to consider ethics, affordances, and limitations of collecting video data. The field of visual studies, and more specifically visual ethnography, is well developed in terms of analytical frameworks (see, for example, Margolis & Pauwels, 2011; Pink, 2012; Rose, 2016). However, the project as a whole collected well over 1,000 videos, and rather than attempting to analyse the entire data set of videos, each video was annotated and subsequently used to develop an understanding of specific contexts, for example related to groups of friends or particular trends that were observed. Multimodal analysis was employed to examine the different modes of play (e.g., talk, bodily-kinesthetic, emotion) and to do more in-depth analyses of select videos for specific pieces of writing (for an introduction to multimodal theory see Burn & Parker, 2003; Kress, 2009).

Playgrounds are often bewildering, noisy, and the setting for numerous, overlapping, and fast-moving activities. Iona Opie, in her book *The People in the Playground*, noted her initial impression of 'uncontrolled confusion' and the difficulty she experienced in making sense of what she saw (1993, p. 2). It was only 'gradually' and often 'with the aid of an interpreter' that she achieved a more assured understanding of what she observed (Opie, 1993, p. 2). It could be argued that a playground is just one, albeit an especially challenging, example of the messy and opaque character of social reality in whatever setting is chosen for research. Law, in *After Method: Mess in Social Science Research*, remarks that "much of the world is vague, diffuse or unspecific, slippery, emotional, ephemeral, elusive or indistinct, changes like a kaleidoscope, or doesn't really have much of a pattern at all". Although Law almost certainly didn't have a school playtime in mind, his views resonate with those that an adult observer new to a school playground might feel after the first, and perhaps the 21st, visit (2004, p. 2). The metaphors associated with understanding – itself a 'pursuit', a 'quest', and a 'challenge' – are familiar enough. The aim of observation might be to 'penetrate' or 'grasp' or 'uncover' the meaning of what is observed. Such metaphors can't be avoided as there is no language of interpretation and analysis without them. But it's worth being well aware of the metaphors in use and what their implications might be, not least because there are always alternatives.

Observation takes time. Some of the precedents are daunting. Shirley Brice Heath (1996) visited the sites discussed in *Ways With Words* from 1969 to 1978. Anna Beresin (2010) worked on *Recess Battles* with her infant son and concluded it when he was old enough to shave. And Iona Opie's visits to her chosen playground in Liss, Hampshire, began in 1960 and continued until 1983. Though most social research cannot be conducted across such extended periods, the implication of such examples is, first, that observation is a commitment – of attention, patience, and presence, and, second, that observation alone is not enough – other ways of knowing are essential and might well include, as is explained below, a variety of forms of interviewing. What the participants themselves have to say about what has taken place in the playground is essential, and in playgrounds the children are the primary participants. Thompson argues, in *Ideology and Modern Culture*, that all social worlds are already "pre-interpreted" by the participant social actors themselves and that further interpretation and analysis is always a "re-interpretation" (1990,

p. 22). To get at social actors' understanding of their own actions requires talk, and facilitating such talk is a key aspect of playground research. Indeed, how otherwise could research document and name the repertoire of media and new media sources on which children frequently draw in their play scenarios?

Beginning with observation, as an outsider, has some advantages. The perhaps unfamiliar array of activities may be more visible to a playground novice, for example, than to those adults and school staff who spend playtimes on duty, day after day, watching. Curiosity and attention are easier to maintain when what is observed retains some degree of novelty. Outsiders may not know what it all means but the profusion of play activities makes asking, albeit puzzled, questions easy enough. But to revisit what has been observed is not easy at all. Memory is not enough. Observation has to be accompanied by the production of some kind of record of what takes place. Keeping a field diary with detailed notes on every playtime observed is essential, but inadequate. A written record might serve as a reminder of what was witnessed but does not make available its detail and nuance. The written account is almost as confined to the time of the event as the event itself, though arguably, it is possible to write more fully immediately after a playtime is over. More importantly, the written record is unlikely to be accessible by, or of much interest to, the participants themselves. Sound recording has some value and has played a significant part in the more language-focussed play research of past decades. Photographs, by contrast, freeze moments stripped of sound. As a focus for conversation about what might have been taking place, photographs can be a productive resource: children may well be willing to talk around still photographic images, but the talk is likely to be relatively speculative. Perhaps the richest source can be found in video recording of children's play. The fully embodied enactment of play is available, unfolding in real time. By themselves, video recordings may well be just as opaque as the events they document, but their value lies in the expansion of the time available to observe and to reflect on what has taken place. A five-minute event might well be a resource for repeated viewing and discussion with the participants, and detailed attention to particular moments, slowed to a frame-by-frame presentation if necessary. The recursive interpretation of video records, in dialogue with one or more of the participants themselves, perhaps most adequately facilitates the work of interpreting events that are already meaningful to and are fully pre-interpreted by the children involved. Further observation is also informed by such discussions; the children's accounts may suggest a new focus of attention or enable the researcher to learn how to 'read' the unfamiliar.

Among many examples, those of apparently lone boys involved in versions of fantasy combat may best illustrate the importance of video recording and the use of subsequent interviews intended to explore the media sources drawn upon in such play. The questions guiding the making of the videos discussed here focussed attention on the media sources for their 'pretend' play: comics, war films, videogames, computer games, or what? It seemed likely that some combination of all of these might be a resource for their more extended play 'fighting' activities. But how exactly did their play relate to its apparent media precedents – was it imitation or something more elaborate than that might imply?

With so much happening all at once in most playtimes, decisions about where to look, and at what, have to be made. For example, it is possible to focus on a single area of a playground for several minutes, documenting what takes place there as children move in and out of the frame. Such an approach has some value where the priority is to examine the variety of ways in which a particular space, or the resources located in it, are used across one or several playtimes. But the examples here follow from a decision to focus on and follow particular boys, in each case a single individual, for as long as possible during extended lunch-time play. In one 20-minute video a boy, seemingly playing alone, ran rapidly across open spaces in the playground, taking cover behind walls, areas of decking, and the few available plants. This was repeated several times.

Only in discussion with him, sitting together watching the video, was it possible to establish any kind of credible interpretation. For him, the presence of playground supervisors was crucial. In his fantasy, it was they who were watching him and whose gaze he had to evade. Open space was thus rendered dangerous and exciting. The assumption that he was alone was contradicted: he insisted that other boys were involved in the same 'agonistic scenario', pretending that the playground was a risky and hazardous space in which they were vulnerable to the threat he attributed to the playground supervisors. The importance of exploring the emotional force of vulnerability – rather than enacting combat, which had recently been banned – slowly emerged as the most plausible and coherent explanation for the actions captured in the video. Similarly another boy, also acting alone, though in this case enacting firing a machine gun and throwing grenades, entirely contradicted the assumption that he was involved in a solitary play scenario. On the contrary, he insisted, there were six boys divided into two teams of three. Again, interpretation depended upon joint viewing and an informal interview conducted in a mostly conversational mode. So the video records were invaluable but also, in themselves, apparently misleading. Almost always, discussion with participants enlarged and complicated what the video record made available. Constructing interpretations thus became a matter of dialogue – with the children who participated and, sometimes, with teachers and playground supervisors – and also of recursive work, on both the video record and the field-notes produced immediately after the event.

A further area of concern turns around the question of research and in what sense participants in the social world of interest – in this case children in playgrounds – have any interest in being 'researched' or in collaborating in researching aspects of their own lives. There is little point in making broad generalisations about the relationships engendered in research projects here, but it is essential to question the assumption that research is welcome and that cooperation will be offered by those participants who are of interest to researchers – or indeed that the explanations given are necessarily reliable. In an article, *Pretty in Pink: Young Women Presenting Mature Sexual Identities*, Gleeson and Frith (2004) remark on the realisation that their participants may not have chosen to be understood and, for example, may have used ambiguity to render themselves unknowable. Perhaps a lot depends on how the research subjects interpret the identity of the researcher and on the institutional or broader social framing of the relationship between them and the research.

In an individual research project conducted in the early 1990s, for example, Richards (1998) investigated the encounter between teacher and taught in the teaching of popular music as an aspect of Media Studies. The research findings were fundamentally reworked around a contrast between how much of themselves students in different schools wished to make visible. Results partly reflected the different backgrounds of participants: one school was highly selective, the other an inner city comprehensive. Interviews and discussions are particular speech genres and may not be familiar, or acceptable, to some research subjects. The relative formality and the variable imbalances of power apparent in these forms of address might well make their use an impediment to the achievement of the kind of knowledge or shared understanding to which research with children might aspire. In the London playground research, interviews and discussions were productive in the context of sustained research with primary school children (ages 5–11), across a two-year period. Familiarity and confidence were established through presence and availability, week after week. In other circumstances, for example in research with teenagers, approaches less anchored in formal modes of questioning would need to be explored.

In conclusion to this discussion of observation and interviewing it needs to be emphasised that very little social research can be extended through decades. Equaling the achievements of the studies cited earlier, in terms of duration, is not realistic. Moreover, all social research is in a sense provisional, work in progress, to be re-read and reconsidered, always open to further reflection and discussion. Some of the children in the playground research (2009–2011) are now adults entering their early twenties and would no doubt be well able to read the published accounts of their childhood media enthusiasms and the play scenarios they elaborated a decade earlier. Such re-visiting of the data might well lead to further interpretations.

Participatory Research Methods

This chapter demonstrates that in building an understanding of children's digital media cultures, researchers need to acknowledge the interpretive aspect of children's practices and the limitations of research in accessing those interpretations. The section above describes the challenges and possibilities afforded by interrelated observations and interviews. A further means of attempting to gain access to children's media cultures in culturally responsive ways is through participatory research methods. With participatory methods, children are involved in various aspects of the research process including designing research, collecting and analysing data, and disseminating findings. This seems promising as a way of researching that respects children's rights and provides insiders' understandings of digital media cultures that might be specific to children, young people, friendship groups, fan cultures, and so on. O'Kane argues that engaging children in participatory techniques enables "children's voices, needs and interests to be articulated and take precedence over adults' research agenda" and further "enables the creation of a more flexible environment in which participants are given more control over the agenda" (2000, p. 152). There have been attempts to develop typologies related to children as participant researchers, with numerous discussions focussing on Hart's (1992) eight-rung ladder which identifies different forms of participation in a hierarchal relationship, ranging from low levels of participation which amount to little more than tokenism, through to projects in which children initiate all parts of projects and share decisions with adults. Debates surrounding these typologies highlight the difficulties in conceptualising children's roles as participatory researchers as well as the feasibility of such participation (Malone & Hartung, 2010). For example, Lomax's (2012) research reveals occasions in which children were excluded in child-led research, and ways in which data collection was limited and shut down through the interventions of child interviewers. For example, in her research, Lomax documented instances when children's taste in popular culture, or "hierarchies of 'cool'", entered into decisions about whose voices were valued by the child researchers (2012, p. 113).

As outlined in the introduction, research in the field of sociology of childhood is interested in theorising children as social actors and finding ways to recognise children's agency as well as the structures through which children are acting. Participatory research methods are designed to provide agency and voice to children. Several researchers have raised questions about assumptions embedded in participatory research projects regarding children's empowerment, however. For example, childhood studies researchers Leslie Gallacher and Michael Gallagher argue that "in some ways, research might be understood as a process of socialisation through which children are taught to conform to adult norms and to value 'adult cultures' over their own" (2008, p. 505). Similarly, Holland, Renold, Ross, and Hillman (2010) argue that participatory research involving children presents itself as more authentic and higher quality due to the participation of children; however, much of this research is highly structured by the researchers who teach children how to research. Further, it tends to assume that children actually want to be researchers. Critics of participatory methods argue against seeing children as experts in their own lives, calling for researchers to be more reflexive when considering epistemological and ontological questions in relation to both child and adult researchers (Gallacher & Gallagher, 2008; Hunleth, 2011; Spyrou, 2011). One example of a more reflexive approach to participatory research is Marsh's (2012) analysis of children as 'knowledge brokers', which focusses on the role of children as mediators of their cultural knowledge (in this case, playground games and practices). Marsh's close analysis reveals ways in which children, in their roles as both insiders and outsiders to playground games, were able to "assess what is knowable and how that knowledge should be presented" as well as maintaining trust and credibility with the researchers and with their peers (2012, p. 511). Rather than assuming that the project provided agency and empowerment to children in the research process, Marsh's analysis demonstrates the complexities of the positions children negotiated as participant researchers.

One of the justifications for including children as participatory researchers is their perceived location as insiders within a child culture (e.g., Kellett, 2010). Arguments made about insider research more broadly claim that insider knowledge of the culture and proximity to participants in terms of social distance are advantageous in developing trust between the participants and researchers. With greater trust, participants are more comfortable, cooperative, and willing to participate, thus improving the quality and quantity of data when compared with data collected from an outsider to a culture (Hodkinson, 2005). Further, where research values an insider's familiarity with particular language and experiences of a culture, a process of dialogue and exchange between the participants and the researchers is more easily established and may be more productive. Insiders are also able to recognise significant elements when collecting data, as Hodkinson (2005) explains: "[insiders] have a significant extra pool of material with which to compare and contrast what they see and hear during the research process" (p. 143). Hodkinson reflects on his position as an insider when conducting ethnographic research on goth culture, having himself identified as a goth when he was a teenager, and immersing himself in the dress, music, social scene, and online spaces of goth culture while conducting his research. However, there is a risk of assuming that an insider's knowledge is shared across a particular culture, that is, assuming that there is a single insider truth; and, further, there is a risk of the insider taking too much for granted and losing objectivity, thus not asking enough questions or limiting the information gained from participants. Whilst children as participant researchers have been viewed as insiders within their peer culture, there is very little discussion of the challenges of this position in relation to child-led research. For example, what constitutes a peer culture in a school is very likely to be contested from a variety of positions, and a child researcher may or may not feel able or willing to align herself or himself with, or represent, such a culture.

One further methodological approach involving children is illustrated by projects employing participatory video methodologies or visual ethnographies with children (e.g., Bloustien, 2003; Lomax, Fink, Singh, & High, 2011). As with participatory video methods more broadly, in these studies there is a desire to give a voice to populations who may be marginalised or whose perspective may be missing from mainstream discourse (Milne, Mitchell, & de Lange, 2012). In relation to children and teens, this literature often focusses on how participants' identities are constructed in relation to and through the videomaking process. Bloustien (2003) discusses ways teenage girls engaged in deep play with visual images and meanings, experimenting with aesthetics and form as they represent themselves in relation to dominant power relations. For example, girls in Bloustien's study created video performances related to pop music which constructed and reconstructed representations around girlhood, exploring dominant discourses connected with age, femininity, and sexuality.

Conclusion

This chapter considers methods of researching children's media cultures, operating upon the assumption that digital media are embedded in children's everyday practices. It can be argued that understanding children's culture requires longitudinal ethnographic studies. Children grow up, however; they are notoriously fickle in their interest in a specific media text, and media modes and cultures are ever-changing. There is clearly value in documenting and analysing broad patterns or processes of engagement with media through a sustained ethnographic approach, and there is value in analysing children's media cultures on a more micro level. Within these limitations, the chapter argues for close attention to be paid to children's interpretations and re-interpretations of digital media. Recognising the child as agentive in making meaning with and through digital media, the methods discussed provide a space in which the child can be a contributor to researchers' interpretive work. The examples of research methodologies discussed here point to a need for reflexivity. It is through careful reflection about the limitations of research, ways to approach children's engagements with digital media in culturally responsive ways, and recognition of the child as a meaning maker that researchers come closer to understanding children's digital cultures.

References

Alderson, P., & Morrow, V. (2011). *The ethics of research with children and young people: A practical handbook* (2nd ed.). London: Sage.

Appadurai, A. (1996). *Modernity at large: Cultural dimensions of globalization*. Minneapolis, MN: University of Minnesota Press.

Beresin, A. R. (2010). *Recess battles: Playing, fighting, and storytelling*. Jackson, MS: University Press of Mississippi.

Bloustien, G. (2003). *Girl making: A cross-cultural ethnography on the process of growing up female*. New York, NY: Berghahn Books.

Burn, A., & Parker, D. (2003). *Analysing media texts*. London: Bloomsbury Publishing.

Gallacher, L., & Gallagher, M. (2008). Methodological immaturity in childhood research? Thinking through 'participatory methods'. *Childhood, 15*(4), 499–516.

Gillen, J., & Cameron, C. (Eds.). (2010). *International perspectives on early childhood research: A day in the life*. London: Palgrave MacMillan.

Gleeson, K., & Frith, H. (2004). Pretty in pink: Young women presenting mature sexual identities. In A. Harris (Ed.), *All about the girl* (pp. 103–114). New York, NY: Routledge.

Hart, R. (1992). *Children's participation: From tokenism to citizenship*. Florence: UNICEF International Child Development Centre.

Headland, N. T., Pike, K., & Harris, M. (Eds.). (1990). *Emics and etics: The insider/outsider debate*. Thousand Oaks, CA: Sage.

Heath, S. (1996). *Ways with words: Language, life, and work in communities and classrooms* (2nd ed.). Cambridge: Cambridge University Press.

Hodkinson, P. (2005). 'Insider research' in the study of youth cultures. *Journal of Youth Studies, 8*(2), 131–149.

Holland, S., Renold, E., Ross, N. J., & Hillman, A. (2010). Power, agency and participatory agendas: A critical exploration of young people's engagement in participative qualitative research. *Childhood, 17*(3), 360–375.

Hunleth, J. (2011). Beyond, on or with: Questioning power dynamics and knowledge production in 'child-oriented' research methodology. *Childhood, 18*(1), 81–93.

James, A., Jenks, C., & Prout, A. (1998). *Theorising childhood*. Oxford: Polity Press.

Johansson, B. (2010). Subjectivities of the child consumer: Beings and becomings. In D. Buckingham & V. Tingstad (Eds.), *Childhood and consumer culture* (pp. 80–93). London: Palgrave Macmillan.

Kellett, M. (2010). Small shoes, big steps! Empowering children as active researchers. *American Journal of Community Psychology, 46*(1–2), 195–203.

Kress, G. (1997). *Before writing: Rethinking the paths to literacy*. London: Routledge.

Kress, G. (2009). *Multimodality: A social semiotic approach to contemporary communication*. London: Routledge.

Law, J. (2004). *After method: Mess in social science research*. London: Routledge.

Leander, K. M., & McKim, K. K. (2003). Tracing the everyday 'sitings' of adolescents on the Internet: A strategic adaptation of ethnography across online and offline spaces. *Education, Communication & Information, 3*(2), 211–240.

Lomax, H. (2012). Contested voices? Methodological tensions in creative visual research with children. *International Journal of Social Research Methodology, 15*(2), 105–117.

Lomax, H., Fink, J., Singh, N., & High, C. (2011). The politics of performance: Methodological challenges of researching children's experiences of childhood through the lens of participatory video. *International Journal of Social Research Methodology, 14*(3), 231–243.

Malone, K., & Hartung, C. (2010). Challenges of participatory practice with children. In B. Percy-Smith & N. Thomas (Eds.), *A handbook of children and young people's participation* (pp. 24–38). New York, NY: Routledge.

Margolis, E., & Pauwels, L. (Eds.). (2011). *The SAGE handbook of visual research methods*. London: Sage.

Marsh, J. (2012). Children as knowledge brokers of playground games and rhymes in the new media age. *Childhood*, *19*(4), 508–522.

Milne, E. J., Mitchell, C., & de Lange, N. (Eds.). (2012). *Handbook of participatory video*. Plymouth: AltaMira Press.

O'Kane, C. (2000). The development of participatory techniques: Facilitating children's views about decisions which affect them. In P. Christensen & A. James (Eds.), *Research with children: Perspectives and practices* (pp. 136–159). New York, NY: Falmer Press.

Opie, I. (1993). *The people in the playground*. Oxford: Oxford University Press.

Pink, S. (Ed.). (2012). *Advances in visual methodology*. London: Sage.

Qvortrup, J., Corsaro, W., & Honig, M. (Eds.). (2009). *The Palgrave handbook of childhood studies*. London: Palgrave Macmillan.

Richards, C. (1998). *Teen spirits: Music and identity in media education*. London: UCL Press.

Rideout, V. (2015). *The common sense census: Media use by tweens and teens*. San Francisco, CA: Common Sense Media.

Rose, G. (2016). *Visual methodologies: An introduction to researching with visual materials* (4th ed.). London: Sage.

Spyrou, S. (2011). The limits of children's voices: From authenticity to critical, reflexive representation. *Childhood*, *18*(2), 151–165.

Thompson, J. (1990). *Ideology and modern culture: Critical social theory in the era of mass communication*. Cambridge: Polity Press.

Thomson, P. (Ed.). (2009). *Doing visual research with children and young people*. London: Routledge.

Uprichard, E. (2008). Children as "being and becomings": Children, childhood and temporality. *Children & Society*, *22*(4), 303–313.

Willett, R., Richards, C., Marsh, J., Burn, A., & Bishop, J. C. (2013). *Children, media and playground cultures: Ethnographic studies of school playtimes*. Basingstoke: Palgrave Macmillan.

5
YOUNG LEARNERS IN THE DIGITAL AGE

Christine Stephen

Introduction

This chapter is about the experiences of young learners as they grow up in home and learning environments where engaging with digital and connected technologies is an established feature of everyday life. Its purpose is to challenge notions of technological determinism and argue for the value of a cultural and critical perspective on children's encounters with digital technologies. The chapter is written from the perspective of an educational researcher, drawing on empirical and theoretical research literature, and adopting a cultural and critical position that sees contemporary experience as the result of historical technological innovation and knowledge evolution (Stephen & Edwards, 2018). The focus is on the early years, typically considered to be from birth to eight years old. While the research considered will reflect the concentration in the educational literature on the lives of children in western societies, the global and situated reach of the digital age is acknowledged. Attending to the specific historical-cultural processes and contemporary situations experienced in other societies would be illuminating but is beyond the space constraints imposed here.

Central to this chapter is the understanding that 21st-century cultural knowledge (conceptual and practical) and cultural tools (including digital tools) have developed in a historic, social, cultural, and value context and that they in turn create the environment in which children currently grow and learn. This cultural-historical perspective prompts attention to children's everyday experiences in their particular cultural setting and to understanding the factors that interact to create the specific environment in which each child grows up.

This chapter begins with a brief consideration of ways of thinking about encounters with digital technologies, followed by a review of the nature of young children's contemporary experience of the digital age. The next section offers an account of the ways in which home experiences shape digital encounters. However, understanding the experience of being a young learner in the digital age also necessitates the account of the impact of individual children's desires, interests, preferences, and social relationships which follows. The chapter concludes with a discussion of the ways in which a situated, critical position can inform the decisions about children's encounters with digital technology that confront parents and educators.

Conceptualising Engagement with Digital Technologies

Digital technologies are frequently conceptualised in a binary way as either beneficial or harmful for young children's development. However, the debate about the potential and perils of children's engagement with tablet computers, digital media, mobile phones, apps, and digital games is increasingly sterile and polarised. On the one hand, digital resources are conceptualised as inappropriate for young children, interfering with 'normal' developmental patterns and challenging traditional values and expectations about play and learning in the early years. Others extol the amplification of mental labour and ease of access to knowledge resources afforded by digital tools, while organisations concerned with health and wellbeing such as the American Academy of Pediatrics (AAP, 2016) offer guidance on ways of safely managing children's encounters with new technologies. Nevertheless, while debates rage in the press and parenting literature about the benefits and dangers of young children spending time viewing screens, playing computer games, participating in social media, and accessing the internet, youngsters are growing up in households where the use of digital resources for managing domestic tasks, communication, and leisure has become an established part of family practices and local culture.

Understanding the digital age as a socio-cultural phenomenon, historically shaped and currently experienced in everyday family life and education, moves the debate away from 'pro' and 'anti' stances to a situated exploration of lived experiences and opens opportunities to consider culturally appropriate and valued forms of response. Selwyn (2010) argues that if understanding is to develop beyond value-laden assertions and generalisations about benefits and harm it is necessary to recognise that encounters with digital technologies are culturally mediated and to focus on the 'state of the actual' in everyday life. Stephen and Edwards (2018) suggest that the attention in research and in the media to the extent to which children, particularly young children, make use of digital technologies and to accounts of negative outcomes is similar to the historical reactions, sometimes characterised as moral panic, following the introduction of other innovative technologies, such as radio and television, into home and educational settings. They argue instead for a perspective on change that sees the contemporary experiences of children, their parents, and educators "as a function of the relationship between individuals and their historically derived social, economic, political and cultural circumstances" (Stephen & Edwards, 2018, p. 93). It is this relationship between children and the circumstances that frame their digital experiences that is the focus of this chapter.

Contemporary Digital Experiences in the Early Years

Digital resources are a ubiquitous feature of the everyday lives of young children (including babies) as they experience the centrality of digital technologies to the working and leisure activities of parents and siblings and make ever more use of these resources themselves. National and multinational surveys (e.g., Chaudron, 2015; Common Sense Media, 2017; Ofcom, 2018), sales figures for digital toys and resources for children (e.g., Euromonitor International, 2015; Juniper Research, 2015) and international press coverage (e.g., Prigg, 2014; Cowan, 2016) repeatedly attest to the growth in young children's ownership of and engagement with digital technologies at home and in educational settings. This trend, often described as a 'proliferation' or 'explosion' was first noticeable in the late 1990s and accelerated with the advent of smart phones and mobile tablet computing in the 21st century. Furthermore, the evidence suggests that as digital technologies have become "embedded in the day to day" (Caldwell, 2000) new cultural norms are evolving in the ways in which children play, learn, communicate, and socialise in the digital age, particularly since mobile digital technology has become widely accessible. Children of all ages now expect to view television and videos on demand and make extensive use of mobile technologies. While waiting or travelling young children commonly watch videos or play games on a smart phone owned by a parent (Nevski & Siibak, 2016). They maintain contact with physically distant family via Skype or Facetime and the Internet of Things means that children are growing up in homes where domestic appliances and playthings may be connected to the internet.

Despite the concerns raised by some writers on parenting and family life (e.g., Palmer, 2006; Teng, 2013; Huffington Post, 2014), and the growth in access to and engagement with digital technologies suggested by the kind of surveys and sales figures referenced above, the literature suggests that spending time interacting with digital technologies is not simply replacing play and learning with traditional playthings. For example, a detailed qualitative study of the place of digital technologies at home found that while digital technologies were part of family life they did not dominate the everyday experiences of young children at home (Stephen, 2011). Digital technologies such as tablet or laptop computers, smart phones, and interactive educational toys were a feature of children's home life, but so too were traditional playthings and toys such as toy train sets, dolls, construction sets, board games, climbing frames, dressing up clothes, craft resources, pencils, and paints. This finding was endorsed more recently by Chaudron (2015), reporting on the digital technology experiences of six- to seven-year-olds in seven countries. Drawing on evidence from parents and children this research concluded that "Even though children loved playing digital games and watching videos ... Digital technology use is balanced with many other activities, including outdoor play and non-digital toys" (Chaudron, 2015, p. 7). In the USA, although use of mobile technologies has increased, the amount of time each day that 0 to 8-year-olds read or were read to remained steady over five years and overwhelmingly it was printed texts rather than e-readers that were being used (Common Sense Media, 2017).

Young children's interactions with digital technology are often described as digital play, without addressing the complexities of defining play, the relationship between the typically taken-for-granted features of play (e.g., natural, normal, a right, fun), and the nature of digital activities or the perspectives held on play and playfulness by the children involved (see Grieshaber & McArdle, 2010). Attention to the "state of the actual" (Selwyn, 2010) of children's everyday play through systematic exploration of naturally occurring play behaviours suggests that it is increasingly difficult to distinguish between traditional play and digital play. Edwards (2014) described young children's play in the digital age as ranging over a continuum from digital to non-digital, illustrating how a popular culture character (Peppa Pig) could be encountered in mediums from the material (soft toys and clothing), through printed text and scheduled television, to apps and YouTube content. As digital activities have sunk into everyday life so too do children's play activities blend together traditional and digital resources and activities. On-line viewing prompts physical pretend play, traditional games are enacted in virtual worlds, and figures for small world play or storytelling are downloaded from internet sites. Further research is needed to understand everyday play, social, and creative experiences in the digital age from the perspective of young children, rather than the technological affordances of the resources.

Digital technologies for young children are marketed as supporting learning as well as play and there is a considerable history of claims about the educational potential of digital games and activities (e.g., Haugland, 1999; Plowman & Stephen, 2003; Daugherty et al., 2014). However, good-quality research about the learning outcomes (particularly long-term outcomes) of digital encounters is more scarce (Bolstad, 2004; Turvey & Pachler, 2016). Digital games and activities may indeed extend the range of play and learning opportunities, but exploration of their content suggests that many offer little that is different from traditional learning tools (Stephen, 2015). Digital games, like traditional activities, typically involve familiar cognitive operations such as matching, categorising, counting, and using phonics skills. Fewer foster exploration, problem-solving, and creative expression. Furthermore, much of the research currently available suggests that learning outcomes from digital activities are conditional on a range of factors, such as the ways in which educators employ digital tools (Couse & Chen, 2010) and the inclusion of specific design features which prompt higher order thinking (Verenikina et al., 2010). A study by Stephen and Plowman (2008) points to differentiated outcomes, conditional on the pedagogic practices that surround children's encounters with digital activities in their educational settings. They found that children acquired a range of operational skills and curriculum or subject knowledge but the outcome most frequently noted by their educators was the development of positive learning dispositions such as growing confidence and willingness to persist. Similar outcomes from three- to five-year-olds' encounters with digital technologies at home were noted, along with their growing capacity to participate in family practices such as reviewing photographs, shared video viewing, and on-line shopping and communication (Plowman et al., 2010). However, the researchers went on to point out that these outcomes were conditional on sensitive and responsive adult support with digital activities if children's experiences were to be positive at home or in their educational setting.

That young children growing up in contemporary times experience digital technologies as a familiar feature of their environment is not in doubt, although these resources have not replaced traditional toys and playthings. However, consideration of the state of the actual suggests that technology-led notions of digital play and claims about digital learning fail to acknowledge the complexities of children's everyday activities and the role of others in their lives.

Home as a Digital Niche: The Influence of Parents and Siblings

The cultural-historical perspective which underpins this chapter draws attention to the ways in which the social and cultural practices, values, and expectations of families create distinct contexts for learning and development (Tudge et al., 2009). Dominant social structural factors such as gender, socio-economic status, and ethnicity make a difference to children's everyday experience with digital technologies, just as they do in other aspects of their lives (Common Sense Media, 2017). More directly, as illustrated by the studies reviewed below, families mediate digital as well as traditional activities through values and expectations and socially mediated behaviours, creating a particular niche for growing up in the digital age.

For young children especially, parents are the gatekeepers to technology use. It is parents who make purchasing decisions, decide where and when technologies can be used at home, and establish family practices with digital technologies, just as they make decisions about other aspects of family life. Parents can decide if digital technologies are to be used for watching educational or entertainment videos, communicating with distant family, or learning science (Kaufman, 2013). Each family has its own definition of suitable content for books or television programmes and this extends to the digital games and apps to which their children are given access. Marsh et al. (2015) found that parents began with a preference for free apps when choosing digital activities for their young children, then decided between the free resources according to what they expected their child to enjoy, ease of use, and the presence of what they considered to be educational outcomes and topics.

Families develop their own distinct boundaries for access to digital technologies. Parents do report being aware of the concerns, raised in the media and by commentators on contemporary society and family life, about digital activities being associated with negative outcomes, such as physical inactivity and social isolation. However, Plowman et al. (2010) report that despite this awareness, families did not consider digital engagement as a threat to contemporary childhood. Rather, parents argue that they make decisions about their children's engagement with digital resources in ways which minimise the risks and maximise what they perceive to be the advantages, and that they typically express fewer concerns for their younger children (Plowman et al., 2010; Holloway et al., 2013). In the UK and across Europe parents talk confidently about the efficacy of the ways in which their household has responded by developing rules for access to digital resources, restrictions on time spent with them and on the nature of the content (Chaudron, 2015; Nevski & Siibak, 2016). However, evidence gathered by Marsh et al. (2015) challenges parental claims that they engage with technologies and apps along with their child, suggesting that parents were typically involved mainly during the initial familiarisation stage with a new app and that thereafter children sought out solo use, albeit with some parental supervision.

Stephen et al. (2013) found that while parents employed a common repertoire of practices to directly support their children's encounters with digital technologies, each child experienced a distinctive domestic niche which was influenced by three factors: parents' views on the educative value of engaging with digital technologies; each parent's typical way of supporting their child's learning; and the nature of family relationships and ways of interacting. For example, in a household which welcomed commercial digital devices marketed as supporting early learning, a digital reading device was incorporated into the parents' practices undertaken to support their son's literacy development before he began primary school. In other homes where explicit preparation for reading was left to the expertise of school teachers, or where parents remained unconvinced of the value of 'reading devices', these resources were little used, even when supplied by the research team. In some households children were encouraged to explore independently the content of computer games, only receiving help when frustrated or annoyed by their digital encounters. Others received careful parental tuition about the function and appropriate use of digital games and devices before commencing their play.

Family schedules influence access to digital technologies too. When there are younger siblings at home access to what are considered expensive or fragile resources may be restricted to times when only the oldest child is present (Stephen et al., 2013). Marsh et al. (2015) discovered that children up to eight years of age were most likely to engage with digital resources at home between 4 p.m. and 6 p.m., a time when there are likely to be other domestic demands on parents and children enjoy leisure time after the preschool or school day. Livingstone et al. (2015) found that even families which made little use of new technologies made exceptions when the children were unable to play outside. Family practices in shared leisure time make a difference to opportunities for digital encounters and the value attached to alternative activities. In some homes engaging with digital games is seen as providing an outlet for a child's competitive behaviours while in other households supportive, collaborative family activities with interactive devices are a regular feature of everyday life (Stephen et al., 2013). Elsewhere children are growing up in households where participating in physical activities such as swimming or cycling at weekends, visiting relatives or participating in creative activities are prioritised by parents, regardless of their access to digital resources. The amount of time that parents spend with digital and print media has been found to be closely associated with the time that their children also spend on various forms of media (Nikken, 2017), suggesting again the influence of family practices and attitudes on children's everyday experiences and expectations.

Siblings are a further influence on younger children's everyday experience of home life in the digital age. Evidence from Verenikina and Kervin (2011), Livingstone et al. (2015), Chaudron (2015), and Stephen et al. (2013) points to the ways in which having older siblings influences both the resources in the household, the kinds of digital activities to which young children are introduced, and the technologies and activities to which young learners ascribe high status. Older siblings pass on digital devices which they no longer want, demonstrate how to engage with Facebook, introduce games and apps which are perceived as both desirable and scary by younger children, set appropriate levels of difficulty, give advice and correct mistakes.

Everyday family digital experiences are sites of positive and negative encounters with siblings; times when brothers and sisters offer help and encouragement or when competition in games and ownership disputes occur. The nature of these experiences is not determined by the technology but rather they are the outcome of family dynamics and practices which are present whether children are engaging with sophisticated new technologies or traditional games or playthings. Ten-pin bowling can cause frustration for younger siblings when played with physical or virtual bowls.

It is clear that families make a difference to children's digital experiences through the distinct developmental niche that evolves, meaning that there can be no assumptions about the experience which each child brings to his or her educational setting or about the determining power of the technologies. But it is not a one-way process; children are active participants in creating the family experiences.

Young Children: Active Agents in the Digital Age

Children themselves are active agents in their home and educational environments (James et al., 1998), making choices and pursuing interests. Children may introduce new technologies into their home through their experiences with friends and in their educational settings. Katz (2010) refers to children as media brokers and points to ways in which parents and children can draw on their comparative skills and understandings to make use of new media sources. While that specific study is concerned with the activities of much older children, the research evidence suggests that the agency of young children is an active factor in developing each family's distinctive niche.

Prensky's (2001) categorisation of children as digital natives has been taken to mean that an interest in and competency with digital technologies is a universal feature of children growing up in the digital age. However, adopting Selwyn's (2010) focus on the state of the actual suggests a more nuanced situation. Although digital resources are important cultural tools in their household, there can be no assumption that any particular child will be attracted to them. Some children growing up in technology-rich households are not attracted to digital play or learning activities while others choose to pursue enduring interests (e.g., vehicles, dinosaurs, pets) across digital and traditional modes (Stephen et al., 2008; Livingstone et al., 2015). Young children refer to digital resources at home as features of their growing up which they engage with, become competent with, and then move on from, just as they expect to do with traditional playthings. They are discriminating users of digital resources, making use of them when they are a source of fun, ignoring them when more tempting activities or social encounters are available, and identifying features that work well or frustrate or bore them (Stephen et al., 2008; Marsh et al., 2015).

Beyond their immediate family children's relationships with their peers, particularly in nursery and school settings, make a difference too, opening up or inhibiting opportunities for play and learning with digital technologies. Positive or negative social relationships between clusters of children engaged with digital or traditional resources can result in excited shared exploration or competitive and excluding behaviour (Kutnick et al., 2016). Despite assertions that play with computer games and other digital technologies fosters collaborative play, the evidence suggests a more mixed outcome. For instance, Brooker and Siraj-Blatchford (2002) found evidence of a range of constructive and collaborative interactions between three- and four-year-olds and that specific aspects of the software were associated with different forms of mutual engagement such as debating a problem or taking turns. On the other hand, no distinct evidence of collaborative behaviour across technological resources was identified by Plowman and Stephen (2003), who observed peers taking control of a game when a child hesitated or asked for help. Ljung-Djärf (2008) demonstrated that three- to six-year-olds adopted three distinct roles as they engaged with games on desk-top computers in their educational setting. Some took the role of owner of the resource (manipulating the hardware and making decisions), some were engaged as active participants contributing to the play, while others were included as spectators only. A study by Arnott (2016) found a further factor influenced the nature of interactions in the playroom and hence the nature of children's engagement with the digital resources provided there. She noted that the social context of the playroom (its rules and expectations) influenced whether peer group relationships when engaged with digital technologies were pro-social, anti-social, or task-driven.

Such evidence reinforces the social and cultural embeddedness of digital technologies and makes evident the need to go beyond technological considerations in order to make sense of the experiences of young children in the digital age.

Parents and Educators Responding to the Digital Age

The technologies which parents purchase for their home, the apps they download, the family practices they endorse, and the rules they set about digital activities are shaped by their relationship with the technologies of the digital age. So too in educational settings, local policy objectives, formal practice guidance, and hardware and software resources all make a difference to children's experience of digital resources. Everyday playroom practices are further influenced by: the educators' own relationship with digital resources; their attitudes towards having digital resources in their playroom or classroom and the play value of digital resources; their understanding of the critical contribution of sensitive pedagogical interactions to ensuring that encounters with digital technologies foster learning; and their experience of professional development opportunities about play and learning with digital technologies (Stephen & Plowman, 2008; Nuttall et al., 2015; Palaiologou, 2016).

Stephen and Edwards (2018) draw attention to three ways of characterising the relationship between people and technological innovations in the digital age. The first is technological determinism which construes the human actor as unable to resist technological developments, the second is a substantive or functional view that focusses on novel technologies as cultural tools which ease domestic or educational life, and the third is a critical position that poses questions about the purposes and values associated with technological innovation and choice-making. Technological determinism is evident in the responses of parents or educators who suggest that children should engage with digital resources because they are necessary for future education and employment (McPake & Plowman, 2010). Furthermore, a technological determinist perspective is likely to result in a focus on mastery of the operational features of the digital resource, rather than on the access to knowledge facilitated or the amplification of mental activity supported. In the context of early years education, Stephen and Edwards (2018) go on to suggest that educators who adopt a technological determinist understanding are likely to experience the demands of the digital age on their provision and practice as challenging, and they feel obliged by the expectations of parents and policymakers to include digital technologies in their settings. Some will accept assertions about the potential of digital resources to support learning but others will have had to overcome their feeling that early years education has little or no place for new technologies.

Parents and educators who hold a substantive perspective are likely to take a more pragmatic approach, driven by the affordances of the resources and focussing on what the technologies allow adults, educators, and children to readily achieve. This outcomes-focussed response is illustrated by the common practice of making extensive use of digital photography to facilitate children and adults to document play and learning in early years settings, sometimes at the expense of time to reflect and respond to the documentation (Bath, 2012).

Stephen and Edwards (2018) argue that, in contrast to a technological determinist or a substantive approach, developing a culturally and socially situated and critical relationship with digital technologies facilitates proactive response-making, allowing for recognition of local contexts, space for value judgements and, in the case of educators, the application of professional knowledge. They contend that while the contemporary digital age creates new conditions for learning and new ways of amplifying mental labour, responding to these opportunities and challenges through a cultural and critical lens can reflect the values and aspirations of families and societies and the cultural niches they develop. These three characteristic approaches to technologies are not intended to be impermeable 'response types' and parents, educators, and policymakers may well move in and out of these characteristic relationships with technology over time, depending on the nature of the digital activity and the centrality of the activity to their perspective on parenting. A qualitative study by van Kruistum and van Steensel (2017) exploring parents' reasons for mediating their children's use of digital technologies revealed a range of core values and emotions underpinning their practices. But within this variability van Kruistum and van Steensel stress the centrality of flexibility, a critical approach which parents employ to make decisions for particular children in particular circumstances – allowing them to do "the right thing at the right time".

Educators and policymakers concerned with educational provision and practices for young children are called upon to make decisions about the alignment of digital activities and the kind of knowledge that matters in the digital age, with views about a 'good childhood', and responsive educational provision. They will seek to foster the curiosity that drives learning, to prompt questioning and problem-solving, develop literacy skills, and skills to interpret digitally available information. However, these challenges are not unfamiliar; educators are already engaged in making decisions about the kinds of materials and ideas that are appropriate for young learners and about how to support children to acquire cultural tools such as reading, number, and quantity concepts. For parents, educators, and policymakers, avoiding technological determinism and adopting a cultural-historical perspective which acknowledges digital technologies as cultural tools to foster knowledge and behaviour that is currently valued and oriented towards expectations of the future leads to decisions that reflect the cultural situation in which young children are growing up at home and in their educational setting.

Conclusion

This chapter has argued for a situated understanding of young children's encounters with digital technologies which recognises these tools as part of the historically evolving and socially and culturally mediated everyday life in which they are growing up at home and in their educational settings. Empirical evidence has been drawn on to challenge commonly cited anxieties about digital resources dominating the lives of young children, suggesting instead a more nuanced approach which acknowledges that children have personalised experiences influenced by their families, peers, and educators, and their own interests and preferences. A cultural and critical perspective on development and education in the digital age recognises the influence of the cultural and social niche in which children are growing up and facilitates proactive decision-making about children's engagement with technological innovations in ways that acknowledge both the opportunities for new ways of knowing and the social and cultural expectations of contemporary societies.

References

AAP Council on Communications and Media. (2016). Media and young minds. *Pediatrics*, *138*(5). Retrieved from: http://pediatrics.aappublications.org/content/pediatrics/early/2016/10/19/peds.2016-2591.full.pdf.

Arnott, L. (2016). An ecological exploration of young children's digital play: Framing young children's social experiences with technologies in early childhood. *Early Years*, *36*(3), 271–288.

Bath, C. (2012). "I can't read it; I don't know": young children's participation in the pedagogical documentation of English early childhood education and care settings. *International Journal of Early Years Education*, *20*(2), 190–201.

Bolstad, R. (2004). *The role and potential of ICT in early childhood education: A review of New Zealand and international literature*. Wellington: New Zealand Council for Educational Research.

Brooker, E., & Siraj-Blatchford, J. (2002). "Click on Miaow": How children of three and four experience the nursery computer. *Contemporary Issues in Early Childhood, 3*(2), 251–270.

Caldwell, J. T. (2000). *Electronic media and technoculture*. New Brunswick, NJ: Rutgers University Press.

Chaudron, S. (2015). *Young children (0-8) and digital technology: A qualitative exploratory study across seven countries*. Luxembourg: Publications Office of the European Union. Retrieved from: http://publications.jrc.ec.europa.eu/repository/handle/JRC93239.

Common Sense Media. (2017). *Zero to eight: Children's media use in America 2013*. Retrieved from: www.commonsensemedia.org/research/the-common-sense-census-media-use-by-kids-age-zero-to-eight-2017.

Couse, L. J., & Chen, D. W. (2010). A tablet computer for young children? Exploring its viability for early childhood education. *Journal of Research on Technology in Education, 43*(1), 75–96.

Cowan, J. (2016, July 20). High tech family life. *The parenting place*. Retrieved from: www.theparentingplace.com/technology/high-tech-family-life.

Daugherty, L., Dossani, R., Johnson, E.-E., & Oguz, M. (2014). *Using early childhood education to bridge the digital divide*. Santa Monica, CA: RAND Corporation. Retrieved from: www.rand.org/pubs/perspectives/PE119.html.

Edwards, S. (2014). Towards contemporary play: Sociocultural theory and the digital-consumerist context. *Journal of Early Childhood Research, 12*(3), 219–233.

Euromonitor International. (2015). Hong Kong toys fair: The rise of technology in toys. *Euromonitor Research*. Retrieved from: http://blog.euromonitor.com/2015/02/hong-kong-toys-fair-the-rise-of-technology-in-toys.html.

Grieshaber, S., & McArdle, F. (2010). *The trouble with play*. Maidenhead: Open University Press.

Haugland, S. W. (1999). What role should technology play in young children's learning? Part 1. *Young Children, 54*(6), 26–31.

Holloway, D., Green, L., & Livingstone, S. (2013). *Zero to eight: Young children and their internet use*. London: LSE, EU Kids Online. Retrieved from: http://eprints.lse.ac.uk/52630.

Huffington Post. (2014, 15 September). How technology is having a serious impact on your child's development. *Huffington Post*. Retrieved from: www.huffingtonpost.co.uk/2014/09/15/children-technology-impact-addiction_n_5821492.html.

James, A., Jenks, C., & Prout, A. (1998). *Theorizing childhood*. Cambridge: Polity Press.

Juniper Research. (2015). Smart toy revenues to hit $2.8BN this year, driven by Black Friday and Christmas Holiday sales. *Juniper Research*. Retrieved from: www.juniperresearch.com/press/press-releases/smart-toy-revenues-to-hit-$2-8bn-this-year

Katz, V. S. (2010). Media connecting family and community. *Journal of Children and Media, 4*(3), 298–315.

Kaufman, J. (2013). Touch-screen technology and children. *Child*. Retrieved from: www.childmags.com.au/child/development/5453-touch-screen-technology-and-children.

Kutnick, P., Brighi, A., & Colwell, J. (2016). Interactive and socially inclusive pedagogy: A comparison of practitioner- and child-orientated cognitive/learning activities involving four-year-old children in pre-schools in England. *European Early Childhood Education Research Journal, 24*(2), 265–286.

Livingstone, S., Marsh, J., Plowman, L., Ottovordemgentschenfelde, S., & Fletcher-Watson, B. (2015). *Young children (0-8) and digital technology: A qualitative exploratory study- national report–UK*. LSE Research Online. Retrieved from: http://eprints.lse.ac.uk/60799/1/__lse.ac.uk_storage_LIBRARY_Secondary_libfile_shared_repository_Content_Livingstone,%20S_Young%20children%200-8_Livingstone_Young%20children%200-8_2015.pdf.

Ljung-Djärf, A. (2008). The owner, the participant and the spectator: Positions and positioning in peer activity around the computer in pre-school. *Early Years, 28*(1), 61–72.

Marsh, J., Plowman, L., Yamada-Rice, D., Bishop, J. C., Lahmar, J., Scott, F., … Winter, P. (2015). *Exploring play and creativity in pre-schoolers' use of apps. Final project report*. Retrieved from: www.techandplay.org.

McPake, J., & Plowman, L. (2010). At home with the future: Influences on young children's early experiences with digital technologies. In N. Yelland (Ed.), *Contemporary perspectives on early childhood education* (pp. 210–226). Maidenhead, UK: McGraw-Hill Education.

Nevski, E., & Siibak, A. (2016). The role of parents and parental mediation on 0-3-year old's digital play with smart devices: Estonian parents' attitudes and practices. *Early Years, 36*(3), 227–241.

Nikken, P. (2017). Implications of low or high media use among parents for young children's media use. *Cyberpsychology: Journal of Psychosocial Research on Cyberspace, 11*(3), article 1. Retrieved from: https://dx.doi.org/10.5817/CP2017-3-1.

Nuttall, J., Edwards, S., Mantilla, A., Grieshaber, S., & Wood, E. (2015). The role of motive objects in early childhood teacher development concerning children's digital play and play-based learning in early childhood curricula. *Professional Development in Education, 41*(2), 222–235.

Ofcom. (2018). *Children and parents: Media use and attitudes report 2017*. Retrieved from: www.ofcom.org.uk/research-and-data/media-literacy-research/childrens/children-parents-2017.

Palaiologou, I. (2016). Teachers' dispositions towards the role of digital devices in play-based pedagogy in early childhood education. *Early Years*, 36(3), 305–321.

Palmer, S. (2006). *Toxic childhood: How the modern world is damaging our children and what we can do about it*. London: Orion.

Plowman, L., McPake, J., & Stephen, C. (2010). The technologisation of childhood? Young children and technology in the home. *Children & Society*, 24(1), 63–74.

Plowman, L., & Stephen, C. (2003). A "benign addition"? Research on ICT and pre-school children. *Journal of Computer Assisted Learning*, 19(2), 149–164.

Prensky, M. (2001). Digital natives, digital immigrants. *On the Horizon*, 9(5), 1–6.

Prigg, M. (2014, February 21). How the iPad replaced the toy chest: Researchers find children play with touchscreens more than traditional toys. *Mail Online*. Retrieved from: www.dailymail.co.uk/sciencetech/article-2565061/How-iPad-replaced-toy-chest-Researchers-children-play-touchscreens-traditional-toys.html.

Selwyn, N. (2010). Looking beyond learning: Notes towards the critical study of educational technology. *Journal of Computer Assisted Learning*, 26, 65–73.

Stephen, C. (2011). *Playing and learning with technologies*. Scottish Universities Insight Institute. Research Briefing, 2. Retrieved from: https://dspace.stir.ac.uk/handle/1893/17643?mode=simple#.XupCZkVKg2w (accessed 17 June 2020).

Stephen, C. (2015). Young children thinking and learning with and about digital technologies. In S. Robson & S. Flannery Quinn (Eds.), *The Routledge international handbook of young children's thinking* (pp. 345–353). Abingdon: Routledge.

Stephen, C., & Edwards, S. (2018). *Young children playing and learning in a digital age: A cultural and critical perspective*. Abingdon: Routledge.

Stephen, C., McPake, J., Plowman, L., & Berch-Heyman, S. (2008). Learning from the children: Exploring preschool children's encounters with ICT at home. *Journal of Early Childhood Research*, 6(2), 99–117.

Stephen, C., & Plowman, L. (2008). Enhancing learning with information and communication technologies in pre-school. *Early Child Development and Care*, 178(6), 637–654.

Stephen, C., Stevenson, O., & Adey, C. (2013). Young children engaging with technologies at home: The influence of family context. *Journal of Early Childhood Research*, 11(2), 149–164.

Teng, A. (2013, June 5). Kids "using gadgets at earlier age being exposed to risks": Study. *The Strait Times*. Retrieved from: www.straitstimes.com/singapore/kids-using-gadgets-at-earlier-age-being-exposed-to-risks-study.

Tudge, J. R. H., Freitas, L. B. L., & Doucett, F. (2009). The transition to school, reflections from a contextualist perspective. In H. Daniels, H. Lauder, & J. Porter (Eds.), *Educational theories, cultures and learning: A critical perspective* (pp. 117–133). London: Routledge.

Turvey, K., & Pachler, N. (2016). Problem spaces: A framework and questions for critical engagement with learning technologies in formal educational contexts. In N. Rushby & D. W. Surry (Eds.), *Wiley handbook of learning technology* (pp. 113–130). Chichester: Wiley-Blackwell.

van Kruistum, C., & van Steensel, R. (2017). The tacit dimension of parental mediation. *Cyberpsychology: Journal of Psychosocial Research on Cyberspace*, 11(3), article 3. Retrieved from: https://dx.doi.org/10.5817/CP2017-3-3.

Verenikina, I., Herrington, J., Peterson, R., & Mantei, J. (2010). Computers and play in early childhood: Affordances and limitations. *Journal of Interactive Learning Research*, 21(1), 139–159.

Verenikina, I., & Kervin, L. (2011). iPads, digital play and preschoolers. *He Kupu*, 2(5). Retrieved from: www.childrensdiscovery.org.au/images/research/Digital_Play.pdf (accessed 17 June 2020).

6
CHILDREN WHO CODE

Jamie C. Macbeth, Michael J. Lee, Jung Soo Kim, and Tony Boming Zhang

Introduction

While an overwhelming majority of children worldwide use the internet, the web, and digital media in their daily lives, few of them have the opportunity to learn even the basics of the underlying hardware and software that make their digital devices work. What ultimately makes digital media dynamic and engaging is the digital computer technology behind the scenes that executes sets of program instructions, commonly called code. Collections of program instructions are also called software, computer programs, or simply programs, while the act of composing these programs is known as computer programming, or simply programming. Digital devices or hardware are computing devices that execute code: sets of instructions that command all of the functions of the device. Code in computer programs can retrieve, manipulate, and store data in the device, or it can instruct the device to interact with the world outside it in some way, for example by sending or retrieving data with other digital devices over a communication network, by playing a sound, by displaying something on the screen, by using the built-in camera and microphone to take a photo or record audio or video, or by responding to user input.

In spite of a long tradition of research efforts to expose children to code and to teach children how to write their own code (Becker, 2001; Bergin, Stehlik, Roberts, & Pattis, 1997; Kelleher & Pausch, 2005; Leutenegger & Edgington, 2007; Papastergiou, 2009; Pattis, 1981), many schools still do not have robust computer science (CS) curricula (Hubwieser et al., 2015). As a result, computer science education activists have launched global campaigns focussed on expanding access to quality computer science education for all children. The Hour of Code is one such campaign, which organises a yearly worldwide event in which millions of school children are exposed to computer programming through a brief online game-based outreach intervention (Lakanen & Karkkainen, 2019; Wilson, 2015). Since its inception, nearly a billion students have participated in the Hour of Code, and Code.org, which promotes the Hour of Code events, has trained computer science teachers, partnered with school districts to increase access to computer science courses, and created a marketing campaign to counter negative stereotypes about computer science.

Studies of the effectiveness of Hour of Code and similar campaigns have focussed largely on how they impact positive attitudes toward the subject of computer science and how they convince children that CS is fun and easier than they expected (Aspray, 2016). Other studies have questioned whether such a brief exposure to coding can teach school-age children 'computational thinking' skills (Wing, 2006) that transfer to other domains (Pea, 1987). However, there has been little research to examine how learning to code might immediately change how children relate specifically to digital media, whether or not they choose to learn more about CS, or even choose to pursue a career in computer programming.

In this chapter the researchers discuss aspects of programming which, when learned by children and young people, may lead to a richer understanding of digital media. The research shows children's responses as they learn that coding is what makes digital media live and interactive, and come to understand how people innovate to create new forms of digital media. An exposure to coding activities demonstrates to children that this is how digital media users achieve the highest levels of personalisation and control over their activities and devices. As a result, children's coding experiences may profoundly change their uses of digital media, with their coding ability making them 'power' users of digital technologies and services, including social media platforms.

Studies of Children Who Code and Their Digital Media

The researchers draw upon two studies that investigated middle school and college students' experiences with coding and examine how these skills may affect young people's perspectives and understanding. Study A collected survey and focus group data from 62 middle school students who participated in coding camps spanning nine consecutive Saturdays (partly described in Lee, 2019b). These students were from various schools within the same school district and were exposed to HyperText Markup Language (HTML) (Kennedy & Musciano, 2017), the Scratch block programming language (Maloney, Resnick, Rusk, Silverman, & Eastmond, 2010), and the Gidget language (Lee, 2015; Lee & Ko, 2015). Study B, completely separate from the first, involved 16 college students taking an introductory computer science course. The aim of this study was to understand and evaluate the influence of their school-aged exposure to coding and programming on their attitudes towards digital devices as adults.

Methodology

Study A

Study A's computer programming camps ran over nine consecutive Saturdays and represented several K-8 public schools in Newark, New Jersey (partly described in Lee, 2019b). Participating school principals recruited students by recommendations from the sixth- and seventh-grade teachers at their respective schools, who made announcements about the camps in their classes. Camps took place at participating middle schools or at a local high school (a centralised location that could accommodate more schools and students). In total, the researchers collected data from 62 middle school students (10–13 years old). The camps included 34 boys and 28 girls (one fifth grader, 28 sixth graders, and 33 seventh graders). All of the students were drawn from underrepresented minorities in science, technology, engineering and mathematics (STEM), identifying as either African American/Black (30 students) or Hispanic/Latino (32 students), and all were eligible for free/reduced cost lunch. This demographic makeup is reflective of the community the school district serves (Lee, 2019a), and the researchers did not specifically recruit for underrepresented minorities (the only recruitment constraint was grade level). The camps were provided at no cost to the student participants and they were not paid for their participation.

Each of the nine Saturday camp sessions consisted of a seven-hour day including breakfast, a morning programming activity, lunch, and an afternoon (block) programming activity. The game/HTML (morning) and block programming (afternoon) activities lasted approximately three hours each, every Saturday. At the end of each camp day, all participating students were asked to participate in a focus group activity. These ten-minute sessions were largely unstructured and asked students to reflect on their computing activities from that day, and to talk about anything they liked, disliked, learned, or anything else they wanted to comment on. The researchers audio-recorded these focus groups and took notes to help them identify the speakers during the subsequent transcription process.

Study B

Sixteen college students took part in Study B, a separate study of students' experiences with coding. Participants were recruited from an introductory computer science course at a small, liberal-arts-focussed university of about 4,000 undergraduate students located in the New York City metropolitan area of the USA. The course met twice a week for 75 minutes per session over a 15-week semester. The researchers offered students a choice of extra credit points for their course grade or $20 (USD) as compensation for participating in the study.

Six of the participants were first-year college students, four were sophomores, and six were juniors. There were 11 male students and 5 female students, and their ages ranged from 18 to 23. Overall, 13 of the 15 participants had declared a STEM subject as either a major or minor. Six had declared computer science as a major, and three had declared computer science as their minor, with two more considering declaring computer science as a minor after the course. Three students were declared as math majors and five more students were declared majors in finance, accounting, and marketing. All students were full-time.

Each participant was interviewed for about one hour at the end of the semester. During the interviews, participants recalled their childhood experiences with computer programming and computer science both inside and outside of school, as well as their experiences in the college course. Interviews were audio-recorded and transcribed.

Data Analysis

Two researchers independently analysed the Study A and Study B transcripts using thematic coding (Boyatzis, 1998), identifying emerging themes, discussing them, resolving inconsistencies, and defining a list of mutually agreed themes. Responses from both these groups of students, speaking of their school-based experiences from the perspective of either their school or college studies, inform the remainder of this chapter. Much of the discussion will use representative quotations from these interviews and focus groups to highlight the subset of themes relating directly to students' thoughts, ideas, and attitudes towards computer programming and coding.

Some aspects of the detailed quotes, including gender, may have been changed as required to protect anonymity. Participants from Study A are referred to as Mxx, where 'M' indicates middle school and xx refers to the respondent number (1–64). Similarly, participants from Study B are referred to as Cxx, where 'C' indicates college and xx refers to the respondent number (1–16).

Customising the Web and Social Media with HTML

Through coding knowledge and experience, children can learn to customise digital media and create their own digital apps and programs. Although many popular social media websites allow users to post content and customise their home pages, it is only through a knowledge of how to use HTML that users can unlock the full range of customisation and personalisation capabilities inherent in the web and social media (Kennedy & Musciano, 2017). Knowing HTML also provides users with a richer understanding of the inner workings of the web and social media, making those users more confident and capable. For example, social media sites and web email services frequently allow users to enhance their messages and posts by including HTML code within them. Further, HTML code allows the user to define the format of text in a web page, writing code to specify things such as font size and section headings and to create paragraphs for different parts of the page.

M3, a participant in the middle school study, recalls her realisation of the role of HTML while navigating a website for the popular video game Minecraft:

> I accidentally clicked on the "[edit] source" button on the Minecraft website, and it showed a bunch of words I didn't understand ... now I know that it's just adding the HTML code to change how the text looks when I click the buttons.
>
> *(M3)*

M3 also recognised that social media sites like YouTube are constructed using HTML, and was excited to use it to compose her own website: "Oh! So the Minecraft website [forum] that I use and YouTube must all be, like, made in HTML since they are all websites ... I want to be able to make sites like these" (M3). Another middle schooler, M15, could immediately see a use for this new knowledge in her life: "so I can use HTML to make my own website or blog? I want to be a wedding planner. I want to make a website for my business" (M15).

One of the middle school study participants was planning for her future as a social media influencer and could clearly see the relevance of coding, not just for creating websites, but for creating images, music, and video content for the web:

> I'm still going to be a YouTuber. But since I know how to code, I can make all the changes myself and also understand all the other programs [applications] better so that I can edit my videos and make effects and stuff. I can also make my own webpage with all my stuff, like Instagram or something.
>
> *(M31)*

This section has described how childhood experiences of coding and programming languages can facilitate a greater appreciation for the building blocks of the web. In a range of cases, an appreciation of how HTML works opens up new possibilities for the students concerned and helps demystify their experiences of interacting with web-based activities, services, and resources. The next section explores how the interactivity of the web and of digital devices depends upon affordances coded into the design of digital services and resources, and that these tools are available to young people if they receive the necessary grounding in code-based education and experience.

How Coding Makes Digital Media Live and Interactive

HTML is not itself an enabler of high-level interactivity. It is a 'markup' language, meaning that it can help users manipulate text and images. HTML code is used to specify how a web page appears when it is accessed via a browser window. HTML allows for the encoding of 'hypertext links' within a page that can open a different page when a user clicks on the link. Other than this, however, in and of itself, HTML is only capable of creating plain web pages that have little to no interactivity (Kennedy & Musciano, 2017).

Because of its comparatively restricted capabilities, HTML coding is distinct from computer programming generally. Some younger coders who know both HTML and general programming languages argue that, while HTML is a useful technology for enhancing their capabilities with digital media, only 'real' programming languages allow them to use the full affordances of digital devices, adding functionality and making them dynamic and interactive. In M45's view:

the next step is to, umm, learn more about programming like Javascript. That's what all the fancy websites seem to, like, be using to get all the advanced stuff to happen on a webpage – like you know, making things move and clickable and getting animations to happen.

(M45)

For many of the middle school study participants, by the end of the nine Saturday camps they realised how ubiquitous code was in their lives, enabling both awareness and a sense of control. Middle school participant M6 talked about his experiences modifying and customising a game written in Scratch, a visual programming language system that allows users to create interactive games by assembling graphical building blocks (Maloney et al., 2010).

I like programming [in Scratch] and making games … so whenever I see something I like [in someone else's program] … I, like, remix it and see how they made it. Then I copy it or try to make it myself and put it into my [own] game.

(M6)

A number of the projects' participants had experienced programming dynamic and interactive digital media outside of the usual digital device contexts. For example, participant C6 in the college-based survey had strong memories of his excitement as a high school student working with robots:

You know those like Lego robotics, like the NXT robots? Well first we started off like learning a code and like all the actions you can do with the code, but after that it gets more complex. You have to build your robot. So like for our final we had to – we used like sensors and we made a claw […] And then with the sensor people like [lay] black tape on the floor so that the robot would follow the sensor to the black tape and then when it would reach the end of the black tape you have to make it stop and then use another sensor to find the bottle and then it's supposed to claw the bottle, take it all the way back around, and drop it at the end of the line […] using a light sensor it detects the black tape and then using another sensor – I forgot the sensor – it sees the bottle, it stops and then you have to program it so it backs up, moves left and right and closes the claw correctly.

(C6)

Clearly the satisfaction of achieving command of a robot and bringing it to life with code was engaging for this student.

Bugs and Debugging Puzzles

People write programs to perform specific tasks and, as the tasks to be performed become more complex, so the programs also need to become more complex (Papadimitriou, 1994). This is true for all programs written for computing devices and digital media. Further, the more complex the programs, the more likely it is that the program instructions will operate in unexpected ways. Unexpected and unplanned programming behaviours are called bugs. Bugs have existed since the dawn of digital computing, and they happen in all kinds of programs (Gill, 1951). Debugging is the activity of finding and fixing bugs in programs to make them run correctly and more reliably (Musa, Iannino, & Okumoto, 1987). The existence of bugs and processes of debugging form important aspects of enhancing children's understanding of digital media through their knowledge and experience of coding.

It was while he was in high school that C5 first realised the importance of learning how to debug:

> In Java, we didn't need to learn but I taught myself it because it helped a lot, like, watching elements and opening declarations and stuff, right. So it really helps – now that I look at it in my current classes, like data structure and stuff, it's like it's such a skill, like not many people know it ... But anyways, what happened is like whenever I get stuck I – debugging, like, I follow the code and it helps me trace it, like what's happening to the variables and everything, so I know what goes wrong.
>
> *(C5)*

Bugs can also be used as effective teaching tools in the right context. The bugs in operating systems software are often exploited by hackers, who break into computer systems, seize control over smart phones and other digital devices, and steal valuable information, often without ever being detected. Children who learn about bugs gain a greater understanding of how digital media and devices are vulnerable to hacking, and the importance of applying security updates and packages to the digital devices they use in order to protect themselves and their data (Moore, Shannon, & Claffy, 2002).

Respondents in the study saw the process of debugging programs as being like solving a puzzle or math problem. The Gidget game is eponymous with the game's central robot character and unique programming language (Lee, 2015). Each level requires players to solve debugging puzzles, increasing in complexity for subsequent levels. One middle school student in the nine-week program particularly liked the puzzle-solving aspect of the Gidget game:

> I like that you have to fix the code to help [Gidget] solve the puzzles. It, like, really makes you think and I like that it gets harder and harder after every level. I like puzzles that make you think logically.
>
> *(M14)*

Another school student, M4, compared program debugging activities favourably with maths.

> I like that [Gidget], you know, since it's a game has to have a right answer. Sometimes when I'm doing math homework, I don't see any way to solve it even though the teacher wouldn't give it [to us] if it didn't have an answer. But since [Gidget] is a game, other people must have finished it right? And that means that I should be able to finish it too.
>
> *(M4)*

When children encounter bugs in their own programs, they understand the time and effort needed to keep the programs and software that they use running correctly.

Code and Children's Digital Futures

What these students make clear is that an understanding of programming can not only help them better understand digital media and digital technologies, it can also help them develop a nuanced appreciation of their chosen life trajectory and assist in refining transferable skills that are valuable in a wide range of contexts.

M33 could see how the skills he had learned in programming were transferable to other contexts:

I'll study to be a lawyer or a judge. But programming, like, it helps you think ... logically ... and also makes you solve puzzles and find out what's wrong, and you have to be really specific. Those are all really important to solving cases and arguing, so programming will help me prepare for stuff like that.

(M33)

Indeed, the impacts of school-based programming and coding experiences are potentially life-changing. Middle school participant M17 greatly enjoyed her experience with the nine-week Saturday coding camp, when she learned HTML, Gidget, and the Scratch block programming language. According to her, the experience cemented her choice of career: "before [learning to program] I didn't know what I wanted to be [when I grow up], but now I want to be a software engineer" (M17). Leaving aside these passionate adopters, however, the most common trend among the middle school students at the end of the nine-week Saturday program was to talk about how their experience with code could enhance or inform their intended career choice. Future wedding planner M15 noted "I can make programs to help me schedule my clients and keep things in order. Keeping things in order is really important for a wedding planner" (M15). M26 did not want to change her career trajectory from becoming a marine biologist, but could see that "coding can definitely help me being a marine biologist because I can make more of the work automatic by coding it when getting data and looking at it and making sense of it" (M26).

Conclusion

Abstractly, one can think of computer code as a form of digital media in and of itself, because it consists of lines of text instructions that are executed by a digital computing device. All the various technological systems that support digital media are executing computer code of various kinds written in various programming languages which can be searched, downloaded, shared, liked, modified, and remixed by users.

An experience of coding has the potential to fundamentally change children's relationships with digital media. Websites, social media applications (apps), games, and other kinds of apps popular with children and teenagers can be changed by making modifications to the original code. Children who code learn that the applications and digital media they download from the web are computer programs that can run on their personal devices. They may also become interested in both customising and tinkering with the programs to explore how changing the code will change the way programs run, and in using what they learn to write and build their own programs. Additionally, learning about bugs and debugging helps make children more aware of both the risks and benefits of downloading apps and files from the web.

Having experienced programming for themselves, these children and young people have realised, in the words of M4, that "programming isn't hard, it's just a challenge" (M4). It is partly because this realisation offers such an important insight into the uses and abuses of digital media that there is a worldwide commitment to try to expose children and adults to code, whether it is for just an hour, or for an entire lifetime.

Acknowledgements

The authors thank the Newark Public Schools for their contributions and participation. This work was supported in part by the National Science Foundation (NSF) under grants DRL-1837489 and IIS-1657160. Any opinions, findings, conclusions, or recommendations are those of the authors and do not necessarily reflect the views of the NSF or other parties.

References

Aspray, W. (2016). Recent efforts to broaden formal computer science education at the K-12 Level. Chapter 4 in W. Aspray, *Participation in computing: The National Science Foundation's expansionary programs* (pp. 103–145). Cham, Switzerland: Springer International Publishing.

Becker, B. W. (2001). Teaching CS1 with Karel the Robot in Java. *ACM SIGCSE Bulletin*, *33*(1), 50–54.

Bergin, J., Stehlik, M., Roberts, J., & Pattis, R. (1997). *Karel++: A gentle introduction to the art of object-oriented programming*. New York, NY: Wiley.

Boyatzis, R. E. (1998). *Transforming qualitative information: Thematic analysis and code development*. Thousand Oaks, CA: Sage Publications.

Gill, S. (1951). The diagnosis of mistakes in programmes on the EDSAC. *Proceedings of the Royal Society of London. Series A. Mathematical and Physical Sciences*, *206*(1087), 538–554.

Hubwieser, P., Giannakos, M. N., Berges, M., Brinda, T., Diethelm, I., Magenheim, J., Pal, Y., Jackova, J., & Jasute, E. (2015, July). A global snapshot of computer science education in K-12 schools. Paper presented at the 2015 Innovation and Technology in Computer Science Education (ITiCSE) on Working Group Reports (pp. 65–83). 10.1145/2858796.2858799.

Kelleher, C., & Pausch, R. (2005). Lowering the barriers to programming: A taxonomy of programming environments and languages for novice programmers. *ACM Computing Surveys (CSUR)*, *37*(2), 83–137.

Lakanen, A. J., & Karkkainen, T. (2019). Identifying pathways to computer science: The long-term impact of short-term game programming outreach interventions. *ACM Transactions on Computing Education (TOCE)*, *19*(3), 1–30.

Lee, M. J. (2015). *Teaching and engaging with debugging puzzles* (Doctoral Dissertation, University of Washington). Retrieved from: https://digital.lib.washington.edu/researchworks/handle/1773/33985.

Lee, M. J. (2019a, July). Exploring differences in minority students' attitudes towards computing after a one-day coding workshop. Paper presented at the 2019 Innovation and Technology in Computer Science Education (ITiCSE) ACM Conference on Innovation and Technology in Computer Science Education (pp. 409–415). 10.1145/3304221.3319736.

Lee, M. J. (2019b). Increasing minority youths' participation in computing through near-peer mentorship. *Journal of Computing Sciences in Colleges (CCSC)*, *35*(3), 47–56.

Lee, M. J., & Ko, A. J. (2015). Comparing the effectiveness of online learning approaches on CS1 learning outcomes. In *Proceedings of the eleventh annual international conference on International Computing Education Research (ICER)* (pp. 237–246).

Leutenegger, S., & Edgington, J. (2007). A games first approach to teaching introductory programming. *ACM SIGCSE Bulletin*, *39*(1), 115–118.

Maloney, J., Resnick, M., Rusk, N., Silverman, B., & Eastmond, E. (2010). The Scratch programming language and environment. *ACM Transactions on Computing Education (TOCE)*, *10*(4), 1–15.

Moore, D., Shannon, C. & Claffy, K. (2002). Code-Red: A case study on the spread and victims of an Internet worm. Paper presented at the Internet Measurement Conference (IMW) 2nd ACM SIGCOMM Workshop on Internet measurement (pp. 273–284). 10.1145/637201.637244.

Musa, J. D., Iannino, A., & Okumoto, K. (1987). *Software reliability: Measurement, prediction, application*. New York, NY: McGraw-Hill.

Papadimitriou, C. H. (1994). *Computational complexity*. New York, NY: Addison-Wesley.

Papastergiou, M. (2009). Digital game-based learning in high school computer science education: Impact on educational effectiveness and student motivation. *Computers & Education*, *52*(1), 1–12.

Pattis, R. (1981). *Karel the Robot: A gentle introduction to the art of programming*. New York, NY: Wiley.

Pea, R. D. (1987). LOGO programming and problem solving. In E. Scanlon & T. O'Shea (Eds.), *Educational Computing* (pp. 155–160). Chichester, UK: Wiley.

Wilson, C. (2015). Hour of code – A record year for computer science. *ACM Inroads*, *6*(1), 22.

Wing, J. M. (2006). Computational thinking. *Communications of the ACM*, *49*(3), 33–35.

7

YOUNG CHILDREN'S CREATIVITY IN DIGITAL POSSIBILITY SPACES

What Might Posthumanism Reveal?

Kylie J. Stevenson

Introduction

This chapter explores the nature of young children's creativity in digital contexts. Taking a broad literature review approach, it draws on creativity theory, in particular the work of Anna Craft (2001) on possibility thinking, to investigate the notion of digital spaces as possibility spaces in which very young children enact Craft's notion of *small c* creativity. The exploration suggests how posthumanism, which is rapidly changing approaches to early childhood education, might inform understanding of the affordances of digital contexts for children's creativity. Whilst not based on any qualitative study itself, this chapter draws on recent research which examines posthuman perspectives of children's engagement with apps, the Internet of Toys, and makerspaces, in order to identify how a posthuman lens may inform understandings of children's real-life practices around technology, play, and creativity, and how such digital play may be perceived as taking place in posthuman digital possibility spaces.

Possibility Spaces

Little c Creativity and Possibility Spaces

The British creativity researcher Anna Craft proposed the notion of children as "digital possibility thinkers" (2011, p. 173), building upon her earlier work about possibility spaces for young children's creativity (1996, 1999, 2001). In her initial research, Craft argued that, as a result of a need to adapt to constant change, "individuals are required to be increasingly self-directed ... One way of describing this quality of self-direction might be 'little c creativity'" (2001, p. 46). Here Craft is referring to her conceptualisation of a continuum of creativity from little c to big C, later expanded by educational psychologists James Kaufman and Ronald Beghetto (Beghetto & Kaufman, 2007; Kaufman & Beghetto, 2009), so that points on the spectrum were made more explicit.

Building upon Vygotsky's (1971) work on the psychology of creativity and Gardner's (1997) work on the creative mind in which he first proposed a new taxonomy of creativity, Craft explained:

> I want to propose that there may be a spectrum of innovation, at one end of which is something which is novel to the agent but not necessarily to the wider world, and at the other end of which is novelty to the wider world.
>
> *(Craft, 2001, p. 50)*

Contrasted with big C creativity, which is typified by the creativity of Gardner's creative genius individuals with extraordinary minds, little c creativity is the other 'end' of the spectrum where the everyday creative actions of the individual are placed, for example the creativity of the exceptional home gardener or hobbyist painter: "'Little c Creativity' (LCC), by contrast, focusses on the resourcefulness and agency of ordinary people, rather than the extraordinary contributions and insights of the few" (Craft, 2001, p. 49). Craft goes on to identify the type of novel thinking typified whilst an individual is engaged in 'little c creativity' as possibility thinking:

> At the core of adaptability and flexibility, which the start of the twenty-first century is demanding of people both young and old is, I have suggested, the notion of "possibility". Thus LCC [little c creativity] involves at its heart the notion of "possibility thinking", or asking, in a variety of ways, "What if?"
>
> *(2001, p. 54)*

New understandings of creativity have incorporated the notion of a creativity continuum and now look towards a 21st-century concept of creativity (Csikszentmihalyi, 1999; McWilliam, 2008; Moran & John-Steiner, 2003; Spencer, Lucas, & Claxton, 2012) that is more interdisciplinary, collaborative, system-contextualised, and learnable. These take into consideration the Vygotskian notion that there is a continuum of creativity and that the creative person may be at any point on this continuum: "Vygotsky's ideas would suggest that he considered little c, or individual inventiveness, and big C, or historical creativity, as dialectically connected" (Moran & John-Steiner, 2003, p. 81).

This concept of little c creativity is particularly important when considering young children's creativity as it foregrounds the individual's attributes and agency as a creative agent unshackled from the formal sanction of the gatekeepers of Big C creativity's validity or importance. However, Craft did not elevate the importance of the individual above a systems view of creativity. Like Csiksentmihalyi's system theory of creativity (1999) in which the system is a dynamic interaction between domain, person, and field, Craft identifies three critical aspects of possibility thinking: "Each of the three parts of the framework – agents, processes and domains – offer a 'frame' or a perspective through which to both observe and also foster creativity. All are necessary parts of the whole" (Craft, 2001, p. 54). In the framework, the individual child has creative agency in their own unique way, applying processes that may include intuitive, non-conscious, and conscious cognition, bounded by domains that encompass all knowledge, "not confined to the arts ... and not simply academic domains but all of life" (2001, p. 56).

Craft's possibility thinking framework illustrates that the child's creativity involves:

> Self-determination and direction ... personal route-finding in life ...
> Innovation ... something which is novel to the child ...
> Action ... an idea is operationalized ...
> Development ... continual development on to a new "place" ...
> Depth ... awareness of convention ... deep concentration on one area ...
> Risk ... the possibility that the intended outcome may not occur.
>
> *(Craft, 2001, pp. 56–7)*

Possibility Spaces in the Material World of the Primary School

Craft worked with Open University and University of Cambridge academics Teresa Grainger (later Cremin) and Pamela Burnard to arrive at "an evidence-based model of possibility thinking" in young children (Grainger, Craft, & Burnard, 2007, p. 8). In this model, the child learner and the teacher are nested in an enabling context, and the entanglement of context, learner, and teacher gives rise to the child's possibility thinking. In this model (pp. 9–10), a child's possibility thinking exhibits the following characteristics:

> POSING QUESTION: The focus on questioning, generating ideas through pondering and positing 'what if' scenarios in the mind.
>
> PLAY AND IMMERSION: Immersion allowed ideas to incubate and questions to merge . . . [what] Winnicott (1974) calls the deep play of childhood was rooted in the body and the senses.
>
> SELF DETERMINATION AND RISK TAKING: By providing more freedom and framing regular "challenges where there is no clear cut solution" (DfES, 2003, p. 9) . . . The children clearly developed the courage to take risks, . . . and they were expected to exercise agency and autonomy.
>
> BEING IMAGINATIVE AND MAKING CONNECTIONS: Few distinctions in terms of subject domains fostered their ability to make unusual connections between, for example, ideas and activities or their own and others' lives.
>
> PEDAGOGY: These [teacher] professionals allowed themselves and the learners time and space to play, to explore, to speculate, to question and to possibility think their way forward.

In 2018, a fieldwork study exploring possibility thinking was carried out at the newly established University of Cambridge Primary School, "a site where possibility 'space', an enabling context for possibility thinking, is embedded in the school's design" (Burnard et al., 2018, p. 253). Burnard et al. (2018) applied an arts-based perceptual ecology framework placing the arts alongside science, technology, engineering, and mathematics, i.e., STEM, as a 'bracketed' concept, STE(A)M (p. 250). In the maths curriculum, they identified possibility spaces in the school evident in the following ways:

> a. experiential possibility spaces where there was direct experience of models and music composing/constructing in mathematics;
> b. intuitive possibility spaces for the use of imagination, intuition and magic in mathematics;
> c. embodying possibility spaces for art-making of composing/constructing in mathematics; and
> d. exploratory possibility spaces for the language of pattern in relation to its detection and recognition in mathematics.
>
> *(p. 276)*

This shows possibility spaces to be relational places of imagination and little c creativity, whereby there is a dynamic relationship between the interior and the exterior worlds of the child and through which the child is transformed and learns. Burnard et al. argue (2018) that, in possibility spaces, the child's "intuition stimulates imagination, acts as an organizing process that creates representations of our learning experiences. Thus, imagination becomes a modelling device through which we can test possibilities and co-create enabling possibility spaces" (p. 277). Craft's research about young children's creativity rapidly evolved as digital technology advanced in the early 21st century and she proposed that, in digital spaces, children could be "digital possibility thinkers posing 'what if?' questions and engaging in 'as if' activity" (2011, p. 173). She argued that, as a result of the digital revolution, there are four key features of the changing nature of childhood which she called the 4Ps – plurality of identities, possibility awareness, playfulness of engagement, and participation (2011, p. 179). She stated:

> The 4Ps have little c creativity inherent within them, each enabling and demanding creativity within and between people ... Understood in this way, it can be seen that the digital play-spaces of children and young people offer inherent opportunities for creativity.
>
> (p. 182)

Whilst Craft's death in 2014 meant the research world was not privy to how she might progress her work on digital possibility spaces nor how she might engage with the burgeoning research about the posthuman child (Murris, 2016), she did begin to evolve her work on creativity in ways that resonate with posthumanist theory, in particular the theory of wise, humanising creativity: "grounded in a reciprocal relationship between the collaborative generation of new ideas and identities, fuelled by dialogues between the participants and the world outside ... [wise, humanising creativity is] an antidote to marketised and individualised creativity" (2011, p. 179).

Posthumanist Possibility Spaces

A posthuman perspective of possibility spaces may extend understandings of agency in possibility thinking. Burnard et al. (2018) allude to a wider view of agency, broadening out from the agency of the little c creative individual, when citing Maxine Green: "landscapes of our interior worlds flow and merge into the landscapes of the exterior world ... [and] can stimulate much needed educational change" (Green, 1978, p. 37, cited in Burnard et al., 2018, p. 253). This merging of the interior and exterior is echoed in children's engagement in virtual spaces, in which the immaterial virtual landscapes of children's creative digital play merge with the materiality of their real-world contexts. Ash (2015) has proffered the term "teleplasty" (2015, p. 23) to describe the way that technology is agentic in shaping the possibilities in digital play. Marsh (2017, p. 5) applies Kuby and Rucker's (2016, p. 17) notion of "togetherness in an entangled moment" to describe children at play with digital environments. She suggests this assemblage of technology and child is "play that crosses virtual/physical worlds, online/offline and digital/non-digital boundaries [which] raises a range of ontological questions" (p. 5). Whilst this chapter does not aim to answer these questions, it does engage with what applying a posthuman lens to the complexities children's creativity in digital possibility spaces might offer.

Posthumanist perspectives decentre the human as an agent in any given context, including the digital. As Kuby and Rucker argue, "posthumanism is rooted in a relational ontology meaning we (humans, nonhumans and more-than-humans) are always already entangled with each other in becoming, in making, in creating realities (the world)" (Kuby & Rucker, 2017, p. 288). Therefore, when considering young children's possibility thinking in the educational space of the primary school or in the interactive virtual space, it is critical in a posthuman perspective that consideration is given to the entanglement of agents, processes, and domains, that is, the entanglement of the person, becoming, being, space, place, things, and knowledges. Chappell (2018) states:

> A dialogue between the inside-out and the outside-in of less boundaried human bodies, other life forms, ideas, objects and environments becomes less partial (whilst still

acknowledging partiality), and allows more perspectives and actants into the creative process, leading to a richer set of possible new ideas.

(p. 290)

Digital possibility thinking could be an encompassing concept for children's digital creativity in which posthumanist entanglements of being and becoming, of the human and nonhuman, are in dynamic inter-relationship. This may offer ways to understand the complex subjectivities that take place when a young child creatively intra-acts in digital spaces.

In Barad's (2003) discussion of discourse and posthumanist traditions, she also identifies that posthumanism is akin to possibilities. Exploring "the mutually constitutive relationship of materials and discourses" (p. 819), Barad argues that discourse in any given context, including the context of children's primary school, is filled with possibilities that arise from the individual and nonhuman agents:

> statements are not the mere utterances of the originating consciousness of a unified subject; rather, statements and subjects emerge from a field of possibilities. This field of possibilities is not static or singular but rather is a dynamic and contingent multiplicity.
>
> *(p. 819)*

The field of possibilities in the University of Cambridge Primary School, in which children were posing questions and play, risk-taking, blurring domains and boundary crossing to make leaps into the unknown, was facilitated through the engagement of the human landscape (child) with the nonhuman (school environment) landscape. This same human–nonhuman entanglement can be found in a child's engagement in digital contexts. Some fields of possibilities for children's dynamic entanglements with digital touchscreen technologies can be found in the examples of 0–5-year-olds' play with iPads in the Toddlers and Tables study, children's creative play with internet-connected toys, and virtual/nonvirtual entanglements in makerspaces, all three of which are addressed later in this chapter.

Posthumanist Digital Possibility Spaces

It is important to acknowledge that the contemporary childhood experience is one in which the human child and the technological are inherently entangled (Marsh et al., 2005; Marsh, 2010; Marsh, 2017). Incorporating posthumanism in conceptualising possibility spaces requires a paradigmatic shift from thinking of human subjects as biological beings to considering them bound in a technological totality:

> Posthuman subjects assume not only the materialist totality of things (i.e., that all matter is One, intelligent and self-organizing), but also that this totality includes technology. This is important because it inscribes the technological apparatus as second nature. Do remember that this "Life" the posthuman subject is immanent to, is no longer "*bios*", but rather "*zoe*": non-anthropocentric, but also non-anthropomorphic. *Zoe* also needs to embrace "geo" and "techno"-bound egalitarianism, acknowledging that intelligence, thinking and the capacity to produce knowledge is *not* the exclusive prerogative of humans alone, but is distributed across all living matter and self-organizing technological networks.
>
> *(Braidotti, 2017, p. 23)*

Thus, before possibility thinking can be reconceptualised from a posthumanist perspective, the child as agent of little c creativity needs to be understood as fundamentally entangled with the material whereby "matter matters" (Barad, 2007, pp. 132–85, cited in Murris, 2016, p. 193). Barad identifies that "'we' are not outside observers of the world. Nor are we simply located at particular places *in* the world; rather, we are part *of* the world in its ongoing intra-activity" (2003, p. 828).

Posthumanist digital possibility thinking challenges the value and assessment of the products (rather than the process) of possibility thinking imposed by a second-generation creativity framework, whereby creativity is "imbued with an economic ethos of being production with others, something which is able to be influenced and encapsulated – plus an understanding that it can be taught, learnt and assessed" (Swist, 2013, p. 146). Third-generation creativity, in Swist's view, is "an authentic and alternative discourse to linear, work-ready and economically driven reductions of [creativity in] education" (p. 147). Positioning children's little c creativity as possibility thinking is one such alternate discourse but further positioning it within children's authentic entanglements in digital contexts leads to the concept of posthumanist digital possibility thinking. Taking a posthumanist perspective on children's creativity and play honours the existing, evolving techno-human assemblages that are the context for 21st-century creativity, what this chapter calls posthumanist digital possibility thinking. Further, these entanglements are made visible in posthumanist digital play.

Posthumanist Digital Play

Posthumanist perspectives of children's possibility thinking may be a challenge for early childhood educators steeped in child-centred pedagogy and the freedom of child-centred (non-technological) play. These are largely drawn from Vygotsky's notion that play is crucial to cognitive development: "play ... is the leading source of development in pre-school years" (Vygotsky, 1933/1976, p. 540). In Vygotsky's view, both child development and children's creativity are seen as the "internalization or appropriation of cultural tools and social interactions" (Moran & John-Steiner, 2003, p. 63). However, this internalisation process is more than just adopting external tools. It is transformative in nature whereby, through a dialectic between the social, cultural, material, and non-material, the child creates new knowledge and ways of being in the world. Similarly, posthumanism "understands the human body as an unbounded organism that exists in an entangled network of human and nonhuman forces. Posthumanism opens up a very different kind of being and knowing" (Murris, 2016, p. 193). Thus, Vygotsky's notion of the metamorphosis of the child from one state of being to another may appear to agree in part with the posthumanism's theorizing of the child:

> The posthuman child is not only discursive, but also material (and/and), including the body that the child not just has, but also is. In a monist universe, all earth dwellers are equal – they are mutually entangled, always becoming, and always intra-acting with everything else. The posthuman child is relational.
>
> *(Murris, 2016, p. 193)*

However, Murris (2016) argues that Vygotskyan assumptions "that children will learn to think for themselves if they engage in the social practice of thinking together" (p. 155) do not equate with a posthuman approach as it is firmly social constructionist. To Murris, such a social constructionist approach "would assume there are bounded subjects and objects 'in' the world moving through space and time" (Barad, 2007, p. 815, cited by Murris, 2016, p. 156). Such children's thinking involves "'internalisation' of the 'outer voices' that build on each other's ideas in a community of enquiry [that] will lead to a richer, more varied 'inner' dialogue, and as a result a better, more reasonable thinking, through 'self-correction'" (Murris, 2016, p. 155). But inner and outer suggest firm boundaries and a subject and other. Murris states:

a relational materialist ontoepistemology does not understand relationships as connections that are made between independently existing ontological units (like the more familiar "inter-action"), ... it is impossible to say where the boundaries are of each child, or the teacher, or the parent, or the gecko on the wall, or the furniture, or the drawings, [or the technology] and so forth (not only from an epistemological, but also from an ontological point of view). For relational materialists, the ontological and epistemological starting points for theorising are the intra-actions – the relations "between" individuals and nonhuman others.

(p. 156)

Thus, posthumanist digital play sees the child in relational engagement with not just humans, but with the nonhuman. This makes sense when one considers the child's play world and the physical toys that are an integral part of children's concrete and imaginary little c creativity. If this notion of the relational to the nonhuman is extended, then it is clear that the virtual toy or game is also a key aspect of the child's creative play world, and that an assemblage of the technological and the human takes place in a child's play interactions with the virtual.

Edwards (2013) described this as converged play, whereby traditional toy play converges with newer forms of digital play, such as virtual apps and games. Ash (2015) identified this process of convergence as teleplasty, "the way in which technologies preshape the possibilities of human activities and sensory experience" (p. 23). He describes these moments of convergence of the physical and the virtual, the human and nonhuman, as interface envelopes: "localized foldings of space-time that work to shape capacities to sense space and time" (Ash, 2010, p. 10). Marsh, however, argues that a different perspective of these convergences of the material and immaterial is needed, one that sees virtual play from a posthumanist perspective: "Given the extent to which the digital is an integral element of young children's play ... there is a need to develop accounts that enhance an understanding of 'ontological entanglements' (Barad, 2007, p. 332) of children and technology" (Marsh, 2017, p. 6).

Marsh gives an account of research by Giddings (2014) in which he observes his sons at play "with Lego across virtual and material planes, [he] notes that they move seamlessly across these domains, and the material and immaterial are interwoven in their imaginatively conceived 'game-worlds'" (Marsh, 2017, p. 15). By viewing the virtual play space as a posthumanist possibility space, and seeing this virtual play as a child's enactment of little c creativity or possibility thinking, the entanglement of the human and nonhuman in digital possibility spaces identify that "his or her sense of presence moves beyond the corporeal to encompass the virtual environment" (Marsh, 2017, p. 6).

Such posthumanist digital play differentiates between a child's *interaction* with the play world, and a child's *intra-action* in an entangled posthuman digital space. As Wohlwend et al. (2017) state:

Interaction is defined as actions that are materially mediated in relations among subjects and objects that constitute social practices in a cultural environment (Scollon, 2001). By contrast, *intra-action* is defined as actions that emerge from within unspecified, entangled and changing phenomena of bodies and give rise to possibilities and transformations (Barad, 2003).

(Wohlwend et al., 2017, p. 453)

They argue that seeing the child's play in the virtual world as intra-actions "reframes materiality from design affordances to a cycling interplay produced by the physicality, fluidity and messiness of entangled bodies, things and places" (p. 447). These posthumanist digital interplay spaces are relational possibility spaces where intuition, imagination, and little c creativity are in dynamic intra-action with the interior and the exterior (including digital) worlds of the child. In its broad review of the field approach, this chapter has not presented primary research conducted by the author. However, below are some instances in which other researchers have viewed children's engagement in digital contexts through a posthuman lens, as the following examples demonstrate.

Digital Possibility Spaces: Examples from the Research

Apps

Arising from the Toddlers and Tablets research project (Holloway et al., 2015; Green, 2019; Green et al., 2019), which investigated family practices related to young children's technology use in the home in Australia and the United Kingdom, Holloway et al. (2019) interrogate skills scaffolding for a young child's use of an app, taking "a broad posthumanist approach" (p. 211). In the child's use of the app, they state, "an instructional assemblage is formed between parental scaffolding, in-built (app) scaffolding, and the child" (p. 210). Here they demonstrate that there is an entanglement between the human (parent and child) and the nonhuman (app) in order for the child to engage fully with the app. To recall Grainger, Craft, and Burnard's (2007, pp. 9–10) model of possibility thinking which encompasses five characteristics – posing questions, play and immersion, self-determination and risk-taking, being imaginative and making connections, and pedagogy – this scaffolding is a kind of pedagogy in which the parent-as-teacher allows the child a possibility space to play and explore the app.

The researchers explain an interaction between parent and two-year-old child Scott whilst using an app. Applying their posthuman perspective, the researchers identify that there is an "entanglement of intra-activity between the three actants [child, parent and app]" (Holloway et al., 2019, p. 216). They demonstrate this intra-activity in which the very young child is engaged in digital play with the app to be a space in which scaffolding supports the child's possibility thinking. Scott is immersed, taking risks at app-led activities outside his skills set, posing questions to his parent about choices, and making connections between his attempts to use the app and his parent's scaffolded suggestions. The child's possibility thinking is facilitated by parental scaffolding and in-built scaffolding within the app. Holloway et al. identify this as "the increasing imbrication or overlap of humans and technology within education [learning] processes" (Holloway et al., 2019, p. 217), highlighting the posthuman nature of the digital possibility space of the child–app engagement, and they call for new ways of considering the child as part of digital assemblages.

Internet of Toys

Arising from the Technology and Play project (Marsh et al., 2015) in which 2,000 parents of young children in the United Kingdom contributed to research about children's use of apps in the home and school, Marsh (2017) constructs a "posthuman and multimodal analysis of connected play" (p. 1) in relation to the Internet of Toys (Chaudron et al., 2017; Mascheroni & Holloway, 2017). Marsh argues that, though Edwards (2013) applies the term converged play "in which traditional play with toys converge with newer forms of digital play" when discussing digital play, Marsh applies the term 'connected play' instead as it more holistically expresses "more peripheral as well as core connections between various aspects of play" (Marsh, 2017, p. 2). This is an important distinction when considering digital play from a posthuman perspective as connections expresses the messy entanglement of the human and nonhuman, rather than a smooth and more stable convergence of the physical and the virtual. Marsh identifies that children's digital play with interconnected toys is comprised of Barad's posthuman "ontological entanglements" (Barad, 2007, p. 332, cited in Marsh, 2017, p. 3), or intra-actions (Barad, 2003) in which the boundaries between the subject/object and material/virtual are in a constant state of forming or 'becoming'.

The important distinction that Marsh makes in relation to children's Internet of Toys play is about children's cardinal orientation. She draws on Ash to explain this as "the spatial orientation given by the structure of the human bodies, rather than in relation to external points in space" (Ash, 2010, p. 416, cited in Marsh, 2017, p. 6). Marsh suggests that a child's engagement with an interconnected toy's touchscreen interface results in a similar "reorganization of the child's cardinal orientation" (p. 6). It is this reorganisation that can be seen as a digital possibility space created though the child's imaginative play, bringing to mind Burnard et al. (2018) on possibility spaces. These Internet of Toys intra-actions are relational spaces of the child's imagination whereby imaginative play is a "modelling device … enabling possibility spaces" (Burnard et al., 2017, p. 277). Possibility thinking's characteristics of play and immersion, being imaginative and making connections are all demonstrated in a child's intra-activity with the Internet of Toys.

Makerspaces

The European Union (EU) has identified the changing nature of children's engagement with technology. Consequently, they funded DigiLitEY (2020), a COST Action concerned with establishing research networks investigating the digital literacy and multimodal practices of young children. Connected to this broad network is the MakEY project – Makerspaces in the Early Years: Enhancing Digital Literacy and Creativity (MakEY). This project is itself a broad network of research projects in seven EU countries (Denmark, Germany, Finland, Iceland, Norway, Romania, and the United Kingdom) and the USA, each of which "explores the place of the rising 'maker' culture in the development of children's digital literacy and creative design skills" (MakEY, 2020).

Though the project does not specifically take a posthuman approach, the term postdigital play (Jayemanne, Apperley, & Nansen, 2015) has been applied to the experiences of young children in makerspaces (Marsh et al., 2017), and this term closely aligns with posthumanism's entanglements of the human and nonhuman. Marsh et al. (2019), in outlining the principles of pedagogy and practice of early childhood makerspaces, state: "The term [postdigital play] emphasizes the way in which the digital is so embedded in everyday play practices that it is no longer meaningful to consider the digital in contrast to the nondigital" (p. 224). They propose that makerspaces enable children to "move seamlessly across digital and nondigital domains in their maker play" (p. 223), again drawing attention to a posthuman interweaving of the material and the immaterial. In this way, makerspaces, like virtual play spaces, become spaces of emergent 'postdigital' possibility thinking.

The MakEY research makes clear that makerspaces encourage little c creativity, or possibility thinking (Blum-Ross, Kumpulainen, & Marsh, 2020). The researchers explain how the MakEY project was concerned with "the kinds of digital literacy skills and creative competences children developed through their participation in makerspaces" (p. 6). A Romanian MakEY case study within the collection is one of the few that positions the makerspace in a posthuman context (Velicu & Mitarca, 2020). The researchers state that they "embraced the hybridised nature of makerspaces (i.e., with their mix of digital and non-digital, art/craft and technology, etc.) but also refer to each particular situation in our project as unique agentic assemblages" (p. 116). It is this notion of the hybridised makerspace that is akin to posthuman assemblages of the agentic human and agentic nonhuman. The child enacts possibility thinking in these makerspace assemblages in which the human child and nonhuman matter (virtual and material) are entangled and have agency.

Conclusion

This chapter has explored the concept of the posthuman possibility space. It makes connections between Craft's (2001) notion of little c creativity and young children's possibility thinking enacted in a digital (and postdigital) world. Consideration has been given to what a posthuman digital possibility space may entail, and the concept of young children's posthuman digital play has been envisioned. It has dipped a toe into the extensive pool of research about very young children and digital contexts to briefly explore what research about apps, the Internet of Toys, and makerspaces reveal about posthuman digital possibility spaces. This chapter's exploration of the literature has revealed that the research field of the digital child is poised for an application of a posthuman lens in order to fully understand the emergent, agentic assemblages of the human child and the digital nonhuman in the postdigital 21st century.

References

Ash, J. (2010). Teleplastic technologies: Charting practices of orientation and navigation in videogaming. *Transactions of the Institute of British Geographers, 35*(3), 414–430.

Ash, J. (2015). *The interface envelope: Gaming, technology, power*. New York, NY: Bloomsbury.

Barad, K. (2003). Posthumanist performativity: Toward an understanding of how matter comes to matter. *Signs Journal of Women in Culture and Society, 28*(3), 801–831. Retrieved from: www.jstor.org/stable/10.1086/345321.

Barad, K. (2007). *Meeting the universe halfway: Quantum physics and the entanglement of matter and meaning*. Durham, NC: Duke University Press.

Beghetto, R., & Kaufman, J. (2007). Toward a broader conception of creativity: A case for "mini-c" creativity. *Psychology of Aesthetics, Creativity, and the Arts, 1*(2), 73–79. doi:10.1037/1931-3896.1.2.73.

Blum-Ross, A., Kumpulainen, K., & Marsh, K. (2020). *Enhancing digital literacy and creativity: Makerspaces in the early years*. Abingdon, UK: Routledge.

Braidotti, R. (2017). Posthuman, all too human – The memoirs and aspirations of a posthumanist. Lecture presented in the 2017 Tanner Lecture Series, Yale University, USA. Retrieved from: https://tannerlectures.utah.edu/Manuscript%20for%20Tanners%20Foundation%20Final%20Oct%201.pdf.

Burnard, P., Dragovic, T., Jasilek, S., Biddulph, J., Rolls, L., Durning, A., & Fenyvesi, K. (2018). The art of co-creating Arts-based possibility spaces for fostering STE(A)M practices in Primary Education. In T. Chemi & X. Du (Eds.), *Arts-based methods on education around the world* (pp. 247–282). Gistrup, Denmark: Rivers Publishers. doi:10.17863/CAM.21144.

Chappell, K. (2018). From wise humanising creativity to (posthumanising) creativity. In K. Snepvangers, P. Thomson, & A. Harris (Eds.), *Creativity policy, partnerships and practice in education* (1st ed., pp. 279–306). Melbourne: Palgrave Macmillan.

Chaudron, S., Di Gioia, R., Gemo, M., Holloway, D., Marsh, J., Mascheroni, G., & Yamada-Rice, D. (2017). *Kaleidoscope on the internet of toys – Safety, security, privacy and societal insights*. Luxembourg: Publications Office of the European Union. Retrieved from: https://publications.jrc.ec.europa.eu/repository/bitstream/JRC105061/jrc105061_final_online.pdf.

Craft, A. (1996). Nourishing educator creativity: A holistic approach to CPD. *British Journal of In-service Education, 22*(3), 309–322.

Craft, A. (1999). Creative development in the early years; Implications of policy for practice. *The Curriculum Journal, 10*(1), 135–150.

Craft, A. (2001). Little c creativity. In A. Craft, B. Jeffrey, & M. Leibling (Eds.), *Creativity in education* (pp. 45–46). London, UK: Continuum Books.

Craft, A. (2011). Childhood in a digital age: Creative challenges for educational futures. *London Review of Education, 10*(2), 173–190.

Csikszentmihalyi, M. (1999). Implications of a system perspective for the study of creativity. In R. Sternberg (Ed.), *Handbook of creativity* (pp. 313–335). Cambridge: Cambridge University Press.

Department for Education and Skills [U.K.]. (2003). *Excellence and enjoyment: a strategy for primary schools*. London: HMSO. Retrieved from: https://webarchive.nationalarchives.gov.uk/20040722022638/http://www.dfes.gov.uk/primarydocument.

DigiLitEY. (2020). The digital literacy and multimodal practices of young children (DigiLitEY). Retrieved from: http://digilitey.eu/about.

Edwards, S. (2013). Post-industrial play: Understanding the relationship between traditional and converged forms of play in the early years. In A. Burke & J. Marsh (Eds.), *Children's virtual play worlds: Culture, learning and participation* (pp. 10–25). New York, NY: Peter Lang.

Gardner, H. (1997). *Extraordinary minds: Portraits of four exceptional minds and the extraordinary minds in us all*. New York: HarperCollins.

Giddings, S. (2014). *Gameworlds: Virtual media and children's everyday lives*. London, UK: Bloomsbury.

Grainger, T., Craft, A., & Burnard, P. (2007). Examining 'possibility thinking' in action in early years settings. Paper presented at the 4th International Conference on Imagination and Education. Vancouver: Simon Fraser University, Imaginative Education Research Group. Retrieved from: www.researchgate.net/profile/Pamela_Burnard/publication/42797985_Examining_possibility_thinking_in_action_in_early_years_settings/links/0a85e52e9fed1cd110000000/Examining-possibility-thinking-in-action-in-early-years-settings.pdf.

Green, L. (2019). Digitising early childhood: An introduction. In L. Green, D.J. Holloway, K.J. Stevenson, & K. Jaunzems (Eds.), *Digitising early childhood* (pp. 1–15). Newcastle, UK: Cambridge Scholars Publishing.

Green, L., Haddon, L., Livingstone, S., Holloway, D., Jaunzems, K., Stevenson, K.J., & O'Neill, B. (2019). Parents' failure to plan for their children's digital futures. *Media@LSE Working Paper Series* (#61). London, UK: London School of Economics and Social Sciences. Retrieved from: www.lse.ac.uk/media-and-communications/assets/documents/research/working-paper-series/WP61.pdf.

Holloway, D., Haddon, L., Green, L., & Stevenson, K. (2019). The parent-child-app learning assemblage: Scaffolding early childhood learning through app use in the family home. In N. Kucirkova, J. Rowsall, & G. Falloon (Eds.), *The Routledge international handbook of learning with technology in early childhood* (pp. 210–218). Abingdon, UK: Routledge.

Holloway, D.J., Green, L., & Stevenson, K.J. (2015). Digitods: Toddlers, touchscreens and Australian family life. *M/C Journal*, 18(5). Retrieved from: http://journal.media-culture.org.au/index.php/mcjournal/article/viewArticle/1024.

Jayemanne, D., Apperley, T., & Nansen, B. (2015). Postdigital play and the aesthetics of recruitment. *Transactions of the Digital Games Research Association*, 2(3), 145–172. Retrieved from: https://e-channel.med.utah.edu/wp-content/uploads/2016/04/digra2015_JAYEMANNE.pdf.

Kaufman, J., & Beghetto, R. (2009). Beyond big and little: The four C model of creativity. *Review of General Psychology*, 13(1), 1–12. doi:10.1037/a0013688.

Kuby, C., & Rucker, T. (2016). *Go be a writer! Expanding the curricular boundaries of literacy learning with children*. New York, NY: Teachers College Press.

Kuby, C., & Rucker, T. (2017). Early literacy and the posthuman: Pedagogies and methodologies. *Journal of Early Childhood Literacy*, 17(3), 285–296. doi:10.1177/1468798417715720.

MakEY. (2020). Makerspaces in the early years: Enhancing digital literacy and creativity (MakEY). Retrieved from: https://makeyproject.eu.

Marsh, J., Brooks, G., Hughes, J., Ritchie, L., Roberts, S., & Wright, K. (2005). *Digital beginnings: Young children's use of popular culture, media and new technologies*. Sheffield: University of Sheffield. Retrieved from: https://esmeefairbairn.org.uk/digital-beginnings.

Marsh, J., Kumpulainen, K., Nisha, B., Velicu, A., Blum-Ross, A., Hyatt, D., & Thorsteinsson, G. (2017). *Makerspaces in the early years: A literature review*. University of Sheffield: MakEY Project. Retrieved from: http://makeyproject.eu/wp-content/uploads/2017/02/Makey_Literature_Review.pdf.

Marsh, J., Plowman, L., Yamada-Rice, D., Bishop, J.C., Lahmar, J., Scott, F., & Winter, P. (2015). *Exploring play and creativity in pre-schoolers' use of apps: Final project report*. Retrieved from: www.techandplay.org.

Marsh, J., Wood, E., Chesworth, L., Nisha, B., Nutbrown, B., & Olney, B. (2019). Makerspaces in early childhood education: Principles of pedagogy and practice. *Mind, Culture, and Activity*, 26(3), 221–233. doi:10.1080/10749039.2019.1655651.

Marsh, J.A. (2010). *Childhood, culture and creativity: A literature review*. Newcastle, UK: Creativity, Culture and Education [organisation]. Retrieved from: www.creativitycultureeducation.org//wp-content/uploads/2018/10/CCE-childhood-culture-and-creativity-a-literature-review.pdf.

Marsh, J.A. (2017). The internet of toys: A posthuman and multimodal analysis of connected play. *Teachers College Record*, 119(12), 1–32. ID Number: 22073. Retrieved from: www.tcrecord.org.

Mascheroni, G., & Holloway, D. (Eds.) (2017). The internet of toys: A report on media and social discourses around young children and IoToys. *DigiLitEY*. Retrieved from: http://digilitey.eu/wp-content/uploads/2017/01/IoToys-June-2017-reduced.pdf.

McWilliam, E. (2008). *The creative workforce: How to launch young people into high-flying futures*. Sydney: University of New South Wales Press.

Moran, S., & John-Steiner, V. (2003). Creativity in the making: Vygotsky's contribution to the dialectic of development and creativity. In R.K. Sawyer, V. John-Steiner, S. Moran, R.J. Sternberg, D.H. Feldman, J. Nakamura, & M. Csikszentmihalyi (Eds.), *Creativity and development* (pp. 61–91). New York, NY: Oxford University Press.

Murris, K. (2016). *The posthuman child: Educational transformation through philosophy with picturebooks*. Abingdon, UK: Routledge.

Scollon, R. (2001). *Mediated discourse: the nexus of practice*. London: Routledge.

Spencer, E., Lucas, B., & Claxton, G. (2012). *Progression in creativity: A literature review*. Newcastle, UK: Creativity, Culture and Education. Retrieved from: www.creativitycultureeducation.org/progression-in-creativity-a-literature-review.

Swist, T. (2013). Third-generation creativity – Unfolding a social-ecological imagination. In M. Peters & T. Besley (Eds.), *The creative university* (pp. 145–160). Rotterdam: Sense Publishers.

Velicu, A., & Mitarca, M. (2020). Types of engagement in makerspaces. In A. Blum-Ross, K. Kumpulainen, & J. Marsh (Eds.), *Enhancing digital literacy and creativity: Makerspaces in the early years* (pp. 116–131). Abingdon, UK: Routledge.

Vygotsky, L.S. (1933/1976). Play and its role in the development of the child. In J.S. Bruner, A. Jolly, & K. Sylva (Eds.), *The collected works of L.S Vygotsky* (Vol. 1, pp. 339–350). New York, NY: Plenum Press.

Vygotsky, L. S. (1971). *The psychology of art*. Cambridge, MA: MIT Press. (1925 dissertation, not published in lifetime).

Winnicott, D. (1974). *Playing and reality*. Harmondsworth, UK: Penguin.

Wohlwend, K., Peppler, K., Keun, A., & Thompson, N. (2017). Making sense and nonsense: Comparing mediated discourse and agential realist approaches to materiality in a preschool makerspace. *Journal of Early Childhood Literacy*, 17(3), 444–462. doi:10.1177/1468798417712066.

8
THE DOMESTICATION OF TOUCHSCREEN TECHNOLOGIES IN FAMILIES WITH YOUNG CHILDREN

Leslie Haddon

Introduction

Over the last two decades there has been a wealth of studies on older children's use of technologies generally and mobile phones and the internet more specifically. But there has also been a separate, smaller literature on pre-school children's experience of ICTs. Touchscreen technologies, principally but not only the tablet and smartphone, have an interface that has now made these ICTs much more physically accessible to this age group (Neumann & Neumann, 2014). Hence, this has generated considerable research interest on their potential role in educational settings (Stephen & Edwards, 2018) and more recently in the home.

While research on parents' and younger children's interaction in relation to technologies is often discussed in terms of children's (especially cognitive) development, it can equally well be framed in terms of a domestication analysis of ICTs. This framework examines the processes by which ICTs find a place in people's routines, sometimes in households generally (Silverstone et al., 1992). Most studies using this domestication approach have focussed on various adults, but some, including the first empirical work in this field (Hirsch, 1992), have taken families as objects of studies, including children. However, these were mostly older children and so there is scope for asking what a domestication analysis might reveal about the dynamics of families with younger children.

This chapter explores how very young, pre-school children – aged 0–5 years old – encounter and experience ICTs and, in particular, how parents of these young children try to manage their use of these technologies. It reports the first findings from the Australia–UK Toddlers and Tablets project, examining the processes by which these technologies are domesticated in the lives of young children.

Literature Review

There is now a body of research on the more general ICT use of pre-school children aged 0–5 in the home (e.g., Plowman et al., 2010a; Rideout, 2011; McPake et al., 2012; Plowman, 2015; see Holloway et al., 2013 for a review). More recently, a somewhat diverse research literature on young children's use of touchscreen technologies in that setting has emerged. Methodologically, this includes surveys of what activities these very young children do with these technologies (Rideout, 2013; Nevski & Siibak, 2016; Pempeck & McDaniel, 2016; Marsh et al., 2015, 2018) as well as surveys examining predictors of their use (Lauricella et al., 2015; Nevski & Siibak, 2016). There have been ethnographic/observational/video studies looking at child–parent interactions around these technologies (Danby et al., 2013; Chaudron, 2015; Neumann & Neumann, 2016; Marsh et al., 2018). Interviews have also been conducted, though more so with parents (e.g., Livingstone et al., 2014).

As regards the theoretical frameworks used, one Human–Computer Interface study examined what children of different ages are capable of doing (Hourcade et al., 2015), and a media studies piece looked at how parents represent children when posting videos of their tablet use (Nansen & Jayamene, 2016). However, reflecting the learning agenda emphasis in research on ICTs more generally (Stephen & Edwards, 2018), one key research interest when looking at touchscreens is children's cognitive development, whether framed in terms of literacy (Neumann, 2014, 2018; Neumann & Neumann, 2014, 2016, 2017), or creativity (Marsh et al., 2018), and how parents support such learning processes.

To provide a wider context, Scottish researchers Plowman et al. (2010a, 2010c) noted a range of moral panics about ICTs more generally that have been expressed in the media, among which are concerns about the negative effects on children's social development as children interact more with technology and less with other people, the addictive nature of such technologies, the inauthentic experience of the digital world compared with the physical one, and how technology fails to stir children's imagination. In contrast to the fear about technology dominating children's lives implicit in some of this negative coverage, these and other researchers (Livingstone et al., 2014; Chaudron, 2015) observe that in practice ICTs are usually not so central to children's routines but are used alongside engagement in other activities.

As regards isolated use, these Scottish researchers and others have observed that parents do sometimes use ICTs as electronic babysitters, occupying young children when parents need their 'free' moments, including those times to deal with non-childcare tasks (Plowman et al., 2008, 2010b, 2010c; Livingstone et al., 2014; for a more extreme example, Bar Lev et al., 2018). However, a UK survey of 0–5-year-olds noted that children were far more likely to be using a tablet with a parent (57%) than alone 35% (Marsh et al., 2015). Based on their various studies, the Scottish researchers also found limited evidence of this isolation (Plowman et al., 2010c). In fact, Stephen et al. (2013) showed the variety of ways in which parents interacted with children, scaffolding their children's experiences in a similar way to the actions of staff in pre-school.

Turning to the domestication framework, this approach often looks at how ICTs are introduced into people's lives and how experience changes over time, trying to make sense of how and why ICTs are used, and what role they play in everyday life (for a review of domestication studies more generally, see Haddon, 2016). This can also include understanding why that role might be limited, sometimes intentionally constrained, or indeed the technologies could be rejected. Research in this tradition often aims to understand this domestication process by appreciating the social context[1] into which these technologies enter, how ICTs fit into the rest of people's daily routines, and how patterns of use emerge from their particular circumstances.

Some domestication studies have focussed on families as the unit of analysis rather than on children, even if older children were present in empirical studies (Lally, 2002; Ward, 2005). Two more recent studies applied a domestication analysis to smartphone use by older children, focussing respectively on parental mediation (Mascheroni, 2014) and how children experienced social constraints on the use of the technology (Haddon, 2018). However, the age of the children makes a difference in various senses, for example in the way that rational negotiation between parents and younger children was made problematic by the children's limited cognitive abilities

(López-de-Ayala-López & Haddon, 2018). In the case of young children, tablets and smartphones are already present in the home, so the question becomes one of how these technologies find a place in these children's lives. As will become clearer, here it is important to understand in particular the motivations of parents and the challenges they face, since how parents approach their children's use of those technologies is so important at this life stage for shaping the children's experience of these technologies.[2]

While much of the early childhood literature focusses on the pedagogical benefits of tablets in particular, it has been noted that there are in fact a variety of diverse reasons why touchscreen technologies first entered children's lives (Marsh et al., 2018). Hence, the domestication analysis starts by exploring how and why young children first encountered these technologies. The influence of parental values on their approach to mediation, parents' approach to parenting in general, and their evaluations of pros and cons of these particular technologies, have been reported in more detail elsewhere (Haddon & Holloway, 2018). In contrast, in this chapter the focus is more on the daily lives of parents and children, especially their diverse interactions with each other that relate to touchscreen technologies – a dimension of frequent interest in domestication analysis. The chapter next deals with certain particular interactions, exploring in a little more depth a practice identified in the literature: how and why parents use touchscreens to occupy their children, but also asking how they feel about this. This section also examines cases where situations unplanned by parents lead to unanticipated roles for these technologies. This is followed by a focus on interactions where parents choose to engage with their children's learning through the use of touchscreens, but noting how this can entail processes over and above specifically supporting or scaffolding their children's technology use. Lastly, the chapter looks at the type of interactions where parents attempt to manage, specifically to control, the place of these ICTs in their children's lives, indicating why parents can be in a stronger position to do this in the case of these very young, as opposed to older, children.

The Toddlers and Tablets Project

Toddlers and Tablets was an Australian–UK project funded by the Australian Research Council's Discovery Programme. This multi-method study looked both at children's practices with touchscreen technologies and the perspectives and actions of key actors in their lives, principally parents, but also grandparents and pre-school staff. The core research involved case studies of families and although these were conducted in both countries this chapter reports specifically on the UK data.

The family studies each entailed an initial interview with one or both parents, depending on the (often busy) timetables of the participants. The parents were then supplied with a videocamera and asked to record some examples of their children's use of tablets and smartphones, with suggestions (e.g., videoing children's use, if they had difficulties, if they received help). During a second visit to pick up the videocamera there was a chance for the researcher to observe the child using the technology and ask further questions. In the case of the UK study this session was also video-recorded. Compared with studies of older children it is often more difficult to hear the child's voice, because even the five-year-olds are less articulate. In practice, there was more reliance on the parents' accounts.

There was a total of nine UK families (plus a pilot study), recruited through diverse sources (e.g., workplaces, social networks, nurseries) but mainly involving snowballing. For example, nursery staff were asked if they could pass on details of this research to the parents of young children. All but one of the families lived in London, the exception living in the commuter belt around London. While the project aspired to produce a range of family circumstances there was a preponderance of middle-class families – only two were from a working-class background, one of which was a lone parent. Gender was balanced, with five boys and five girls aged 0–5. There were three 0–1-year-olds, three 2–3-year-olds and four 4–5-year-olds. Older siblings were present in some families, but only one family had two children in the 0–5 age range of the project. The cosmopolitan nature of the country, and London in particular, was reflected in the fact that quite a few of the parents had been born in other countries: the Tosettis were Italian, Klara Brown was a Slovak, the Jameson parents were Australian and French and the Mansi parents were Canadian-Indian and Russian.

The families filled in consent forms and their identities were anonymised. The analysis of the interviews and video material was in part informed by reacting to the literature on young children outlined above. But it was also based on approaches found in other domestication studies – e.g., how and why touchscreens first entered children's lives, identifying various forms of interaction between parents and children relating to the technologies. Emerging themes, including summaries and quotes, were organised into different sections forming the basis for a variety of publications on the different facets of parents' approaches to and young children's experiences of touchscreen technologies.

Findings

Initial Encounters with Touchscreens

Even though the children were still young, some of the parents found it difficult to remember the details of how their children first encountered touchscreen technologies. But it is clear that routes varied, and were not necessarily simply for encouraging educational literacy. Sometimes there were specific occasions when the parents first decided they needed to occupy the child such as on flights and a long car journeys or when preparing the baby's meals. But there were also motivations for introducing the child to touchscreen technologies based on parents' evaluations of perceived benefits. A number of the families thought it was useful for their children to interact with relatives, and temporarily absent parents, using the videochat facility on devices such as Facetime and Skype (noted also in previous research by McClure et al., 2015). Linda Palmer had first downloaded nursery rhymes onto the tablet so she and daughter Leela could sing them together. And Mirabella Tosetti had been showing son Leopoldo things on the tablet since he was a few months old because she thought it was easier for him to relate to moving images and sounds rather than pictures in books. Although that would be an example of seeing educational potential, Mirabella also found what she considered to be a 'good app' that meant her son had to turn off the lights to make cartoon animals go to bed. This became part of his own going-to-bed ritual.

Whatever parents' intended approach to parenting, the child had agency in this process. For example, children with older siblings had grown up seeing their siblings use the technologies and hence wanted to access the devices themselves. And there were sometimes factors specific to the child that affected parents' decision. Daughter Ellen Brent had a disorder that affected her language-learning abilities, so mother Elisabeth had, since Ellen was very young, left a TV channel on all day that showed someone signing. Elisabeth hoped her daughter would pick this up through such exposure. Later Elisabeth downloaded an assisted and augmented communication app onto the smartphone and then onto a tablet to provide Ellen with another way to communicate.

Occupying and Distracting Children with Touchscreens

Even if touchscreens were not originally introduced into children's lives to occupy them, eventually many parents at some stage used them for that purpose. The most common example given was letting the children use the technologies on long journeys to stop them getting bored, but also to keep them quiet and so provide some peace for the parents. But touchscreens could also fulfil this role on shorter outings. Here there is a new departure from the previous studies reviewed because either the child's tablet or smartphone were carried outside the home for this purpose, or parents let the children use their own personal devices when outdoors. For example, the Mansis carried an old smartphone in the pram for one-year-old Sergei to use. Trish Greenfield was willing to let one-year-old Andrew play with her own smartphone when they were out of the home. Sometimes the aim was to occupy children at particular times or in particular spaces, such as when a relative was visiting the home, or when at the hairdresser or the doctor. Stella Kramer even downloaded extra apps in preparation for some of these occasions. And as Elisabeth Brent pointed out, whereas she might give her older children something to read to occupy them, since Ellen could not yet read letting her use the tablet was the alternative.

It is worth adding, however, that parents had differing views about resorting to these technologies for this purpose at times and spaces that had a specific symbolic meaning. The Spinners took the tablet with them when they occasionally went to a restaurant, "in case of an emergency" – i.e., if daughter Imelda suddenly wanted to go home. But even they stressed that usually Imelda would be offered an alternative first, like something to colour in, where the tablet was the back up. Various comments like this remind us that restaurants are spaces where parents can feel that they are publicly on show to others, and being judged by them:

STELLA KRAMER: "I just thought that it would be better to try and teach the children as early as possible how to behave in a restaurant rather than risk having a child who can only entertain themselves with a phone or a tablet ... [adding later in the interview] ... it is a pet hate when I see other people who just fall back on it as the quick and easy option to entertain a child and I didn't want to fall into that habit."

There were other times when it was the child's situation that prompted parents to provide a touchscreen technology as a distraction – when it was not just an electronic babysitter, but a means to cope with a problem. For example, when Sergei was upset or ill Rohan and Nadia Mansi sometimes allowed their son to play on the tablet. Leopoldo Tosetti sometimes had nightmares and, while still semi-asleep, looking at pictures of the family on the smartphone was a way to calm him down. Simon Brown had a genetic disorder that meant he did not want to eat. So, as part of the major effort at mealtimes, the Browns found it was useful to let Simon watch the tablet since it distracted their child while they fed him. Similarly, Ellen Brent suffered from constipation, so Elisabeth let her watch the tablet once again as a distraction while she gave Ellen some medicine for this condition hidden in fruit puree. In fact, Elisabeth was happy to let Ellen take the tablet to the toilet because "as long as she's got that with her she'll sit there quite happily and not try and get off".

These examples often entailed discovering a use for the devices. The researcher had, early in the interviews, asked parents to remember what type of approach to parenting they had originally planned. While they might describe some parenting style, it is clear that usually they had not anticipated the issues discussed in this section. Sometimes parents felt guilt, or at least ambiguity, specifically when occupying children with technologies (in some social situations more than others). But it was nevertheless recognised as being a 'practical' decision at times to allow parents to carry out other activities while coping with the presence of (potentially demanding) children. Meanwhile, using the touchscreens as distractions were part of the parents' solutions to problems faced by the child.

Parents Engaging with Children's Touchscreen Use

It is easy to see why the case of occupying children with ICTs can feed into those concerns about children being isolated with technology rather than interacting with people. However, it is worth noting that even when children are doing something alone with the screen, parents (and siblings) can check up on them intermittently, as was also noted in Marsh et al. (2015). Indeed, the next section shows how this often happens specifically because parental help is requested.

In addition, and in contrast to, the 'isolated with technology' fear, many of these parents at various points chose to use the technology as a chance to engage with their children. In fact, they did so in the same way as they might talk to them about a book or about any non-technological activity in which the child was involved. Just as in the research by Stephen et al. (2013) and Neumann and Neumann (2016), this could mean suggesting what the children could do next when using an app, explaining why some tactic in a game was not working, asking about the decisions the children made when trying to solve a problem or asking children what[3] they thought was happening in a storyline (i.e., getting them to articulate their perceptions and decisions), and congratulating the children when they were successful in the apps. But beyond this scaffolding of children's use, there were also many instances of parents going beyond the task in the app to ask tangential questions that came to mind. In other words, playing with technology could be a springboard to interaction where what was happening on the screen provided the stimulus for more general parental involvement with their children.

Although this was a predominantly middle-class sample, with many mothers based at home part-time or full-time, these interactions occurred at some points in nearly all the families. Sometimes, from the child's perspective, it seemed that the children appreciated that interaction with the parent as well as, or indeed as much as, the interaction with the technology.

Parents' Management of Their Children's Use of Touchscreens

The last form of interaction to consider is parents' efforts to control their children's use of touchscreens. To put this into context, the amount of control that parents wanted to exercise varied. The Browns observed that they did not restrict Simon much – they let him use the tablet whenever he asked for it. The Tosettis were also happy for Leopoldo to use the tablet anytime. This did not mean that the children who were granted such access actually used the technologies often. For instance, Imelda Spinner went through phases when she did not use the tablet at all, and others when she did. For some, like Leela Palmer, use was more seasonal, in the winter when there was less chance to go out. In general, for a number of parents, the main restriction was not on the total time spent using devices but it was that the children should not use these digital technologies in the evening when the parents wanted the children to calm down before sleeping.

Even though some parents observed that it was occasionally difficult to get the children to put the technologies away, that they could get a bit grumpy, on the whole managing their children's use was not so much of an issue. This is because there are various factors that differentiate the engagement of younger children with these technologies from that of older children. One is that these younger children would often forget about the technologies if they were not visible. Hence, sometimes parents simply put the devices out of sight. This was even easier when young children with limited attention spans would move between these technologies and other toys. The relatively fixed structure of younger children's routines was also a factor. In the evening there were often winding-down-for-bed routines (e.g., baths) so the children did not really have time then to think about technologies. Either because of going to some pre-school facilities (nurseries, toddlers' groups) or because mothers especially took them out or engaged in activities with them in the home, there were many occasions when the children were (happily) doing something else rather than using tablets or smartphones.

These young children, even the five-year-olds, were also to varying degrees more dependent on their parents when trying to use the technologies compared with older children (also noted in

Livingstone et al., 2014; Marsh et al., 2015). This again made parental management easier. The youngest among them could not engage digitally at all unless the parents set things up and reminded the children how to navigate or explained the purpose of an app and what the children were expected to do in relation to any one screen. Even then, the children, including more skilled ones, regularly ran into problems (as was especially clear in the videos of children playing with tablets and smartphones) where they needed the parents to sort things out. Examples included when the children could not understand the written instructions because they could not read, when they accidently got lost and could not navigate back to the page they wanted, when an advert came up that they could not remove, when a password was needed, or when the children needed advice about where to touch the screen or how heavily to touch it. Hence, not only did parents in general often keep an eye on what the children were doing, as well as engage with them intermittently, but they were often actually summoned to help out.

Conclusion

There is always scope for additional qualitative studies to provide more insights into the material covered here, providing more examples, identifying more processes, perhaps finding more to say on the difficulties that parents can face when trying to manage their children's technologies. Meanwhile quantitative studies on these topics could provide a better sense of their prevalence: for example, how often and when parents use touchscreen technologies to occupy children (as opposed to times when children choose independently to use them). Nonetheless, even this small-scale study can help to sensitise us to certain issues.

Since much of the literature on young children is interested in processes supporting cognitive development – whether through play and creativity or literacy – one first contribution was to explore some of the diverse reasons for introducing children to touchscreen technologies, apart from educational ones. Often in domestication studies, ICTs find a variety of routes into people's lives and in this study it is clear that the case of young children is no exception. Sometimes it is not even the parent who initiates the process, but it was the younger children copying others. At other times, the parents are reacting to a situation. And while parents may think a particular app is good for the child, this is not only because of literacy considerations – for instance, it might help the child to get into routines.

Although previous studies mention parents occupying children with technologies, this has not previously been explored in any depth. Since domestication analysis does not have a particular developmental focus, it has a potentially equal interest in how parents manage the non-parental aspects of their lives, when they are not interacting with the child. This study shows how wider societal discourses about good parenting can also make them limit this occupying 'use' of the technology or make parents feel guilty about the practice. Meanwhile, the (unanticipated) use of technology to distract children is using it as part of solutions to ameliorate or work around problems separate from the cognitive development agenda.

The section on parents interacting around technology shares more common territory with many previous studies of young children. Some of the latter play down differences between the digital and non-digital domains of children's lives, noting how the children move between or combine them (e.g., Marsh et al., 2018). In the Toddlers and Tablets study there were examples of how parents' scaffolding of technology use is not so different from their interactions with children relating to non-technological experiences such as playing with things or looking at books. Indeed, conversations with children about touchscreens can turn into conversations about other topics. This provides a less techno-centric appreciation of what is happening.

As regards managing and monitoring children's use of the technology, the third section of this chapter explored how parents of young children are able to mediate technology use, reflecting the limited capabilities of young children and their routines. This section also reminds us (as was clear in Marsh et al.'s (2015) list of what children of different ages cannot do) that while touchscreen technologies may provide an easier interface to use than the PC's mouse and keyboard, it by no means follows that all barriers to young children's use disappeared.

Finally, the domestication approach more generally allows some reflection on the specific agency of both young children and their parents. Although this theme was not developed so much, the children obviously have agency in terms of what they want to do, what interests them, who and what they copy. But that agency is also present in the summoning of parental help and, in a different form, through children's problems that require parents to find solutions. Compared with the case of older children, there are various ways in which these parents clearly have considerable influence on when, how, and why children first experience touchscreen technologies and how their use by young children is subsequently mediated.

Notes

1 Although not a domestication study, research on young children that refers to the 'cultural ecology' of families captures the idea that we need to be attentive to this context (Plowman & Stevenson, 2013).
2 The different type of domestication analysis of younger and older children, using the Toddlers and Tablets finding as one case study, is explored more systematically in Haddon (2020).
3 For a more detailed examination of these scaffolding processes from the Toddlers and Tablets project, see Holloway et al. (2018).

References

Bar Lev, Y., Elias, N. & Levy, S. (2018). Development of infants' media habits in the age of digital parenting. In G. Mascheroni, C. Ponte & A. Jorge (Eds.), *Digital parenting: The challenges for families in the digital age* (pp. 103–112). Gothenburg: Nordicom.
Chaudron, S. (2015). *Young children (0–8) and digital technology: A qualitative exploratory study across seven countries*. Report EUR 29070. Ispra (VA), Italy: Joint Research Centre.
Danby, S., Davidson, C., Theobald, M., Schrive, B., Cobb-Moore, C., Houen, S. & Thorpe, K. (2013). Talking activity during young children's use of digital technologies at home. *Australian Journal of Communication*, 40(2), 83–99.
Haddon, L. (2016). Domestication and the media. In P. Rössler (Ed.), *The international encyclopedia about media effects, Vol.1* (pp. 409–417). London: John Wiley and Sons.
Haddon, L. (2018). Domestication and social constraints on ICT use: Children's engagement with smartphones. In J. Vincent & L. Haddon (Eds.), *Smartphone cultures* (pp. 71–82). Abingdon: Routledge.
Haddon, L. (2020). Domestication analyses and the smartphone. In R. Ling, L. Fortunati, G. Goggin, S.-S. Lim & Y. Li (Eds.), *Oxford handbook of mobile communication culture*. Oxford: Oxford University Press.
Haddon, L. & Holloway, D. (2018). Parental evaluations of young children's touchscreen technologies. In G. Mascheroni, C. Ponte & A. Jorge (Eds.), *Digital parenting: The challenges for families in the digital age* (pp. 113–123). Gothenburg: Nordicom.
Hirsch, E. (1992). The long term and the short term of domestic consumption: An ethnographic case study. In R. Silverstone & E. Hirsch (Eds.), *Consuming technologies: Media and information in domestic spaces* (pp. 208–226). London: Routledge.
Holloway, D., Green, L. & Livingstone, S. (2013). *Zero to eight: Young children and their internet use*. London: EU Kids Online.
Holloway, D., Haddon, L., Green, L. & Stevenson, K. (2018). The parent-child-app learning assemblage: Scaffolding early childhood learning through app use in the family home. In N. Kucirkova, J. Rowsell & G. Falloon (Eds.), *The Routledge international handbook of playing and learning with technology in early childhood* (pp. 210–218). Abingdon: Routledge.
Hourcade, J., Mascher, S., Wu, D. & Pantoja, L. (2015). "Look, my baby is using an iPad!" An analysis of YouTube videos of infants and toddlers using tablets. *Proceedings of CHI 15*. New York: ACM Press, pp. 1915–1924.
Lally, E. (2002). *At home with computers*. Oxford: Berg.
Lauricella, A., Wartella, E. & Rideout, V. (2015). Young children's screen time: The complex role of parent and child factors. *Journal of Applied Developmental Psychology*, 36, 11–17.

Livingstone, S., Marsh, J., Plowman, L., Ottovordemgentschenfelde, S. & Fletcher-Watson, B. (2014). *Young children (0–8) and digital technology: A qualitative exploratory study national report – UK*. Luxembourg: Joint Research Centre, European Commission. Retrieved from: http://eprints.lse.ac.uk/60799.

López-de-Ayala-López, M. & Haddon, L. (2018). *The parental mediation strategies of parents with young children*. London: Media@LSE Working Paper #50. Retrieved from: www.lse.ac.uk/media-and-communications/assets/documents/research/working-paper-series/WP50.pdf.

Marsh, J., Plowman, D., Yamada-Rice, J., Bishop, C., Lahmar, J. & Scott, F. (2018). Play and creativity in young children's use of apps. *British Journal of Educational Technology, 49*(5), 870–882.

Marsh, J., Plowman, L., Yamada-Rice, D., Bishop, J., Lahmar, J., Scott, F., ... Winter, P. (2015). *Exploring play and creativity in pre-schoolers' use of apps*. Final project report. Retrieved from: www.techandplay.org/reports/TAP_Final_Report.pdf.

Mascheroni, G. (2014). Parenting the mobile internet in Italian households: Parents' and children's discourses. *Journal of Children and Media, 8*(4), 440–456.

McClure, E., Chentsova-Dutton, Y., Barr, R., Holochwost, S. & Parrott, G. (2015). "Facetime doesn't count": Video chat as an exception to media restrictions for infants and toddlers. *International Journal of Child-Computer Interaction, 6*, 1–6.

McPake, J., Plowman, L. & Stephen, C. (2012). Pre-school children creating and communicating with digital technologies in the home. *British Journal of Educational Technology, 44*(3), 421–431.

Nansen, B. & Jayamene, D. (2016). Infants, interfaces, and intermediation: Digital parenting in the production of "iPad Baby" YouTube videos. *Journal of Broadcasting and Electronic Media, 60*(4), 587–603.

Neumann, M. (2018). Using tablets and apps to enhance emergent literacy skills in young children. *Early Childhood Research Quarterly, 42*, 239–246.

Neumann, M. & Neumann, D. (2014). Touch screen tablets and emergent literacy. *Early Childhood Education Journal, 42*, 231–239.

Neumann, M. M. (2014). An examination of touch screen tablets and emergent literacy in Australian pre-school children. *Australian Journal of Education, 58*(2), 109–122.

Neumann, M. M. & Neumann, D. L. (2016). An analysis of mother-child interactions during an iPad activity. In K. Alvarez (Ed.), *Parent-child interactions and relationships: Perceptions, practices, and developmental outcomes* (pp. 133–148). Hauppauge, NY: Nova Science Publishers Inc.

Neumann, M. M. & Neumann, D. L. (2017). The use of touch screen tablets at home and pre-school to foster emergent literacy. *Journal of Early Childhood Literacy, 17*(2), 203–220.

Nevski, E. & Siibak, A. (2016). The role of parents and parental mediation on 0–3-year olds' digital play with smart devices: Estonian parents' attitudes and practices. *Early Years: An International Journal, 36*, 227–241.

Pempeck, M. & McDaniel, B. (2016). Young children's tablet use and associations with maternal well-being. *Journal of Child and Family Studies, 25*, 2636–2647.

Plowman, L. (2015). Researching young children's everyday uses of technology in the family home. *Interacting with Computers, 27*(1), 36–46.

Plowman, L., McPake, J. & Stephen, C. (2008). Just picking it up? Young children learning with technology at home. *Cambridge Journal of Education, 38*(3), 303–319.

Plowman, L., McPake, J. & Stephen, C. (2010a). The technologisation of childhood? Young children and technology in the home. *Children & Society, 24*(1), 63–74.

Plowman, L., Stephen, C. & McPake, J. (2010b). Supporting young children's learning with technology at home and in preschool. *Research Papers in Education, 25*(1), 93–113.

Plowman, L., Stephen, C. & McPake, J. (2010c). *Growing up with technology. Young children learning in a digital world*. London: Routledge.

Plowman, L. & Stevenson, O. (2013). Exploring the quotidian in young children's lives at home. *Home Cultures, 10*(3), 329–347.

Rideout, V. (2011). *Zero to eight: Children's media use in America*. San Francisco, CA: Common Sense Media.

Rideout, V. (2013). Zero to eight: Children's media use in America 2013: A Common Sense Media research study. Retrieved from: www.commonsensemedia.org/research/zero-to-eight-childrensmedia-use-in-america-2013#.

Silverstone, R., Hirsch, E. & Morley, D. (1992). Information and communication technologies and the moral economy of the household. In R. Silverstone & E. Hirsch (Eds.), *Consuming technologies: Media and information in domestic spaces* (pp. 15–31). London: Routledge.

Stephen, C. & Edwards, S. (2018). *Young children playing and learning in a digital age*. London: Routledge.

Stephen, C., Stevenson, O. & Adey, C. (2013). Young children engaging with technologies at home: The influence of family context. *Journal of Early Childhood Research, 11*(2), 149–164.

Ward, K. (2005). Internet consumption in Ireland: Towards a "connected" life. In R. Silverstone (Ed.), *Media, technology and everyday life in Europe* (pp. 107–123). Aldershot: Ashgate.

9

GRANDPARENTAL MEDIATION OF CHILDREN'S DIGITAL MEDIA USE

Nelly Elias, Dafna Lemish, and Galit Nimrod

Introduction

Given the complex challenges families face today, one cannot overestimate the major role grandparents play in their grandchildren's lives. Recent surveys in various Western countries reveal that about half of grandparents look after at least one grandchild, typically at a frequency of once a week or more (Di Gessa, Glaser, & Tinker, 2015; Hank, Cavrini, Di Gessa, & Tomassini, 2018; Horsfall & Dempsey, 2015). Grandparental care often involves tending to their grandchildren's physical needs, driving them from one place to another, or helping them with their homework. No less important, however, is the role played by the grandparents in their grandchildren's leisure activities, such as going to the park, reading, baking, and using various media (Kornhaber, 1996; Share & Kerrins, 2009).

Recent research shows that watching television and playing digital games account for a large proportion of the time children spend under their grandparents' care (Dunifon, Near, & Ziol-Guest, 2018; Öztürk & Hazer, 2017). Yet, no studies prior to the authors' on-going research project have explored grandparents' mediation of their grandchildren's media uses, such as limiting the grandchild's screen time, selecting appropriate content, or using the digital devices together. This chapter, which is part of a larger project, aims to explore patterns of grandparental mediation of their grandchildren's digital media uses. By conducting a parallel exploration of both *non-interactive* (e.g., watching any kind of screen content) and *interactive* media uses (e.g., playing digital games, using software/applications, etc.) and focussing on grandparents of children aged two to seven years, who are especially in need of adult mediation, it fills a significant gap in the existing body of knowledge.

Literature Review

Mediation of Children's Media Use

Since nothing is known of grandparents' mediation role, this section will explore major parental mediation strategies that have been a topic of intensive academic inquiry for more than two decades. Valkenburg, Krcmar, Peeters, and Marseille (1999) outlined three key mediation strategies of television viewing that served as the basis for much of the research that followed:

'restrictive' mediation, 'instructive' (also known as active) mediation, and 'social co-viewing'. Parents who engage in restrictive mediation set rules for viewing or prohibit the viewing of certain content; instructive mediation refers to the parental discussion of certain aspects of programmes with children during or following the viewing; and co-viewing describes situations in which parents and children share the viewing experience without necessarily discussing it.

With the advance of the internet and the growing presence of interactive digital devices in children's lives, researchers have begun to suggest new mediation strategies. One pioneering study in this field by Livingstone and Helsper (2008) claims that internet use is highly different from television viewing and consequently demands the development of new parental mediation categories. Their findings point to a new strategy of 'active co-use' that contains a mixture of practices previously included in instructive mediation, restrictive mediation, and co-viewing, as well as to a 'monitoring' strategy that consists of checking children's online activities following computer use.

Other researchers, however, have found no confirmation for the active co-use mediation strategy and even argued that existing mediation strategies apply to television viewing and digital media alike. Indeed, four mediation strategies appeared as meaningful constructs in most of the recent studies on interactive media uses, three of which are similar to television viewing strategies: restrictive mediation, instructive/active mediation, and co-use. Furthermore, these studies suggest a new category of mediation, 'supervision', that includes parents' attempts to remain proximal to the child when they engage in media use and to keep an eye on the screen (Li & Shin, 2017; Nikken & Jansz, 2014; Nikken & Schols, 2015; Smahelova, Juhová, Cermak, & Smahel, 2017; Sonck, Nikken, & de Haan, 2013). This literature provided the grounding for exploring grandparents' mediation of their grandchildren's media use in the current study (Elias, Nimrod, & Lemish, 2019; Nimrod, Elias, & Lemish, 2019).

Grandparents' Use of Media with Their Grandchildren

Most of the studies on grandparents' media use with their grandchildren focus on technological affordances that allow remotely located grandparents to communicate across distances and not on shared media consumption of physically close grandchildren and grandparents. These studies found that pre-school children and their grandparents use Skype as their favourite platform to communicate and even to play physical games such as jumping and virtual hide and seek (Busch, 2018). In addition, collaborative web applications such as StoryVisit enable long-distance grandparents to engage in simultaneous book reading with their pre-school grandchildren, thus cultivating a sense of togetherness between them (Raffle et al., 2011). These video-chats allow the grandparents greater involvement in their grandchildren's lives and even improve the quality of in-person visits. Similarly, young children's formative relationships with distanced grandparents are often mediated by a screen (McClure, Chentsova-Dutton, Holochwost, Parrott, & Barr, 2017) and therefore grandchildren do not perceive their grandparents to be remote relatives (Forghani & Neustaedter, 2014; Lin & Harwood, 2003).

Another field of research that deals with the role of media in grandparent–grandchild relations focusses on teenage grandchildren's attempts to help their grandparents learn how to use new media devices. In this regard, the literature suggests that grandparents who wish to communicate with their grandchildren through various online platforms and devices are more satisfied when learning to use technology (Hunt, 2012). Moreover, grandparents report a newly acquired sense of empowerment and self-competence in surfing the internet due to knowledge exchange with primary school grandchildren (Gamliel & Gabay, 2014). Interestingly, grandparents' potential to improve their grandchildren's digital skills was never the subject of academic inquiry despite children's possible need for adult assistance.

Finally, only a few studies examined (in a very partial manner) how grandparents and grandchildren use media together. Smith (2005) has revealed that as grandchildren get older, grandparents typically shift their childrearing practices from participating in outdoor activities, such as going to the playground, to engaging in indoor activities, such as watching television. Moreover, Öztürk and Hazer (2017) found that shared television viewing was the most common activity between grandchildren and their grandparents, even identifying this as a key feature of a strong grandparent–grandchild relationship.

No less important is the issue of young children's media consumption under their grandparents' watch. In this regard, the authors found that young children aged two to seven tended to use various media for extensive periods of time while being watched by their grandparents. Namely, the grandchildren's screen time reached nearly two hours per average 'caregiving event' and accounted for almost half the total time the grandchildren and grandparents spent together (Elias et al., 2019). Given the children's very young age and the high amount of media exposure, these findings emphasise the importance of grandparental mediation and how it is applied to various media uses. Accordingly, this chapter aims to fill this gap in knowledge by answering the following research questions:

1   What is the level of grandparents' familiarity with the different media that their grandchildren use?
2   What are the grandparents' attitudes towards their grandchildren's media uses?
3   To what extent do grandparents mediate their grandchildren's media uses?
4   And how do their current mediation practices, when applied towards their grandchildren, compare with the way they mediated the use of media with their own children in the past?

It is worth noting that the social context in which this study has taken place provides a fruitful ground for conducting such an investigation. First, Israeli society is characterised by a strong family-oriented culture. Geographical distances are short, and many extended families live in proximity to each other. Second, the vast majority of children participate in mandatory schooling – pre-schools, kindergartens, and elementary schools. However, the school day is short (commonly 8:00–14:00), with very expensive day-care offerings beyond these restricted hours. As a result, many families rely on alternative childcare support, especially the voluntary help of grandparents. Finally, Israeli families are characterised by a high penetration of mobile digital devices and online viewing platforms (especially YouTube), which are available to young children as well (Elias & Sulkin, 2017).

Methods

Data from two complementary studies – a quantitative survey and qualitative interviews – were used to answer the above questions. The first study was based on an online survey of 356 Israeli grandparents of young children aged two to seven years who reported taking care of their grandchildren at least once a week. They were recruited by a commercial firm that operates an online panel of 50,000 internet users, who were randomly sampled from panellists aged 50 and over and then contacted via email with a link to the survey. Among other questions (measures detailed below), study participants were asked whether their grandchildren typically used various media when they took care of them, and if so, how much time they usually spent using each type of media. Only grandparents who reported the use of interactive digital media, defined as "playing computer games, using software or applications, visiting websites for purposes other than watching videos, and so forth", were included in the current analysis.

The sub-sample size was 213. Participants' ages ranged from 50 to 80, with a mean of 62.9 years (SD = 6); 66.7% were women, and 54.5% had an academic degree. Half the participants reported having a higher than average income and 19.7% lower than average; 46% were retirees and 32.4% worked full-time. A majority of participants (88%) took care of their grandchildren between one to three times a week, and the rest more frequently. The average 'caregiving event' lasted four hours. All survey participants reported that their grandchildren were engaged with non-interactive and interactive media use when they were watching them, with an average of 87 minutes of viewing (SD = 68) and 69 minutes of digital media use (SD = 61).

The second study was based on a series of in-depth interviews with 23 dyads (46 interviews) of mothers and grandmothers of children aged two to seven years. Participants were recruited via snowballing involving the participation of trained students, each recruiting and completing one set of dyad interviews. The interviews with both women were conducted separately, lasted about one and a half hours, and focussed on parental and grandparental mediation practices applied towards television viewing and digital media use. For this chapter, only those grandmothers who reported that their grandchildren use digital media when they take care of them were selected, i.e., 16 out of the 23 grandmothers. Their socio-demographic characteristics strongly resembled those of the survey participants, as a majority were educated women belonging to the middle and upper-middle classes.

Results

RQ1: How Familiar are Grandparents with Children's Media?

The grandparents who participated in the survey were asked to assess how familiar they were with four types of media common among children on a five-point Likert scale ranging from one ('not familiar at all') to five ('very familiar'). While 58% declared that they were sufficiently familiar ('quite familiar' and 'very familiar') with children's television programmes and 54.5% were sufficiently familiar with online viewing platforms popular among children, only 44% reported familiarity with educational software and 38.5% with digital games. Hence, a significant group of grandparents (about half of the sample) was not sufficiently familiar with children's chosen media, especially with digital games and apps.

Likewise, with means ranging between 3.15 and 3.62, results indicated an overall average familiarity with the various media (see Figure 9.1). Yet, the results also showed that the grandparents' self-rated familiarity with children's TV programmes and online viewing platforms was significantly higher ($p < .001$) than their self-perceived knowledge of digital games and educational software, websites and applications.

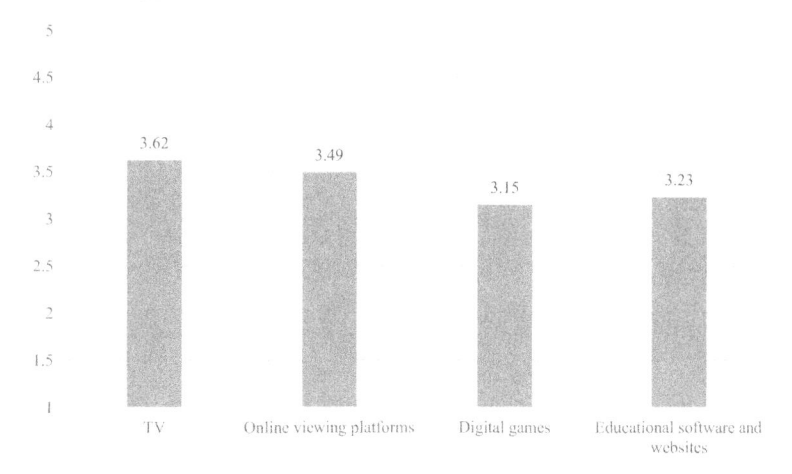

Figure 9.1 Familiarity with children's media: mean scores.

The qualitative interviews suggested that grandparents' lower familiarity with interactive media may be explained by their relatively poor digital literacy. For example, Sandra (79 years old, middle class, high-school education) confessed:

> I have to admit, my husband and I don't ... we weren't born to these things, to this generation. It is so complicated sometimes, all these devices, it's ... if her [granddaughter's] brothers or parents are with us, they help her if she needs help. I don't have any idea what to do with it, my husband a bit more, but not a lot either.

This lack of confidence was expressed by older and younger grandparents, as well as by persons with various socio-economic backgrounds. Dvora, for example (59 years old, upper-middle class, academic education), said in reference to her seven-year-old grandson: "he has a very high level of technological literacy, he often teaches me how to use the computer and to surf the internet ... My technological skills are deficient". Unlike Sandra, however, she felt she could also help when her grandson needed assistance with operating digital devices.

RQ2: What Do Grandparents Think about Children's Media?

The survey participants were also asked to report their opinion about the impact that each type of media use has on child development on a five-point Likert scale ranging from one ('very harmful') to five ('very beneficial'). Results indicated significant differences in their perception of the various media (Figure 9.2): whereas their appreciation of TV and online viewing platforms was similar, they ranked digital games as significantly more beneficial to child development than the viewing of screens ($p < .01$). Moreover, their appreciation of educational software, websites, and apps was significantly higher than that of digital games ($p < .001$).

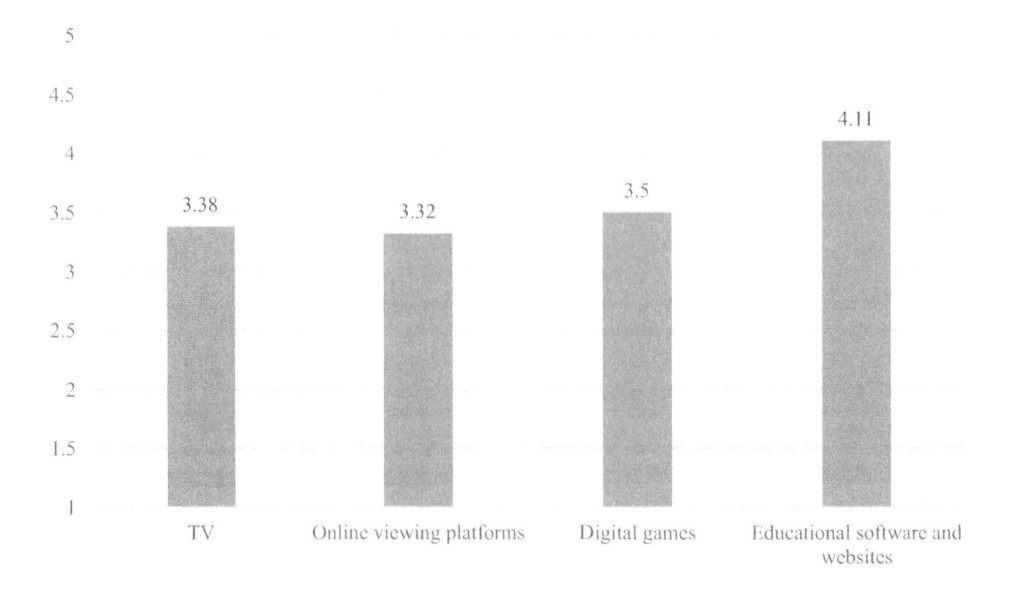

Figure 9.2 Attitudes toward children's media: mean scores.

Additional analysis indicated significant positive associations (1.70 < Pearson correlations < 2.62, p < .05) between grandparents' familiarity with children's media and their appreciation of that media. Hence, the more that grandparents felt they were familiar with a certain medium, the more they valued it. The only exception was educational software, websites, and apps that were highly valued regardless of grandparents' familiarity with those media.

The link between the perceived educational value of a certain medium or content and its appreciation was also well-reflected in the qualitative interviews. Generally, the grandparents expressed a desire that their grandchildren would spend less time using media. Specifically, they were critical of a perceived over-use of smartphones that are difficult to control in terms of access, and age-inappropriate content, as well as certain TV content that was described by Ronit (62 years old, upper-middle class, academic education) as "shallow, very popular" and as having an overwhelming pace that "trains children's mind to move too quickly from one thing to the other". Michal (64 years old, middle class, high school education) even described TV content as having "no filters – lots of negativity, lots of violence, lots of nonsense, all this reality TV, it is so useless, really, so void of all content".

Simultaneously, however, the grandparents highly valued TV content that they perceived to have educational value (e.g., National Geographic programmes) and a positive impact on children's language skills: "here is a three-year-old boy already singing the [English] ABCD ... He may not understand the meaning, but slowly, as he grows up, we will explain to him and he will have the beginning of another language", shared Rivka (63 years old, middle class, academic education).

In contrast to their ambivalent attitude toward TV content, some grandparents were highly supportive of digital media, especially if it was perceived as having educational value, as can be seen in the following examples:

> I think children today accumulate a lot of knowledge through these devices. They can search for information about everything, with no problem at all. Everything is accessible to them ... they don't need to go to encyclopedias – they can search their devices and know everything. It provides lots of information, enriches their lives.
>
> *(Sandra)*

> One can make fantastic use of the tablet. I can see that here, they work with tablets for special education needs, which is amazing. There are things that you can make very good use of it, very educational.
>
> *(Michal)*

RQ3: How Do Grandparents Mediate Their Grandchildren's Media Use?

A scale developed and validated by the authors was used to assess the survey participants' involvement in mediation. This 16-item scale includes two subscales: one for interactive and one for non-interactive media use. Each subscale refers to four mediation strategies (restrictive mediation, instructive mediation, supervision, and co-use), with two items per construct. Sample items include: "specify when and for how long your grandchild can watch films, videos and TV programs" and "Talk with your grandchild about something specific s/he does with digital media". Respondents were asked to rate the frequency with which they were involved in the various mediating actions when they took care of their grandchildren on a five-point Likert scale ranging from one ('never') to five ('always'). The same procedure was applied to non-interactive as well as interactive media use (see Nimrod et al., 2019 for the full scale).

The analysis demonstrated almost similar patterns of mediation for non-interactive and interactive use (Table 9.1). In both types of media use, the most salient mediation was 'supervision', followed by 'restrictive' and 'instructive' mediation, with 'co-use' of digital media being the least common. The difference between each pair of means in each column was significant ($p < 0.01$), with one exception: the reported involvement in 'restrictive' and 'instructive' mediation of non-interactive use was similar.

Overall, participants took a significant interest in the mediation of their grandchildren's media use, but the total score for mediation of non-interactive use was somewhat higher than that for

Table 9.1 Grandparental mediation.

	Non-interactive use		Interactive use	
	Mean	(SD)	Mean	(SD)
Restrictive	3.63	(1.16)	3.53	(1.29)
Instructive	3.56	(1.03)	3.32	(1.02)
Supervision	4.08	(0.82)	3.96	(1.03)
Co-use	3.14	(0.91)	2.92	(1.10)
Mediation index	14.36	(2.96)	13.35	(3.72)

Note: The mediation index for each participant was calculated by summing up the four construct means.

interactive use (14.36 versus 13.35, respectively). The paired-samples T-tests conducted for participants who reported both types of media use showed that this difference was significant ($p < 0.01$) not only for the total score but also for each type of mediation. The one exception was 'restrictive' mediation, where the scores did not significantly vary between non-interactive and interactive use.

These differences can also be illustrated through comparisons between frequencies of two particular mediation practices, which were more frequently applied towards non-interactive media. Thus, 72.2% of participants declared that they often or quite often ask questions (e.g., 'supervision' mediation strategy) when grandchildren consume non-interactive media content, compared with 49% who do so with regard to interactive media. Likewise, only 34.8% join their grandchildren (often or quite often) when they use interactive media, compared with 56% who do so regarding screen viewing.

Similarly, many grandparents reported in the interviews that they regularly keep an eye on what their grandchildren are doing, thus reinforcing the dominance of the supervision mediation strategy. "He uses the tablet on high volume, so I know what he is watching" (Dvora); "I look at what she is watching" (Ronit); "The TV is on volume so I hear the series that he is watching and I am also always around, sometimes doing some errands next to him so I can see" (Rivka). In contrast, watching television with grandchildren was much less common, and playing digital games and apps alongside grandchildren even less so. The minority of interviewees who did make an effort to use media with their grandchildren reported a sense of involvement in their grandchildren's world, which helped the two generations to feel closer to each other, as described by Dvora:

> When I take care of my grandchildren I stay close to them while they are watching television. It is important for me to be with them. It is important for me to watch with them the series that they like so they can include me in the content of their world, so they will feel that I am interested, that I am involved.

Interestingly, the application of 'restrictive' mediation typically resulted from rules set by the grandchildren's parents. Some grandparents, however, refused to follow the parents' instructions in order to achieve the grandchildren's cooperation in a more peaceful way. Ronit, for example, explained:

> we don't keep the rules they have at home ... we just go with the flow. If there is a tense atmosphere in the room then there is the iPhone, the tablet. If things are more relaxed then there is playing in the room.

Similarly, Meirav (78 years old, academic education, middle class) testified:

> I have learned that since they don't obey by the rules anyway, I don't forbid and I don't try to educate them ... There is a separation between Grandma and Mom. As a mother, I had rules. As a grandmother, I am here to spoil.

RQ4: Are Grandparents' Current Mediation Practices Associated with Their Habits as Parents in the Past?

Survey participants were asked to think about the time when their children were about the same age as their grandchildren, and to evaluate their then-involvement in the four mediation practices. In this case, no distinction was made between non-interactive and interactive media uses, and respondents were asked to relate to TV and computers alike. Results (see Figure 9.3) indicated that, like today, the application of 'supervision' in the past was significantly higher than that of all other mediation strategies ($p < 0.05$). However, no significant differences were found among the latter three strategies.

Moreover, the analysis indicated strong positive associations between grandparents' reports of parental mediation in the past and their grandparental mediation in the present of both non-interactive and interactive media use (Table 9.2). Hence, individuals who reported high

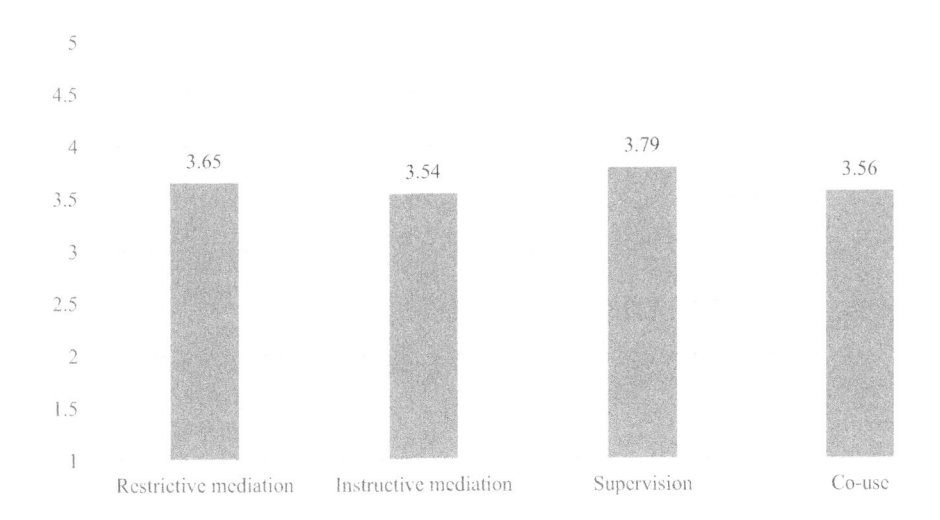

Figure 9.3 Involvement in mediation in the past (as parents): mean scores.

- Restrictive mediation: 3.65
- Instructive mediation: 3.54
- Supervision: 3.79
- Co-use: 3.56

involvement in a certain type of mediation as parents were also inclined to report the application of this practice in mediating their grandchildren's media use.

It is important to consider the possibility that grandparents were projecting their current attitudes back to their early years of parenting. However, the interviews demonstrated that they were also able to distinguish between the two. For example, Rachel (65 years old, middle class, high-

Table 9.2 Pearson's correlations between past and current involvement in mediation.

Mediation type		Correlation of past involvement with the current mediation of…	
		Non-interactive use	Interactive use
Restrictive	Pearson	.494★★	.548★★
	N	193	188
Instructive	Pearson	.455★★	.453★★
	N	198	195
Supervision	Pearson	.395★★	.462★★
	N	194	191
Co-use	Pearson	.336★★	.236★
	N	194	200

Notes: ★p < 0.01. ★★p < 0.001.

school education) thought that her daughter was "too tough" with her children: "I didn't limit my own children … [but] I apply the rules [the daughter sets]. I don't necessarily agree with them always, but respect them. I am not going to violate her education and the agreements they have".

In addition, some grandparents argued that more mediation is necessary nowadays, because of the much richer environment of media devices and contents, as expressed by Michal: "I think there wasn't much of a need to restrict media use in the past. It wasn't an issue. See, the world has changed". Similarly, Ronit explained:

> When our children were young there were only two hours of [television] broadcast a day, so there wasn't much to deal with. Today it is so accessible and on such high intensity, such high levels of stimuli and content, that there is a need to mark and sort and make decisions about what to see and what not to see … It is the role of the parents to create boundaries, and it is not an easy role.

Conclusion

This pioneering study, which combined quantitative and qualitative methods, investigated grandparental involvement in their grandchildren's use of various media. The findings suggest that grandparents apply a complex set of knowledge, attitudes, and behaviours to grandchildren's media use while caring for them.

First, the findings point to a clear distinction between non-interactive and interactive media use common among children. Whereas many grandparents reported considerable familiarity with TV programmes and online viewing platforms for children, they were less familiar with the digital world available to children today in the form of games, software, and apps, and admitted to lacking the level of digital literacy necessary to help their grandchildren. Accordingly, their lower familiarity with interactive media may be related to their relatively poor digital literacy. In addition, as the use of such media is typically solitary, their low familiarity with interactive media may be explained by the fact that grandparents and grandchildren are rarely able to use such media together. This explanation is supported by the finding which indicates that 'co-use' of digital media is the least common mediation strategy among grandparents.

This finding is important given the fact that grandchildren spend a significant amount of time using digital devices under their grandparents' watch, which could preclude the two generations from spending time on shared activities. On the other hand, those interviewees who made the effort to share the media preferences of their grandchildren felt a sense of closeness and better understanding, which is very important for maintaining close ties with their grandchildren as they grow.

The distinction between non-interactive and interactive media was also reflected in grandparents' attitudes toward children's media. Generally, grandparents tended to place more value on the media they knew better. However, they seemed to hold mixed views about the benefits and risks that media use has for their grandchildren. On one hand, they appreciated the accessibility of information and the enrichment potential provided mainly by digital media and educational programming. On the other hand, they expressed concerns over exposure to inappropriate and/or shallow content, over-stimulation, and too much time spent with smartphones.

When asked about their strategies for mediating their grandchildren's media use, grandparents offered diverse approaches, ranging from trying to implement instructions and rules specified by their grandchildren's parents to not intervening at all, perceiving that their main role was to 'spoil' their grandchildren rather than educate them. Supervising children's media activities (e.g., keeping an eye on what they are doing while remaining in close proximity) was the most common mediation strategy they felt comfortable in executing. Although this tendency was reflected in both the qualitative and the quantitative data, the survey findings also highlighted a more intense involvement in the mediation of non-interactive media use compared with interactive use. This finding suggests consistency between attitudes and behaviour: similar to parents (Nikken & Schols, 2015; Valkenburg et al., 1999), grandparents less frequently mediate media use that they perceive contributes to child development. Moreover, 'keeping an eye' on children while doing other things is more easily implemented than actually spending time with the grandchildren, which demands a greater obligation and more spare time.

Finally, in spite of strong positive correlations between grandparents' reports of parental mediation in the past, and their grandparental mediation of both non-interactive and interactive media in the present, grandparents argued that there was much less need to intervene in the past due to fewer television offerings and no digital devices. Overwhelmed by the current rich media environment and holding ambivalent attitudes about its potential impact on child development, they thought that children's media use should be mediated but were reluctant to take this role – especially regarding its restrictive component – considering this to be the parents' responsibility. These findings call for closer attention to the intergenerational dynamics of mediating children's media uses, which seem to be shaped by both parents' and grandparents' worldviews and values together.

The present study confirms that overseeing grandchildren's media use is an integral and important aspect of grandparenting activities and is a source of concern for many grandparents. Moreover, for the first time, it exposes the complex challenges that grandparents currently confront when taking care of their grandchildren. While the generational gap of familiarity with digital technology plays an important role in explaining the results, the perception of the nature of the role of grandparenting also influences how the study participants approach the topic.

Although the grandparents in this study were mostly middle and upper-middle class, and well-educated seniors, which might limit the generalisability of the findings, the study adds weight to the possibility that an age-related digital divide exists, even among highly educated older adults. The next phase of this on-going project explores more diverse populations in a cross-cultural framework, as well as a host of additional related aspects of grandparenting and children's media use. Clearly, mediating young children's media use by all caregivers – be they parents, grandparents, or educators – poses a comprehensive challenge across all the media environments children currently occupy.

Acknowledgements

This work was supported by Ageing + Communication + Technologies (ACT), a research project funded by the Social Sciences and Humanities Research Council of Canada and housed at Concordia University in Montreal, Canada. All authors contributed equally to this chapter.

References

Busch, G. (2018). How families use communication technologies during intergenerational skype sessions. In S. J. Danby, M. Fleer, C. Davidson, & M. Hatzigianni (Eds.), *Digital childhoods: Technologies and children's everyday lives* (pp. 17–32). Singapore: Springer.

Di Gessa, G., Glaser, K., & Tinker, A. (2015). The health impact of intensive and nonintensive grandchild care in Europe: New evidence from SHARE. *Journals of Gerontology Series B: Psychological Sciences and Social Sciences, 71*(5), 867–879.

Dunifon, R. E., Near, C. E., & Ziol-Guest, K. M. (2018). Backup parents, playmates, friends: Grandparents' time with grandchildren. *Journal of Marriage and Family, 80*(3), 752–767.

Elias, N., Nimrod, G., & Lemish, D. (2019). The ultimate treat? Young children's media use under their grandparents' care. *Journal of Children and Media*, 1–12. 10.1080/17482798.2019.1627228.

Elias, N., & Sulkin, I. (2017). YouTube viewers in diapers: How toddlers' online viewing is related to child and parents' characteristics, parental perceptions, mediation styles and parenting media practices. *Cyberpsychology: Journal of Psychosocial Research on Cyberspace, 11*(3). doi:10.5817/CP2017-3-2. Retrieved from: https://cyberpsychology.eu/article/view/8559/7739.

Forghani, A., & Neustaedter, C. (2014). *The routines and needs of grandparents and parents for grandparent-grandchild conversations over distance*. Paper presented at CHI conference, Toronto, Canada, 26 April–1 May 2014. Retrieved from: http://clab.iat.sfu.ca/pubs/Forghani-Grandparents-CHI.pdf.

Gamliel, T., & Gabay, N. (2014). Knowledge exchange, social interactions and empowerment in an intergenerational technology program at school. *Educational Gerontology, 40*(8), 597–617.

Hank, K., Cavrini, G., Di Gessa, G., & Tomassini, C. (2018). What do we know about grandparents? Insights from current quantitative data and identification of future data needs. *European Journal of Ageing, 15*(3), 225–235. doi:10.1080/03601277.2013.863097.

Horsfall, B., & Dempsey, D. (2015). Grandparents doing gender: Experiences of grandmothers and grandfathers caring for grandchildren in Australia. *Journal of Sociology, 51*(4), 1070–1084.

Hunt, D. S. (2012). *Technology and the grandparent-grandchild relationship: Learning and interaction* (Master's Thesis). University of Toledo, Toledo, OH. Retrieved from: https://pdfs.semanticscholar.org/3311/160be7f5a862cf9ad763f313d7c96253421f.pdf.

Kornhaber, A. (1996). *Contemporary grandparenting*. Thousand Oaks, CA: Sage.

Li, B., & Shin, W. (2017). Parental mediation of children's digital technology use in Singapore. *Journal of Children and Media, 11*(1), 1–19.

Lin, M. C., & Harwood, J. (2003). Accommodation predictors of grandparent-grandchild relational solidarity in Taiwan. *Journal of Social and Personal Relationships, 20*(4), 537–563.

Livingstone, S., & Helsper, E. J. (2008). Parental mediation of children's Internet use. *Journal of Broadcasting & Electronic Media, 52*(4), 581–599.

McClure, E. R., Chentsova-Dutton, Y. E., Holochwost, S. J., Parrott, W. G., & Barr, R. (2017). Look at that! Video chat and joint visual attention development among babies and toddlers. *Child Development, 89*(1), 27–36.

Nikken, P., & Jansz, J. (2014). Developing scales to measure parental mediation of young children's internet use. *Learning, Media, and Technology, 39*(2), 250–266.

Nikken, P., & Schols, M. (2015). How and why parents guide the media use of young children. *Journal of Child and Family Studies, 24*(11), 3423–3435.

Nimrod, G., Elias, N., & Lemish, D. (2019). Measuring mediation of children's media use. *International Journal of Communication, 13*(2019), 342–358.

Öztürk, M. S., & Hazer, O. (2017). The intergenerational activities: Perspectives of young grandchildren. *Dumlupinar Universitesi Sosyal Bilimler Dergisi, 53*, 55–71.

Raffle, H., Revelle, G., Mori, K., Ballagas, R., Buza, K., Horii, H., ... Spasojevic, M. (2011). *"Hello, is grandma there? Let's read!" StoryVisit: Family video chat and connected e-books.* Paper presented at CHI 2011 conference, Vancouver, Canada, 7–12 May 2011. Retrieved from: www.nataliefreed.com/wp-content/uploads/2012/01/p1195-raffle.pdf.

Share, M., & Kerrins, L. (2009). The role of grandparents in childcare in Ireland: Towards a research agenda. *Irish Journal of Applied Social Studies, 9*(1), 33–47.

Smahelova, M., Juhová, D., Cermak, I., & Smahel, D. (2017). Mediation of young children's digital technology use: The parents' perspective. *Cyberpsychology: Journal of Psychosocial Research on Cyberspace, 11*(3). Retrieved from: https://cyberpsychology.eu/article/view/8561.

Smith, P. K. (2005). Grandparents & grandchildren. *The Psychologist, 18*, 684–687.

Sonck, N., Nikken, P., & de Haan, J. (2013). Determinants of internet mediation: A comparison of the reports by parents and children. *Journal of Children and Media, 7*(1), 96–113.

Valkenburg, P. M., Krcmar, M., Peeters, A. L., & Marseille, N. M. (1999). Developing a scale to assess three styles of television mediation: "Instructive mediation," "restrictive mediation," and "social coviewing." *Journal of Broadcasting & Electronic Media, 43*(1), 52–66.

PART II

Digital Media Lives

10
YOUNG CHILDREN'S HAPTIC MEDIA HABITUS

Bjørn Nansen

Introduction

Young children's contemporary engagements with digital media are embodied relations shaped with and through the interfaces, materiality, and mobility of haptic media technologies. This chapter explores these embodied dimensions of young children's digital media use, drawing on research from ethnographic observation in family homes, and from analysis of user interface and mobile app developer literature, and in particular the 'Event Handling Guide for iOS', which encodes touchscreen interaction through the design constraints and possibilities of gesture input techniques. Connecting this research and analysis with phenomenologically informed cultural theory, particularly as it relates to research on mobile technologies, haptics, and everyday life, this chapter describes the emergence of what could be described as a *haptic habitus*. That is, the cultivation of young children's embodied dispositions, conduct, and competence towards haptic media.

As explored below, children's haptic habitus can be seen to take shape through the media environments they inhabit, and the processes by which they habituate to mobile touchscreen interfaces. These are situated within the materialities of domestic media spaces and family life. Within these contemporary habitats, children are both interfacing with and habituating to mobile devices (tablets and smartphones) in ways that appear to diverge from, but also resonate with residual media's directed modes of interaction. These are explored through themes of encounter, enculturation, and embodiment of haptic and mobile media. Yet, this research also reveals how children's haptic habitus is configured – enabled and constrained – by the commercial and design operations of mobile media, in which relays between cultural contexts of use, user interface studies of children's developmental capacities for gestural interaction, and the modulation of touchscreen gestures by technology companies can be seen.

Researching Children and Haptic Interfaces

There is relatively little research on young children's everyday play with or use of digital media, which is in one sense unsurprising given young children's historically limited engagement with, or capacity to use, older desktop devices and their associated interfaces. However, developments in haptic media through touchscreen interfaces and their widespread adoption following Apple's launch of the iPhone and later iPad in the 2000s have challenged these historical conditions, making digital media accessible to wider demographics of users, including young children. These conditions have prompted emerging strands of research into young children's haptic media play, including research from the social sciences working on media and communications to quantify the devices, activities, and time spent by young children with mobile and touchscreen devices (e.g., OfCom, 2013; Rideout, 2013), including some preliminary research trying to understand some of the qualities of these playful and embodied relations (Marsh et al., 2018; Nansen & Jayemanne, 2016; Nevski & Siibak, 2016).

Alongside this social and cultural research is a growing body of more political-economy-inflected research that seeks to critically understand the design and marketing of children's mobile devices, applications, and software products (Burroughs, 2017; Chiong & Shuler, 2010; Shuler, 2009). At the same time, researchers working in interaction design and user experience design (UX) are exploring young children's gestural capacities to interact with touchscreen interfaces (Buckleitner, 2011; Hourcade et al., 2015) in order to inform user interface (UI) developments for child-friendly mobile software applications. Here, the term 'Minimum User Competency' (MUC) has been coined to characterise the lowering of usability thresholds to ever-younger populations of users for gestural and touchscreen interfaces – down to approximately 12 months of age, from the previous two-and-a-half years for keyboard and mouse interfaces.

These strands of research provide some insights into the cultural and economic contexts of young children's mobile and touchscreen media use. Yet, there is scope for more situated and theoretically informed research, exploring how technologies and bodies intersect in the formation of young children's media practices. Drawing on published research from the author (Nansen & Jayemanne, 2018; Nansen & Wilken, 2019), this chapter focusses on these intersections and entanglements by applying insights drawn from phenomenologically informed cultural theory in the contexts of media studies approaches that seek to understand everyday media use. This analysis helps to reveal how mobile technologies, haptic interfaces, and media dispositions are operationalised within young children's contemporary digital cultures.

The Phenomenology of Haptic Media

Understood as the acquisition and embodiment of dispositions or forms of conduct, the concept of habitus has been developed across anthropological and sociological literature to address the relations that emerge between bodies and technologies in everyday life (Bourdieu, 1977; Mauss, 1973). Marcel Mauss, for example, located habitus at the intersection of bodily practices, object designs, and cultures of use, noting how particular forms of movement, from walking, swimming, sitting, and digging, were entrained and organised over time within specific cultural contexts through forms of repetition, interaction, and imitation. Pierre Bourdieu's social analysis understood habitus less in terms of micro analysis of bodily movements, but still as a significant element at the intersection of culture and embodiment, in which dispositions are culturally shared and shaped through class-based activities and experiences. Phenomenology, with its focus on the body's place, performance, and expression of material culture, has productively contributed to this concept of habitus and its intersection with media technology. From this work, body techniques have come to be understood as "culturally and contextually specific – taught, learnt, and dynamically evolving" (Richardson & Wilken, 2009, p. 24). In phenomenological terms, the way in which body–technology relations become part of our habitus, our "corporeal schema" (Richardson, 2012, p. 135), "expresses the power we have of dilating our being in the world, or of altering our existence through incorporating new instruments" (Merleau-Ponty, 2012, p. 145). For Merleau-Ponty, whose focus was on analogue technologies, habitus was not simply an involuntary or rigid pattern of behaviour, but, rather, an empowering relationship between bodies and artefacts that expressed capacities to adopt and adapt to technologies, to embody them in order to act in the world. Merleau-Ponty identified multiple layers of habitus, which incorporated physical bodies, repeated use, learnt movements, and cultures of use. So, for example, the typing body habituated to keyboard use when the corporeal schema was distributed in the fingers, performed through their dexterity, and learnt through cultural norms, such as touch-typing (2012, p. 145).

Such reflections have been taken up by more recent variants of phenomenology, such as 'post-phenomenology', which seeks to understand the situated negotiations and multi-stable qualities of human–technology relations. Here, the influential work of Don Ihde (1990, 1993), which understands embodied relations as one type of interrelation form – alongside alterity, hermeneutic, background – has provided a productive lens for considering various technologies and their embodied dimensions, including mobile media and haptic interfaces (Wellner, 2016). This, in turn, connects to a broader 'material turn' in media and communication studies, especially the study of mobile and touch-based interfaces (Mowlabocus, 2016; Parisi et al., 2017; Richardson & Hjorth, 2017), which orient us to the histories, senses, and experiences of contemporary haptic media. One trajectory of analysis and theorising of such forms of habitus is labelled 'cultural phenomenology' (Connor, 2000; Csordas, 1999; Richardson & Third, 2009). Cultural phenomenology "resituates embodiment and materiality within sociocultural contexts" by turning our attention to "the body–technology relations that emerge from particular cultural milieu and collective habits" (Richardson & Wilken, 2017, pp. 120−1). In bringing together both phenomenological and cultural studies traditions, this approach has been deployed to "critically account for the perceptual and sensory dimensions of everyday material culture" (Richardson & Third, 2009, p. 49), including the hapticity and embodiment of mobile devices (Richardson, 2012; Richardson & Wilken, 2017). Such phenomenological reflections have also been taken up within the contexts of human–computer interaction (HCI) research, documenting how appropriating gestural interfaces requires levels of physical ability, learned and controlled bodily movements as input, and situated meanings of use (e.g., Loke & Robertson, 2011; Nansen et al., 2014).

Clearly, phenomenologically informed cultural theory around habitus and body–technology relations forms a productive way of understanding young children's encounters, enculturation, and embodiment of touchscreen media. This orientation towards habitus as both mediated by technologies and embedded in culture contexts is valuable in turning our attention to everyday media practices and their situated contexts. More specifically, it highlights the importance of attending to the specificity of haptic interfaces, the conduct of young bodies, the ecologies of media spaces (both mobile and residual), the cultural practices surrounding and shaping these activities, and the wider communities of interest accommodating, representing, designing, or commodifying these relations.

In order to explore the haptic habitus of young children, this chapter draws on qualitative research and ethnographic observation of young children's mobile media practices in family homes conducted with children aged from birth to 5 years old ($n = 41$) in their domestic media settings in Melbourne, Australia, during 2016–2017; and analysis of UI and mobile app developer literature, and in particular the 'Event Handling Guide for iOS', which encodes touchscreen interaction through the design constraints and possibilities of gesture input techniques. Combining these theoretical and empirical lines of inquiry, this chapter explores the cultivation of young children's embodied dispositions for touchscreen conduct and competence – their *haptic habitus*. The following analysis is structured around the relational processes of *encounter, enculturation,* and *embodiment*. These are situated within the materialities of domestic haptic media spaces and family relations in which haptic media use unfolds. The analysis is also concerned with how, in turn, these spaces and practices are enfolded into wider communities of design, development, and commercialisation, in which relays can be seen between cultural contexts of use, user interface studies of children's developmental capacities for gestural interaction, and the modulation of touchscreen gestural events by children's app developers.

Cultivating Young Children's Haptic Media Habitus

It is now commonplace for young children to inhabit household media environments characterised by dense ecologies of digital media, including wi-fi infrastructures, the presence of multiple and mobile touchscreen devices, along with residual media technologies such as televisions and desktop computers. The domestication of and dwelling within these contemporary media habitats facilitates young children's *encounters* with media technologies: *We've got an iPad, which just floats around anywhere.*[1] In particular, the mobility of tablet computers and mobile phones, no longer located in a fixed place but circulating around the home through routines of use and disuse, has prompted children's early and regular encounters: *They just kind of picked up the things that were laying around.*

Haptic media, then, come to inhabit homes in ways that become readily available but also appealing for young children through the affordances of the interface responding to touch with screens lighting up, and gestural movements activating applications: *He notices when the lights, the bright light. A little bit, little bit moth to a flame, you know.* These routinised encounters with touchscreen devices habituate young children to the availability and interactivity of haptic media. These media habitats and touchscreen encounters were not purely an outcome of spatial arrangements and mobilities of haptic media, but also are culturally encoded or *encultured* in the ways parents make available, model behaviour, and mediate their children's media interactions. For example, young children observed their parents embodied, distracted, or intimate relations with their phones and tablets (see Mowlabocus, 2016): *I, I suppose indirectly he's fascinated ... he notices when our attention is drawn by it.* Through these observations, children become enculturated into understanding the cultural value of mobile screens in contemporary life, and they embody such values through imitation: *The other day he found ... he got his mum's phone and starting going, "Lala-lala", talking.*

In addition to such indirect forms of habituation, parents identified more deliberate practices of providing children with mobile devices, so-called "passing-back" (Chiong & Shuler, 2010), in order to 'pacify' them in situations where they were otherwise occupied, such as driving, working, or socialising, and thus they deploy mobile devices as a tool of distraction or management within the routines of family life: *... on my phone and she'll watch a show if I'm out somewhere. It's usually a ... I use it like a tool to entertain her.* Yet, such parental provision of devices was not simply an expression of what Mowlabocus (2016, n.p.) describes as the hail of smartphones "reminding us to be productive ... as workers, students, parents, friends, consumers, and producers", in which "their constant notifications interpellate us into the contemporary political-economic structure from an ever-earlier age". Instead, such attachments also reflected the value placed by families on children's digital play, learning, and social interaction, in which the everyday and ordinary usage of haptic media slowly seeped down to younger children's everyday media practices: *We had my son's birthday and there were some photos, some footage of us singing happy birthday and the little one just wants to watch it over and over again.*

Young children's haptic media habitus is, then, embodied through the affordances and materiality of mobile devices for being held, touched, and carried: *The phone is 100% instant and it's little, they can carry it around, so I think that's part of the attraction as well.* Haptic media encounters are animated by touchscreen interfaces that are responsive to simple gestural actions of young children: *They can grab it and start playing with it. It just shows that it's so much part of their world ... to swipe something.* And these haptic media relations are habituated over time through cultural contexts of provision and performance as part of their "individual and collectively realized corporeal schema" (Richardson, 2012, p. 135). Arguably, the *swipe* emerges as the key gesture of a haptic habitus: *She knew from quite a young age to swipe a photo on the phone.* Yet, the swipe is not immediately part of haptic conduct, but emerges as critical in the transition from simple and intuitive discrete interaction to more encoded multi-touch gestural styles. Like Merleau-Ponty's keyboard habitus, it is expressive of young children's internalisation of a particular mode of gestural input for corporeal conduct as part of a wider haptic habitus.

The swipe speaks to the formation of young children's haptic habitus and embodied capacities for and relations with media being shaped through the dominance of a particular interfacial mode of engagement, touch. This, then, guided interactions and expectations with media more generally, including interfacing with "residual media" (Acland, 2007): *It's funny because when she was younger she would go up the T.V. and she would try swiping the T.V. to turn the channel*. The 'failure' of legacy media to respond to touch was seen as underscoring the intuitive qualities of haptic media, located in the generational naming of 'natural user interfaces' within the product design and manufacturer communities (e.g., Norman, 2010): *He has been using an iPad before he was 1. He could unlock it. He could open things with it. Play games. Choose apps. Before he could talk or walk. It's such an intuitive interface*. Such embodied dispositions highlight how young children's means of conceptualising digital media are driven by modes of interfacing: *The, the keyboard in my office is a big novelty . . . So, it's a novelty, that, I think that they actually don't see the computer and the tablet as similar devices*. A haptic habitus is, then, not just cultivated by relations of encounter, enculturation, or embodiment, but critically constrained and guided by codified regimes of interaction involving product design and development.

Configuring Haptic Habitus through Interface Design

As the discussion of young children's touchscreen habitats and habituation above suggests, the formation of young children's touchscreen *habitus* emerges through their embodiment and enculturation of dispositions towards touchscreen media shaped by direct experience, by rich household media environments, and through relations of mimesis and mediation. Here, the haptic interface is understood not solely as the point at which the user interfaces with the computer screen, but, as Cramer and Fuller (2008) argue, the interface becomes a site of exchange which operates below the level of the user interface through hardware, software, and code within computer systems, as well as beyond the screen through shared practices and norms operating at the level of culture.

At the level of the screen, touchscreen gestures must be registered by and map onto a predefined and limited range of common UI gesture types (tapping, pressing, swiping, dragging, scrolling, pinching, spreading, rotating). These gesture types are designed, detailed, and determined by product manufacturers such as Apple, and made available for software developers through APIs and documentation such as Apple's developer manual for gestural input, the 'Event Handling Guide for iOS'.

But, these gestural interactions and encodings are, in turn, informed by recursive examples of UX research that draw on cultural resources. YouTube videos of young children playing with iPads, for example, have been used as a resource by interaction design researchers to understand young children's capacities to use touchscreen interfaces *and* mobile applications (Buckleitner, 2011). Analysing YouTube videos of young children's embodied interactions with touchscreen devices is used to inform the ongoing development of touch design in commercial mobile apps. Through such circuits of cultural production children's haptic habitus within wider economies of play is becoming a commercially valuable resource for informing interaction design, and haptic software product development can be located:

> A perfectly flat, glassy surface is magical all by itself. It doesn't exist in nature . . . and when it's covered with fog or a slippery oleophobic coating, it gets even more interesting to your fingers . . .

> The Minimum User Competency (MUC) has dropped from around 2½ years (for the mouse) to around 12 months (for the iPad) . . .
>
> This presents new opportunities for children's interactive media developers; nothing short of a new era in computing, as the user interface becomes increasingly invisible.
>
> *(Buckleitner, 2011, p. 10)*

This research highlights a common and not unexpected observation that children's initial modes of haptic interaction involve actions such as jabbing, swatting, licking, and smearing (e.g., Buckleitner, 2011). While "looking, tasting, smelling, and hearing" – alongside jabbing, swatting, and smearing – "are all variants of 'handling' the world" (Richardson & Third, 2009, p. 154), in design terms such haptic interface exploration can be understood as a form of gestural excess (Apperley, 2013; Simon, 2009), insomuch as these gestures exceed and therefore are not clearly registered within the codified regime of touchscreen interface design. For young children, touchscreens (and mobile devices more generally) require subtle yet significant reformulations of, adjustments to, and disciplining of, gesture. With children, this gestural literacy involves learning through doing – whether their fingers have moved far or fast enough, or in a straight enough line – to activate on-screen actions. That is, they must discover and then adjust their actions to map onto movements incorporated within predefined gesture recognition lists. And yet, young children's capacities to deliberately interact with touchscreens are fairly quickly acquired. Beginning from around the age of 12 months, children demonstrate abilities for simple discrete types of single-fingered gestural interaction such as tapping and swiping (or flicking) (Cristia & Seidl, 2015; Hourcade et al., 2015). More complex and multi-touch gestures, such as dragging or pinching, are, whilst slower to develop, displayed from around 18 months and steadily increase over time (Hourcade et al., 2015).

Children's haptic habitus, then, becomes a site of interest for UX and interaction design researchers aiming to build applications for play and learning that accommodate these capacities through programmed tolerances for gestural input techniques. Whilst designing for bodily interaction is an implicit dimension to UX and human-centred design traditions (e.g., McCarthy & Wright, 2004), it is in the design and development of haptic interfaces that the notion of a habitus emerges in a more explicit and significant aspect of design research. HCI and media scholars have noted that haptic media and gestural interfaces are not unique to our current moment of digital mobile media (Norman, 2005; Parisi et al., 2017), drawing on past regimes of interaction such as GUI (graphical user interface). They are, nevertheless, part of an apparatus that imagines a renovated experience of computer interaction by incorporating people's natural modes of physical communication and movement – natural user interfaces (NUIs). The NUI paradigm of interaction has, however, been critiqued for the assumption that such interfaces are somehow intuitive, universal, and immediately usable (Norman, 2010). Rather than a mode of interaction that comes naturally, Donald Norman and others have noted that gesture systems still require designing a grammar of interaction that follows well-defined modes of expression and navigation. Thus, like any other mode of interfacing, haptic media are still subject to entanglements of design protocols and learnt user practices in which specific gestures must become habituated.

In turn, phenomenologically informed cultural theory of mobile media emphasises as part of the enculturation of technology that gestural interfaces are "culturally specific and materially contextual" (Richardson & Third, 2009, p. 155). Despite efforts to naturalise this habitus, whether that naturalness is located in the child or the gestural interface – accompanied by claims to either digital natives (Prensky, 2001) or natural modes of computer interaction (e.g., Widgor & Wixon, 2011) – young children's haptic media habitus cannot be disentangled from the site of its cultural production, material performance, and economic exploitation. Designing for young children's haptic habitus may appear to be a task in which UI designers simply codify children's gestural capacities onto touch-based user interfaces. Yet, as this research highlights, haptics are both specific to and produced within different bodily, technological, and cultural contexts. The ability to use touchscreen devices is not simply determined by children's developmental capacities, as this operates within feedback loops involving forms of encounter, enculturation, and embodiment described above. Parents deliberately assemble the interface between child and touchscreen through the provision and promotion of mobile devices and applications (Nansen & Jayemanne, 2016).

Similarly, the so-called 'Minimum User Competency' (MUC) of touchscreen interfaces is not simply a product of touchscreens automatically lowering thresholds of computational usability to ever-younger populations. Instead, children's capacities for gestural interaction are closely mapped, fostered, and fed back into UI development in order to inform the design of child-friendly software applications *and* extend the commercial market of potential users (Buckleitner, 2011). Within such political economies of media haptics minor variations of gesture type and tolerance spread across various mobile applications, operating systems, and device manufacturers. Commercial efforts to own particular gestures like the swipe to unlock or the pinch to zoom have featured in the long-running patent wars between Apple and Samsung, and yet legal settlements of these differences signal to the standardisation of touchscreen gestures, enrolling media haptics within a wider platform imperialism (Yong Jin, 2015). The result is a kind of "ergonomic branding" (Parisi, 2015), in which the material design of branded touchscreen interfaces inscribes bodies with a haptic habitus that codifies the feel and performance of gestures. Whilst this may maximise the efficiency of gestural interaction, and lower thresholds of usability, it comes at the "cost of the autonomy of gesture" (Zehle, 2012), delimiting the possibilities of children's haptic media technologies, experiences, and cultures.

Conclusions

This chapter has applied phenomenologically informed cultural theory to technology relations as a way to approach young children's formation of an embodied disposition or haptic habitus towards touchscreen interfaces. This habitus is produced through young children's increasing use of mobile and touchscreen media, cultivated by encounters, enculturation, and embodiment of haptic media in domestic and family life, and appropriated by haptic user interface designers and product manufacturers. It can be seen that UX and interaction design researchers are implicitly interested in how developmental capacities intersect with forms of encounter, enculturation, and embodiment as part of the dominant interface now reconfiguring children's media habitus.

With young children growing up in media environments defined by haptic media experiences, parents of young mobile media users reflecting on the phenomenological significance and implications of such changing media interfaces can be seen: *I think that in some ways it (touchscreen) makes them feel more connected to the device, like they're more part of what they're doing*. Such observations highlight shifting but shared media subjectivities entrained through an emergent haptic habitus in terms of dispositions and expectations for immediacy, for availability, and for connectivity in the operation of digital media. Paradoxically, whilst such reconfigurations enable new modes of experience not available through older interfaces, the touchscreen interface also installs anxieties about the erasure of sensory engagement afforded by more traditional modes of physical play and learning: *With the iPad, you don't get texture. You don't sort of feel, you know, if you're using sand, or if you're using tissue paper, or you're using Play-Do, or whatever, you're actually getting different textures to feel. It's definitely missing a sensory input to it.*

These tensions around the redistribution and revaluation of sensory experience structured through young children's every-day and embodied touchscreen interfacing are, in turn, folded into broader economies of media haptics. On the one hand, acquiring capacities for using touchscreen interfaces equips young children with embodied resources for relating to and through digital media, whilst, on the other hand, touchscreens inscribe bodies with codified gestures for manipulating interfaces (Parisi, 2015; Zehle, 2012), thus delimiting the potentials for children's haptic habitus. These contradictions raise important questions about the significance of a culturally dominant interface form in reconfiguring dispositions, especially for young children growing up in media environments defined by increasingly intimate and entangled haptic media experiences. And they call for understandings of children's digital media informed by, and accounting for, relays between everyday media practices, cultural norms, and economies of design.

Acknowledgements

This research was supported through funding from an Australian Research Council (ARC) Discovery Early Career Researcher Award (DE130100735).

References

Acland, C.R. (Ed.). (2007). *Residual media*. Minneapolis: University of Minnesota Press.
Apperley, T.H. (2013). The body of the gamer: Game art and gestural excess. *Digital Creativity 24*(2), 145–156.
Bourdieu, P. (1977). *Outline of a theory of practice*. Cambridge: Cambridge University Press.
Buckleitner, W. (2011). A taxonomy of multi-touch interaction styles, by stage. *Children's Technology Review 18*(11), 10–11.
Burroughs, B. (2017). YouTube kids: The app economy and mobile parenting. *Social Media + Society 3*(2), n.p.. Retrieved from: https://journals.sagepub.com/doi/full/10.1177/2056305117707189.
Chiong, C., & Shuler, C. (2010). *Learning: Is there an app for that? Investigations of young children's usage and learning with mobile devices and apps*. New York: The Joan Ganz Cooney Center at Sesame Workshop.
Connor, S. (2000). Making an issue of cultural phenomenology. *Critical Quarterly 42*(1), 2–6.
Cramer, F., & Fuller, M. (2008). Interface. In M. Fuller (Ed.), *Software studies: A Lexicon* (pp. 149–153). Cambridge: MIT Press.
Cristia, A., & Seidl, A. (2015). Parental reports on touch screen use in early childhood. *PLoS ONE 10*(6), 1–20.
Csordas, T.J. (1999). Embodiment and cultural phenomenology. In G. Weiss & H.F. Haber (Eds.), *Perspectives on embodiment: The intersections of nature and culture* (pp. 143–162). New York: Routledge.
Hourcade, J.P., Mascher, S.L., Wu, D., & Pantoja, L. (2015). Look, my baby is using an iPad! An analysis of YouTube videos of infants and toddlers using tablets. In *Proceedings of the CHI 15* (pp. 1915–1924). New York: ACM Press.
Ihde, D. (1990). *Technology and the lifeworld: From garden to earth*. Bloomington: Indiana University Press.
Ihde, D. (1993). *Postphenomenology: Essays in the postmodern context*. Evanston: Northwestern University Press.
Loke, L., & Robertson, T. (2011). The lived body in design: Mapping the terrain. In *Proceedings of the OZCHI '11* (pp. 181–184). New York: ACM Press.
Marsh, J.L., Plowman, D., Yamada-Rice, J., Bishop, C., Lahmar, J., & Scott, F. (2018). Play and creativity in young children's use of apps. *British Journal of Educational Technology 49*(5), 870–882.
Mauss, M. (1973). Techniques of the body. (B. Brewster, Trans.). *Economy and Society 2*, 70–88.
McCarthy, J., & Wright, P. (2004). *Technology as experience*. Cambridge: MIT Press.
Merleau-Ponty, M. (2012). *The phenomenology of perception*. (D.A. Landes, Trans.). London: Routledge.
Mowlabocus, S. (2016). The 'mastery' of the swipe: Smartphones, transitional objects and interstitial time. *First Monday 21*(10). Retrieved from: http://journals.uic.edu/ojs/index.php/fm/article/view/6950/5630.
Nansen, B., & Jayemanne, D. (2016). Infants, interfaces, and intermediation: Digital parenting in the production of 'iPad Baby' YouTube videos. *Journal of Broadcasting and Electronic Media 60*(4), 587–603.
Nansen, B., & Jayemanne, D. (2018). écrans tactiles, accoutumances et habitus des jeunes enfants [Young children's touchscreen habitats, habituation, and habitus]. In M. Loicq, A. Seurrat, & I. Dumez et Féroc Eds., *Les cultures médiatiques de l'enfance et de la petite enfance* (pp. 114–125). Paris: Booke-e.
Nansen, B., Vetere, F., Downs, J., Robertson, T., Brereton, M., & Durick, J. (2014). Reciprocal habituation: A study of older people and the Kinect. *Transactions on Computer-Human Interaction (ToCHI) 21*(3), Article 18, 1–20.

Nansen, B., & Wilken, R. (2019). Techniques of the tactile body: A cultural phenomenology of infants and mobile touchscreens. *Convergence 25*(1), 60–76.

Nevski, E., & Siibak, A. (2016). The role of parents and parental mediation on 0-3-year olds' digital play with smart devices: Estonian parents' attitudes and practices. *Early Years: An International Research Journal 36*(3), 227–241.

Norman, D. (2005). *Emotional design*. New York: Basic Books.

Norman, D. (2010). Natural user interfaces are not natural. *Interactions* May-June, 6–10.

OfCom. (2013). *Children and parents: Media use and attitudes report*. London: OfCom.

Parisi, D. (2015). A counterrevolution in the hands: The console controller as an ergonomic branding mechanism. *Journal of Games Criticism 2*(1). Retrieved from: http://gamescriticism.org/articles/parisi-2-1.

Parisi, D., Paterson, M., & Archer, J.E. (2017). Haptic media studies. *New Media & Society 19*(10), 1513–1522.

Prensky, M. (2001). Digital natives, digital immigrants. *On the Horizon 9*(5), 1–6.

Richardson, I. (2012). Touching the screen: A phenomenology of mobile gaming and the iPhone. In L. Hjorth, J. Burgess, & I. Richardson (Eds.), *Studying mobile media: Cultural technologies, mobile communication, and the iPhone* (pp. 133–151). New York: Routledge.

Richardson, I., & Hjorth, L. (2017). Mobile media, domestic play and haptic ethnography. *New Media & Society 19*(10), 1653–1667.

Richardson, I., & Third, A. (2009). Cultural phenomenology and the material culture of mobile media. In P. Vannini (Ed.), *Material culture and technology in everyday life: Ethnographic approaches* (pp. 145–156). New York: Peter Lang.

Richardson, I. and Wilken, R. (2009). Haptic vision, footwork, place-making: A peripatetic phenomenology of the mobile phone pedestrian. *Second Nature: International Journal of Creative Media 2*(1), 22–41.

Richardson, I., & Wilken, R. (2017). Mobile media and mediation: The relational ontology of Google Glass. In T. Markham & S. Rodgers (Eds.), *Conditions of mediation: Phenomenological perspectives on media* (pp. 113–123). New York: Peter Lang.

Rideout, V. (2013). *Zero to eight: Children's media use in America 2013*. San Francisco: Common Sense Media.

Shuler, C. (2009). *iLearn: A content analysis of the iTunes app store's education section*. New York: The Joan Ganz Cooney Center at Sesame Workshop.

Simon, B. (2009). Wii are out of control: Bodies, game screens and the production of gestural excess. *Loading 3*(4). Retrieved from: http://journals.sfu.ca/loading/index.php/loading/article/view/65/59.

Wellner, G. (2016). *A postphenomenological inquiry of cell phones: Genealogies, meanings, and becomings*. Lanham: Lexington Books.

Widgor, D., & Wixon, D. (2011). *Brave NUI world: Designing natural user interfaces for touch and gesture*. Burlington: Morgan Kaufmann.

Yong Jin, D. (2015). *Digital platforms, imperialism and political culture*. New York: Routledge.

Zehle, S. (2012). The autonomy of gesture: Of lifestream logistics and playful profanations. *Distinktion: Journal of Social Theory 13*(3), 340–353.

11
EARLY ENCOUNTERS WITH NARRATIVE
Two-Year-Olds and Moving-Image Media

Cary Bazalgette

Introduction

This chapter starts from the premise that all people have learned, very early in life, how to understand moving-image media, meaning any moving-image material, from short sequences in apps, games, and advertisements to full-length television programmes and films. It may seem strange to insist that viewers have had to learn to understand these media. From its earliest days in the late 19th century, the movie industry has promoted itself as the most 'lifelike' medium, and much of the extensive literature on children and moving-image media takes this for granted. The famous – and probably exaggerated (Loiperdinger, 2004) – accounts of audiences recoiling or screaming when in 1896 or soon afterwards they saw the Lumière brothers' 50-second movie *L'arrivée d'un train en gare de La Ciotat* formed, as Loiperdinger argues, the 'founding myth' of moving-image media: that viewers are supposed to instinctively believe they are watching 'real life'. But moving-image media are now a distinctive, long-established art form that has been developing for more than a century. They are full of rhetorical devices that do not reproduce daily perceptual experiences: for example, jump-cuts, parallel montage, shot/reverse-shot sequences, non-diegetic sound. These terms may be familiar only to film buffs and movie professionals, but moving-image audiences can effortlessly 'read' the features they refer to: if they could not, they would not be enjoying what they watch! Because these audiences do not remember learning to interpret these features, they think that they never had to.

But when does this learning happen? Broadcasters and film-makers know that three- and four-year-olds can be expected to follow and enjoy many feature films and programmes that older age groups like as well. If evidence of the prior learning that has enabled them to do this is sought, it is necessary to look at younger children. This chapter proposes that two-year-olds' engagement with moving-image media is a socially and culturally important process of learning how to understand the medium itself, alongside – and inherently bound up with – their efforts to follow narratives. This approach challenges two preoccupations that currently dominate academic research about children and moving-image media. First, there is an overriding concern with the risk that these media may present a threat to children's well-being. Second, most research on children and media in the 21st century has concentrated on digital technologies rather than on the different types of content that these technologies enable viewers to consume and create (Carlsson, 2010; Lankshear & Knobel, 2008; Livingstone & Sefton-Green, 2016).

Research on Young Children and Media

Most Anglophone research in this area takes place within an inherently anticipatory 'risks and benefits' paradigm that seeks to identify the psychological, cognitive, and social effects of these media on children's later development. Within this paradigm, scholars either emphasise the supposed risks of 'too much' viewing (Palmer, 2006; Vandewater, Bickham, Cummings, Wartella, & Rideout, 2005; Zimmerman, Christakis, & Meltzoff, 2007), or they argue for its benefits. These may relate to language acquisition or print literacy (Kendeou, Bohn-Gettler, White, & Broek, 2008; Lemish & Rice, 1986; Marsh, 2000; Robinson & Turnbull, 2005), or they may point to the educational or sociocultural value of media content (Davies, 1989; Lauricella, Gola, & Calvert, 2011; Marsh et al., 2005).

Very little research takes an informed approach to the specificities of moving-image media. For example, the stylistic devices media makers employ to convey meanings; their densely multimodal structures; their enormous stylistic and generic variation, both historically and globally; the fact that they are not merely visual but also aural; and that, as in music, movies' management of sound track duration, rhythm, and pace is an essential dimension of meaning-making. The tendency has been to regard television as a visual (rather than audiovisual) medium, whose defining features reside in the technology – in particular, the screen – rather than in the institutional or aesthetic features that distinguish, for example, different genres and intended audiences (e.g., Anderson & Hanson, 2010; Gola & Calvert, 2011). In addition, critics make little reference to children's own interests in re-viewing material, and discussions of 'response' and 'attention' focus largely on gaze, with little consideration of features such as bodily tension, posture, gesture (apart from pointing) and choice of position in relation to the screen (Pempek, Kirkorian, Richards, Anderson, & Lund, 2010).

The period around the third year of life (approximately 18–40 months) is an immensely important time for learning. This period – known in Anglophone cultures as the 'terrible twos' but in German and Danish as the 'age of autonomy' – is when children learn to speak, become much more mobile and dexterous, and make huge progress in understanding their social and cultural surroundings. However, as Rowe and others indicate, ethnographic studies of two-year-olds are rare (2008), and rarer still in research on children and moving-image media. This gap in the research was noted by Collins as long ago as 1979, but has persisted: Lealand (1998) points out that "among the thousands of research studies and policy statements on children and television, viewers under five years old are usually underrepresented and often ignored" despite general acceptance of the idea that the early years are the most formative (p. 4). Such studies as there are inevitably involve difficult "practical and logistical considerations, including gaining access, involving children as active research participants and negotiating consents" (Plowman & Stevenson, 2013, p. 330). One way of overcoming these difficulties is for researchers to study their own children or grandchildren. A few well-known studies of this nature have resulted in key insights on toddlers' learning (Britton, 1970; Darwin, 1877; Edmiston, 2008; Halliday, 1975; Piaget, 1928; Weir, 1970).

Research that has depended on information from parents or carers (Certain & Kahn, 2002; Schmidt, Rich, Rifas-Shiman, Oken, & Taveras, 2009; Vandewater et al., 2005), or that has only gathered data through periodic and relatively short visits to homes – the problems of which are discussed by Jordan (2006) – cannot claim to provide confident interpretations of the idiosyncratic ways in which individual children, especially those under three, express their responses to the moving-image media they engage with; or to capture the subtleties of the social contexts in which much viewing may take place. Dafna Lemish's 1987 paper, "Viewers in diapers" stands out as an important study of this type, given that it followed 16 children for six to eight months, covering an age range from 6.5 to 36 months, aiming "to discover and describe the process through which babies become television consumers" (1987, p. 54). However, each family was visited only four or five times, and the research depended as heavily on parental viewing logs and diaries as it did on researcher observation. The children's viewing was also dominated by *Sesame Street*, the long-running programme from the US-based Children's Television Workshop. Lemish herself points out that the study "is only one step towards a better understanding of young children's television viewing" (p. 56). Many changes in moving-image media, technologies, and family life have occurred since 1987, and it is unfortunate that few researchers since then have attempted to undertake similar studies of this age group or to use more intensive observational methods. Two notable exceptions in the UK context are Briggs' study of his own family's relationships with the TV series *Teletubbies* (2006) and Robinson and Turnbull's (2005) case study of a child's literacy development – including her relationship with films and TV – from birth to age six; but again, neither addresses the question of how these children learned to understand the medium itself.

The author's own interest in addressing this question was originally motivated by her professional experiences in developing education about moving-image media, which included persuading teachers that children's ability to make inferences and predictions about narratives, to recognise generic features, and to appreciate and enjoy stories is enhanced by their film and television viewing. Primary school teachers who overcome their worries about institutional or parental disapproval and start teaching about moving-image media in the classroom are almost invariably amazed by the apparent transformation of their pupils' knowledge and abilities that results. They tend to infer that the moving-image media have acted as a trigger or accelerator for children's learning, whereas what has arguably happened is that teacher training and the school system, in general, have failed to recognise or value the prior learning about moving-image media that children bring with them to nursery and reception classes.

This chapter draws on a 20-month observational study of the author's own grandchildren (Connie and Alfie: dizygotic twins), focussing in particular on the 22–36-month phase (Bazalgette, 2018). Through more frequent (at least weekly) extended and closer contact and familiar surroundings (the author's home and theirs, separated by only 30 minutes' travel time), this study collected more material than visiting researchers usually achieve. Research data amounted to over 12 hours of video (taken on an unobtrusive and familiar device: an iPhone), 90 sets of observation notes and over eight hours of parental interviews. A grounded theory approach to analysis of these data (Charmaz, 2006; Glaser, 1967) led to the author drawing upon insights from the broad and evolving field of embodied cognition (Coegnarts & Kravanja, 2015; Damasio, 2000; Daum, Somerville, & Prinz, 2009; Gallese & Sinigaglia, 2011; Trevarthen & Aitken, 2001). In this process, the researcher was in many ways a participant observer who often had to slip between the roles of observer and grandmother. As with other studies of children by family members, the findings may be somewhat subjective due to familiarity with the participants, but they may still provide insights with important implications for future debate and research. The potential ethical issues in the research were discussed with the family, and the project was considered and approved by the relevant university ethics committee.

The Social Context of Viewing

Parents who enjoy moving-image media are likely to share this enjoyment with their children, often starting by the time their babies are three months old (Marsh et al., 2005). Many parents soon find that leaving the baby to watch a television programme or DVD enables them to get on with essential household tasks, even though they may feel anxious in case the baby watches for 'too long' (Blum-Ross & Livingstone, 2018).

Thus babies quickly become accustomed to their family's moving-image media viewing practices: the devices family members use, the times and places where they watch, and how they watch. Ofcom's 2018 report *Children and Parents: Media Use and Attitudes* provided a snapshot, from the middle of the century's second decade, of how UK children's viewing habits were changing, which included some data on three- to four-year-olds. They found that, although viewing broadcast programmes on a TV set was in overall decline, 96% of three- to four-year-olds watched TV on a TV set for an average of 14 hours per week, while 30% watched moving-image media on other devices, mainly on a tablet, much of which would have entailed watching YouTube for animated movies, funny videos, or pranks. While most of these figures increased substantially for older age groups, it was still the case that watching movies on a TV set, although declining slowly but steadily overall, remained an important activity for three-year-olds. Judging by anecdotal evidence on social media, and by the digital practices described by Bar Lev, Elias, and Levy (2018), it is possible to infer that two-year-olds and even infants also play frequently with portable devices such as smartphones and tablets and that this is likely to include opportunities to view moving-image media.

Modes of watching will differ between or even within families. Some family members may be doing other things while they watch, while others may sit and watch intently from beginning to end; some may comment frequently to each other, while others may maintain an attentive silence. Some families will have their televisions on continually for much of the day, others will not. Some audiovisual phenomena will not be entirely new to those neonates who have already heard many theme tunes, sound effects, and audience reactions while they were still in the womb (Johansson, Wedenberg, & Westin, 1992).

How Two-Year-Olds Watch Moving-Image Media

The author's research indicated that two-year-olds' engagements with moving-image media follow a similar pattern to their other daily activities. There may be a lot of 'milling about' as they explore the spaces they inhabit and search for things that will be interesting to investigate. When they do find something promising, they will give it absolute attention for as long as they can. A movie playing on a flat-screen television may be one of the things in their environment, but they will only pay it attention when they want to, often stimulated by sound-track elements that attract them. Their attention may also be stimulated by a co-viewer, as in "ooh, look at that!" but only if a glance at the screen confirms that it is more interesting than what they are already doing. In other words, like most other things that toddlers do, their attentiveness – and their learning – is largely self-directed, and to interfere with this can result in screams of rage: hence the parental frustrations that have given rise to the unfortunate label 'terrible twos'.

A close look at how rapt attention in a two-year-old manifests itself reveals an enormous investment of energy. Gazing at a screen is different from, say, investigating the cutlery drawer, in that the hands may not be so active – but they are used to grip on to something if, as often happens, the child is standing up to watch the screen. A toddler's centre of gravity is higher than an adult's (Huelke, 1998); if they want to pay attention to a large screen they will want to get as close to it as they can and may need to 'brace' themselves against a piece of furniture in order to maintain a steady gaze and follow on-screen movement by moving their heads. Alternatively, if they are not quite so close to the screen, they may simply leave their hands where they were when their attention was first seized, and maintain almost complete stillness as they watch.

Pleasure, Re-Viewing, and 'Using It Up'

An initial viewing of a media text may well not reveal pleasure. The child may frown, chew her cheek, purse her lips, and perhaps grip a table or chair tightly as she watches. The toddler's perennial runny nose may ensure that her mouth stays open, so she will periodically lick her lips and perhaps hastily wipe her nose on her sleeve, maintaining her gaze at the same time. If she is drinking from a bottle or cup she will hold it to one side as she does so, in order not to miss anything on the screen. If she sees, hears, or even anticipates anything alarming in the movie, her bodily tension will increase: shown perhaps through clenched fists, raised shoulders, and deeper breathing.

When a child has bestowed this much attention on a movie, she is likely to ask for 'more' as soon as it finishes. She may excitedly anticipate the bits she remembers, point to the screen and shout out the name of the character or thing that is going to appear, touch the screen to identify an object of interest, grin knowingly as an action that she understands well plays out as expected; and her pleasures here will be enhanced when co-viewers respond appreciatively. By considering a child's intense – and sometimes maddening – desire to constantly re-view a selected movie as a learning process, one may be better able to respect the child's choices. And when she no longer wants to re-view it, this is not necessarily because she is 'bored' or 'fed up' with it but because she has used it up: she has extracted all she can from it and is ready to move on to the next thing.

The twins often gave their greatest attention, and most demands for re-viewing, to moving-image media that not only appealed to them but were also 'at the edge' of their ability to understand. For example, when they were 28 months old they shifted their attention from short and relatively simple TV episodes such as the eight-minute *Baby Jake* (Darrall Maqueen Ltd/JAM Media, CBeebies, 2011–2012), which appeals to toddlers, to *Tree Fu Tom* (CBeebies/Fremantle Media/Blue-Zoo Production, 2012–2016), a 28-minute narrative programme aimed at 'up to five year olds' featuring live-action and CGI animation and a complex mix of arthropod, vegetable, and human characters. This programme was considerably more demanding than anything they had watched before, and yet the toddlers maintained their interest in it for five months. Extended periods of re-viewing or series loyalty, then, related to material whose complexity took a long time for them to 'use up'.

An Embodied Cognition Perspective on Movie-Watching

Conventional ideas about two-year-olds' movie-watching fall broadly into three modes of thought. First, there is the mode signalled by using the language of affect, as in "he just **loves** *In the Night Garden*" or "*Peppa Pig* is her absolute **favourite**". Second, the use of pop-psychology language reveals, even if only light-heartedly, anxieties about the risks of movie-watching, as in "she's completely **obsessed** by *Waybuloo*" or "he's really **addicted** to *Paw Patrol*". Third, there is the perspective adopted by many broadcasters and production companies, as in "if children aren't able to follow the story, they won't be interested" (Steemers, 2010, pp. 127–30). All three modes focus on supposed deficits in the two-year-old's brain.

Embodied cognition offers a different approach to two-year-olds' movie-watching. A broad field that draws upon many academic disciplines including neurosciences, evolution, and philosophy (Shapiro, 2012), this perspective challenges cognitivist approaches to learning and Cartesian dualism's separation between mind and body. Instead, it proposes that cognition (in animals as well as in humans) is intricately bound up with the body's motor and perceptual systems and how they interact with the physical world and with other creatures. It is a reminder that the extraordinary brains of *homo sapiens* evolved in dangerous and demanding environments and that people still carry the instinctive behaviour and modes of thought that were essential to group survival in those environments (Panksepp, 2004). It thus enables a fresh approach to the study of very young children and their "entry into the sociocultural world" (Trevarthen & Aitken, 2001, p. 20), leaving room for the hypothesis that babies and toddlers, confronted by the intense multimodality of moving-image media, are far from being baffled but will often rise immediately to the challenge of figuring out what the texts they are watching mean.

Emotion and Cognition

The power of moving-image media to affect people emotionally has a long history and is an intrinsic element of the wariness with which Anglophone culture has treated the medium. Given the widespread assumption that emotions are something that toddlers have to learn to bring under control, it is understandable how anxieties about the risks of 'exposure' to moving-image media have arisen and why they have focussed particularly on the assumed vulnerabilities of young children (AAP, 1999).

According to neuroscience, emotions are vitally important systems that help to motivate both thought and action and are deeply embedded in people's brains. 'Primitive' emotions like fear and rage may have been essential in the environmentally dangerous lives and close social inter-dependence of early humans, but what Panksepp calls the 'seeking' emotion was just as important. It generates anticipation and investigation, and by helping individuals perceive causal connections, enables the formation of ideas (Panksepp, 2004, pp. 144–9). An important insight into the role of emotions in social interactions comes from research into mirror neurons and how these enable interpretation of and response to the actions and motivations of others (Gallese, 2001). Gallese explains how the mirror neuron system not only impels people to imitate the actions of others (like smiling back when smiled at) but also functions as an important basis for empathy.

Bearing these arguments in mind, when observing two-year-olds viewing and re-viewing a movie, it is clearer how their intense attentiveness has an emotional force that is more than simply 'enjoying it'. In seeking meaning, very young children are not only learning how to interpret the expressions and actions of characters but also how to assemble causal connections and, therefore, how to follow a narrative. This can be inferred in several different ways.

Expectations of Significance

Much of toddlers' efforts to understand moving-image media are self-driven. Watching TV is not like shared reading of picture books; it is not mediated by an adult or caregiver. The multimodal density of moving-image media offers many 'ways in' to potential meanings that the child can latch on to by herself. But co-viewers can still mediate, if in different ways. Through their engagements with any media – books, pictures, computer games, radio, mobile phone calls and texts, music, and of course moving-image media – adults and older siblings unconsciously communicate the importance they ascribe to media content. Lancaster's (2001) analysis of a two-year-old making drawings with her father describes how a shared activity communicates what she calls "an expectation of significance about the semiotic objects encountered" (p. 136). The two-year-old doesn't, at this point, learn how to draw a cat that looks like a cat, but she does discover the importance of drawing as a mode of communication and understands that mark-making can be meaningful. Shared viewing of moving-image media contributes to a child's determination to crack the codes of moving-image media because she knows that moving-image media are important to her co-viewers.

Co-viewers' contributions to the movie-watching environment may be deliberate and even didactic, as in "Oh, look at the poor cat! He's sad, isn't he?", etc. More often, they are unconscious. When adults watch moving-image media with little children, especially if it's something they hope the children will like, their spontaneous exclamations such as "oh!" or "wow!" or "uh-oh!" may cue responses from the children. But even the comments adults may make to each other during the movie, or the bodily tensions or chuckles that may be felt by a child sitting on an adult's lap, can act as clues to meaning for the less experienced child viewer.

Diakresis: Selecting the Salient

Moving-image media use images, movement, colour, voice, sound effects, music, and the duration, transitions, and juxtaposition of shots in constructing and conveying meaning. How does anyone, let alone a two-year-old, take all this in at once? Dehaene (2014) claims that even adults can really only deal with one thought at a time because their consciousness imposes a narrow bottleneck on the multiple perceptions that their daily experiences – including moving-image media – present to them. Drawing on Dehaene, Wojciechowski suggests that in watching a movie, "we perform continual acts of diakresis – a *separating out* of information that is salient enough to enter into our conscious awareness, and the distinguishing of the salient from everything else" (Wojciechowski, 2015, p. 124). The more extensive the movie-watching experience, the more skilled children are at drawing on their experiences of narratives and genres in the use of diakresis. As two-year-olds repeat-view, they pile up their diakretic selections until they have assembled enough of a coherent whole to satisfy their desire for significance. And because diakresis is a highly individual process, it is difficult for adults to predict just what an individual child may find interesting, or frightening, or baffling.

The beginnings of diakresis can be observed in very young children, starting with the apparently irrational terror that can be sparked off by innocuous material in children's moving-image media; a phenomenon that is often discussed on social media.[1] The diakresis theory would suggest that in these cases, the salience of the disturbing element of the scene overrides what is intended to be gentle and amusing programme content. This corresponds with Kagan's observation that one-year-olds "are sensitive to events that appear to contrast with those which adults have indicated are proper" like broken toys or clothing that's damaged or stained (1981, pp. 47–8). But in movie-watching, it is often the narrative that establishes what has 'gone wrong', not the family's social rules: so these odd fears can be a sign that a child actually is beginning to follow stories.

A later example of diakresis at work appeared when the twins were watching *Finding Nemo* (Stanton, 2003) for the first time, aged just three. Connie was unable to 'correctly' interpret the death of Nemo's mother Coral; not just because the actual death is not shown, but also because she could not countenance it emotionally. Instead, she constructed what was, for her, an alternative narrative enigma – Coral has disappeared somewhere, and they have to find her. Connie held on to the narrative until the end of the movie when she was surprised to discover that Coral had simply been replaced by Dory. She had yet to get hold of the generic knowledge and the concomitant awareness of convention that would enable her to accept that Coral was dead and gone, but she was using diakresis to identify a situation she found to be emotionally salient and helpful in constructing her own narrative expectations.

Modality Judgements: 'Real' and 'Pretend'

Hodge and Tripp's concept of 'modality judgements' (Hodge & Tripp, 1986) is taken directly from linguistics and does not equate with the later connotations of 'modality' within multimodality theory. It simply refers to what the assumed truth or reality status of a movie is supposed to be, thus making the important assertion that the appearances of 'truth' and 'reality' can be highly questionable or at least uncertain. In the context of this chapter's argument, modality judgements can also be usefully linked to the ways in which children operate their rules about 'real' and 'pretend' in play; these can be arbitrary but hold good for the duration of the game. Anxieties about the risks of movie-watching often include the mantra that "children cannot distinguish between fantasy and reality" but, as Woolley points out, children are not fundamentally different from adults in their ability to distinguish fantasy from reality, and that everyone operates "a continuum of ontological commitment to what we think the world is really like" (Woolley, 1997, p. 991): the 'fake news' phenomenon provides ample demonstration of this.

Two-year-olds are as interested as anyone in what is or is not meant to be real but, being small and relatively vulnerable, their threshold for fearful reactions is set sensibly lower than that of larger, stronger, and more experienced people, and they are more likely to be frightened by characters or events that appear to claim a high modality status; in other words, that seem to be meant to be real. For example, Alfie (at 34 months) remained uncertain for some time about whether there really was a 'big bad mouse' in *The Gruffalo's Child* (Welland & Heidschtter, 2011), exorcising this fear through many games of running through the woodland in the local park with Connie, waving a stick and screaming "Monsters!" Thinking about and negotiating the modality status of moving-image media, especially where this involves potentially frightening things, is thus an important part of learning how to understand moving-image media and, by extension, narratives in general. It is important to recognise that two-year-olds can, to some extent, do this for themselves.

Conclusion

The argument of this chapter is founded on the principles, first, that moving-image media are not 'transparent' and instantly accessible to the novice viewer, but instead employ complex, multimodal devices to convey meanings, and second, that these multimodal devices have to be learned, usually very early in life. These principles distinguish the research reported here from themes that have long dominated the study of children and moving-image media, such as the over-arching concern with the risks and benefits of children's 'exposure' to audiovisual material, and the growing tendency to focus on technology – digital media for example – rather than on the specificities of different types of content, and how and why children engage with them.

The research findings on which this chapter is based are drawn from the author's 20-month study of her twin grandchildren's viewing practices between the ages of 22 and 42 months, focussing particularly on when they were two: an age range relatively neglected in academic research, given the difficulties of access and methodology that it presents. Two aspects of their viewing behaviour were described: social contexts such as family viewing, in which co-viewers' utterances and physical behaviour formed part of the children's experience; and the phenomenon of focussed attention, which provided evidence of the enormous investment of energy that children can make when a film or television programme engages their interest. By recognising two-year-olds' "expectations of significance" (Lancaster, 2001) it is possible to see their attentiveness and demands for re-viewing as evidence of learning processes at work, rather than as idiosyncratic desires. Their changing preferences about what they watch may often be grounded in the desire to move on to more challenging material rather than merely 'becoming bored'.

Insights drawn from the developing field of embodied cognition help to illuminate these findings further. Children's instinctive emotional responses to what they watch may be the starting point for how they interpret and reflect upon a scene: identifying aspects that they judge to be salient, for example, and trying to assess how 'true' or 'real' a character or setting is intended to be.

Moving-image media have been an important part of human culture for more than a century. They are now made and shared in ways that, only 20 years ago, most commentators could not imagine. An appreciation that learning to understand these media is a significant achievement for most two-year-olds may enable a deeper understanding of children's personal, cultural, and social development.

Note

1 See, for example, www.netmums.com/coffeehouse/being-mum-794/toddlers-1-3-years-59/1180634-2-year-old-suddenly-scared-fav-tv-shows-random-adverts.html (retrieved 25 July 2018).

References

AAP. (1999). Media education. *Pediatrics*, *104*(2), 341–343, Recommendation 3.
Anderson, D. R., & Hanson, K. G. (2010). From blooming, buzzing confusion to media literacy: The early development of television viewing. *Developmental Review*, *30*(2), 239–255.
Anderson, D. R., & Pempek, T. A. (2005). Television and very young children. *American Behavioral Scientist*, *48*(5), 505–522.
Bar Lev, Y., Elias, N., & Levy, S. T. (2018). Development of infants' media habits in the age of digital parenting. A longitudinal study of Jonathan, from the age of 6 to 27 months. In G. Mascheroni, C. Ponte, & A. Jorge (Eds.), *Digital parenting: The challenges for families in the digital age* (pp. 103–112). Goteborg: Nordicom, University of Gothenburg.
Bazalgette, C. (2018) *Some secret language: How toddlers learn to understand movies* (Doctoral dissertation). UCL Institute of Education, London.
Blum-Ross, A., & Livingstone, S. (2018). The trouble with "screen-time" rules. In G. Mascheroni, C. Ponte, & A. Jorge (Eds.), *Digital parenting: The challenges for families in the digital age* (pp. 179–187). Goteborg: Nordicom, University of Gothenburg.
Briggs, M. (2006). Beyond the audience: Teletubbies, play and parenthood. *European Journal of Cultural Studies*, *9*(4), 441–460.
Britton, J. (1970). *Language and learning*. Harmondsworth: Penguin Books.
Carlsson, U. (Ed.). (2010). *Children and youth in the digital media culture*. Goteborg: The International Clearinghouse on Children, Youth and Media.
Certain, L. K., & Kahn, R. S. (2002). Prevalence, correlates, and trajectory of television viewing among infants and toddlers. *Pediatrics*, *109*(4), 634–642.
Charmaz, K. (2006). *Constructing grounded theory* (2nd ed.). London: Sage.
Coegnarts, M., & Kravanja, P. (Eds.). (2015). *Embodied cognition and cinema*. Leuven: University of Leuven Press.
Collins, W. A. (1979). Children's comprehension of television content. In E. Wartella (Ed.), *Children communicating: Media and development of thought, speech, understanding* (pp. 21–52). Beverly Hills, CA: Sage.
Damasio, A. (2000). *The feeling of what happens*. London: Vintage.
Darwin, C. (1877). A biographical sketch of an infant. *Mind*, *2*, 285–294.
Daum, M. M., Somerville, J. A., & Prinz, W. (2009). Becoming a social agent: Developmental foundations of an embodied social psychology. *European Journal of Social Psychology*, *39*(7), 1196–1206.
Davies, M. M. (1989). *Television is good for your kids*. London: Hilary Shipman Ltd.
Dehaene, S. (2014). *Consciousness and the brain*. New York, NY: Viking Press.
Edmiston, B. (2008). *Forming ethical identities in early childhood play*. Abingdon: Routledge.
Gallese, V. (2001). The "shared manifold" hypothesis. From mirror neurons to empathy. *Journal of Consciousness Studies*, *8*(5–7), 33–50.
Gallese, V., & Sinigaglia, C. (2011). What is so special about embodied simulation? *Trends in Cognitive Sciences*, *15*(11), 512–519.
Glaser, B. (1967). *The discovery of grounded theory*. Chicago, IL: Aldine.
Gola, A. A. H., & Calvert, S. (2011). Infants' visual attention to baby DVDs as a function of program pacing. *Infancy*, *16*(3), 295–305.
Halliday, M. A. K. (1975). *Learning how to mean: Explorations in the development of language*. London: Arnold.
Hodge, B., & Tripp, D. (1986). *Children and television: A semiotic approach*. Cambridge: Polity Press.
Huelke, D. F. (1998). An overview of anatomical considerations of infants and children in the adult world of automobile safety design. *Annual Proceedings of the Association for the Advancement of Automotive Medicine*, *42*, 93–113.
Johansson, B., Wedenberg, E., & Westin, B. (1992). Foetal heart rate response to acoustic stimulation in relation to foetal development and hearing impairment. *Acta obstetricia et gynecologica Scandinavica*, *71*(8), 610–615.
Jordan, A. (2006). Make yourself at home: The social construction of research roles in family studies. *Qualitative Research*, *6*(2), 169–185.
Kagan, J. (1981). *The second year: The emergence of self-awareness*. Cambridge, MA: Harvard University Press.

Kendeou, P., Bohn-Gettler, C., White, M. J., & Broek, P. V. D. (2008). Children's inference generation across different media. *Journal of Research in Reading*, *31*(3), 259.

Lancaster, L. (2001). Staring at the page: The functions of gaze in a young child's interpretation of symbolic forms. *Journal of Early Childhood Literacy*, *1*(2), 131–152.

Lankshear, C., & Knobel, M. (Eds.). (2008). *Digital literacies: Concepts, policies and practices*. Oxford: Peter Lang.

Lauricella, A. R., Gola, A. A. H., & Calvert, S. (2011). Toddlers' learning from socially meaningful video characters. *Media Psychology*, *14*, 216–232.

Lealand, G. (1998). Where do snails watch television? Preschool television and the New Zealand curriculum. In S. Howard (Ed.), *Wired-up: Young people and the electronic media* (pp. 1–17). London: UCL Press.

Lemish, D. (1987). Viewers in diapers: The early development of television viewing. In T. R. Lindlof (Ed.), *Natural audiences: Qualitative research of media uses and effects* (pp. 33–57). Norwood, NJ: Ablex.

Lemish, D., & Rice, M. L. (1986). Television as a talking picture book: A prop for language acquisition. *Journal of Child Language*, *13*, 251–274.

Livingstone, S., & Sefton-Green, J. (2016). *The class: Living and learning in the digital age*. New York, NY: NYU Press.

Loiperdinger, M. (2004). Lumiere's arrival of the train: Cinema's founding myth. *The Journal of the Association of Moving Image Archivists*, *4*(1), 89–118.

Marsh, J. (2000). Teletubby tales: Popular culture in the early years language and literacy curriculum. *Contemporary Issues in Early Childhood*, *1*(2), 119–133.

Marsh, J., Brooks, G., Hughes, J., Ritchie, L., Roberts, S., & Wright, K. (2005). *Digital beginnings: Young children's use of popular culture, media and new technologies*. Report of the "Young Children's Use of Popular Culture, Media and New Technologies" Study, funded by BBC Worldwide and the Esmée Fairbairn Foundation Literacy Research Centre, University of Sheffield. doi:10.2304/ciec.2000.1.2.2.

Palmer, S. (2006). *Toxic childhood: How the modern world is damaging our children and what we can do about it*. London: Orion.

Panksepp, J. (2004). *Affective neuroscience*. Oxford: Oxford University Press.

Pempek, T. A., Kirkorian, H. L., Richards, J. E., Anderson, D. R., & Lund, A. F. (2010). Video comprehensibility and attention in very young children. *Developmental Psychology*, *46*(5), 1283.

Piaget, J. (1928). *The child's conception of the world*. London: Routledge and Kegan Paul.

Plowman, L., & Stevenson, O. (2013). Exploring the quotidian in young children's lives at home. *Home Cultures*, *10*(3), 329–347.

Robinson, M., & Turnbull, B. (2005). Veronica: An asset model of becoming literate. In J. Marsh (Ed.), *Popular culture, new media and digital literacy in early childhood* (pp. 39–54). Abingdon: Routledge.

Rowe, D. (2008). Social contracts for writing: Negotiating shared understandings about text in the preschool years. *Reading Research Quarterly*, *43*(1), 66–77, 79–95.

Schmidt, M. E., Rich, M., Rifas-Shiman, S. L., Oken, E., & Taveras, E. M. (2009). Television viewing in infancy and child cognition at 3 years of age in a US cohort. *Pediatrics*, *123*, 370–375.

Shapiro, L. A. (2012). Embodied cognition. In E. Margolis, R. Samuels, & S. P. Stich (Eds.), *The Oxford handbook of philosophy of cognitive science* (pp. 118–146). Oxford: Oxford University Press.

Stanton, A. (Director, Co-Writer). (2003). *Finding Nemo* [Movie]. Emeryville, CA: Pixar Animation Studios [Walt Disney Pictures].

Steemers, J. (2010). *Creating preschool television*. Basingstoke: Palgrave Macmillan.

Trevarthen, C., & Aitken, K. J. (2001). Infant intersubjectivity: Research, theory, and clinical applications. *Journal of Child Psychology and Psychiatry*, *42*, 3–48.

Vandewater, E. A., Bickham, D. S., Cummings, H. M., Wartella, E. A., & Rideout, V. J. (2005). When the television is always on: Heavy television exposure and young children's development. *American Behavioral Scientist*, *48*(5), 562–577.

Welland, J. & Heidschtter, U. (Directors). (2011). *The Gruffalo's Child* [Movie]. London, UK: Magic Light Pictures.

Weir, R. H. (1970). *Language in the crib*. The Hague: Mouton.

Wojciechowski, H. C. (2015). The floating world: Film narrative and viewer diakresis. In M. Coegnarts & P. Kravanja (Eds.), *Embodied cognition and cinema* (pp. 115–138). Leuven: Leuven University Press.

Woolley, J. D. (1997). Thinking about fantasy: Are children fundamentally different thinkers and believers from adults? *Child Development*, *68*(6), 991–1011.

Zimmerman, F. J., Christakis, D. A., & Meltzoff, A. N. (2007). Associations between media viewing and language development in children under age 2 years. *Pediatrics*, *161*(5), 364.

12
SIBLINGS ACCOMPLISHING TASKS TOGETHER

Solicited and Unsolicited Assistance When Using Digital Technology

Sandy Houen, Susan Danby, and Pernilla Miller

Introduction

Children are immersed in digital worlds at home with family members, including parents and siblings. They engage in a range of digital practices that include social gaming, information searching, and digital communication such as video conferencing. Almost 20 years ago, Sonia Livingstone (2002) recognised the home as a site for digital media culture and, since then, the global phenomenon of family use of digital technologies has permeated many aspects of family life. It is nearly impossible nowadays to observe everyday family practices without observing family members engaging in digital technologies (Ayaß, 2012). As such, studies of everyday family life involve taking into account the social interactions of family members with each other and with digital technologies. 'Close looking' at digital practices in family life makes possible detailed investigations of particular digital cultural practices as they unfold moment by moment (Marsh & Bishop, 2012).

In everyday life, people help each other to accomplish tasks that may be problematic or unachievable without assistance. Kendrick and Drew (2016) define assistance as "actions by one person that may resolve troubles or difficulties in the progressive realisation of a practical course of action by another" (p. 2). For example, shopkeepers help customers to locate items on the shelf; parents assist toddlers to clean their teeth; siblings help each other when playing games. Young people, older adults, strangers, peers, children, or family members can provide assistance. This chapter illuminates how sibling assistance is sought, offered, provided, and managed in relation to a task underway. The focus is how siblings recruit and provide assistance to each other, showing how assistance is managed *in situ* as they engage with digital technology. It contributes new understandings about how siblings seek assistance from each other, identifying the nature of the assistance provided, and the influences of this assistance in relation to their continued engagement with digital technology and with each other.

Studies of family interactions involving digital technologies have focussed mostly on informal relational networks undertaken through digital media (Marsh et al., 2005; Marsh, Hannon, Lewis, & Ritchie, 2015; Plowman, Stephen, & McPake, 2010). For example, Tiilikainen and Arminen (2017) explored how family members negotiate their expectations and behaviours within the family interactional space of digital media practices. Even with the rapid and worldwide uptake of digital practices in families, there is a comparative absence of studies that seek to understand the actual practices of young children's participation with digital technologies and others in family settings. There are studies that investigate intergenerational everyday practices, often involving parents, children, and grandparents, including family members negotiating digital game play (Aarsand & Aronsson, 2009) and the use of Skype to maintain family contact (Busch, 2018). There are also studies of older children, usually friends, engaged in digital gaming (Piirainen-Marsh, 2012).

Understanding sibling relationships with each other offers the potential for learning about how to co-exist in a shared social world, and often provides the first contexts for learning about social and cognitive worlds (Howe & Recchia, 2014). Absent from many studies of digital life in families is a specific focus on the digital activities of siblings, although there are exceptions. For example, an EU Kids Online study investigated the impact of sibling status to find that older siblings had the effect of increasing the scope and number of online activities with some consequences for exposure to risk online (Olafsson, Green, & Staksrud, 2017). Young children, including siblings, engage and interact with digital technology such as digital gameplaying and edutainment software in order to aid task completion (Danby, Evaldsson, Melander, & Aarsand, 2018; Davidson, 2012). Davidson (2012) shows how "help was mutually accomplished" (p. 196) through siblings using directives to (i) complete a specific action and (ii) provide a list of instructions to achieve upcoming problematic tasks. The social nature of digital activities means that children coordinate their actions to accomplish a task at hand, such as working together to destroy enemies, to enter passwords to enable game play, and to help an inexperienced player engage with the game (Danby et al., 2018). Instructions are a key resource for children, as is collaboration and monitoring others' actions to find a solution. Without an adult present, siblings can experiment and explore the possibilities of digital devices and games, in ways not possible when an adult is present. These digital activities promote independent exploration through use of trial and error, copying and demonstrating (Plowman, McPake, & Stephen, 2008; Wong, 2015). Studies of these activities reveal children's competence in providing assistance when navigating problems associated with using digital technologies. In this chapter, knowledge of young children, who are siblings, and their use of digital technology is extended by describing how they offer assistance, and manage that assistance, as they engage with digital technologies in their home environment.

The approach taken is one that recognises children's *in situ* competences. Competence, from an ethnomethodological perspective, refers to the understanding that children are "competent interpreters in the world" (Mackay, 1991, p. 31). Ethnomethodological and conversation analysis approaches (Heritage, 1984; Sacks, 1992) reveal strategies that siblings use to support each other's digital activities. Ranging in age from two to nine years, siblings at times were participants in a mutually shared digital activity; at other times, while engaged in their own digital activities, they intervened to offer support to their sibling. For instance, there were examples of siblings calling out for help, and receiving solicited (or unsolicited) guidance through verbal and non-verbal means. Also, strategies of problem solving and collaboration were evident across these social interactions.

Recruiting Assistance

In social interaction, assistance involves "recruitment" (Kendrick & Drew, 2016, p. 1). Persons requiring assistance can seek it, while others can volunteer if they infer that help to accomplish a practical action is required. Recruitment of assistance can occur through direct and indirect means, using verbal and semiotic strategies (Kendrick & Drew, 2016, p. 1). Kendrick and Drew (2016, p. 11) conceptualise a continuum of recruitment ranging from direct to indirect methods.

Direct ways are usually explicit verbal requests (e.g., "Can you please get the suitcase down from the top shelf for me?") and reports of trouble (e.g., "I can't reach the suitcase"). Trouble alerts (e.g., "Oh No!") fall between direct and indirect methods as they do not explicitly describe the trouble but allude to problems completing a task at hand. Conversely, indirect ways are not overt and can involve hints, embodied displays of trouble, and others' foreseeing trouble. These indirect ways can prompt an offer or the provision of help (Haugh, 2017; Kendrick & Drew, 2016).

The Study

The data are drawn from approximately 200 hours of video recordings of children's situated activities in home and school collected as part of an Australian longitudinal ethnographic study that investigated young children's use of digital technologies (Danby, 2017; Danby & Davidson, 2019; Danby et al., 2018). Families were purposely selected to include those residing in urban and regional areas of Queensland, and families with different income and educational backgrounds. Parents were asked to video record their children's and family's activities while engaging in digital technologies.

This chapter focusses on sibling interactions from three families as they use digital technology. The siblings are of different age combinations (family one – children aged five and three years; family two – children aged nine and five years; family three – children aged three years and 18 months) and are recorded trying to accomplish an activity that was not pre-determined, rather the activity evolved as the interaction unfolded. Data include dyad sibling interactions that are (i) working cooperatively to progress through levels of a game on the iPad (family one), (ii) collaborating to win a virtual game of tennis (family two), and (iii) locating the cartoon character Peppa Pig (family three).

Conversation analysis was employed to examine data extracts from these families. Conversation analytic research involves creating detailed transcripts that capture verbal (e.g., words spoken, prosody, etc.) and non-verbal aspects of talk (e.g., gaze, gestures, etc.). While these fine-grained transcripts might be difficult to follow at first, their inclusion is necessary due to the analytic claims asserted in the chapter and for critiquing these claims. Table 12.1 details the key transcription conventions employed in this chapter (Hepburn & Bolden, 2017; Jefferson, 2004). Further explanation about conversation analytic transcription practices can be found in published papers (cf. Hepburn & Bolden, 2017; Jefferson, 2004). All participant names in the transcripts are pseudonyms.

The next section presents analyses of five data fragments. *Fragment 1*, *Fragment 2* and *Fragment 3* focus on how siblings offer and manage unsolicited assistance, and *Fragment 4* and *Fragment 5* focus on solicited assistance. Together, these show how siblings manage offers of and requests for assistance and what this means for accomplishing tasks together using digital technology.

Unsolicited Assistance

This section presents three fragments to explore how unsolicited assistance is given. *Fragment 1* and *Fragment 2* are from an extended interaction between siblings from family one (Tina – five years of age and Trae – three years of age) playing the game *Spider: Rite of the Shrouded Moon*, which had been downloaded from the App Store. During this interaction, Tina and Trae are lying side by side, each have their own device and play the same game, but separately, not interactively (see Figure 12.1).

Table 12.1 Key transcription conventions employed in this chapter.

Tin:	Denotes speaker label: Tina
Tra:	Denotes speaker label: Trae
((swipes Trae's screen))	Double parentheses represent physical actions
Tin: [turn on that] Tra: [((lifts arm]	Square brackets indicate overlap – either an overlap of talk or an overlap of physical action. Left square brackets indicate the onset of the overlap and the right indicating the offset of the overlap.
>when< (0.2) ↑aargh:::	A number within parentheses refers to silence, measured to the nearest tenth of a second.
I don't know.	A full stop indicates falling intonation at the end of a unit of talk.
got ya feast first,	A comma indicates slightly rising intonation.
tennis racquet¿	An inverted question mark indicates moderately rising intonation.
↑you're six points more	↑ arrow pointing upwards indicates an intonation spike.
points more than ↓me	↓ arrows pointing downwards indicates an intonation dip.
Maa::arm?	A question mark indicates rising intonation.
ar hum_	An underscore symbol indicates level intonation.
Oh NO!	An exclamation mark indicates animated tone
li:ght	Underlining indicates emphasis in the talk.
argh:::	Colons indicate elongation of the immediately preceding sound. Multiple colons indicate prolonged elongation.
(I don't)	Words encased in single parentheses indicate the transcriber's best guess of an utterance that was unclear to the transcriber.
°that way°	Talk encased in degree symbols indicates whisper talk.
<ar hum_>	Talk encased in <> indicates talk that is spoken slowly.
>ar hum_<	Talk encased in >< indicates talk that is spoken quickly.

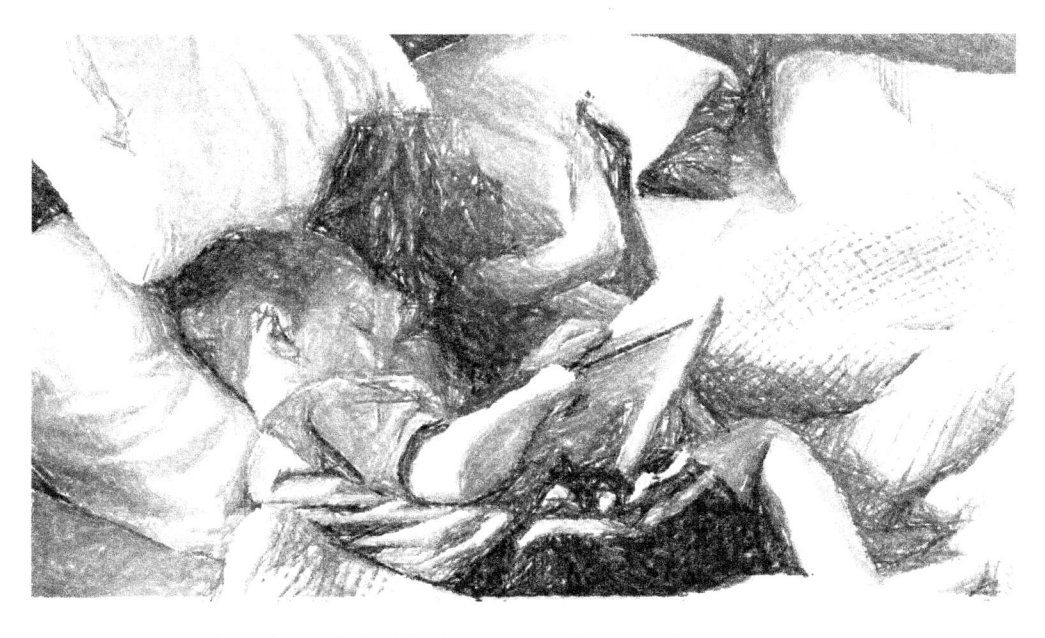

Figure 12.1 Tina and Trae lying side by side playing with their own devices.
Source: see Acknowledgements.

The game involves controlling a spider that searches for, captures, and eats bugs. The first fragment occurs approximately eight minutes into the interaction when Trae's spider is trapped in a cage. He tries three times to release the spider without success. Although he does not explicitly ask for help to rescue the spider, Tina responds to Trae's embodied display of trouble (Kendrick & Drew, 2016) and provides assistance.

```
ARCFF_TXX_270114_00019_10min43-11mins50
103    Tin:    I know how to get [out of the cage             ]
104    Tin:                      [((swipes Trae's screen))]
105    Tra:                      [((watches Tina        ))]
106    Tin:    [((swipes screen, releases spider from cage))]
107    Tra:    [((Trae watches.                             ]
108    Tra:    ((Pushes Tina's hand away=))
109    Tin:    =pt- (°dair you go°)
110            (3.0)((Trae plays game, Tina watches Trae))
```

Fragment 1 Rescuing Trae's trapped spider.

Tina first claims knowledge (Koole, 2010) about how to get the spider out of the cage (line 103). Tina's claim is followed by a demonstration of that knowledge (Koole, 2010) when she swipes the screen and releases the spider from the cage (line 106). While a demonstration might assist Trae to learn how to rescue the spider from the cage, Tina's physical assistance also means that she is in control of the iPad, instead of Trae. Once the spider is released, Trae pushes Tina's hand away from the iPad, signposting that her assistance is no longer required (line 108). Tina accepts Trae's resistance to further help and acknowledges that the task of rescuing the spider is complete by saying, *dair you go* (line 109). She hands Trae control of the device, and he continues playing while Tina watches on.

Fragment 2 occurs just after *Fragment 1*. Here, Tina assists Trae to turn on a light to catch bugs.

```
ARCFF_TXX_270114_00019_10min43-11mins50
116            (3.1)((Trae - swipes screen. Tina watches Trae))]
117    Tin:    do you want to get into the cage
118    Tra:    (°no:: I want to get some bugs°)
119            (1.2)((Trae - swipes screen. Tina watches Trae))]
120    Tra:    (I don't)
121    Tin:    you make a web
122            ((Trae - swipes screen. Tina watches Trae))
123            ((Both Trae and Tina-swipe screen))
124    Tin:    we'll turn on that light=
125    Tin:    [=((presses screen    ))]
126    Tra:    [ ((Trae watches Tina))]
127            (2.1)((Tina presses twice, Trae pushes Tina's hand away))
128    Tra:    ((swipes screen))
129    Tin:    [turn on that              ))] li:ght
130    Tin:    [((lifts arm out of Trae's hold))]
131            (5.0)((Trae plays game, Tina watches Trae))
132    Com:    ((Light turns on screen))
133    Tra:    °mmuck-°
134    Tin:    now you can catch some easy
135            (9.2)(((Trae plays game, Tina watches Trae))
136    Tra:    [((continues playing own game                  ))]
137    Tin:    [((returns gaze at own screen and plays own game))]
```

Fragment 2 Making a web, turning on a light helps to catch bugs.

After watching Trae (line 116), Tina displays her understanding of Trae's focus by asking if he wants to get into the cage (line 117). Trae disagrees and informs her of his current task; to get some bugs (line 118). Here, their differing understandings of the task at hand are revealed. Once Tina is familiar with Trae's goal, they coordinate their subsequent talk to the task of catching some bugs.

Tina first watches Trae swipe the screen for 1.2 seconds. When he does not catch any bugs, she treats this as problematic by issuing a directive to make a web (line 121). As directed, Trae swipes the screen in a manner that looks like he is creating a web (line 122), although, at this point, he seems to be unsuccessful. In response to this embodied display of trouble, Tina upgrades her assistance from a verbal instruction to providing physical support by swiping Trae's screen in tandem with him (line 123). She presents the task as a joint activity, saying, *we'll turn on that light* (line 124). Trae watches while Tina manipulates the screen, but she too fails to activate the light. After 2.1 seconds, Trae manages Tina's assistance by pushing and holding her hand away, indicating that her turn to turn on the light is over, and that he now wants to reclaim the iPad (line 127). In response, Tina downgrades her physical aid to verbal support via a directive telling him to turn on that light (line 129). Trae swipes the screen continuously and activates the light (line 132). Tina then provides an upshot formulation (Antaki, 2008; Baraldi, 2014), *now you can catch some easy* (line 134). The upshot formulation assesses the past action of turning on the light with future action; that catching bugs will be easy, because the bugs are presumably attracted to the light, bringing closure to this sequence. Tina watches Trae as he plays the game for 9 seconds before returning focus to her own screen (line 136–137). This action indicates that Trae no longer needs assistance to catch bugs.

The next fragment, *Fragment 3*, is of siblings from family two in the lounge room of their family home (see Figure 12.2), who collaborate to enable the brother to win a virtual game of tennis. The motion-sensing console allows users to control their avatar using body movements; for instance, when the child jumps, their avatar also jumps.

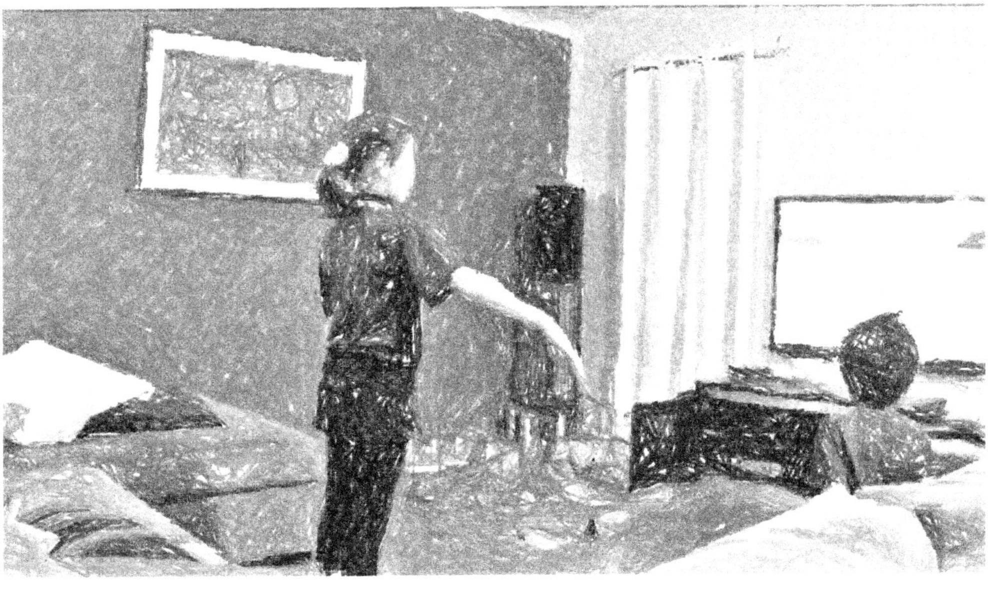

Figure 12.2 Siblings playing a motion-sensor-based virtual tennis game.
Source: see Acknowledgements.

The extract commences 12 minutes into an interaction between siblings Jett and Lara who wait for the screen to display the previous game's scorecard. Once displayed, a new game begins loading. As the game loads, Lara offers unsolicited assistance to Jett to help him win the game. While it is unclear why Lara is willing to let Jett win, it might be because she is playing consecutive games, and not taking the game play in turns, as is done typically.

```
ARCFF_JXX_150914_00016_12min37-14mins20
501  Lar:      Jett >do ya want me to ↓win< fa you?
502             (0.5)
503  Jet:      >ar hum_<
504             (0.3)
505  Lar:       okay ((squats with hands on knees))
506             (1.6)
507             [(2.3)                                                 ]
508  Lar:      [(( as game loads makes noises, reaches hands through legs))]
509             (1.0)
510             [(1.5)                                                 ]
511  Jet:      [((waves hands in front of tv, makes noises as game loads))]
512  Lar:      °move backwards.°
513             [(1.1)                                                 ]
514  TV :      [((character appears as count down to start of game occurs))]
515  Lar:      Jett move_ ((waves hand to indicate to Jett to move away))
516  Jet:      ((sits back on couch))
517  Lar:      >°that way_°<
518  Jet:      ((jumps up and down once on couch, sits back on the couch))
519  Lar:      ((holds arm horizontal to floor))
520  Jet:      >when<(.2)↑argh::: ↓almost wred.
521            ((games commences - virtual tennis ball approaches Lara)
522  Lar:      ((swings arm to hit the virtual tennis ball))
523  Jet:      I don't know when you'll- (0.5) neva (wed pen).
524             (2.7)
525  Lar:      ((swings arm forward))
526  Jet:      >why do you have >>a red<<< tennis racquet¿
527  Lar:      ((swings arm forward - hits virtual ball))
528  Lar:      I don't know.
529             [(7.6)            ]
530  Lar:      [((swings arm twice))]
531  Jet:      ((leaves room to find his mother to ask for some milk))
  .           [(40.9)((interaction stops while Jett leaves the room.
(40.9)  }     Lara continues playing the game while Jett is out of the
              room.   ))]
532  Lar:      [((Lara keeps playing, swinging her arm to hit tennis balls))]
533            ((game ends. processing score card))
534  Jet:      ((off camera)) (>wahya< did not_)
535             [(0.85)                    ]
536             [((scorecard to be displayed))]
537  Lar:      ((gazes towards Jett)) okay (.) >let's see< who'll win.
538  Jet:      ((re-enters camera shot))
539             [(0.4)            ]
540  TV :      [((displays score card))]
541  Lar:      ((drops on couch, makes pretend crying sounds))=
542  Lar:      ya:↑how:::::::::↓ow::: ↑you're six points more than ↓me:.
543             (1.1)
544  Lar:      are you (cazsh)with that¿
545  Jet:      ah ha ((nods yes))
546  TV :      ((games loads new sport to play))
547  ???:     °wait°
548  ???:     This time you can swim by yourself_
```

Fragment 3 Winning the virtual tennis game.

Lara names Jett as the recipient of her offer of assistance aimed at winning the game by asking, *Jett >do ya want me to ↓win< fa you?* (line 501). Although Lara's assistance is unsolicited, Jett accepts her offer (line 503). Lara uses the change of state token, *okay* (line 505), to acknowledge his acceptance and to agree that their current focus is on Jett winning the game.

While the game loads, Lara and Jett make noises, reach their hands through their legs and wave their hands in front of the television (lines 506–511). Just before the game loads, Lara quietly instructs Jett to move backwards (line 512). This instruction may have been in response to previous technical trouble they encountered when Jett was standing too close to Lara, and the game console picked up Jett's movements instead of Lara's. When Jett does not move, Lara names Jett as the recipient and tells him to move (line 515). This time, Jett follows her instruction and moves slightly out of the way. Lara motions with her hand and quietly instructs him to move *that way* (line 517). He sits further back on the couch. Lara anticipates play by holding her arm horizontally (line 519). As the game commences, Lara swings her arms to control the onscreen tennis racket. While she plays, Jett asks her why she has a red tennis racket (line 526). Lara responds to Jett's question saying, *I don't know* (line 528), perhaps suggesting she does not want to engage in a general discussion at present. This non-engagement might have something to do with her current focus on winning the game for her brother.

Jett leaves the interaction and returns 40 seconds later, as the game processes the score card (line 536). Lara gazes towards Jett and again uses the change of state token, *okay* (line 537) to connect the prior action of playing the game with the focus of winning the game for Jett (line 537). Jett re-enters the camera view as the scorecard is displayed. Next, we see Lara flop onto the couch (line 541) and pretend to cry, *ya:↑how:::::::::↓ow:::* (line 542). She announces to Jett that he is six points ahead of her and she asks if he is *cazsh* (okay) with that (line 544). Here it emerges that the competition to win is between Jett and his sister rather than Jett and the game. He confirms that he is okay with that. This additional information might suggest that Lara's offer to help Jett win might have been a strategy employed by her to gain an additional turn to play the game. She does this in a way that secures Jett's affiliation and alleviates potential conflict relating to turn taking.

The first three fragments in this chapter show how unsolicited assistance is provided by siblings to support accomplishment of a task at hand. The next section uses two fragments to show how siblings solicit and respond to assistance requested.

Solicited Assistance

Two fragments (*Fragment 4* and *Fragment 5*) are used to capture siblings' solicitations for assistance. *Fragment 4* is a continuation of *Fragment 2* where Tina has established that catching bugs is easy to do with a light on. They continue to play *Spider: Rite of the Shrouded Moon*.

```
ARCFF_TXX_270114_00019_11mins50-13mins
140              (5.3)((both play game on own device))
141     Tra:     [where's that li:↓ght.          ]
142              [((both gaze at own devices))]
143              (0.2)((both play game on own device))
144     Tra:     [(°°Tina°°) °<where's that li:↓ght.>°]
145              [((both play game on own device))   ]
146     Tra:     (xxxx)
147     Tin:     [((gazes at Trae's screen      ))]
148     Tra:     [((continues playing game      ))]
149     Tin:     I >show °you°< ((moves to hold Trae's iPad and point))
150     Tra:     [>nn↑argh-<.          ]
151     Tra:     [((pushes Tina's arm))]=
```

```
152   Tin:    =[>De light< is back °dair.°]
153   Tra:    [holds left arm up            ]((RH continues playing game))
154   Tin:    [°°the°° li:ght isn't over here,      ]
155   Tra:    [((continues swiping screen      ))]
156           (4.1)((Tina watches Trae play game))
157   Tin:    [(°>have you<°)got ya feast first,   ]
158   Tin:    [((watches Trae's screen   ))]
159   Tra:    [((continues playing game))]
160           (2.1)((Tina watches Trae play game))
```

Fragment 4 Finding another light, locating a feast and catching bugs.

As they play individual games on their own devices, Trae solicits Tina's assistance to find another light to catch more bugs. He asks, *where's that light?* (line 141). Shortly after, he reinitiates his call for help, naming Tina as the recipient of his request (line 144). First, Tina offers physical assistance, saying, *I'll show you* (line 149), and moves to take the iPad from him (line 149). Tina's physical aid could result in her taking control of the iPad and Trae halts playing the game. Trae declines her offer by saying *nnargh* (line 150) and pushing her arm away (line 151). Next, Tina downgrades her assistance from a physical demonstration to a verbal telling, informing him where he may find the light (line 152). The upshot of this verbal assistance means that Trae maintains control of the iPad and can continue playing the game. It also means that Trae can either accept or decline the verbal assistance offered by Tina. Trae continues swiping the screen, does not follow Tina's directions (line 155), and fails to find it. Tina reformulates her verbal assistance and tells him that the light is not where he is (line 154). She watches Trae play for 4.1 seconds before initiating a sequence of talk that focusses not on finding the light, but on getting a feast of bugs first (line 157). Finding a feast becomes their new focus. Although not captured in the extract, the interaction continues with Trae finding a feast. Amid the feast, he locates a light that attracts many bugs. Tina provides further instructions about making a web to catch them. After trial and error, Trae makes a web and captures some bugs.

Fragment 5 captures a younger sibling assisting his older brother. While Emanual (three years of age) has solicited help from his mother to locate Peppa Pig, it is Emanual's younger sibling Zavier (18 months of age) who assists in accomplishing the task at hand. Zavier is located nearby using a touchscreen laptop located in the family lounge room (see Figure 12.3). He is scrolling through the menu on the YouTube Junior website. As he swipes the screen, different sounds and voices play. Emanual is off camera, but can be heard asking his mother to find Peppa Pig.

```
ARCFF_DBX_2013_00005_50sec to 1min30
001           (2.0)((younger brother swipes laptop screen with LF scrolling
002           Youtube menu)
003   Ema:    Maa::arm?
004           (1.0)((Zav: swipes left-moves through You Tube catalogue))
005   Ema:    MU:M_
006           (1.4)[((Zavier: swipes screen to the left))]
007   Zav:         [vaa::rp                             ]
008   Ema:    Wis maa:::  [peppa pig     ]fing.
009   Zav:                [((turns head))]((continues swiping screen))
010   ???:    nnno.
011   Zav:    ((swipes screen))
012   Com:    ((catalogue displays a Peppa Pig image))
013   Zav:    dai↑r::?=
014   Zav:    =((points at Peppa Pig image gazes around))
015   Zav:    ((gazes back at screen))
016   Ema:    ((stands beside brother))
```

Siblings Accomplishing Tasks Together

```
017   Com:     fr::(.)[og(.)    ]
018   Ema:            [°press it°]=
019   Ema:     =((presses Peppa Pig image))
020   Com:     ((displays Peppa Pig hyperlink))
021   Com:     ((Starts playing Peppa Pig clip))
022   Com:     [frog]
023   Zav:     [Her↑][ar:: >erpa< pig.            ]
024   Zav:            [((raises hands above head))]
```

Fragment 5 Locating Peppa Pig.

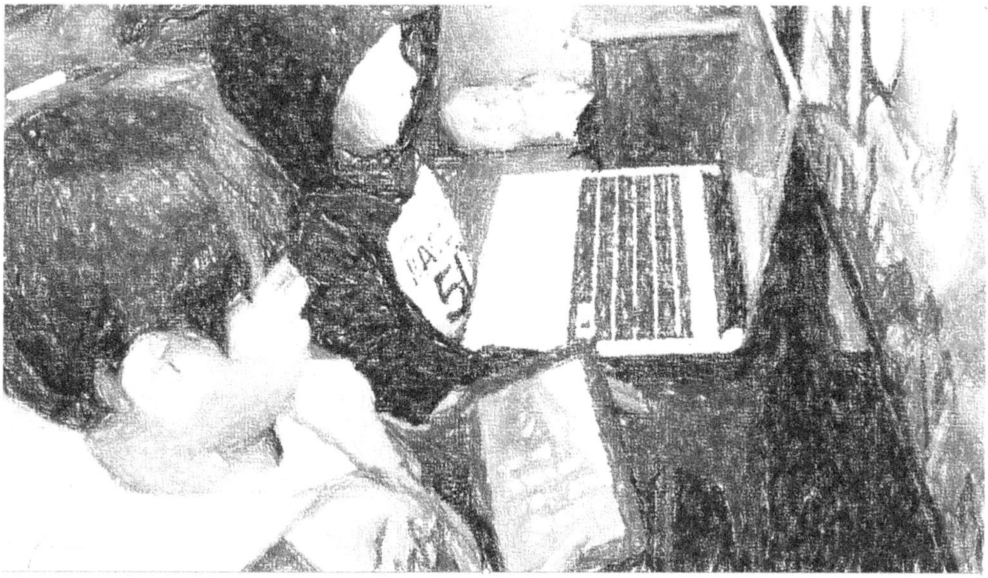

Figure 12.3 Siblings navigating YouTube Junior.
Source: see Acknowledgements.

Fragment 5 commences with Emanual seeking assistance to find Peppa Pig. Although Emanual's query is directed at his mother (lines 3 and 4), his younger brother Zavier gazes (line 9) towards Emanual when he asks about Peppa Pig's location (line 8). This gaze suggests that Zavier overhears Emanual's request for help (line 8). Zavier's focus returns to the computer screen and he continues swiping through the YouTube menu. While it is unclear whether the younger brother intentionally sets out to find Peppa Pig, when one is displayed on the screen he announces, *Dair* (line 13), and points to the Peppa Pig image (line 14). Having located Peppa Pig, Zavier has accomplished assisting Emanual. Emanual accepts the assistance when he stands beside his younger brother (line 16) and says, *press it* (line 18). At first, Emanual's turn looks to be an instruction for his younger brother, but it is Emanual who quickly presses the image to play the clip. The two brothers stand beside each other when the clip begins to play. Zavier displays his excitement by raising his hands above his head saying, *Her↑//ar:: >erpa< pig* (line 23).

In this fragment, the task of finding Peppa Pig was accomplished when a younger sibling volunteered and successfully provided aid to his older sibling after overhearing Emanual's request for help; a request that was initially directed towards their mother.

Discussion

The family setting is an ideal context for understanding how siblings engage with each other and with digital technology. These data fragments and accompanying analysis show that siblings' digital activities include instances where they are engaged socially. A close analysis of children's social interactions shows how they collaboratively achieved a task when they build upon shared knowledge, and produce different kinds of digital practices. Across all of the interactions discussed, recruiting and accepting assistance led to a shared social enterprise (Danby et al., 2018). Verbal strategies that seek and offer assistance can happen via a variety of interactional means, such as "requesting", *would you/could you* (Curl & Drew, 2008) and *do you want me to* (Curl, 2006). Davidson (2012) specifically looked at the social organisation of help during young siblings' use of the computer to reveal that, in addition to talk such as issuing instructions, assistance also could be achieved through multimodal actions, for example pointing a finger at the relevant point on the computer screen.

The siblings' offering and seeking assistance from each other occurred through talk and multimodal action. Solicited assistance was achieved via questions, such as "where's that light" (*Fragment 4*) or "where's my Peppa Pig" (*Fragment 5*). Unsolicited assistance was offered in response to observed potential, or embodied displays of, trouble in accomplishing the task at hand. Most assistance was offered through verbal strategies, such as issuing directives, but physical strategies were also used, such as swiping the screen or taking the device to accomplish the task at hand. *Fragment 1*, for instance, showed Trae taking 1.2 seconds without accomplishing the task of rescuing the spider, which prompted Tina to treat this as an embodied display of trouble. She responded by trying to assist him by swiping the screen. In this case, physical assistance required the original game player to hand over control of the device. There is always a risk of handing over control of the device as this may result in (i) disengagement with the task at hand or (ii) losing the device to the other sibling, which may require the original player to do additional work to re-establish control of the device. For example, when Lara (*Fragment 3*) played the game so that Jett could win, Jett left the room, seemingly no longer engaged. He returned as the game ended and the scorecard was displayed. In *Fragment 1*, Trae managed Tina's physical assistance by pushing her hand away, ensuring control of the device remained with him.

In returning to the data fragments discussed in the previous section, *Fragment 2* is now reused to illustrate how assistance giving is modified based on the siblings' prior turns of interaction. Using *Fragment 2*, we developed Figure 12.4 to provide a diagrammatic summary of how assistance was modified based on the other sibling's uptake (or not) of assistance, either verbal or nonverbal.

At the start of *Fragment 2*, when Trae was initially unsuccessful, Tina modified her assistance in three ways. First, she presented the task as a joint activity, using the pronoun "we'll" (line 124). Second, she modified her instruction to "we'll turn on that light" (line 124) and third, she provided physical assistance by tapping the screen. This physical assistance provided Trae with a demonstration of what he should be doing. After Trae pushed her hand away, he showed that he no longer needed physical assistance and, instead, he copied her demonstration. Recognising that Trae was still unsuccessful, Tina tried another strategy, which was to revert back to offer assistance verbally by issuing a modified instruction. This strategy was ultimately successful.

In these sibling interactions, the provision of assistance, whether solicited or unsolicited, was negotiated and managed as part of the unfolding interaction. This was the case even when the assistance provided was unsuccessful or rejected. Assistance, whether offered or requested, successful or not, is negotiated and managed through a co-constructed accomplishment of social interaction including talk and non-verbal actions.

```
Verbal assistance offered via an instruction to Trae
```

```
121    Tin:    you make a web
```

Assistance, via instruction, was unsuccessful. Trae did not make a web.

```
Assistance is modified, modifying both the instruction and upgrading her assistance from
verbal to physical. Additionally, Tina presents the task at hand as a joint one ('we'll turn
                                  on that light').
```

```
124    Tin:    we'll turn on that light=
125    Tin:    [=((tapping screen))]
126    Tra:    [((watches Tina        ))]
127    Tin:    ((Tina presses twice, Trae pushes Tina's=
                =hand away))
```

Physical assistance is managed by Trae who after 2.1 seconds pushes Tina's hand away.

```
While Tina's physical assistance was unsuccessful in turning on the light, it provided Trae
with a demonstration of what he should be doing. Trae manages Tina's assistance by
pushing her hand away indicating that he no longer needs her physical assistance.
```

```
128    Tra:    ((swipes screen))
```

Trae copies Tina's actions, but is still unsuccessful at turning on the light.

```
Tina once again modifies the type of assistance provided and reverts to verbal assistance
                      by issuing a modified instruction
```

```
129    Tin:    [turn on that             ))] li:ght
130    Tin:    [((lifts arm out of Trae's hold ))]
131            (5.0) ((Trae plays game, Tina watches Trae))
132    Com:    ((Tina presses twice, Trae pushes Tina's hand away))
```

Figure 12.4 Revisiting *Fragment 2*: the management and negotiation of assistance.
Source: the authors.

Conclusion

There is a common assumption that children do not need to be taught about technology; rather parents often suggest that children "automatically pick it up" (Plowman et al., 2008). Plowman et al. (2008) point out that parents often do not explicitly tutor their children in digital engagement, but that it is through family practices that children acquire digital literacy skills, how to find information, and the cultural practices of digital life in families. This chapter has extended these descriptions of family life to show how siblings do not just pick up skills and dispositions when using digital devices and digital games. As demonstrated in close detail through analysis of siblings engaged in different kinds of digital activity, children take on roles and interactions, both verbal and nonverbal, that provide participatory spaces to observe and interact with each other when using digital devices. Here, the siblings' acts of assistance, both solicited and unsolicited, and requests for assistance, make possible the introduction and demonstration of a range of technical digital literacy skills. Just as important, though, is that sibling participation make possible relationships that support familial social and emotional closeness.

In contributing to understandings of sibling interactions as they engaged with digital technology in home environments, this chapter shows how siblings sought and provided assistance in their social interactions with each other. To complete the digital task at hand, the siblings used a variety of interactional strategies that provided assistance. There is no suggestion that interactional strategies that solicit or provide unsolicited assistance are unique to sibling interactions. Even so, within the home context, children who also happen to be siblings may engage with digital technology without adults present, while socially producing their sibling relationship.

Acknowledgements

Susan Danby was awarded an Australian Research Council Future Fellowship (FT120100731) for this study. Ethical approval by Queensland University of Technology's Human Research Ethics Committee. Children's images were taken from the video footage. Picture formatting and artistic effect tools in MS PowerPoint™ were used to convert the image to a sketch, making participants de-identifiable. We sincerely thank the children and families for their participation in this study.

References

Aarsand, P. A., & Aronsson, K. (2009). Gaming and territorial negotiations in family life. *Childhood*, *16*(4), 497–517. doi:10.1177/0907568209343879.
Antaki, C. (2008). Formulations in psychotherapy. In A. Peräkylä, C. Antaki, S. Vehviläinen, & I. Leudar (Eds.), *Conversation analysis and psychotherapy* (pp. 26–42). Cambridge: Cambridge University Press. doi:10.1017/CBO9780511490002.003.
Ayaß, R. (2012). Introduction: Media appropriation and everyday life. In R. Ayaß & C. Gerhardt (Eds.), *The appropriation of media in everyday life* (pp. 1–15). Amsterdam: John Benjamins Publishing Company.
Baraldi, C. (2014). Formulations in dialogic facilitation of classroom interactions. *Language and Dialogue*, *4*(2), 234–260. doi:10.1075/ld.4.2.04bar.
Busch, G. (2018). How families use video communication strategies during intergenerational Skype sessions. In S. Danby, M. Fleer, C. Davidson, & M. Hatzigianni (Eds.), *Digital childhoods: Technologies and children's everyday lives* (pp. 17–32). Singapore: Springer.
Curl, T. S. (2006). Offers of assistance: Constraints on syntactic design. *Journal of Pragmatics*, *38*(8), 1257–1280. doi:10.1016/j.pragma.2005.09.004.
Curl, T. S., & Drew, P. (2008). Contingency and action: A comparison of two forms of requesting. *Research on Language & Social Interaction*, *41*(2), 129–153. doi:10.1080/08351810802028613.
Danby, S. (2017). Technologies, child-centred practice and listening to children. In L. Arnott (Ed.), *Digital technologies and learning in the early years* (pp. 127–138). London: Sage. doi:10.4135/9781526414502.n11.

Danby, S., & Davidson, C. (2019). Webs of relationships: Young children's engagement with web searching. In R. Flewitt, O. Erstad, B. Kümmerling-Meibauer, & I. Pires Pereira (Eds.), *Routledge handbook of digital literacies in early childhood* (pp. 402–415). London: Routledge.

Danby, S., Evaldsson, A.-C., Melander, H., & Aarsand, P. (2018). Situated collaboration and problem solving in young children's digital gameplay. *British Journal of Educational Technology*, *49*(5), 957–972. doi:10.1111/bjet.12636.

Davidson, C. (2012). The social organisation of help during young children's use of the computer. *Contemporary Issues in Early Childhood*, *13*(3), 187–199. doi:10.2304/ciec.2012.13.3.187.

Haugh, M. (2017). Prompting offers of assistance in interaction. *Pragmatics and Society*, *8*(2), 183–207. doi:10.1075/ps.8.2.02hau.

Hepburn, A., & Bolden, G. B. (2017). Getting started with transcription. In A. Hepburn & G. B. Bolden (Eds.), *Transcribing for social research* (pp. 13–20). London: Sage. doi:10.4135/9781473920460.n2.

Heritage, J. (1984). *Garfinkel and ethnomethodology*. Cambridge: Polity Press.

Howe, N., & Recchia, H. (2014). Sibling relationships as a context for learning and development. *Early Education & Development*, *25*(2), 155–159. doi:10.1080/10409289.2014.857562.

Jefferson, G. (2004). Glossary of transcript symbols with an introduction. In G. H. Lerner (Ed.), *Conversation analysis : Studies from the first generation* (pp. 13–31). Amsterdam and Philadelphia, PA: John Benjamins Publishing Company.

Kendrick, K. H., & Drew, P. (2016). Recruitment: Offers, requests, and the organisation of assistance in interaction. *Research on Language and Social Interaction*, *49*(1), 1–19. doi:10.1080/08351813.2016.1126436.

Koole, T. (2010). Displays of epistemic access: Student responses to teacher explanations. *Research on Language & Social Interaction*, *43*(2), 183–209. doi:10.1080/08351811003737846.

Livingstone, S. (2002). *Young people and new media: Childhood and the changing media environment*. London: Sage.

Mackay, R. W. (1991). Conceptions of children and models of socialization. In F. C. Waksler (Ed.), *Studying the social worlds of children: Sociological readings* (pp. 23–37). London: Falmer Press.

Marsh, J., & Bishop, J. (2012). Rewind and replay? Television and play in the 1950s/1960s and 2010s. *International Journal of Play*, *1*(3), 279–291. doi:10.1080/21594937.2012.741431.

Marsh, J., Brooks, G., Hughes, J., Ritchie, L., Roberts, S., & Wright, K. (2005). *Digital beginnings: Young children's use of popular culture, media and new technologies*. University of Sheffield, Literacy Research Centre. Retrieved from: https://esmeefairbairn.org.uk/digital-beginnings.

Marsh, J., Hannon, P., Lewis, M., & Ritchie, L. (2015). Young children's initiation into family literacy practices in the digital age. *Journal of Early Childhood Research*, *15*(1), 47–60. doi:10.1177/1476718X15582095.

Olafsson, K., Green, L., & Staksrud, E. (2017). Is big brother more at risk than little sister? The sibling factor in online risk and opportunity. *New Media & Society*, *20*(4), 1–18. doi:10.1177/1461444817691531.

Piirainen-Marsh, A. (2012). Organising participation in video gaming activities. In R. Ayaß & C. Gerhardt (Eds.), *The appropriation of media in everyday life* (pp. 197–230). Amsterdam: John Benjamins Publishing Company.

Plowman, L., McPake, J., & Stephen, C. (2008). Just picking it up? Young children learning with technology at home. *Cambridge Journal of Education*, *38*(3), 303–319. doi:10.1080/03057640802287564.

Plowman, L., Stephen, C., & McPake, J. (2010). *Growing up with technology: Young children learning in a digital world*. London: Routledge.

Sacks, H. (1992). *Lectures on conversation, Volumes I and II*. Oxford: Blackwell.

Tiilikainen, S., & Arminen, I. (2017). Together individually. In A. R. Lahikainen, T. Mälkiä, & K. Repo (Eds.), *Media, family interaction and the digitalization of childhood* (pp. 155–172). Cheltenham: Edward Elgar.

Wong, S. S.-H. (2015). Mobile digital devices and preschoolers' home multiliteracy practices. *Language and Literacy*, *17*(2), 75–90.

13
CHILDREN AS ARCHITECTS OF THEIR DIGITAL WORLDS

Joanne O'Mara, Linda Laidlaw, and Suzanna So Har Wong

Introduction

Given current sweeping changes in digital literacies, children need to acquire knowledge and proficiencies to navigate a constantly changing, complex digital world (Berger et al., 2001). Across the globe, a general consensus exists that classrooms need to shift the 20th-century models upon which they were originally designed and remain predominantly structured, in response to these changes. School systems worldwide are addressing new digital challenges (Burnett & Merchant, 2016; DEEWR, 2012; Gov't of Alberta, 2016; Sahlberg, 2015), and beginning to acknowledge, understand, and address the ways in which children's own digital agency, usage, and proficiency are also shifting.

Recent developments in mobile device technologies enable young people to access and contribute to digital media and the social worlds around them from early childhood. They are able to extend their play across digital and physical worlds in ways that were not previously possible (Marsh, 2010; Rowsell, Saudelli, McQuirter-Scott, & Bishop, 2013). This chapter's authors have been investigating how the relationships across language, literacy, and literature in the curriculum have been impacted in the digital era. This work finds that young people constantly shift between/across/through these communication forms as they text/design/produce/phone/play games/talk with each other, often simultaneously. The children and young people focussed on have shifted their textual dispositions, mirroring Carrington's (2017) research suggesting that the boundaries between the digital and 'offline' realms are blurring, and that the metaphors for online/offline may no longer be valid. Moving from the stability of the printed word to the ephemerality of digital texts, textual genres are constantly morphing and young people are developing both new and traditional digital literacy and design skills through their digital play (Laidlaw & Wong, 2016; O'Mara, 2017; O'Mara & Laidlaw, 2011; Rowsell, 2014; Yelland, 2015) as they become architects of their digital worlds.

This chapter considers how children can become architects of their digital worlds and the ways that the adults around them might support this. It draws on three case studies from Australia and Canada to illustrate ways in which young people aged 5 to 10 years old design and create within open-ended applications, and describes how schools might utilise young people's engagement with these applications to develop digital literacy, design, and coding skills.

The term 'digital literacies' is used to refer to literacy practices that are digitally and technologically mediated, as children access, use, analyse, produce, and share texts and other artefacts

(Marsh, 2005; Merchant, 2015; Pahl & Rowsell, 2010; Sheridan & Rowsell, 2010; Walsh, 2011), drawing from the maker movement to inform this research. The maker movement refers to an approach that embraces creative production by providing the technologies, resources, and materials to make texts and objects through experimentation and problem-solving (e.g., Halverson & Sheridan, 2014; Peppler & Bender, 2013). Students engage in 'making' and producing different kinds of texts and objects, and then reflect upon their processes. These processes inform new ways of thinking about literacy learning and teaching, particularly where children and youth are able to respond to the affordances of digital media to produce, design, and even make widely public their own digital texts and products. The metaphor of 'the architect'[1] is used to represent the requirements for effective digital literacy learning – where students are cast in the role of designers, producers, problem-solvers, and innovative thinkers, and can be working to develop spatial literacies and concepts in three-dimensional spaces, and with a range of materials and media, both virtual and actual.

Unboxing Dot and Dash: Creating Imaginary Worlds through Coding and Digital Play

The first example draws from a case that is part of a longitudinal study of home and 'out of school' literacy practices. In this case, Suzanna began observing and gathering literacy data from a set of twin girls in Canada when they were three years of age. The authors have continued to follow the girls' digital literacy interests and engagements, and, in the example focussed on here, they are now ten years old. Olivia and Hannah have been active and curious users of a range of technologies (iPods, iPads, laptop computers) from the time Suzanna began observing them when they were younger and perhaps even earlier. While older now, they have remained interested in creating and producing their own play materials, both digital and traditional print based. As three-year-old children they owned individual iPods and before the end of the initial study phase, which followed them for two years, they also began to use iPads. Their mother gave them a small amount of pocket money every month for buying apps (applications) and they learned to pool their resources and share the games and apps they purchased to increase their play options. Fast forward to more recent times and the girls continue to show resourcefulness, interest, and curiosity about 'making' and technology. Their mother is a library technician for a city library 'maker space' and former teacher. The girls are being home schooled due to their mother's interest in teaching and her belief that she can support their engagement and deep learning. Home schooling or 'parent directed learning' is an option that receives support and funding from the local school district, with a significant portion of participating families choosing this option due to the desire for flexible instruction. Both girls also attend some classes at a school district centre that offers support for home-schooled children.

The following vignette occurred when Olivia and Hannah were invited to visit Linda and Suzanna's literacy lab at the University of Alberta to try out some new robotic and 'maker' resources. They chose to 'unbox' the 'Wonder Pack' that contained the small robots Dot and Dash and 'challenge cards' for beginning to use coding to work with the robots (www.makewonder.com). Dash is a small interactive and mobile robot than can be programmed to respond to voices and sounds, while Dot can be programmed to create a range of different interactive games. The girls commented that Suzanna and Linda should make a video of their 'unboxing' (see Marsh, 2016 for further description of the 'unboxing' phenomena) and were keen to have their robotic activities recorded. While Olivia and Hannah had extensive experience working with iPads and a range of computer games, they had never worked with robotics previously, and the 'Dot and Dash' robots were new to them. They were keen to work in the role of 'testers' for these new activities. Their 'unboxing' and initial activities were filmed as part of data gathering and also because the girls were keen to have their experiences recorded.

After they open the kit, Hannah and Olivia intently examine the interface on the two iPads (Suzanna and Linda had previously uploaded the Wonder app (www.makewonder.com/apps/wonder):

> Hannah decided she would work with 'Dash', while Olivia was in charge of 'Dot'. They explore, poke, tap on the iPads and review information on the coding cards. They make some changes to personalise the robots, modifying their eye colours, and give the robots new names. After observing and testing out how the robots can respond to simple commands via the iPad, Hannah sets Dash on the floor in order to explore the little robot's capabilities – playing with movement and sound options. Hannah makes Dash roll quickly down the long hallway alongside Linda and Suzanna's department colleagues' offices. Hannah explores the sound options and learns how to make Dash bark like a dog, and make other animal sounds, but no adults come out to investigate the curious sounds outside their closed office doors. 'Hmmm,' reflects Hannah, 'You know, we could record someone knocking on the door and see if *that* gets someone's attention . . .'. She brings the little robot to our work space and records herself knocking loudly on the door. With a mischievous smile, she sends Dash gliding back down the hallway, where he 'knocks' on a colleague's door. Eventually there is a response from a neighbouring office, and an adult peers out in response to the 'knocking'. Hannah, in a fit of giggles, hurries back into the literacy lab, making Dash run behind, before our confused colleague can sort out what has just taken place.

While this first 'case' example is a simple one – two young girls who are exploring coding through the 'Dot' and 'Dash' robot characters – it was selected as a representation of how easily and quickly children can begin to design and create an imaginary 'world' through digital play. For these girls, the experience was connected to exploration of a new digital device (the robots) 'having a bit of fun' and playing a trick on the adults. For them, learning some new digital skills (simple coding) was secondary to working with the devices in a way that extended their own social and play preferences, with Hannah actively trying to engage others in her 'game' with Dash, and Olivia working individually to program Dot to play a game she would show later to her sister and mother. As they learned how the robots operated and explored some of the possibilities through coding on the 'challenge cards', they brought their own interests and capabilities to the activities, and subsequently have communicated with Suzanna that they would like to return to test out some new ideas they have for working with the robots.

As Marsh (2016) suggests, the relationship between children's online and offline practices deserves consideration, which can be extended further to digital and non-digital learning and play in this example. The realm of digital learning – that of interpreting basic coding instructions and working with the iPads to operate the robots – for the two girls was interconnected with their desire to engage in mischievous play, and also perhaps to engage in a 'performance' to show the adults (researchers, parent, and the colleagues 'down the hall') that they had agency and control over what the robots could do. The girls' 'unboxing' and exploration of the devices and the capacities of the robots quickly shifted to social engagements, with each other and also extending an invitation for others (even outsiders) to play by luring them to open their office doors. Significantly, the ten-year-old children rapidly figured out how to engage with the robots and get them to perform particular tasks, and they learned how to use the coding instructions very quickly. This was in stark contrast to observations of a group of teachers invited to test out the Dot and Dash; the adults took much longer to figure out how to work very basically with the robots and, unlike the two children, spent much longer reading instructions before getting started and were more hesitant about physically touching and engaging with the devices.

Designing a Sustainable Present: Teachers Enabling *Minecraft* Worldmaking

Along with the introduction of robotics such as Dot and Dash in schools, there has been an increase in schools using open-world digital games where players can create virtual worlds and interact with the world in the classroom. These games, such as *Minecraft* (Mojang, 2011), are readily adaptable to a wide range of curriculum usages, whereas linear games are often less adaptable to classroom usage. In *Minecraft*, players build using blocks – designing, creating, and making their own world. There are many different modifications in the game, enabling some customisation, and also a huge array of materials that can be mined, grown, and sourced. As well as being persistently and overwhelmingly popular with young people, having reportedly over 91 million players per month (Statistica, 2019), *Minecraft* offers multiple affordances to schools with a wide array of curriculum possibilities. It has been used in maths to create a scale replica of a school and to make scale models of rooms, in history to create a replica of historic locations such as the Globe Theatre and ancient Rome, and to create designs for sustainable housing. The ways in which the game's affordances might be drawn upon, particularly the passion and dedication many young people have to the game, and the possibility of drawing on this to create impassioned learning (Dezuanni & O'Mara, 2017), enables children to operate as literal architects in creating collaboratively a digital world.

Jo researched the development of a *Minecraft* unit with a group of over 130 Grade 5/6 students in an Australian primary school. In this unit the students worked collaboratively to design a new, sustainable virtual world in *Minecraft*. The teachers designed this unit (approximately 80 hours altogether over 10 weeks) following a 'Spaceship Earth'-styled scenario (see, for example, Morgan & Saxton, 1989), where the Earth is destroyed and there is an opportunity create a new, utopian version. In this case, the planet is in chaos due to the effects of human-induced climate change: loss of food and drinking water, and an exponential increase in the rate of natural disasters lead to civil unrest, poverty, and spread of disease. Throughout this unit, the students were given opportunities to 'terraform', design and create the new planet, and the design included both structural and societal aspects of life there. In preparation for leaving Earth, everyone designed a spaceship. In doing this, the young people drew upon their knowledge from both science and science fiction, merging the scientific and the fictive together in their designs, and drawing on their imaginings of what they might need for the journey – how to prepare, what they might need to bring to the new planet, and what was important to them. This activity deepened the inquiry through enabling students to imagine both possibilities and restrictions of leaving Earth. Classes then conducted a drama exercise where the chairs were placed according to the rocket design selected, the students acted out packing the rocket, the farewells to friends and family, and the lift-off to the new planet. When the rocket landed, everyone held onto their seats and imagined themselves zooming into *Minecraft* and entering the new planet, which was the *Minecraft* server. Laptop lids were opened and the students shifted between the dramatic virtual world and the digital virtual world, imagining themselves landing on the planet in *Minecraft*. Jo was present and participated in one of these classes. She noted that the students shifted the play from the dramatic virtual world to the digital virtual world seamlessly.

While teachers framed the design of the unit, they tried to work so that students could collaborate and work creatively together to make the decisions for how the new world would operate. Teachers provided an overview structure where students worked on different districts or sections of the *Minecraft* world, each with a specific purpose: Industry, Agriculture, City and Culture,

Discovery and Education, and Recreation. Additionally, a weekly 'All Citizens Meeting' was held in the school hall. Initially the meetings were teacher-led, with new questions and prompts given to the students. Later, students worked in their districts, with reports from each district about issues that were occurring given to everyone. Over the duration of the project, the teachers stepped back and the students took increasing control of organising the meetings. At the end of the unit, students presented their findings more broadly at a large summit to younger students at the school, parents, and invited external guests.

For the teachers involved in the *Minecraft* unit, the development of high-level IT skills and teaching styles that worked with this kind of project were key. One of the teachers, Bec, commented:

> You have to be comfortable with changing your style of teaching. I think that for some teachers it's difficult because it is very much a 'facilitator' role and not a 'dictator' role, and you have to be comfortable with that. You have to be comfortable with the fact that the kids are going to know a heap more than you, and you have to trust them ... there is a lot of fear of the unknown.

She described the skills for teachers as 'additional, not different' to skills used in everyday practice. She said, "it's another tool. You're not replacing existing strategies. You are enhancing through the use of gaming".

In addition to developing new teaching skills, working with parents is integral to the success of a curriculum unit like this one. Parents can sometimes be suspicious of 'open' curriculum work, and the school was constantly dealing with 'moral panics' connected to technology, particularly when additional technology was introduced into the curriculum. In this unit, most parents were impressed with the quality of the work the students achieved and were generally supportive of the work. However, there were some parental complaints about the killing of animals in *Minecraft*, and the school had complaints about the "clearing the land of creatures that live there". Bec expressed her frustration at this. She iterated that the teachers were not "sending messages to children to hurt the land animals ... They weren't animals! They were shapes! They are pixelated shapes!"

In this unit, in order to enable the students to have the freedom to design, teachers' practices had to change significantly, they had to trust the students, and they needed to work carefully in communicating clearly with parents.

Digital Game Making in School

This chapter now considers how schools and teachers might work with young people to enable them to be architects of their digital world. It is becoming more common for students to design, code, and make their own games in school, particularly with the focus on STEM subjects in both Canada and Australia. Jo has worked with several teachers who have been developing their programmes and practices over an extended period of time, finessing them as they offer game making year after year to their students. One of these high school teachers, who has guided his classes through game making with GameMaker™ from YoyoGames for over ten years, noted that one of the great pleasures of this work is that every student designs, makes, and codes a playable game that they can play and share with friends (O'Mara & Richards, 2012). At his school there were many examples of the student-made games being played extensively by others. In one case, Jo researched a small group of students who had made a very successful game in class. After the class game making unit finished, the students continued building levels on the game, accepting ideas and even levels made by students outside the group. A large group from across the year level designed an informal 'Championship Series', where young people competed against each other to become the champion player of the game. The game architecture the students designed in this case extended from the production of the game itself into the social aspects of its usage – the playability, the ability to be reconfigured and re-designed, and a shaping around the purposes of play – the championship itself.

It is only recently that more opportunities have been provided for children to make games in elementary/primary school, and we noticed that this has occurred in conjunction with the rise of provision of 1:1 computing in elementary schools (O'Mara, Laidlaw, & Blackmore, 2017). Kon, a teacher at a government primary school in Melbourne, worked over a three-year cycle with the 8–10-year-old children in his class making their own digital games using *Scratch*, free 'visual' programming software developed by the Lifelong Kindergarten Group (2003) at the MIT Media Lab.[2] The *Scratch* website is designed to be both a resource and a community, and is highly accessible for usage with young people. Resnick et al. (2009) describe it as "more tinkerable, more meaningful and more social than other programming environments" (p. 2). *Scratch* has blocks of computer instructions that can be moved around to create commands. Marji (2014) describes programming in *Scratch* as "snapping those color-coded blocks together as you would puzzle pieces or *LEGO* bricks" (p. 21).

The students in Kon's class worked in teams, positioned as software architects and designers, running their own digital game design lab, taking on and sharing different production roles. The work was integrated more deeply into the curriculum as Kon came to understand the game making processes and affordances more deeply himself. By the third year of running the game making unit with his students, Kon worked much more extensively to prepare the students for making the games than he did when he first ran the unit, so that extensive critical literacy and analysis work were linked into the making process. Students began by reviewing commercial games. They analysed digital game storylines and how they worked, considered that some games have multiple possible ways of being played and that some games have sequential levels, and how all the elements of a game come together to produce the experience of gameplaying. The unit also focussed on the marketing of games and the usage of 'in app' purchases. Students then designed their own narratives, storyboarding, and characters, and wrote a prequel to the game. Games were programmed using *Scratch*, with character drawings and narrative elements built into the game. Once a game was coded, it would be tested by other students, with feedback provided about the clarity of the instructions and the 'playability' of the game. The games were saved onto CDs and the students designed logos and box covers for the games, as well as an in-box game booklet.

In an interview with Kon at the end of the project, he described the final game pack as having everything in it: "to show the journey, beginning with nothing, and then to the end product". He described the improvements made to the game making unit over the three years:

> The first year was building an interactive game. Because that was the first year, it was more about getting games working and having sort of a rough story. And the second year was more consolidating that and getting all that literacy stuff like character design and character profiles and stories and trying to get it together. And then this year, actually, we have been getting it all together … This year they were able to build a game, build a game booklet, and then like a DVD case that went with it … They have actually produced a product like you would buy in the shop. So, we finally got it to where we wanted it. So, it feels like we have accomplished more this year than ever before.

Students were further enabled to become game producers as Kon's familiarity and skills with both the game making and the teaching and learning cycle around the game making unit increased. Lankshear, Snyder, and Green (2000) note the importance of teachers being adept users of technology, arguing for 'teachers first' when introducing digital technologies in the classroom. Nearly 20 years later, this same principle is in action again with Kon, an expert user of technology and an expert teacher incorporating technology into the teaching and learning cycle – and that as his specific knowledge around the unit increases, the design of the curriculum becomes more nuanced and provides more opportunities for students to become architects of their digital worlds.

Children as Architects of Their Digital Worlds

These three examples illustrate the ways in which young people can be provided with opportunities to be producers rather than consumers of digital knowledge. In each of the three cases the children and young people are positioned as planners and designers, with the opportunities to imagine and create. As architects report that they do in their work (Leclerc, 2018), the young people in the three examples were also planners, problem-solvers, non-linear thinkers, who made connections within their immediate contexts and 'worlds'.

Importantly in each case, the young people were given the opportunity, support, and freedom to develop and create their own digital worlds. Olivia and Hannah have been supported and encouraged throughout their lifetime in their experimentation, usage, and creation using digital technologies, so they were open, knowledgeable, and imaginative in their approach to Dot and Dash. The school-based examples required the teachers to provide more openness to the students and, as Bec put it, to shift from 'dictator' to 'facilitator'. While many different approaches to teaching and a range of practices are available, teachers and adults working with children must work as enablers and facilitators, with young people provided with the time, space, opportunity, and supports to create and design as architects of their digital worlds.

Notes

1 We acknowledge a presentation by architect Eleonore Leclerc which has further informed our use of this metaphor.
2 You can watch a short video of Kon and his students through this link here: https://youtu.be/aTOf99I50P8.

References

Berger, B., Costello, D., Demers, P., Graham, D., Hutcheon, L., McClatchie, S., ... De Groote, T. (2001). The humanities in 2010: Alternative worlds the humanities in 2010. Retrieved from: www.sshrc-crsh.gc.ca/about-au_sujet/publications/humanities_report_e.pdf.
Burnett, C., & Merchant, G. (2016). Boxes of poison: Baroque techniques as antidote to simple views of literacy. *Journal of Literacy Research*, *48*(3), 258–279.
Carrington, V. (2017). How we live now: "I don't think there's such a thing as being offline". *Teachers College Record*, *119*(12), 1–24.
DEEWR (Department of Education, Employment & Workplace Relations). (2012). *Digital education revolution*. Retrieved from: www.deewr.gov.au/SCHOOLING/DIGITALEDUCATIONREVOLUTION/Pages/default.aspx.
Dezuanni, M., & O'Mara, J. (2017). Impassioned learning and Minecraft. In C. Beavis, M. Dezuanni, & J. O'Mara (Eds.), *Serious play: Literacy, learning and computer games* (pp. 36–48). New York, NY: Routledge.
Government of Alberta. (2016). *The guiding framework for the design and development of future kindergarten to grade 12 provincial curriculum*. Edmonton, AB: Ministry of Education.
Halverson, E. R., & Sheridan, K. M. (2014). The maker movement in education. *Harvard Educational Review*, *84*(4), 495–504.

Laidlaw, L., & Wong, S. (2016). Complexity, pedagogy, play: On using technology within emergent learning structures with young learners. *Complicity: An International Journal of Complexity and Education, 13*(1), 30–42.

Lankshear, C., Snyder, I., & Green, B. (2000). *Teachers and techno-literacy: Managing literacy, technology and learning in schools*. Sydney: Allen & Unwin.

Leclerc, E. (2018). Architecture: A (non)linear path [PowerPoint presentation]. (E. Leclerc, personal communication, February 4, 2019).

Lifelong Kindergarten Group. (2003). Scratch, MIT Media Lab. Retrieved from: http://scratch.mit.edu (Accessed 28 February, 2019).

Marji, M. (2014). *Learn to program with scratch: A visual introduction to programming with games. Art, science, and math*. San Francisco, CA: No Starch Press.

Marsh, J. (2005). *Popular culture, new media and digital literacy in early childhood* (pp. xiii, 245). London: Routledge.

Marsh, J. (2010). Young children's play in online virtual worlds. *Journal of Early Childhood Research, 8*(1), 23–39.

Marsh, J. (2016). 'Unboxing' videos: Co-construction of the child as cyberflaneur. *Discourse: Studies in the Cultural Politics of Education, 37*(3), 369–380. doi:10.1080/01596306.2015.1041457.

Merchant, G. (2015). Keep taking the tablets: IPads, story apps and early literacy. *Australia Journal of Language & Literacy, 38*(1), 3–11.

Mojang. (2011). Minecraft. Retrieved from: https://minecraft.net (Accessed 18 June 2020).

Morgan, N., & Saxton, J. (1989). *Teaching drama: A mind of many wonders*. Cheltenham: Stanley Thornes.

O'Mara, J. (2017). Narratives come to life through coding: Digital game making as language and literacy curriculum. In C. Beavis, M. Dezuanni, & J. O'Mara (Eds.), *Serious play: Literacy, learning and digital games* (pp. 102–114). New York, NY: Routledge.

O'Mara, J., & Laidlaw, L. (2011). Living in the iWorld: Two literacy researchers reflect on the changing texts and literacy practices of childhood. *English Teaching: Practice and Critique, 10*(4), 149–159. Retrieved from: http://edlinked.soe.waikato.ac.nz/research/journal/view.php?article=true&id=754&p=1.

O'Mara, J., Laidlaw, L., & Blackmore, J. (2017). The new digital divide: Digital technology policies and provision in Canada and Australia. In C. Burnett, G. Merchant, A. Simpson, & M. Walsh (Eds.), *The case of the iPad: Mobile literacies in education* (pp. 87–104). Singapore: Springer Nature. doi:10.1007/978-981-10-4364-2_6.

O'Mara, J., & Richards, J. (2012). A blank slate of potential: Using GameMaker to create computer games. In C. Beavis, J. O'Mara, & L. McNeice (Eds.), *Digital games: Literacy in action* (pp. 57–64). Kent Town, South Australia: Wakefield Press.

Pahl, K., & Rowsell, J. (2010). *Artifactual literacies: Every object tells a story*. New York, NY: Teachers College.

Peppler, K., & Bender, S. (2013). Maker movement spreads innovation one project at a time. *Phi Delta Kappan, 95*(3), 22–27.

Resnick, M., Maloney, J., Monroy-Hernández, A., Rusk, N., Eastmond, E., Brennan, K., & Kafai, Y. (2009). Scratch: Programming for all. *Communications of the ACM, 52*(11), 60–67.

Rowsell, J. (2014). *Working with multimodality: Rethinking literacy in a digital age*. New York, NY: Routledge.

Rowsell, J., Saudelli, M., McQuirter-Scott, R., & Bishop, A. (2013). iPads as placed resources: Forging community in online and offline spaces. *Language Arts, 90*(5), 351–360.

Sahlberg, P. (2015). *Finnish lessons: 2.0: What can the world learn from educational change in Finland?* New York, NY: Teachers College Press.

Sheridan, M., & Rowsell, J. (2010). *Design literacies: Learning and innovation in the digital age*. London: Routledge.

Statistica. (2019). Sourced on February 20, 2019. Retrieved from: www.statista.com/statistics/680139/minecraft-active-players-worldwide.

Walsh, M. (2011). *Multimodal literacy: Research classroom practice*. Newton, NSW: PETA.

Yelland, N. (2015). Playful explorations and new technologies. In J. Moyles (Ed.), *The excellence of play* (pp. 225–236). Milton Keynes: Open University Press.

14
TEENS' ONLINE AND OFFLINE LIVES
How They Are Experiencing Their Sociability

Sara Pereira, Joana Fillol, and Pedro Moura

Introduction

Sociability – or, to put it simply, "association for its own sake" (Simmel, 1949, p. 254) – has long been a recurrent subject of study. Despite being traditionally present in research on teenagers' relationship with the media, it has been gaining renewed interest in the digital and online communication era due to the proliferation of new technologies which open up possibilities for the creation of new forms of sociability. This concept, according to Haddon (2017, p. 244), has been used "to capture the nature of our interactions, our communications, and our relationships" with others. Fortunati, Taipale, and de Luca (2013, p. 895) add that "sociability takes place in cooperation with others and necessitates movement as well as communication".

Sociability has always been dependent on different kinds of constraints and the history of social ties is also the history of the fall of different technological barriers. Over time, numerous inventions determined different forms of mutual interaction (handwriting and paper, transport and post, to mention just a few), helping humans to model new ways to connect and to communicate with one another – with family, friends, acquaintances, and strangers. Each new technology, in its time, meant a small revolution, eliminating time and/or space constraints, facilitating the maintenance or the creation of social bonds; in sum, enriching sociability possibilities.

In the last (almost) three decades (Fortunati et al., 2013), digital media has brought the technical possibilities of new forms of communication, interaction, and participation, giving people the opportunity to speak, to write, to share what is happening in their lives for the first time combining three crucial factors: time (anytime), place (almost anywhere), and affordability (at minimal cost). However, there is no consensus regarding the consequences of this panorama since both apocalyptic and enthusiastic perspectives have been voiced, particularly regarding its impact on young people. On the one hand, it is argued that digital communication can merely promote superficial ties, decreasing the time people have for face-to-face relations – an argument known as the displacement hypothesis (Valkenburg & Peter, 2011) – and fostering shallow relationships and different kinds of risks, from excessive exposure to online harassment. On the other hand, a more optimistic perspective – the stimulation hypothesis (Valkenburg & Peter, 2011) – underlines the promotion and the reinforcement of social interactions, saying that digital media help youngsters "to conduct the social psychological task of adolescence" (Livingstone, 2008, p. 396), engaging in some risks and taking opportunities to present and manage their – now online and offline – personae while learning to make sense of social situations (Lim, 2013, p. 325). The latter "has received more support than the displacement hypothesis", as summarised by Valkenburg and Peter (2011, p. 124). However, both sides present valid arguments: as the teenagers' world cannot be read only in black and white tones, and since their media practices are heterogeneous (Hasebrink, 2012; Vanden Abeele, 2016), both risks and opportunities could be present (Livingstone, Mascheroni, & Staksrud, 2018; Valkenburg & Peter, 2011) when associating digital/online communication with sociability.

Studies of media and adolescents' sociability conducted in the last decade (e.g., Haddon, 2017; Lim, 2013; Ling & Bertel, 2013; Mesch, 2013; Mesch & Talmud, 2006; Valkenburg & Peter, 2011) stress precisely the newer and more complex tones with which digital media has imbued sociability. According to these studies, young people are experiencing new forms of sociability in which digital media and social networks assume a prominent place. As pointed out by Mesch (2013, p. 292), digital media, in most cases, are promoting "existing social contacts with friends from school, connecting adolescents into local, rather than global, networks". Operating in a "logic of anytime-anyplace connectivity" (Vanden Abeele, 2016, p. 90), social networks – and the devices where they are based, such as mobile phones – foster a connected presence (Nag, Ling, & Jakobsen, 2016) which might not have a major purpose besides "simply being together and acknowledging the other in one's life" (Lüders, 2011, p. 454).

Based on such topics discussed by earlier studies and having drawn on data provided by the Portuguese branch of the European research project Transmedia Literacy, this chapter is guided by the following research question: how are digital and online media contributing to teenagers' sociability? Floridi's onlife concept (2007, 2015), presented below, will anchor this discussion.

Teenagers' 'Onlife' Sociability

Gustavo Mesch (2013), who has conducted extensive research on adolescents and sociability, but also Sun Sun Lim (2013) and Ralph Schroeder (2016), emphasised the increasing fading of the boundaries established between offline and online lives. Mesch stated that "with the passage of time the online/offline comparison is becoming a faded and even false dichotomy" (2013, p. 293). The views of these authors concerning media and sociability are mirrored in the broader concept of 'onlife' coined by Luciano Floridi, which is focussed precisely on the blurring of the concepts of online and offline in human lives. For this researcher and philosopher this is what the current younger generations are already experiencing as he considers his own generation to most likely be the last "to experience a clear difference between onlife and online" (Floridi, 2007, p. 62). This transformation is, from Floridi's point of view, more than a simple shift, it is a "revolution", the fourth in terms of philosophical anthropology, after Copernicus, Darwin, and Freud (Floridi, 2015, p. 21). It opens up a new era, given the strong impacts ICTs have on the human condition that reverberate in different domains and also on the concept discussed herein: sociability. As mentioned in *The Onlife Manifesto*, subscribed to in 2013 by 15 scholars from different areas:

> ICT are not mere tools but rather environmental forces that are increasingly affecting: 1. Our self-conception (who we are); 2. Our mutual interactions (how we socialise); 3. Our conception of reality (our metaphysics); and 4. Our interactions with reality (our agency).
>
> *(Floridi, 2015, p. 2)*

Simon and Ess (2015, p. 157) summarise the onlife concept noting that it designates the "transformational reality that in contemporary developed societies, with few exceptions, our offline and online experiences and lives are inextricably interwoven". Regarding teenagers' mutual interactions, data presented below clearly show that young people are living in an 'onlife-world' experiencing an 'always on' sociability (Baron, 2008) with their peers, which corroborates Floridi's perspective.

Being Young and Socialising in the Digital Era

Methods

The media practices of Portuguese youngsters who participated in the Transmedia Literacy project are at the centre of this chapter. Lasting from 2015 to 2018, this project, funded by the European Commission, involved eight countries and sought to exploit teenagers' transmedia skills and informal learning strategies to improve their formal education.

Teenagers from all the countries were involved in fieldwork comprising three phases: 1) administration of a questionnaire to obtain information about teens' socio-cultural backgrounds and media access, uses, and perceptions; 2) two participatory workshops to explore, in an immersive way, the teens' transmedia practices and informal learning strategies while engaging them in media production and gameplay; 3) in-depth interviews with a sample of participants in the workshops (who were also challenged to complete a one-week media diary) to get to know their doings and sayings as regards media, social networks, and videogames. These methodological procedures were part of a triangulation effort in an ethnographic-inspired study based on short-term approaches (Pink & Ardevòl, 2018).

The Portuguese sample was recruited in two different public schools, one from an urban area and the other from a rural one. In each school, two classes were chosen: one from the national 7th grade (12–14 year-olds) and the other from the 10th grade (15–16 year-olds). In total, 77 students completed the questionnaire, 78 participated in the workshops, and 40 were interviewed. Table 14.1 summarises the constitution of the Portuguese sample.

Drawing on the data of the three research phases mentioned above, this chapter looks at the role of digital media in teenagers' sociability. Approaching the topic from their own practices and voices, it addresses the aforementioned research question: how are digital and online media contributing to teenagers' sociability?

How are Digital and Online Media Contributing to Teenagers' Sociability?

It clearly emerged from this study that this is a connected generation, which is not in fact a novelty, considering the results of other national (Pereira, Pinto, & Moura, 2015; Simões, Ponte, Ferreira,

Table 14.1 Number and gender of the youngsters by school and class.

Class	Urban school (boys/girls)	Rural school (boys/girls)	Total (boys/girls)
7th grade	18 (8/10)	18 (8/10)	36 (16/20)
10th grade	25 (10/15)	17 (6/11)	42 (16/26)
Total (boys/girls)	43 (18/25)	35 (14/21)	78 (32/46)

Source: Sara Pereira, Joana Fillol, and Pedro Moura.

Doretto, & Azevedo, 2014) and international research (Ling & Bertel, 2013; Livingstone et al., 2018). Data highlighted teenagers' ubiquitous media access to devices such as mobile phones, computers, internet and TV. Social network sites – mostly Facebook's Messenger and YouTube – are accessed daily by the majority (n= 68), but television also comes close behind, with 64 teenagers reporting they watch it every day. Most of them also reported using Instagram (56), Snapchat (52), and WhatsApp (48). It is very rare for a teen to use only one medium: their practices are transmedia, which is also reflected in their sociability. This simultaneity could be observed in these testimonials, in which the online conversations with friends are very visible:

> I watched videos on YouTube while I was speaking with schoolmates through Messenger and while I was watching TV.
>
> *(12-year-old boy)*

> I was watching a series on television while looking at my friends' posts.
>
> *(15-year-old girl)*

> I was on Twitter for an hour and a half and at the same time I was listening to music on Spotify.
>
> *(15-year-old girl)*

> Before I got up I went on Facebook, I chatted with my friends and played 8 Ball Pool on my mobile phone.
>
> *(15-year-old boy)*

Data from questionnaires revealed that being on social media and communicating/talking to friends is what students say they like the most on the internet (45). Going on social media and checking notifications/messages is also the first thing students do when they connect to the internet (55) and this happens throughout the day. Texting and talking to friends is an activity they do very regularly and, on many occasions, simultaneously with other activities. They are permanently in touch with each other when they are not co-present, and technologies link them even when friends share the same physical space. That is, even when together they tend to connect to some device:

> During the break I watched videos on YouTube with friends.
>
> *(15-year-old boy)*

> Sometimes, here at school, I'm in a certain place and a classmate of mine is in another and we're playing [8 Ball Pool].
>
> *(15-year-old girl)*

Technologies are at the core of the socialising process, wherever it takes place: at school, at home, but also when teens meet up at each other's houses. According to a five-point Likert scale, watching videos (M= 3.51) and series (M= 3.26), playing videogames (M= 3.45) and making videos (M= 2.77) are quite common practices when they go to friends' houses, as the excerpt below from the interview with a 16-year-old boy illustrates:

[Researcher]: Do you usually play videogames with your schoolmates?
[Félix]: Yes, yes. Last Friday, before "Braga Romana" [a public event], we went to my house. We should have gone out at nine, but we ended up going out just at 11 o'clock as we

	had been playing PES [Pro Evolution Soccer]. What matters is playing with friends. When we have friends visiting us we try to play as much as we can.
[Researcher]:	When your friends visit you is it to play videogames?
[Félix]:	No, it's about spending time with friends. But, of course, we always play videogames and joke around. It's always like this.

Non-face-to-face contact mediated by technologies takes on two dimensions: it occurs mainly with real-life friends while a minority establish contact with people they just know from the virtual sphere and with whom they share some entertainment or cultural interests. It is with their everyday friends that they develop closeness and build a sense of intimacy, which resonates with what was stated by Mesch (2013) regarding the prevalence of local, rather than global, networks in teenagers' sociability.

Portable technologies have allowed the extension of media use to times and spaces where they were once absent. The media are everywhere and available all the time in teenagers' lives. Socialising is an act that nowadays does not exist disconnected from technologies. More than an overlap between teenagers' online and offline worlds, online communication is complimenting, extending and reinforcing sociability. Online communication is teenagers' mode of everyday communication with peers, and media content and their own media practices are a regular topic in their conversations.

This online world, so important for teenagers' sociability, is sparsely inhabited by adults and is even considered to be off-limits to them. At the time this study was conducted, teenagers were abandoning Facebook because their parents had begun to use it. They did not eliminate their profiles and they continue to operate on this platform, but more as discrete observers than active participants. At that time, they began to resort more often to Instagram, a social network that keeps them away and safe from the eyes of their parents. Thus, there is a world in teenagers' online communication that they share only with their peers, where adults are cut off from this domain. This does not mean that teenagers do not communicate online with adults, such as parents, other relatives, and teachers, but with them they establish other types of conversation. Since in adolescence there have always been spaces, places, and conversations which are out of bounds for adults, these findings are neither new nor surprising. What does merit close attention, however, is whether the time spent by children and young people (and adults as well) on their mobile devices, the time spent on their screens, is keeping them away from their family.

An aspect that digital technologies have promoted concerns the exchange of information regarding school. Social networks are now a medium used to share general information, to ask questions about some subjects, to share texts and other materials. This is also an important form of sociability, which involves the entire class and is beneficial for all students.

Another insight that emerges from the analysis of the data concerns the importance digital technologies have had in reducing the inequalities among students from different geographical areas. This study was conducted in an urban and in a rural area and no significant differences were found with regard to connectivity and access. This could be a general benefit of being connected online. Digital technologies allow them to belong and to participate in the social activities and exchanges of their peer groups and to expand their relationships. For those who live in an isolated geographical area (as is the case of the participants from the countryside), this is undoubtedly a great benefit, although it does not erase all inequalities. As was the case in a previous study carried out in Portugal with children aged between eight and ten years old (Pereira, Pereira, & Melro, 2015), in which the geographical area variable was also considered, the differences found were not in access, but rather in their capacity to critically analyse, interpret, and understand messages. In the case of these students, what differentiates those from the urban area from those of the countryside is teenagers' and their friends' cultural capital (Bourdieu, 1986) and media repertoires. The media repertoires of the rural students were more limited and this was due to the more restricted information circulating among peer groups, which was much broader among students in the urban area.

Finally, on the recurring question of whether mediated communication leads to fewer face-to-face meetings or to a diminishing of their importance, teenagers replied that digital technologies, especially the smartphone, that they carry and access easily everywhere, enable them to be in near-permanent contact with friends, enhancing their sociability. But these teenagers consider that such mediated communications do not replace face-to-face relationships. In any case, the analysis of the data shows that mediated sociability is reinforced but not necessarily extended to a larger circle of people. They tend to follow, to contact, and to talk to their close circle of friends, the ones they also speak with in their offline lives.

Conclusion

As young people move beyond the nuclear family, peers play an increasingly central role (Lim, 2013; Nag et al., 2016). Valkenburg and Peter (2011, p. 122) state that one of the fundamental tasks assigned to adolescence is to develop "the abilities that are necessary to form, maintain, and terminate close, meaningful relationships with friends". Various authors have pointed to the importance of everyday friends – as well as family, teachers or neighbours, albeit to a lesser extent (Livingstone & Haddon, 2012; Nag et al., 2016) – as the main interlocutors within adolescents' sociability, underlining the digital media capacity for expanding the geographic reach of relationships (Livingstone et al., 2018; Mesch, 2013; Pereira, Moura, Masanet, Taddeo, & Tirocchi, 2018).

Despite the intrinsic and diverse social features of the media (Baym, 2015; McQuail, 1997), digital platforms, such as social networks, have undoubtedly opened up new possibilities, different in nature and intensity and providing distinctive affordances (Hall, 2018) for interpersonal mediated communication. They are simultaneously content providers and platforms for some sorts of communication (Lim, 2013). Teens establish a continuous dialogue among themselves in a permanent fusion of online and offline lives, materialising Floridi's concept of "onlife", which suggests the "very distinction between online and offline will become blurred" (Floridi, 2007, p. 61).

While media and adolescents' culture have always been closely connected (Arnett, 1995), they now seem to be umbilically linked. But while friends are omnipresent in a variety of ways – from public displays of interaction to committed private chats and mere connected presences – adults are many times avoided or, at least, filtered out. For adolescents, social networks are particularly important to share 'private experiences', create 'spaces of intimacy' (Livingstone, 2008, p. 11) and also 'affinity spaces', that is, "a place or set of places where people can affiliate with others based primarily on shared activities, interests, and goals" (Gee, 2004, p. 67). These are spaces mostly inhabited by members of a 'walled community' (Ling & Haddon, 2008, p. 146), which leads us to question if teens are taking advantage of all the opportunities that technologies give them in terms of sociability or if they are creating a 'filter bubble' (Pariser, 2011) by reinforcing the relationships and the conversations with people they already know or with whom they share the same interests, ideas, and opinions, keeping away or avoiding contacts and contents that do not fit their profiles. When analysing the media practices of the Portuguese sample, but also those from Italy and Spain (Pereira et al., 2018), it is possible that the preference for a close circle of friends in their online sociability could also be a way to protect their privacy as it avoids greater exposure to risk and makes the experience pleasurable.

Teenagers' online behaviour is not homogeneous and having access to the digital world or even interacting there does not equate to wise use. In this study, the results on teenagers' sociability are somewhat in line with the findings on media production practices and competences (Pereira & Moura, 2018). In the same way that having access to the media does not mean they produce content and participate in the digital public sphere, contacting others and friends online does not mean that they go beyond their close circle of friends and expand social ties and horizons. The experience reported above by the adolescents themselves conveys a strengthening of their existing social ties, showing that those with whom they socialise in the virtual sphere are mostly their everyday friends. The process of self-disclosure in this mediated sociability sphere "becomes an ever-evolving cycle through which individual identity is presented, compared, adjusted, or defended against a constellation of social, cultural, economic, or political realities" (Papacharissi, 2011, p. 304). In the study reported here it was not possible to verify the premise of Valkenburg, Peter, and Schouten (2006, p. 589) that "positive feedback enhanced adolescents' self-esteem, and negative feedback decreased their self-esteem", but it was clear that teenagers regularly follow and monitor the posts that they, and others, share on social media and that they appreciate positive feedback on their posts, they count the likes obtained (for example, eliminating a photo that does not reach the number of likes they expect) and these make them happy, at least.

Online sociability may not be free of risks (for instance, talking to strangers, revealing personal data, being tricked), however this was not a major concern among adolescents and did not figure much in their discourses. In fact, they said they feel confident and informed about such things. Online risks and their prevention are issues that draw schools' attention and therefore training sessions are usually held for students. In the schools participating in the study and throughout most of Portugal, this is, indeed, the media literacy topic that is most discussed and addressed in the school context, and sometimes the only one.

To conclude, it may be argued that sociability is a subject of study that will never be exhausted. On the one hand, the lives of children and adolescents are dynamic, and, on the other hand, digital technologies and the internet, besides being dynamic as well, will continue to influence and affect how people communicate and interact with each other. Topics such as the risk of isolation and of being 'alone together' (Turkle, 2012), the fear of substitution of face-to-face interaction by online relationships, and sociability during vacation time, when teenagers do not regularly meet up with their schoolmates, need to be further studied. This chapter, based on results involving a small sample of Portuguese adolescents, has brought to light some contributions to understand better how sociability is experienced in a hyperconnected era, having the advantage of making the voices of the young people themselves known. The major conclusion is undoubtedly that teenagers' sociability is deeply mediated by technologies that complement, expand, and reinforce forms of co-present sociability, but that it is also clearly different (Schroeder, 2016) in terms of the way they pay attention and how they verbally and non-verbally react one to another. When they interact and communicate online and when they share mundane events from their everyday life, they do not always intend to create or reinforce social bonds, they simple want to foster an 'online togetherness', that is, "a sense of being together online" (Schroeder, 2016, p. 5634) in an increasingly 'onlife' world, always on.

References

Arnett, J. J. (1995). Adolescents' uses of media for self-socialization. *Journal of Youth and Adolescence*, 24(5), 519–533.
Baron, N. (2008). *Always on: Language in an online and mobile world.* New York, NY: Oxford University Press.
Baym, N. K. (2015). Social media and the struggle for society. *Social Media + Society*, April–June, 1–2.
Bourdieu, P. (1986). The forms of capital. In J. Richardson (Ed.), *Handbook of theory and research for the sociology of education* (pp. 241–258). Westport, CT: Greenwood.
Floridi, L. (2007). A look into the future impact of ICT on our lives. *The Information Society*, 23(1), 59–64.
Floridi, L. (Ed.). (2015). *The onlife manifesto: Being human in a hyperconnected era.* Cham, Switzerland: Springer.
Fortunati, L., Taipale, S., & de Luca, F. (2013). What happened to body-to-body sociability? *Social Science Research*, 42, 893–905.

Gee, J. P. (2004). *Situated language and learning. A critique of traditional schooling.* New York, NY: Routledge.

Haddon, L. (2017). Sociability, smartphones, and tablets. In A. Serrano Tellería (Ed.), *Between the public and private in mobile communication* (pp. 243–261). New York, NY: Routledge.

Hall, J. A. (2018). When is social media use social interaction? Defining mediated social interaction. *New Media & Society, 20*(1), 162–179.

Hasebrink, U. (2012). Young Europeans' online environments: A typology of user practices. In S. Livingstone, L. Haddon, & A. Görzig (Eds.), *Children, risk and safety on the internet* (pp. 127–139). Bristol, UK: The Policy Press.

Lim, S. S. (2013). Media and peer culture: Young people sharing norms and collective identities with and through media. In D. Lemish (Ed.), *The Routledge international handbook of children, adolescents and media* (pp. 322–328). Abingdon, UK: Routledge.

Ling, R., & Bertel, T. (2013). Mobile communication culture among children and adolescents. In D. Lemish (Ed.), *The Routledge international handbook of children, adolescents and media* (pp. 127–133). Abingdon, UK: Routledge.

Ling, R., & Haddon, L. (2008). Children, youth and the mobile phone. In K. Drotner & S. Livingstone (Eds.), *The international handbook of children, media and culture* (pp. 137–151). London, UK: SAGE Publications.

Livingstone, S. (2008). Taking risky opportunities in youthful content creation: Teenagers' use of social networking sites for intimacy, privacy and self-expression. *New Media & Society, 10*(3), 393–411.

Livingstone, S., & Haddon, L. (2012). Theoretical framework for children's internet use. In S. Livingstone, L. Haddon, & A. Görzig (Eds.), *Children, risk and safety on the internet* (pp. 1–14). Bristol, UK: The Policy Press.

Livingstone, S., Mascheroni, G., & Staksrud, E. (2018). European research on children's internet use: Assessing the past and anticipating the future. *New Media & Society, 20*(3), 1103–1122.

Lüders, M. (2011). Why and how online sociability became part and parcel of teenage life. In M. Consalvo & C. Ess (Eds.), *The handbook of internet studies* (pp. 452–468). Chichester, UK: Wiley-Blackwell.

McQuail, D. (1997). *Audience analysis.* Thousand Oaks, CA: SAGE Publications.

Mesch, G. (2013). Internet media and peer sociability. In D. Lemish (Ed.), *The Routledge international handbook of children, adolescents and media* (pp. 287–294). Abingdon, UK: Routledge.

Mesch, G., & Talmud, I. (2006). The quality of online and offline relationships: The role of multiplexity and duration of social relationships. *The Information Society, 22*(3), 137–148.

Nag, W., Ling, R., & Jakobsen, M. H. (2016). Keep out! Join in! Cross-generation communication on the mobile internet in Norway. *Journal of Children and Media, 10*(4), 411–425.

Papacharissi, Z. (2011). A networked self. In Z. Papacharissi (Ed.), *A networked self: Identity, community, and culture on social network sites* (pp. 304–318). New York, NY: Routledge.

Pariser, E. (2011). *The filter bubble: What the internet is hiding from you.* London, UK: Penguin Books.

Pereira, S., & Moura, P. (2018). Production skills. In C. A. Scolari (Ed.), *Teens, media and collaborative cultures—Exploiting teens' transmedia skills in the classroom* (pp. 22–32). Barcelona: Universitat Pompeu Fabra. Retrieved from: http://hdl.handle.net/10230/34245.

Pereira, S., Moura, P., Masanet, M.-J., Taddeo, G., & Tirocchi, S. (2018). Media uses and production practices: Case study with teens from Portugal, Spain and Italy. *Comunicación y Sociedad, 33*, 89–114.

Pereira, S., Pereira, L., & Melro, A. (2015). The Portuguese programme one laptop per child: Political, educational and social impact. In S. Pereira (Ed.), *Digital literacy, technology and social inclusion: Making sense of one-to-one computer programmes around the world* (pp. 29–100). Vila Nova de Famalicão, Portugal: Húmus.

Pereira, S., Pinto, M., & Moura, P. (2015). *Níveis de literacia mediática: Estudo exploratório com jovens do 12.º ano.* Braga, Portugal: CECS. Retrieved from: http://hdl.handle.net/1822/40488.

Pink, S., & Ardèvol, E. (2018). Ethnographic strategies for revealing teens' transmedia skills and practices. In C. A. Scolari (Ed.), *Teens, media and collaborative cultures: Exploiting teens' transmedia skills in the classroom* (pp. 108–117). Barcelona: Universitat Pompeu Fabra. Retrieved from: http://hdl.handle.net/10230/34245.

Schroeder, R. (2016). The globalization of on-screen sociability: Social media and tethered togetherness. *International Journal of Communication, 10*, 5626–5643.

Simmel, G. (1949). The sociology of sociability. *American Journal of Sociology, 55*(3), 254–261.

Simões, J. A., Ponte, C., Ferreira, E., Doretto, J., & Azevedo, C. (2014). *Crianças e meios digitais móveis em Portugal: Resultados nacionais do projeto Net Children Go Mobile.* Lisbon, Portugal: CESNOVA. Retrieved from: http://hdl.handle.net/10362/23687.

Simon, J., & Ess, C. (2015). The ONLIFE Initiative—a concept reengineering exercise. *Philosophy and Technology, 28*(1), 157–162.

Turkle, S. (2012). *Alone together: Why we expect more from technology and less from each other.* New York, NY: Basic Books.

Valkenburg, P. M., & Peter, J. (2011). Online communication among adolescents: An integrated model of its attraction, opportunities, and risks. *Journal of Adolescent Health, 48,* 121–127.

Valkenburg, P. M., Peter, J., & Schouten, A. P. (2006). Friend networking sites and their relationship to adolescents' well-being and social self-esteem. *Cyber-Psychology and Behavior, 9*(5), 584–590.

Vanden Abeele, M. M. P. (2016). Mobile youth culture: A conceptual development. *Mobile Media & Communication, 4*(1), 85–101.

15

TEENS' FANDOM COMMUNITIES

Making Friends and Countering Unwanted Contacts[1]

Julián de la Fuente and Pilar Lacasa

Introduction

This chapter is dedicated to digital fan communities (Duffett, 2013). Of particular interest are online practices that allow teenagers to build a community of interest around an idol and thus establish friendships (Chambers, 2013). The analytical framework of contact management is applied, understood to be types of people's relationships and the voluntary selection of these through direct or indirect strategies (Hinton & Hjorth, 2013). Usually, these practices come about through the creation of multimodal discourses that mark the belonging to or exclusion from the community through the fanfiction remix (Navas, Gallagher, & Burrough, 2015).

Taking into account these principles, the main goals within this research are as follows:

1. To explore how teenagers use social networks, and where they select their contacts from by looking for common interests to participate as active citizens in the fan community;
2. To analyse how they build friendship between fans, when interaction processes are established between the fan community framework and the personal relationships that followers maintain;
3. To examine the role of multimodal texts in the formation of the community insofar as they become instrumental in the engagement between fans in online and offline contexts.

For this research, a three-year ethnographic study was carried out from digital creation workshops that took place in a city lab, and which grouped together young people between 8 and 14 years of age. In this chapter, the focus is on a group of girls who regard themselves as fans of celebrities, such as One Direction or Harry Styles, as an example of a relationships community. These fangirls were selected by their active participation and the public commitment to their music idols. As a result of the analysis of their mobile phone contents and in-depth group interviews, their material practices can be connected with the meanings created around the fan community. In this chapter, the mechanisms these communities use to guide contacts management will be explored.

Theoretical Framework

The theoretical framework of the research allowed an approach to fans' internet practices (Ito, 2010; Marwick & boyd, 2014) that explored the interaction between macro and micro communities (Hinton & Hjorth, 2013), and strategies that fans carry out to manage their contacts (Chambers, 2013). The research refers to desired contacts when there is a positive selection of them, in online and offline contexts. It refers to countering mechanisms for unwanted contacts, alluding to those relationships between people who avoid each other or relationships which finally fail to be established.

Fan Communities as a Source of Contacts

The activity of young people on the internet is marked by the use of social networks (Cortesi et al., 2015) that allow them to interact with people beyond the family or the school as physical places of socialisation. In many cases, this is where teens explore and get access to new contacts. Searching for information or content creation are preferred activities that lead young people to participate through social networks (Hinton & Hjorth, 2013). Fan communities appear within this context as interest groups who share a hobby or admiration for an idol.

If, originally, fans were regarded as a transgressive minority (Fiske, 1992), more recently these communities have been gaining more prominence in digital media and can be considered an increasingly common context for adolescent relationships. To reach this point, fandom studies have gone through several stages: from a focus on the fan community as interpreters of texts (Jenkins, 1992/2013), to a perspective based on social practices (Barton & Lampley, 2013), and then to a more individual analysis focussed on the identity established between the idol and their follower (Duffett, 2013).

Regarding the focus of this study, the interaction between the fans from musical groups has previously been studied by authors such as Kibby (2000), and especially the friendship relations developed between musical fans by Beer (2008). There are also numerous studies that link these fan communities with age and gender groups like fangirls (Trier-Bieniek, 2015).

Moreover, although it is primarily a certain idol, such as a celebrity or hobby, that brings these fans together, their community progressively develops and becomes more complex in terms of the contacts participants establish with each other (Gray, Sandvoss, & Harrington, 2017). As a result, each case must essentially be studied in great detail in order to understand the dynamic participation strategies occurring in communities of fans and particularly those among young people.

The researchers, therefore, understand that fan communities are not just cultural phenomena, since their activities range from civic engagement (Jenkins, Ito, & boyd, 2015) to social learning (Holland & Lave, 2009). These activities are closely related to the strategies with which community participants establish relationships among their members. To understand how these relationships come about, the practices that are carried out through social networks will now be examined.

Relationship Practices between Fans

The practices within a community of fans must be addressed in relation to the public and private activities of its members, which are characterised by connecting the online and offline worlds (Ito, 2010; Miller, 2016). Therefore, this research is interested in the community activities that extend beyond social networks and private relationships maintained by the fans. In this sense, friendship practices (Chambers, 2013) are particularly significant as is countering unwanted contacts (Marwick & boyd, 2014).

To describe these practices, first a definition of their role within the fandom is presented. For this, Mizuko Ito (2010) proposes the concept of 'genre of participation', connecting this category of textual analysis with social activity. She explains how the context of the media is in itself a model of community involvement and therefore contact selection. In fact, two modes through which this participation is organised are established.

The first genre of participation is characterised by personal interests, which leads many children to seek contacts through social networks (Willett, 2017). This means, in practice, participation in communities that at first have nothing more in common than the interests that bind them as fans, but that over time develop personal relationships that often translate into offline contacts.

The other genre of participation centred on friendship refers to communities that transfer relationships established in the offline world to social networks. Therefore, the decision to accept a contact or not conditions the nature of the sociability that the children perform, but, at the same time, encourages more intense and continuous friendships (boyd, 2014).

The community can also be approached from macro or micro perspectives (Hinton & Hjorth, 2013). In the first case, the focus of interest is placed on culture, in the second on personal relationships. In both, these forms of participation lead to mediatisation of a fan community (Chambers, 2013) that suddenly becomes a list of contacts to manage. Now, which discourses enable this participation process in the fan communities are examined.

Fans Engagement through Multimodal Discourses

It has already been demonstrated that social networks are the preferred expression space for fan communities (Burton, 2017). Within these networks, young people use different language modes to communicate, whether through text, images, videos, sound, or emoticons. The creation of messages using these different languages together is called multimodality (Kress, 2010; Rowsell, 2013) and is configured as a preferred form of discourse within the fan communities, used to strengthen engagement between members of this community.

This multimodal discourse used by young people to build messages in fan communities and establish engagement among participants is called remix (Navas & Gallagher, 2014). It is a practice of appropriation of content distributed over the network, preferably images, texts, or songs that are easily edited and redistributed through social networks. But at the same time, the mere recontextualisation of these contents generates new meanings (Knobel & Lankshear, 2010) that are interpreted as completely new messages by the fans. In this way, the fans not only relate to each other, but also generate discourse models that predefine the content created by followers who want to join the community.

Among those types of multimodal discourses that use the remix to create new material are memes, fanarts, or fanfictions. In this study, special attention is paid to fanfiction, as a community-mediating element that contributes to engagement between fans (Hellekson & Busse, 2014). These discourses start from the elements exhibited in the canon of the idol, from which they explore narrative worlds that often connect with personal experiences, their own cultural traits, or shared desires in the community (Thomas, 2006).

Multimodal discourses are the means of participation not only in the fan community, but also in moving the fans' initiative out of the community (Daugherty, Eastin, & Bright, 2008). This is how social learning and civic engagement arise from fandom, and this is particularly reflected among the young (Soep, 2014).

The researchers have found fan communities which, thanks to friendship and countering practices, develop strong engagement that allows them to tackle challenges that would otherwise be impossible to carry out in offline spaces such as in the family or at school. Social networks allow young people to build their own identity (Lacasa et al., 2017) and develop meaningful participation in their interests.

Methodological Approach

The researchers adopted an ethnographic approach (Pink, 2012) for this study which allowed them to specifically locate the fan communities they wanted to study in online and offline scenarios (Boellstorff, 2012). The interaction between these two worlds is facilitated by technology, the use of multiple platforms and profiles, as well as the special protection required by the privacy rights of young people (Livingstone & Bovill, 2013).

Fangirls around One Direction and Harry Styles

This research looked at the One Direction and Harry Styles fan community. One Direction is a British band that rose to fame in 2010 thanks to a television contest and whose presence through social networks is particularly prominent. The band announced their temporary separation in 2016, which has not prevented any of its members from continuing their solo career. Such is the case of Harry Styles, actor and singer, who has brought together many of the One Direction fans.

The fan phenomenon of this boy band has been the subject of numerous studies (Direction, 2013; Korobkova, 2014), standing out especially for its particular commitment to celebrity, to the point of identifying with separate names those fans who participate in the community as 'directioners' and those who simply declare themselves followers of the group as 'directionators'. This is an example of a fan community where it is not enough to identify with the celebrity, one is also required to establish relationships with other fans. For this, there are multiple strategies that force the 'directioners' to participate in those activities that are considered essential to demonstrate that they are true One Direction fans. Otherwise, the tendency is to exclude themselves as 'directionators'. All of the above makes this community a particularly significant example for analysis of the processes through which participants seek or exclude contacts.

For this longitudinal study, a group of girls between 13 and 14 years of age were selected when the study began in 2015 and they have continued to be in the study to this day. They go to the same school and regard each other as friends (Lacasa, Méndez, & de-la-Fuente, 2016). All of them have participated in digital creation workshops around the fandom developed in a city lab called 'Matadero Madrid'[2] (Spain). These workshops were carried out by researchers to collect data by creating content around popular idols. Those participants who regarded themselves as fans and agreed to share their activity through social networks were selected. Their online evolution was observed over a period of three years (Gair & Van Luyn, 2017; Pink, 2012), whilst at the same time periodic interviews were also simultaneously conducted to explain their offline relationships. In the interviews, which took place in informal contexts closely connected to everyday life, the researchers monitored the girls' development and shared their 'zone of proximal development' in order to get closer to what was of interest to the girls at any given moment (Holzman, 2010). This approach allowed the researchers to relate the activities of the fans' community to their interpersonal relationships, offering a model of practices that will be analysed next.

The Analysis Process: Unit and Levels of Practices

Analysis of the girls' activity inside and outside the fan community, relating to the strategies that facilitate the establishment or the containment of contacts, enabled the researchers to reconstruct their practices holistically. For this, an interpretive paradigm was used (Bourdieu, 1972; Flick, 2018) that led the researchers to superimpose successive levels of analysis from the practice concept unit. They were able to extend with this unit of analysis (Matusov, 2007) from the context, through the activity, until they reached the discourse:

1   The first level of analysis focusses on the socio-cultural context, that is, on social networks as spaces for socialising available to teenagers to build fan communities (Gray et al., 2017). In this case, the researchers analysed how they carry out contacts within this community and what rules are followed to maintain these relationships;
2   The second level involves analysing the activities that girls develop inside and outside the community, as genres of participation (Ito, 2010). For this, the analysis focussed on the interpersonal relationships that arise between fans and how they specifically occur in the offline world;
3   The third level is dedicated to discourses, especially the use of the remix as a multimodal discourse that helps to build the identity of the idol and the social engagement of the community (Duffett, 2013). The selected examples refer to the creation of fanfictions and the rules that govern their distribution through social networks.

The tool used to process all this data was NVIVO software, which enabled analysis of the audiovisual recordings of the workshops, the audio recordings of the in-depth interviews, and the investigators' reports, all on the same platform. The participants' own interpretation of their activities and the evolution in these data over time was particularly important for node classification. This method (Lacasa, Martinez-Borda, & Mendez, 2013) allowed the researchers to create a narrative and, at the same time, a conceptual explanation of the results which is presented below.

Results

Young fans participate in the community by establishing contacts through social networks. This practice involves the selection of these contacts directly or indirectly. This chapter discusses processes and genres of participation in social networks (Chambers, 2013; Ito, 2010; Marwick & boyd, 2014) as a starting point to analyse engagement with the community through diverse communication settings, immersed in specific social and cultural contexts and mediated by multimodal discourses. As indicated, this study's data comes from musical communities, whose participants share interests around One Direction, when the study began in 2015, and currently around Harry Styles.

Social Networks and Fans: Interest, Friendship, and Commitment

The process of seeking and excluding contacts among teens when they participate in the community, associated with the use of certain cultural instruments – social networks in this case – will now be looked at. We will look at a community of practice understood as a social environment mediated by technology, in which people unfold their daily lives, sharing common goals and interests (Holland & Lave, 2009).

Friendship and Interest Practices between Fans

In the example below, in transcript 1, the researcher asked about people with whom the fans maintained contacts because they shared common interests. Teenagers do not explicitly refer to exclusion mechanisms, but they point out the selection criteria used to include other participants among their contacts. In this regard, boyd (2014) refers to the construction of what she considers 'networked publics', partly supported by technology and partly by the fan communities. Feelings of tolerance and respect towards others may develop there.

Transcript 1 The meaning of a contact (2015).

Ana: So for example, I follow an account and if you retweet something, I get into your account, take a look, and see what it is like, what it is that you like, what opinion you have about that relationship and all that ... Of course, in the real world, it is more complicated ....
Researcher: ... but you have reached those virtual friends because you are both fans.
Luisa: Yes, of course, because we had something in common.
Ana: But then you do not talk to them just about One Direction or some other celebrity ... in the end you end up talking about your opinions about other things. I mean, in the end it's not just that, you start talking about that.

To interpret this transcription, researchers identified the need for interaction between the two participation processes proposed by Mizuko Ito (2010), alluding to 'interest driven' and 'friendship driven' processes. The first process would take place in the fan communities themselves, the second leads to forms of interaction that can be considered as personal. Both forms of participation interact, establishing a continuous feedback between them so that relationships can be established with the same people in the two participation genres.

The online world gives fans the possibility to choose between people who would be difficult to approach in offline situations. This chapter has first shown that social networks are an instrument to establish genres of participation, and now this chapter will explain how these genres are immersed in other types of practices. The researchers were interested to know how the participants interpret their participation in a fan community.

Contacts, Participation, and Social Engagement

Taking into account several studies (Burton, 2017; Soep, 2014), the focus here is on the strategies that lead young people to select certain social networks they participate in, and which will condition who they will establish contacts with. More specifically, in this case, Rosa relates civic engagement to the obligations of those who have to maintain the commitment to their audiences on the network. Once again, positive rather than exclusive implications of this participation in the network are sought. The transcript below refers to a writer they follow who writes fanfiction:[3]

Transcript 2 Community engagement and fanfiction (2018).

Researcher: And why do you think she does it?
Ana: Well, I think she likes writing a lot and of course she likes Harry too! Because she's a fan of Harry.
Researcher: Because she's a fan of Harry, right?
Rosa: I don't know, she likes to write, it's her hobby, but there comes a point when if you have an audience of 9,000 followers, you cannot stop posting photos, you have that commitment.

The researchers are interested in exploring the girls' opinions about an author related to fanfiction as a form of citizen participation (Korobkova, 2014; Soep, 2014). In the case of the author mentioned by Rosa, the commitment is to the author's audience, evidently fans of One Direction.

This author, on the other hand, contributes to the fact that adolescents can select their contacts in that community where they expect to find other people with similar interests. It is a positive selection of contacts, of people with whom they will interact on the internet.

Interpersonal Friendship and Countering Relationships

The focus of this section will be on analysing how girls move in another universe of personal relationships, which Ito (2010) calls 'friendship driven' and which has been analysed in depth by other authors (Chambers, 2013). In this case, it is about relationships that they maintain with friends and peers in both online and offline environments. In some instances, they support each other and use strategies to strengthen the community, both by seeking or establishing new contacts and excluding others, generally indirectly.

Social Media Profiles and Relationships

The girls talk about a relatively common practice among them which is that of maintaining different accounts in social networks. In transcript 3, Ana is explicit about the differences between her fan profile and another one she considers personal. She prefers to keep what she calls her 'fan profile' well away from her usual contacts. In this profile, she expresses her feelings towards Harry and it even sometimes becomes a diary of personal feelings and experiences that she wishes to keep in a private setting (Marwick & boyd, 2014). On the other hand, in the profile that she considers personal, she identifies herself, she mentions her usual friends who are mostly her schoolmates, and she also recounts her daily activities.

Transcript 3 Relationships between accounts (2015).

Researcher: Do you follow the same people that you have in one place in another?
Ana: No, not the same but ....
Researcher: So the messages that you post are different?
Ana: Sure.
Ana: In that account (personal) I am more, because I do not know ... (stops).
Researcher: In which one?
Ana: Well, who I am and things like that. I mean, if I'm meeting up or something, then I'll say that I'm doing that and say who I've arranged to meet up with.
Researcher: In your profile?
Luisa: In the real one.
Ana: In the personal one.

It is clear that Ana maintains two independent worlds that try to exclude each other. In each, there are clear differences between the contents that are published or explored and also the people at whom it is aimed. Chambers (2013) points out how technology allows this intimacy, shortening barriers in space and time. But what is perhaps more relevant is that each communication channel has a set of attributes that makes it more suitable for conveying one message or another, and they are selected based on those characteristics.

The 'Hangouts' and the Presence in the Physical World

Various studies have insisted on the fact that physical contact contributes properties to human relationships that are not present in online life (Turkle, 2011). In this case, the researchers observe how offline relationships are established in the macro and micro communities, and how they are maintained in differentiated areas, although it is difficult to establish any separation between them.

In transcript 4 Luisa and Ana differentiate between two types of relationships that take place in offline spaces. The first ones are what they call 'prestige hangouts', which have been organised by staff directly related to One Direction. In those meetings that are accessed through a contest, the fans listen to music, play, or exchange objects.[4] The fans are selected in such a way as to increase their interest in attending the events. Other ways to physically interact among fans is what they call 'hangouts of people', implying that the selection is made by those who follow a particular fan account through Twitter, and from which contacts are subsequently established through WhatsApp. These smaller groups can physically interact with one another if they live in the same city, but, in any case, they establish personal friendships between participants:

Transcript 4 Friendships and relationships in the offline world (2015).

Researcher: And what are these hangouts like?
Luisa: Some are prestigious, so to speak, because they are for draws.
Ana: Oh yeah!
Luisa: Like the one Ana and I went to, and then there are others that are hangouts but with people . . . .
Researcher: And how do you know about them?
Ana: On Twitter.
Luisa: There was the big group and then another smaller group and then those of us who did a lot, a lot, more friends.
Ana: Sometimes someone says, do you want to make a WhatsApp group? Or you say tell is there any WhatsApp group to get into?
Ana: They put it on Twitter, the fan account says who wants to make a WhatsApp group, then you say, yes, I want to follow it back.

Luisa explained clearly how participants are selected in a fan group who are also friends, by simply privately sending phone numbers and following the person proposing the creation of that group. It should be kept in mind that, at that time, to send private messages to someone it was necessary for both people to follow one another on the social network. In this sense, it is obvious that the communication channels will condition the messages sent by them.

Multimodal Texts as Mediators in the Fan Community

If anything has been clarified so far it is that the relationships that are established through the community are mediated by multimodal texts (Kress, 2010), including those that contain multiple expressive written, visual, or sound signals. The next section discusses some examples of how the use of these texts also contributes to generating links between those who participate in the community, and how they can also indirectly generate inclusion and exclusion processes when establishing engagement (Owens, 2015).

Fanfictions in Wattpad

The first focus is on texts produced through the Wattpad application, in which teenagers create and reconstruct stories related to fan communities. This application facilitates the self-publication of texts similar to novels, written in chapters and narrating the adventures of the character. Participants become followers of certain texts, keeping up with new contributions by the author. In this way, fans not only establish contacts but also commit to their relationship. Transcript 5 includes comments[5] from Lucia, author of a number of chapters on Wattpad. Lucia had started writing in 2014 and has 43 followers, among whom are schoolmates and some participants in fan communities.

Transcript 5 Fanfiction in Wattpad (2015).

Lucia:	Have you seen my book?
Researcher:	I loved it! I've seen that you had three or four chapters! I saw it recently.
Lucia:	No, I have 17 chapters . . . .
Researcher:	And how did you come to write it?
Lucia:	It's because I like to read, and I guess I wanted to try. If everyone does it, well, why not me?

This fragment highlights the importance of multimodal discourses and fanfiction in particular (Hellekson & Busse, 2014; Thomas, 2006) to strengthen relationships between fans. Lucia shows her commitment to the community when producing these texts that allow her to expand her number of contacts, as well as to deepen her relationships and status within the community.

Remix: Twitter and Instagram

The narratives around the idol are also built around audiovisual discourse. Kress (2010) noted that the image is displacing other forms of expression in public domains. The girls refer to an author who appears in different social networks with the user name 'hsxallthelove'. Again, the discourse is a narrative whose character is Harry Styles, who had previously been a band member of One Direction. This is now not just a remix of images, but more of a contribution with a text on the escapades of the characters who belonged to the band. The author has 8,298 followers in a closed account to which it is necessary to be accepted, although she only follows the official account of Harry Styles.

Transcript 6 Remix on Instagram (2018).

Researcher:	Well, tell me a little bit about it.
Rosa:	Well, this girl writes stories and the characters in the stories are Harry, Liam . . . .
Rosa:	As you can see each picture is like a part of the story, then if you look here, each picture is like a piece of text.
Researcher:	She does not write very long text, does she?
Rosa:	No, no . . . .
Researcher:	That's what I was going to say, there is great coherence here.
Rosa:	It's really good, because not only does she really work on the story, it is very good because it is all . . . you see here there are messages and also pieces of news and things like that, you know? Which is all highly consistent with the story.

The girls also explain how the coherence of the story is achieved, when the chapters take place or another book is started. The author plays with the typology or even with the colours, from real photographs of the characters (Navas et al., 2015). In addition, the author uses diverse strategies to achieve audience immersion, for example by allowing the person to become the protagonist of the story and even including his or her own name. For this, each time the protagonist is mentioned the name is blanked out.

These data demonstrate how fanfiction and remix represent a form of expression that helps to strengthen the One Direction community. Harry Styles followers have selected a cultural production generated by a member of the community with whom they share values, knowledge, and feelings. This research has identified ways of engagement that cause the selection of community contacts between fans.

Conclusions

The conclusions of this study focus on how adolescents who participate in fan communities organised around musical celebrities establish their contacts through certain strategies that also contribute to the maintenance and transformation of the aforementioned communities.

First, the fan communities to which young people belong rely on the social networks that are projected in online and offline areas. Within these networks, contacts are sought by exploring the information provided by the participants in these two areas. It is this information that allows them to select who they want to interact with or which containment mechanisms they can use to avoid certain participants.

Second, the strategies that allow fans to establish contacts with other people, whom fans have considered as 'wanted contacts', rely on friendship and shared interests. However, these contacts can be established on a double level, which the researchers have called macro and micro. The macro level focusses on the broader fan community and the micro level deals with the interpersonal relationships, with interaction taking place between the two levels.

Third, the countering practices that teens establish can be related to the concept of 'unwanted contacts' and include at least three processes. First, certain practices lead them to focus attention on those who share interests, excluding the rest. Second, the way online social networks work guides their exploration and selection of contacts to those with similar interests. Finally, the lack of an offline relationship or even a change in one's interests is also a mechanism that may inhibit contact.

The fourth conclusion is that the creation of multimodal texts mediate the relationships established between fans. In this case, it is necessary to go beyond the reconstruction of canonical texts. New meanings are generated through remix that allow fans to associate their own contexts with the celebrity. The creation of fanfiction is an example of participation and contact management. In this way, the engagement of the participants with the community is reaffirmed, helping to establish ties among the fans and thus further affirm the teen fandom community.

Notes

1 This work has been funded by the Ministry of Science, Innovation and Universities (Spain) and the Department of Research and Universities of the Regional Government of Castilla La Mancha. All participants in the research gave their written consent, as did their legal representatives. Our thanks to the girls and their families, without whom this study would not have been possible. www.mataderomadrid.org.
2 www.mataderomadrid.org.
3 Her account can be found at www.instagram.com/hsxallthelove/?hl=en.
4 http://los40.com/los40/2013/08/15/del40al1/1376602298_006150.html.
5 Lucia's participation in social networks can be found in several pages of her account in Wattpad:
   www.wattpad.com/user/Lucialds7
   www.wattpad.com/user/Lucialds7/following
   www.wattpad.com/list/91077228-Lucialds7s-reading-list.

References

Barton, K. M., & Lampley, J. M. (2013). *Fan culture: Essays on participatory fandom in the 21st century.* Jefferson, NC: McFarland.

Beer, D. (2008). Making friends with Jarvis Cocker: Music culture in the context of Web 2.0. *Cultural Sociology, 2*(2), 222–241.

Boellstorff, T. (2012). *Ethnography and virtual worlds: A handbook of method.* Princeton, NJ: Princeton University Press.

Bourdieu, P. (1972). *Outline of a theory of practice.* Cambridge, UK: Cambridge University Press.

boyd, d. (2014). *It's complicated: The social lives of networked teens.* New Haven, CT: Yale University Press.

Burton, J. T. D. (2017). *Making space on the digital margin: Youth fandom communities on tumblr as spaces for making the self and re-making society.* Camden, NJ: Rutgers University-Camden Graduate School.

Chambers, D. (2013). *Social media and personal relationships: Online intimacies and networked friendship.* Basingstoke: Palgrave Macmillan.

Cortesi, S., Gasser, U., Adzaho, G., Baikie, B., Baljeu, J., Battles, M., & Burton, P. (2015). *Digitally connected: Global perspectives on youth and digital media.* Harvard: Berkman Centre.

Daugherty, T., Eastin, M. S., & Bright, L. (2008). Exploring consumer motivations for creating user-generated content. *Journal of Interactive Advertising, 8*(2), 16–25.

Direction, O. (2013). *Meet one direction.* London, UK: HarperCollins.

Duffett, M. (2013). *Understanding fandom: An introduction to the study of media fan culture.* New York, NY: Bloomsbury.

Fiske, J. (1992). The cultural economy of fandom. In L. A. Lewis (Ed.), *The Adoring audience: Fan culture and popular media* (pp. 30–49). London and New York, NY: Routledge.

Flick, U. (Ed.). (2018). *The Sage handbook of qualitative data collection.* London and Thousand Oaks, CA: Sage Publications Ltd.

Gair, S., & Van Luyn, A. (2017). *Sharing qualitative research: Showing lived experience and community narratives.* Abingdon, Oxon and New York, NY: Routledge.

Gray, J., Sandvoss, C., & Harrington, C. L. (Eds.). (2017). *Fandom. identities and communities in a mediated world* (2nd ed.). New York, NY: New York University Press.

Hellekson, K., & Busse, K. (2014). *The fan fiction studies reader.* Iowa City, IA: University of Iowa Press.

Hinton, S., & Hjorth, L. (2013). *Understanding social media* (1st ed.). Los Angeles, CA: Sage Publications Ltd.

Holland, D., & Lave, J. (2009). Social practice theory and the historical production of persons. *Actio: An International Journal of Human Activity Theory, 2*(1), 1–15.

Holzman, L. (2010). Without creating ZPDs there is no creativity. In M. C. Connery, V. John-Steiner, & A. Marjanovic-Shane (Eds.), *Vygotsky and creativity: A cultural-historical approach to play, meaning making, and the arts* (pp. 27–40). New York, NY: Peter Lang.

Ito, M. (Ed.). (2010). *Hanging out, messing around, and geeking out: Kids living and learning with new media.* Cambridge, MA: MIT Press.

Jenkins, H. (1992/2013). *Textual poachers: Television fans and participatory culture* (2nd ed). (Updated 20th anniversary ed.). New York, NY: Routledge.

Jenkins, H., Ito, M., & boyd, d. (2015). *Participatory culture in a networked era: A conversation on youth, learning, commerce, and politics.* Cambridge, UK and Malden, MA: Polity Press.

Kibby, M. D. (2000). Home on the page: A virtual place of music community. *Popular Music, 19*(1), 91–100.

Knobel, M., & Lankshear, C. (2010). *DIY media: Creating, sharing and learning with new technologies.* New York, NY: Peter Lang.

Korobkova, K. A. (2014). Schooling the directioners: Connected learning and identity-making in the one direction fandom. *Digital Media and Learning Research Hub, 1,* 39.

Kress, G. R. (2010). *Multimodality: A social semiotic approach to contemporary communication.* London and New York, NY: Routledge.

Lacasa, P., de-la-Fuente, J., García-Pernía, M., & Cortés, S. (2017). Teenagers, fandom and identity. *Persona Studies, 2,* 51–65. Retrieved from: https://bit.ly/2Ym6zjX.

Lacasa, P., Martinez-Borda, R., & Mendez, L. (2013). Media as practice: Narrative and conceptual approach for qualitative data analysis. *Studies in Media and Communication, 1*(1), 132–149. Retrieved from: https://bit.ly/2Lo8ooC.

Lacasa, P., Méndez, L., & de-la-Fuente, J. (2016). Fandom, music and personal relationships through media: How teenagers use social networks. *Journal of the International Association for the Study of Popular Music, 6*(1), 44–67. Retrieved from: https://bit.ly/2maP7e5.

Livingstone, S., & Bovill, M. (2013). *Children and their changing media environment: A European comparative study.* Abingdon, UK: Routledge.

Marwick, A., & boyd, d. (2014). Networked privacy: How teenagers negotiate context in social media. *New Media & Society, 16*(7), 1051–1067.

Matusov, E. (2007). In search of 'the appropriate' unit of analysis for sociocultural research. *Culture & Psychology, 13*(3), 307–333.

Miller, D. (2016). *How the world changed social media.* London: UCL Press.

Navas, E., Gallagher, O., & Burrough, X. (2015). *The Routledge companion to remix studies.* New York, NY: Routledge.

Navas, E., & Gallagher, O. (2014). *The Routledge companion to remix studies.* London: Routledge.

Owens, T. (2015). *Designing online communities: How designers, developers, community managers, and software structure discourse and knowledge production on the web.* New York, NY: Peter Lang.

Pink, S. (2012). *Situating everyday life: Practices and places* (1st ed.). Thousand Oaks, CA: Sage Publications Ltd.

Rowsell, J. (2013). *Working with multimodality: Rethinking literacy in a digital age.* London and New York, NY: Routledge.

Soep, E. (2014). *Participatory politics: Next-generation tactics to remake public spheres.* Cambridge, MA: MIT Press.

Thomas, A. (2006). Fan fiction online: Engagement, critical response and affective play through writing. *The Australian Journal of Language and Literacy, 29*(3), 226–239.

Trier-Bieniek, A. (2015). *Fan girls and the media: Creating characters, consuming culture.* Lanham, MD: Rowman & Littlefield.

Turkle, S. (2011). *Alone together: Why we expect more from technology and less from each other.* New York, NY: Basic Books.

Willett, R. (2017). "Friending someone means just adding them to your friends list, not much else": Children's casual practices in virtual world games. *Convergence, 23*(3), 325–340.

16
IDENTITY EXPLORATION IN ANONYMOUS ONLINE SPACES

Mary Anne Lauri and Lorleen Farrugia

Introduction

Adolescence is characterised by the individuals' ongoing self-exploration of their physical, cognitive, and social characteristics. While these developmental processes remain consistent across generations, online technologies have significantly impacted both the context and how they take place. Social networking sites (SNS) have changed people's lives in dramatic ways, perhaps more so for adolescents.

Social platforms such as Ask.fm, Sarahah, Secret, Roastme, Whisper, Tumblr, Anomo, After School, Psst! Anonymous, and others, offer the possibility of anonymous social interaction. This facilitates self-expression and communication without the need to reveal one's identity. Stories about young people using such platforms have been in the international press a number of times, often after the incidence of a tragedy like the suicide of Hannah Smith in 2013. The rhetoric surrounding these platforms is negative (Binns, 2013; Vaughan, 2013). Media panics about this technology are similar in many ways to those which occurred about other forms of communication such as television (Drotner, 1999). Many platforms, including the ones which allow anonymous communication, are used by young people who may not be fully aware of the effects these could have on their developmental process, the development of their identity and their emotions (Peter & Valkenburg, 2013). This chapter investigates how many young people use sites which support anonymous communication and what characteristics users have in common. It also explores the reasons behind communicating anonymously or using pseudonyms.

Social Networking Sites Supporting Anonymous Communication

Raskauskas and Stoltz (2007) recommend that the study of adolescent development needs to take into consideration the internet as a 'place' where personal and social identities are being developed (p. 571). The online and offline worlds converge to such a high degree that all aspects of psychological and sociological development are impacted. This change presents a challenge to psychologists working with children, adolescents, and adults. The search for personal identity is no longer restricted to physical, interpersonal interactions with family and the peer group. It is now wider and takes place in the negotiated reality of the online world (Livingstone & Bovill, 2001; Moinian, 2006).

While the physical world restricts one's identity with bodily features such as stature, age, and race, the cyber world provides the user with opportunities for exploring different identities (Huffaker & Calvert, 2005). Through their profiles, adolescents create their own and their group's identities (boyd, 2007).

Adolescents mostly use platforms such as Ask.fm for fun and because the anonymity provided by the site helps them avoid awkward face-to-face conversations (Binns, 2013; Farrugia, Lauri, Borg, & O'Neill, 2018). They offer the possibility to communicate either anonymously or under a pseudonym. Post (1996) describes a message with a pseudonym as one that does not provide the name of the sender but contains some information about the identity of the originator of the message. These could be single individuals, groups, or organisations. An anonymous message does not provide these clues. The effect of using a pseudonym on the receiver is very similar to an anonymous message when the receiver cannot recognise whom the pseudonym is representing (Post, 1996).

Online communication and mainly anonymous interactions lack many of the clues and signs that are part of face-to-face interaction. This lack of identifiers and information is both a limitation and a resource, making certain kinds of interaction more challenging but also providing room to explore one's identity (Smith & Kollock, 1999). Users can describe themselves or say things which are not necessarily true about themselves. They can give correct, incorrect, or fake information. The feedback they receive is processed and noted.

As the popularity of such sites among adolescents has increased, these sites received significant adverse publicity due to their association with cyberbullying incidents. Anonymity allows adolescents to control what to reveal about themselves and how to do so. Simultaneously, the disinhibition associated with anonymity can easily lead to online harassment and cyberbullying (Suler, 2004; Valkenburg & Peter, 2011; Vásquez, 2014). Such behaviour was also associated with up to five teenage suicides in the UK, Ireland, and the USA (Blake, 2015; Vaughan, 2013). This type of behaviour, now termed *cyberbullycide*, is extreme and does not often happen even if cyberbullying is frequent (Chadwick, 2014). There is no conclusive evidence that anonymity gives rise to cyberbullying; however, the disinhibition effect of anonymity and the lack of confrontation can be enablers of this harmful behaviour (Valkenburg & Peter, 2011).

Identity Exploration

In the mind of many adults, anonymous posts and messages are synonymous with hurt, harassment, and bullying, but for some young people they are perceived as exciting and fun. They use SNS sites, including those sites where they can remain anonymous, for entertainment or to escape boredom. Adolescents also join because their friends are there and they want to feel that they belong to their group of peers (boyd, 2007, 2014; Farrugia et al., 2018). They also want to find out more about how others see them and possibly how they see themselves. Identity exploration is at the core of the use of these platforms and self-knowledge is among the motivations for media use (Roberts, Henriksen, & Foehr, 2004). Adolescents depend on social media to understand what identities are acceptable, to identify with their peers, and to express their new-found autonomy (Padilla-Walker, 2007).

The theory of psychosocial development (Erikson, 1963) presents identity development as a core task of adolescence. Through their social interactions, both online and offline, adolescents seek who they are and what they want to be. This can help the adolescents become more aware of their traits, but it also can give rise to identity confusion where the individual's sense of self is impaired (Reid & Boyer, 2013). When anonymous messages are positive and playful, young people feel good about themselves, and this may help their self-esteem. However, when anonymous messages have negative motives, young people can be severely damaged (Sticca & Perren, 2013).

Vásquez (2014) argues that profiles are not the only way through which adolescents present themselves online. Conversations such as chats also provide an opportunity for self-presentation. This identity is a discursive one. It is created by the user and acknowledged by online peers. Peter and Valkenburg (2013) argue that through five features of online media – anonymity, asynchronicity, cue management, accessibility, and retrievability – adolescents can manage the way they present themselves and what to disclose. The positive and negative implications of these five features pose to the adolescent opportunities but also risks.

Many users are savvy and use these sites to their advantage. To protect their privacy, adolescents engage in cost–benefit analyses when deciding whether to share information online. If they perceive benefits, they disclose readily, but if they perceive risks as being more significant than the benefits, they withhold information (Youn, 2005). In deciding whether to disclose information to a website, teens often perceive benefits rather than the risks involved. This is unsurprising, given that this age is characterised by risk-taking and experimentation (Casey, Jones, & Hare, 2008).

Withholding one's identity on anonymous platforms allows the adolescent to choose and control what to reveal about themselves. This facilitates the process of identity experimentation, self-disclosure, making new connections, and sexual exploration. Social media becomes the space in which adolescents in particular, "co-develop their identities and start their biographies" (Andrade, 2011, as cited in Rizzi & Pereira, 2013, p. 22).

The following two studies explore the use of anonymous platforms and look for patterns among users. Study one is about the anonymous platform Ask.fm while study two is about anonymous platforms in general.

Method

The first qualitative exploratory study has been published in Farrugia et al. (2018). Data was collected from four individual interviews and four focus groups carried out in 2013. These data were collected as part of a cross-national research project investigating European children's understanding of problematic situations online (see Šmahel & Wright, 2014 for details).

Focus Groups and Interviews

During the data collection for EU Kids Online, the researchers became aware of the popularity of the Ask.fm platform among Maltese participants. Ask.fm is a platform which invites its users to ask and reply to questions made by other anonymous users. Those replying to these questions also have the choice to do so anonymously. Instances when Ask.fm was mentioned in the Maltese interviews and focus groups were analysed in order to understand their motivations for using this site. Table 16.1 shows the participants' ages and gender. The participants were a convenience sample selected from eight different schools, two independent schools, two state schools and four church schools within the Northern, Northern Harbour, Central, and Western demographic regions of Malta.

Table 16.1 Participants in interviews and focus groups.

	Boys	Girls	Ages
Focus Group 1		5	11–12
Focus Group 2	4		12–13
Focus Group 3		4	14–16
Focus Group 4	5		14–16
Interview 1	1		13
Interview 2		1	15
Interview 3	1		16
Interview 4		1	16

Source: Figure generated from the 2013 EU Kids Online Malta Dataset.

The qualitative data were coded using thematic analysis after carrying out inductive and deductive coding, as discussed by Braun and Clarke (2006). Table 16.2 outlines the four themes resulting from this analysis with sample quotes that portray the themes. The findings indicate that participants used Ask.fm to have fun, to be accepted by their peers, to get feedback about themselves, and to experiment with the possibilities offered by anonymity.

One of the reasons given by participants for using Ask.fm was for its intriguing and entertaining value. It provided them with a way to kill time while having fun reading, answering, and asking questions. Participants enjoyed answering questions put to them anonymously as they could experiment with different identities online through the answers they gave. Since content on Ask.fm is often cross-posted to other platforms, this provided further opportunities for others to comment, adding to the entertainment they sought.

Participants often mentioned the need to be accepted by their peers as a reason why they joined Ask.fm. Some participants felt that having an Ask.fm account enabled them to connect with peers, and they continued using it even though they were aware that it distracts them from their studies. Participants' need to belong was also fulfilled through the question and answer interactions. When they felt they were not being asked the same number of questions as other users, it made them question why this was so and whether and why they were less popular. The pressure to belong and conform was also evident when participants admitted that they still answered unpleasant or inappropriate questions, even when it made them feel uncomfortable.

According to participants, receiving anonymous feedback was less risky both for the person asking for feedback and the one giving it. Through answering questions, they got to know more about themselves and what others thought of them. Such questions often focussed on their likes, dislikes, and personal opinions about a range of topics including personal characteristics as well as opinions on issues. Participants were also asked questions about their relationships, such as whom they were dating. They also received compliments from admirers. Participants mentioned that sometimes they were also asked to discuss their sexual history on these sites, and they disliked this because they felt it was inappropriate.

The use of Ask.fm often shifted beyond the original scope of asking and answering questions. Participants mentioned several instances where Ask.fm was used to circulate links with sexual, pornographic, or scary content. Cyberbullying was also present in the form of hate messages, insults, awful comments, provocation, and harassment. Some of them perceived anonymity as dangerous since users could get hurt and would not know the identity of the person insulting them. They were also aware that having an account on Ask.fm exposed them to those who wanted to insult them, but they were willing to take the risk because of the strong desire to find out what others thought about them.

Table 16.2 Motivations for using Ask.fm.

Themes	Clustered codes		Codes	Sample quotes
Whiling away the time, fun, intrigue	Fills time. Answering questions. Make the day better. Avoid boredom. Intrigue. Thrill.	Fun. Questions. Enjoy. Fascination. Interest. Facebook. Pastime.	Funny questions. Enjoyed seeing answers to questions. The unknown Challenge Game.	I enjoy seeing them ask me (Boy, 14). It's exciting to be asked questions anonymously (Boy, 15). I like not knowing who will ask me (Girl, 14).
The need to be accepted	Connecting with others. What is wrong with me? Being popular. Feeling excluded.	Fulfilled. Belong. Peer influence. Sharing information. Be noticed. Compelled. Connect. Tormented. Answering anyway.	Left out. Popularity. Being liked. Social media norms. Online community. Genuine questions. Pressure to fit in. Passing fad.	You start questioning "why aren't they asking me?".... You start wondering "what is it that they see in others that they don't see in me?" (Boy, 16).
Identity exploration	How others see them. Comments. Feedback. Role experimentation. Exploring identity.	Ask questions. Reply to questions. Personal questions. Self-disclosure. Negative comments. Showing off.	Roles. Dating. Relationships. Sexuality.	They ask you about your crushes (Girl, 14). I like the fact that they can ask me and I can reflect before I answer (Boy, 16).
The risks of anonymity	Asking for it. Inappropriate content. Inappropriate contact. Arguments. Positive and negative.	Anonymous questions. Avoiding confrontation. Insults. 'Hate'. Bullying. Suicide. Dangerous.	Mentioning the past. Hurt. Anger. Double bind. Disempowered. Facebook. Jealousy.	As soon as the anonymous people start asking you, you wouldn't know who they are, and you have to say "I asked for it" (Boy, 14). Let's say God forbid something bad happens to his family and they [his friends] would go to Ask.fm and start insulting him about it (Boy, 14).

Source: Table reproduced with permission of SAGE from Farrugia, L., Lauri, M. A., Borg, J., & O'Neill, B. *Have you asked for It? An exploratory study about Maltese adolescents' use of Ask.fm* (2019, Table 2, p. 746).
Note: Dataset: interviews and focus groups carried out in Malta in 2013 for the EU Kids Online Project.

Survey

The second study sought to find out the prevalence of children who use these sites, whether these children have characteristics which distinguished them from non-users and the reasons and motivations for using these platforms. To collect this data, a section with questions on anonymous sites was included as part of the EU Kids Online IV Survey – a European project researching children and the internet. The data collection took place between February and May 2018. Using stratified sampling, 20 schools from the six geographic regions in Malta took part. Consent was obtained from the Directorate for Learning and Assessment Programmes, the heads of schools, parents, and students. Participants were recruited in state, church, and independent schools in urban, suburban, and rural areas of Malta. This ensured that the sample was representative of the population of students aged 12 to 16 years. The survey was administered in classrooms by teachers who were briefed and trained by the researchers. A total of 993 questionnaires were collected.

Participants were presented with nine statements and an open-ended question (j) about platforms and apps through which one can communicate anonymously (see Figure 16.1).

Ask.fm, Sarahah, and Whisper were given as examples of such sites. These statements were based on qualitative findings presented in the first study. Respondents had to reply 'Yes' or 'No' to each statement, (a) to (i). The first statement (a) asked the participants whether they use anonymous platforms. Statements (d) and (g) dealt more directly with the young participants' sense of identity, while questions (b) and (i) touched on the issue of peer pressure. Statements (e) and (f) asked respondents whether they think that such sites are risky, while statements (c) and (h) asked about whether they enjoy using these sites.

Table 16.3 gives the percentages of those who use these sites and those who do not and their demographics.

Separate chi-squared tests between the responses to the anonymity statements and gender showed no significant associations except with the responses to statement (h) (chi-squared = 4.4856, df = 1, p =

PLEASE TICK YES or NO ON EVERY LINE

		Yes	No
a)	I use one of these platforms to talk to others anonymously	☐	☐
b)	I use these anonymous platforms because my friends do so	☐	☐
c)	I enjoy spending time talking to others anonymously	☐	☐
d)	I get to know more things about myself when I answer questions put to me anonymously	☐	☐
e)	I feel it is risky to communicate with others anonymously	☐	☐
f)	Those who use anonymous sites are inviting trouble	☐	☐
g)	I prefer getting feedback about myself from others anonymously	☐	☐
h)	It is fun to communicate online anonymously	☐	☐
i)	I would feel left out if I do not use these apps like my friends do	☐	☐
j)	Give one word you would use to describe anonymous sites		

Figure 16.1 Survey instrument investigating users' responses to platforms and apps that allow anonymous communication.

Table 16.3 Demographics of respondents.

	Number	Gender F	Gender M	Gender No answer	Age 11–12	Age 13–14	Age 15–17	Age No answer
Used anonymous sites	230	44%	54%	2%	2%	54%	43%	1%
Did not use anonymous sites	580	36%	61%	3%	2%	56%	41%	1%
Did not answer the section on anonymous sites	183	36%	62%	2%	0%	69%	27%	4%

Bases of percentages: users of anonymous sites, non-users and those who did not respond.

0.03418) and statement (i) (chi-squared = 13.455, df = 1, p = 0.00024). In both cases, boys tended to answer 'yes' to the statement more than girls, but the effect was more noticeable for statement 9. So, from these questions, it seems that boys, more than girls, think that it is fun to communicate via anonymous platforms and, even more so, they feel that they will be left out if they do not use such platforms. A similar chi-squared analysis showed that there was no significant association between the age of the participants and their response to any of the statements.

In order to gain more insight into how the responses to these statements categorise the participants, a multivariate technique, Latent Class Analysis (LCA), was used. This type of analysis hypothesises that, based on their responses to statements (b) to (i), participants can be categorised into a small number of latent classes and it calculates, for each participant, the probability that he or she is in any of the classes. In LCA this is done by creating a small number of new latent variables. Participants, based on their responses, are assigned a probability of being in a particular class. In a sense, LCA can be described as factor analysis for categorical variables. LCA enables the researcher to reduce the dimensionality of the data by classifying the respondents into a small number of meaningful categories giving a better understanding of the characteristics of the sample.

Finally, a regression analysis was carried out with the dependent variable being membership in these classes and the predictor (independent) variable being whether participants used anonymous sites. (For a discussion of LCA refer to Chapter 8 in Finch & French, 2015.) The LCA analysis was carried out using the poLCA package of the R programming language (Linzer & Lewis, 2011). The acronym poLCA stands for 'Polytomous variable Latent Class Analysis'. The poLCA program is given the observed response variables and the number of latent variables which the researcher wants to extract. In this case four models were extracted with two, three, four, and five latent variables respectively. The programme also calculates the value of BIC for each model. The lower the value of BIC the better the model. BIC stands for 'Bayesian Information Criterion' and it gives a measure of how likely the model is the true model while penalising model complexity. The model which gave the largest estimate of the maximum log-likelihood (-2655.716) and the least value of the BIC (5565.92) was the one with four latent classes. This was taken as the final model. The poLCA procedure estimated the sizes of each class, as given in Table 16.4.

Table 16.4 Estimated class shares.

	Class 1	Class 2	Class 3	Class 4
Estimated share	39%	22%	5%	34%

Base of percentages: sample of 813 participants who responded to the statement whether they use anonymous platforms.

Table 16.5 gives, for each of the four latent classes, the proportion of participants who would answer 'Yes' to each of the eight statements making up the manifest variables.

Table 16.5 The four latent classes emerging from the model.

Statement	Class 1	Class 2	Class 3	Class 4
(b) Use these sites to be like friends	1%	0%	97%	38%
(c) Use these sites because they enjoy it	1%	0%	100%	51%
(d) Use sites to get to know more about themselves	0%	7%	89%	55%
(e) Think communicating via these sites is risky	5%	87%	81%	45%
(f) Think these sites invite trouble	3%	94%	82%	39%
(g) Use sites to get feedback about themselves	1%	20%	87%	54%
(h) Think communicating anonymously is fun	1%	6%	100%	55%
(i) Feel left out if they did not use these sites	1%	4%	85%	37%

Bases for percentages: members of each respective class.

The poLCA program also carried out a logistic regression analysis to test how the concomitant variable use (whether the participant uses anonymous platforms) predicted membership of these classes. This procedure produced the results shown in Table 16.6. This table shows that using anonymous sites was a significant predictor for membership of each of Classes 2, 3, and 4 relative to the base Class 1.

Using Formula 12 of Linzer and Lewis (2011), the predicted probabilities that a respondent in each of the classes uses anonymous sites can be calculated from the regression coefficients given in Table 16.6, and these probabilities are presented in Table 16.7.

Interpretation of Results

From this model, it seems that participants can be classified in one of two main groupings based on whether they are users or non-users of anonymous platforms. The non-users would mostly be found in Class 1 with a probability of 53.9% or in Class 2 with a probability of 29.2%. These

Table 16.6 poLCA logistic regression model with USE as a predictor of class membership.

Class 2 vs Class 1

	Coefficient	Std. Error	t value	Pr(>|t|)
(intercept)	2.36689	1.41087	1.678	0.095
Use	-1.49041	0.70859	-2.103	0.037

Class 3 vs Class 1

	Coefficient	Std. Error	t value	Pr(>|t|)
(Intercept)	22.76939	0.30938	73.596	0.000
Use	-20.47185	0.30938	-66.171	0.000

Class 4 vs Class 1

	Coefficient	Std. Error	t value	Pr(>|t|)
(Intercept)	8.56789	1.18699	7.218	0.000
Use	-4.86225	0.60334	-8.059	0.000

Bases for percentages: members of each respective class.

Table 16.7 For each respective class, the probability that respondents are in that class if they are users/non-users of anonymous platforms.

	Class 1	Class 2	Class 3	Class 4
Probability of being in class if a user of anonymous sites	1.85%	4.4%	18.4%	75.3%
Probability of being in class if not user of anonymous sites	53.9%	29.2%	0.0%	16.9%

Base of percentages: users/non-users of anonymous sites.

classes are estimated to contain, between them, 61% of the participants (Table 16.4). On the other hand, users of anonymous sites are mostly found in Class 3 with a probability of 18.4% or in Class 4 with a probability of 75.3%. These two classes are estimated to contain between them 39% of the participants (Table 16.4). The characteristics of members of these four classes will be discussed using the data given in Table 16.5.

From Table 16.5, it would seem that for most members of **Class 1** – here labelled the *Indifferent Users* – participants answered 'No' to all statements. They do not feel peer-pressure to use these sites, they do not think these sites are dangerous or risky, they do not think they are fun to use, and they do not think they have benefits of imparting some self-knowledge. They seem to have no opinion in favour or against using anonymous sites. The members of Class 1 are estimated to contain 39% of the sample (Table 16.4).

Most members of **Class 2** – the *Guarded Users* – do not see much fun in using these sites, they do not experience peer-pressure to use them, they are not very much convinced that these sites can help them acquire self-knowledge, but most of them think that using anonymous sites is risky and invites trouble. The members of this class contain an estimated 22% of the sample.

Most members of **Class 3** – the *Avid Users* – hold the most extreme views of such sites. The majority of those in this group know that these platforms are risky, but all enjoy using such sites and most also feel pressure from their peers to be users. Most members of this class also believe that anonymous platforms help them know themselves better. So, although they know the risks, they are swayed by the benefits they see in such sites and by peer-pressure. Class 3 forms a very small group, estimated to claim only a 5% share of the sample.

Finally, the profile of **Class 4** – the *Moderate Users* – is similar to that of Class 3, but their opinions are not as widely held. Thus, only between 51% and 55% of respondents in this class think that using these sites is fun or enjoyable, around 38% feel peer-pressure in favour of using such sites, and between 39% and 45% of participants in this class think that using these sites is risky or invites trouble. Around 55% of members of this class think that these sites help them to know more about themselves. This class is estimated to contain 34% of the sample.

Therefore, most predicted users can be found in Class 4 (a user of anonymous sites has a 75% chance of being in this class). They are the Moderate Users. This class best represents the typical profile of a young user of anonymous sites.

Discussion

The survey indicates that anonymous websites are used by only 28% of the participants and only 2% were between the ages of 11 and 12. The results from these two studies point to four main findings. The first finding is that most of the users of anonymous platforms know that it is risky to use such platforms. For some users, the fear of social isolation is greater than the fear of getting hurt. Participants are aware that anonymous sites, perhaps more than other sites, can give rise to cyberbullying. They know that sometimes this could result in an elevated risk of suicidal thoughts, attempted suicide, and, in rare cases, completed suicides.

The second main finding is that, despite knowing the risk involved, some young people enjoy using anonymous sites and describe them as fun, cool, challenging, playful, fascinating, and funny. They are interested to know how others perceive them. Participants spoke about the excitement of engaging in such activities, the thrill they experienced and the intrigue about the unknown persons on the other side.

The third main finding is that for a group of young people, experimenting with anonymous social media platforms is viewed as an important part of belonging to a group. Peers exert covert pressure to use these sites and not using them creates anxiety in some participants for fear of not being considered as part of the in-group. Although pseudonyms are sometimes used, an in-group would have clues about who is writing what and who is not participating in this exchange of messages. Knowing that they can be identified and scapegoated if they do not participate creates fears of appearing to be weak and not tough enough to take up the challenge.

The fourth and perhaps most important finding is that exploring identities is very important for adolescents and anonymous online platforms seem to provide the space where young people can experiment with self-presentation. They can receive feedback about what they disclose and this may help them develop self-awareness and self-knowledge. Social media becomes the space in which adolescents develop their identity.

This fourth finding needs further exploration since there are many unanswered questions in this area. What role do social media play in the development of self-awareness, both private and public? How does feedback, even when given anonymously, lead to self-knowledge and how does it influence self-esteem? What type of self-comparison is at play online and what strategies are used to enhance the social self? Does the presence of social media change aspects of Social Identity Theory? Identity development in developmental psychology and social psychology has to be revisited to explore how important, long-standing, classic theories are impacted by the presence of the internet and smartphones in young people's lives. This chapter merely explored this topic at surface level and highlighted the need for more in-depth studies.

Conclusion

When the media report cases of cyberbullying leading to suicide, social media, and especially platforms supporting anonymous communication, are targeted and branded as very dangerous. This media panic does not seem to be justified as many users of these platforms know the danger involved and look upon their use as an activity in which they are in control and which they can take in their stride. Participants in this study who engage in anonymous communication seem to be resilient enough to cope with negative messages. Those who think they are too risky are very cautious and only use them guardedly. The number of casualties cannot be ignored and parents and teachers must encourage safe use of the internet through formal media education and informal sharing of information about safe social media practices. A safety net must be in place to make it easy for those experiencing distress to be able to report abuse and get help quickly. Safety features should be present in these platforms and updated periodically. Curtailing the use of anonymous sites is not possible, therefore discussing the dynamics and the effects these sites can have on users should become a crucial part of education and socialisation in general.

The authors would like to thank the Malta Communications Authority, the University of Malta and the Directorate for Learning and Assessment Programmes for financing and coordinating the data collection.

References

Binns, A. (2013). Facebook's ugly sisters: Anonymity and abuse on Formspring and Ask.fm. *Media Education Research Journal, 4*(1), 27–41. ISSN 2040-4530.

Blake, J. (2015). Ask.fm owners "considered shutting down" social network. Retrieved from: www.bbc.co.uk/newsbeat/31249209.

boyd, d. (2007). Why youth (heart) social network sites: The role of networked publics in teenage social life. *MacArthur Foundation Series on Digital learning–Youth, Identity, and Digital Media Volume*, 119–142. Retrieved from: https://ssrn.com/abstract=1518924.

boyd, d. (2014). *It's complicated: The social lives of networked teens*. Yale: University Press.

Braun, V., & Clarke, V. (2006). Using thematic analysis in psychology. *Qualitative Research in Psychology, 3*, 77–101. doi:10.1191/1478088706qp063oa.

Casey, B., Jones, R. M., & Hare, T. A. (2008). The adolescent brain. *Annals of the New York Academy of Sciences, 1124*(1), 111–126. doi:10.1196/annals.1440.010.

Chadwick, S. (2014). *Impacts of cyberbullying, Building social and emotional resilience in schools*. New York, NY: Springer Science & Business Media.

Drotner, K. (1999). Dangerous media? Panic discourses and dilemmas of modernity. *Paedagogica Historica, 35*(3), 593–619.

Erikson, E. (1963). *Childhood and society* (2nd ed.). New York, NY: Norton.

Farrugia, L., Lauri, M. A., Borg, J., & O'Neill, B. (2018). Have you asked for it? An exploratory study about Maltese adolescents' use of Ask. fm. *Journal of Adolescent Research*, 1–19. Advance online publication. doi:10.1177/0743558418775365.

Finch, W. H., & French, B. F. (2015). *Latent variable modelling with R*. New York, NY: Routledge.

Huffaker, D., & Calvert, S. (2005). Gender identity, and language use in teenage blogs. *Journal of Computer-Mediated Communication, 10*(2), n.p. doi:10.1111/j.1083-6101.2005.tb00238.x.

Linzer, D. A., & Lewis, J. B. (2011). poLCA: An R package for polytomous variable latent class analysis. *Journal of Statistical Software, 42*(10), 1–29.

Livingstone, S., & Bovill, M. (Eds.). (2001). *Children and their changing media environment: A European comparative study*. Mahwah, NJ: Lawrence Erlbaum Associates.

Moinian, F. (2006). The construction of identity on the internet. Oops! I've left my diary open to the whole world. *Childhood, 13*(1), 49–68. doi:10.1177/0907568206058610.

Padilla-Walker, L. M. (2007). Developmental needs of adolescence and media. In J. J. Arnett (Ed.), *Encyclopedia of children, adolescents and the media* (Vol. 1, pp. 2–5). Thousand Oaks, CA: Sage.

Peter, J., & Valkenburg, P. M. (2013). The effects of internet communication on adolescents' psychological development. In A. N. Valdivia (Ed.), *The international encyclopaedia of media studies* (pp. 678–697). Hoboken, NJ: Blackwell Publishing Ltd. doi:10.1002/9781444361506.wbiems136.

Post, D. G. (1996). *Pooling intellectual capital. Thoughts on pseudonymity and limited liability in cyberspace*. Chicago, IL: University of Chicago Legal Forum.

Raskauskas, J., & Stoltz, A. D. (2007). Involvement in traditional and electronic bullying among adolescents. *Developmental Psychology, 43*(3), 564–575. doi:10.1037/0012-1649.43.3.564.

Reid, G. G., & Boyer, W. (2013). Social network sites and young adolescent identity development. *Childhood Education, 89*(4), 243–253. doi:10.1080/00094056.2013.815554.

Rizzi, C., & Pereira, A. G. (2013). Social networks and cyberbullying among teenagers. *Publications Office of the European Union, Luxembourg*. Retrieved from: http://publications.jrc.ec.europa.eu/repository/bitstream/JRC80157/lbna25881enn.pdf.

Roberts, D. F., Henriksen, L., & Foehr, U. G. (2004). Adolescents and media. In R. M. Lerner & L. Steinberg (Eds.), *Handbook of adolescent psychology* (2nd ed., pp. 487–521). Hoboken, NJ: John Wiley & Sons Inc.

Šmahel, D., & Wright, M. F. (Eds.). (2014). *Meaning of online problematic situations for children. Results of qualitative cross-cultural investigation in nine European countries*. London: EU Kids Online, London School of Economics and Political Science. Retrieved from: http://eprints.lse.ac.uk/id/eprint/56972.

Smith, C., & Kollock, P. (1999). *Communities in cyberspace*. London: Routledge.

Sticca, F., & Perren, S. (2013). Is cyberbullying worse than traditional bullying? Examining the differential roles of medium, publicity, and anonymity for the perceived severity of bullying. *Journal of Youth and Adolescence, 42*(5), 739–750.

Suler, J. (2004). The online disinhibition effect. *Cyberpsychology & Behaviour, 7*, 321–326. doi:10.1089/1094931041291295.

Valkenburg, P. M., & Peter, J. (2011). Online communication among adolescents: An integrated model of its attraction, opportunities, and risks. *Journal of Adolescent Health, 48*(2), 121–127.

Vásquez, C. (2014). "Usually not one to complain but ...": Constructing identities in user-generated online reviews. In P. Seargeant & C. Tagg (Eds.), *The language of social media* (pp. 65–90). London: Palgrave Macmillan UK.

Vaughan, R. (2013). Technology – Girls suffer on site "made for bullying". *The Times Educational Supplement Scotland, (2332)*, 14–15. Retrieved on 3 August 2014 from: http://search.proquest.com/docview/1444758894?accountid=27934.

Youn, S. (2005). Teenagers' perceptions of online privacy and coping behaviours: A risk–benefit appraisal approach. *Journal of Broadcasting & Electronic Media, 49*(1), 86–110.

17
SUPERVISED PLAY
Intimate Surveillance and Children's Mobile Media Usage

William Balmford, Larissa Hjorth, and Ingrid Richardson

Introduction

Contemporary homes have become environments within which appropriate times, spaces, and places for the use of screen interfaces are constantly contested and (re)negotiated. Mobile media further complicates these practices, as they are intimate and playful devices that are carried on the body (thus often with no designated place within the home), and their networking and social media capability renders them potentially risky for young users. This chapter focusses on parental monitoring of their children's mobile media practices, contributing to extant scholarship that has explored the role of mobile media in redefining place (de Souza e Silva & Frith, 2012), surveillance practices (Humphreys, 2011), privacy (Gazzard, 2011), and the impact of mobile technology on corporate and governmental surveillance in an age of Big Data (e.g., Andrejevic, 2006, 2013; Cincotta et al., 2011; Farman, 2011; Lupton, 2016). The authors suggest that new forms of social surveillance (Marwick, 2012) are becoming part of everyday life in domestic and familial settings, adding another – and, to date, under-researched – component to the practices of care and supervision of children in the home (Fitchard, 2012; Clark, 2013; Burrows, 2017; Leaver, 2017). Little research has been conducted into the friendly, informal modes of surveillance that take place within the family (Leaver, 2017; Hjorth et al., 2018), and especially across the range of different social and hierarchical relations that exist in domestic contexts.

Care has always had a complex relationship to surveillance (Bellacasa Puig de la, 2012), as it involves paradoxical notions of constraint, control, guardianship, and concern. Digital and mobile media complicates this imbrication further. Mobile technologies are frequently deployed as ambient forms of surveillance between family members (Matsuda, 2009; Clark, 2013). Misa Matsuda discusses such a phenomenon in her work on the use of *keitai* (mobile phones) (2009). Matsuda argues that alongside the growth of *keitai* in Japan, the Japanese family "now makes optimal use of the *keitai* in order to maintain their familial bonds" while engaging in other daily tasks (Matsuda, 2009, p. 62).

Likewise, Clark engages notions of the ambient to explore how mobile media allows for unobtrusive remote contact or what she terms "respectful connectedness" through more subtle surveillance, as an alternative to more conspicuous modes of monitoring teenagers' mobile (and other media) usage, which she describes as "helicopter parenting" (2013, p. 205). Other forms of child surveillance have also been of interest to scholars, including research into school surveillance (Shade & Singh, 2016) and intergenerational 'friendly surveillance' (Hjorth et al., 2018). These studies effectively recalibrate how we conceptualise surveillance, yet there is still more work needed to understand these quotidian modes of care and supervision as they are woven into and through the mobile media practices of children and parents.

This chapter seeks to explore the informal ways in which friendly, intimate, and careful surveillance plays out in domestic mobile media practices. How are parents and children deploying media in forms of ambient watching? And what do these current practices suggest in terms of future implications for the field?

The chapter draws on ethnographic fieldwork conducted as part of the Games of Being Mobile (GoBM)[1] project. Over three years, the researchers conducted in-home interviews, participant observation, and play sessions in 60 households across five major cities around Australia. In what follows, the chapter begins with an overview of the GoBM study and a discussion of current debates around everyday surveillance and media. Then, drawing on the project's findings, the chapter provide examples of how this is shaped in and by parents' and children's mobile media practices. The authors argue that the dynamic relationship between families and media use involves complex notions of intimacy, care, mediated sociality, and media literacy.

Contextualising the Study

The GoBM study was funded by the Australian Research Council (ARC) and is the first Australia-wide and longitudinal study of mobile gaming practices in the home. The project investigated Australian mobile gaming to better understand how mobility, play, and location are entangled in digital and networked media usage, particularly in domestic contexts. Ethnographic fieldwork was conducted over three years in 60 participant households across five cities (Sydney, Melbourne, Adelaide, Perth, and Brisbane). Throughout this chapter the authors draw on the experiences of several key participants that offer a variety of insights into the changing conceptions of informal surveillance in Australian homes. Throughout the GoBM project three key ethnographic methods were employed: informal interviews, play sessions, and participant observation.

Interviews were informal and semi-structured, most often conducted within participants' households. Each household was interviewed on three occasions, in which their history with and ongoing use of mobile media was explored. Follow-up interviews often included 'play sessions', which involved playing videogames with participants, predominantly on mobile devices. Participants chose the games to be played and the sessions were crucial in highlighting intersections between device use and being-at-home and capturing typical scenarios of media practice. Through the play sessions researchers were able to informalise their position as researchers and better observe ambient mobile usage within the home. The other key method used during the GoBM fieldwork was participant observation – viewing and engaging in activities with participants. Although the play sessions conducted were a form of participant observation, other activities, such as family dinners, board game nights, or 'no screen' occasions, were also observed as a way to extend the authors' ethnography into the everyday routines of the participants' lives.

Each of these techniques were deployed across one or more of three key meetings with participant households, which included an introductory meeting, a return meeting six to 12 months later, and a final meeting another six to 12 months after that. Recruitment for GoBM consisted of a plain language statement (PLS) and accompanying call for interest on social media platforms such as Facebook and Twitter. Digital communities such as Reddit and Gumtree (an online community marketplace) were also engaged, with potential participants being contacted through direct messaging. Potential participants were also 'snowballed' from existing social networks. As the GoBM project sought to engage with a variety of age and literacy demographics, a simplified PLS was written for participants who were under the age of 18. In these more vulnerable participant cases, a simplified PLS was especially useful to ensure ongoing informed consent. These accommodations allowed research to be conducted with a variety of groups including families with younger children – an important focus of this chapter.

Understanding Informal Surveillance

Practices of monitoring media use within domestic settings – or everyday, interpersonal, careful, and caring modes of surveillance – require a rethink of what surveillance means outside traditional corporate or governmental contexts. Lee Humphreys identifies three kinds of surveillance within social media practice: the voluntary panopticon ("voluntary submission to corporate surveillance"), lateral surveillance ("asymmetrical, nontransparent monitoring of citizens by one another"), and self-surveillance (monitoring oneself through technology) (2011, p. 577). These various forms of surveillance correspond in various ways to the different styles of intimate and careful parental monitoring of children's mobile media usage that will be explored later in the chapter.

While surveillance is often immediately thought of as something carried out by government bodies or large companies, there are many more types of surveillance – horizontal and vertical, benevolent and malevolent – that move in and out of daily practices. These practices are indicative of new forms of social surveillance (Marwick, 2012) within families that are creating additional – and to date under-researched – layers (Clark, 2013; Shade & Singh, 2016). Where Clark's *The Parent App* (2013) explores how families are adapting to the growing presence of digital technology (with mobile phones being a particular focus), Shade and Singh discuss the growing trend of student social media surveillance by schools in the United States (2016). These two works both explore how contemporary media are layering new formal and informal modes of surveillance across everyday life contexts. The emergence of this ongoing surveillance is potentially problematic, with Shade and Singh arguing that "surveillance of young people can erode their trust in parents, authority figures, schools, and the state; it can stifle the development of autonomy, resilience, and agency" (2016, p. 9). Due to such potential risks, many stakeholders (including families) are seeking less blatant forms of social surveillance.

For Alice Marwick, 'social surveillance' is distinguished from traditional forms through three axes – power, hierarchy, and exchange. Utilising Foucault's notion of capillaries of power, Marwick argues that social surveillance assumes "power differentials evident in everyday interactions rather than the hierarchical power relationships assumed in much of the surveillance literature" (2012: p. 378). Marwick identifies some of the common notions of surveillance such as lateral (Andrejevic, 2006), participatory (Albrechtslund, 2008), social searching (Lampe et al., 2006), and social (Joinson, 2008; Tokunaga, 2011). Where lateral surveillance refers to the observation of peers, participatory modes invite a more playful framing, understanding surveillance as potentially 'positive and empowering' (Marwick, 2012, p. 381). Social searching – the use of social media to learn more about one's family and friends – is one example of how participatory surveillance can be perceived in a more positive light (Marwick, 2012). As Marwick notes, social surveillance differs from traditional models insofar as it is focussed around micro-level, decentralised, reciprocal interactions between individuals.

The parent–child surveillance relationship has been extensively written about in popular media, particularly in terms of digital and online privacy, and is commonly referred to as 'internet parenting' (Bakardjieva, 2005; Valcke et al., 2010). The terminology refers to the myriad of approaches parents take to protect, teach, and manage the online media consumption of their children (Bakardjieva, 2005). As Sonia Livingstone has argued, the issue of risky media engagement by children has become ever more difficult to monitor as interfaces have shifted from stationary positions within 'collective family space' to mobile and online devices that are used in "individualised, personalised, and, for children, unsupervised spaces" (2009, p. 156).

Leaver discusses the perceptions and manifestations of such surveillance, arguing that parental monitoring both of and through media usage is contributing to the "normalisation of intimate surveillance, where to monitor, mediate, and publicly share media about infants become markers of good parenting and culturally appropriate levels of care" (2017, p. 8). Likewise, Hjorth, Heather Horst, and Sarah Pink have written about the ongoing shift towards intimate surveillance, paying particular attention to the idea of 'friendly surveillance' (2018). Friendly surveillance speaks to the geographies of care that infuse everyday life with benevolent modes of watching (Mol, 2008; Marwick, 2012) and the use of technology to enable care from a distance.

It is this body of research concerning 'friendly' and intimate surveillance to which this chapter contributes. Through an exploration of parental surveillance in Australian households, the authors argue that mobile media engages discourses and practices of 'friendly' and 'careful' surveillance in new and ambient ways. The following sections provide detailed scenarios of use, with a particular focus on the ways these routines of surveillance involve both 'ambient presence' through social mobile media and networked gameplay, and the co-located implementation of usage boundaries within the physical space of the home.

Checking In and Friending: Ambient Surveillance

Margaret, aged 50, often worries about her 17-year-old daughter Chrissy[2] while she is out of the house. Living in Melbourne's outer suburbs with her husband Frank, Margaret has noticed that over the school holidays Chrissy spends most of her time out and about with friends in Melbourne's inner-city areas. Fearful of "overwatching" her daughter (as Chrissy put it) she instead tries to carefully surveil Chrissy through the mobile games they play together. When Chrissy was younger the mother and daughter would often play *Scrabble* on family holidays or during quiet weekends. Now both have smartphones, through which they play the *Scrabble*-like game *Words With Friends*. The game enables them to play at a distance, a capability Margaret often takes advantage of. As she explained during one interview, she will play a word while Chrissy is out, feeling that "really it is just saying 'well hey I'm here', without actually having to make a phone call".

Alongside her turn in the game, Margaret will also frequently send a short message through the game's chat function. She explained she does this because it is less overt and intrusive than a text message. She described this form of communication with her daughter as "a sort of secret corridor", a private communication line to her daughter. Many of the participants referred to what is termed the phatic nature of their communication in mobile social games – micro-social interactions such as sending a gift, taking one's turn in a game, or messaging "Hi" – as a means of verifying that the channel of communication is open and working, or as a way to say "I'm here (for you)" (Jakobson, 1960). The use of mobile and social media as enablers of phatic or ambient communication, through texting, online communication, playful mobile apps, and gameplay is well recognised (Kirman et al., 2009; Hjorth & Richardson, 2014; Balmford & Davies, 2019). For Margaret, phatic communication with her daughter through *Words With Friends* is an instance of both ambient play (Hjorth & Richardson, 2020) and ambient surveillance.

The way in which Margaret uses *Words With Friends* also echoes ideas of "geographies of care" and "care at a distance" (Mol, 2008; Marwick, 2012). Through the act of game playing she is able to reach out and make contact with her daughter, displaying affection and a kind of low-stakes or unobtrusive concern through the application. This app-negotiated surveillance is similar to the scenarios of use Leaver details, however it plays out in a different manner (2017). Where Leaver explores parental mediation through image sharing and texting – often through very public "influencer" accounts (2017) – Margaret's intent was to enact subtle and careful surveillance, seeking to register contact with her daughter to "let her know I'm here (if she needs me)", without exposing this concern to her daughter's wider social circle. This careful negotiation was important as Chrissy, nearly 18, desired a certain amount of freedom from her mother's oversight.

Likewise, Margaret wanted to promote such independence in her daughter while still ensuring her safety. To this extent Margaret admitted there was an element of subterfuge in her surveillance. Rather than the explicit purpose of communicating through a text message, her communication through *Words With Friends* was obfuscated through a layer of play. In this way her surveillance was more ambient – interwoven with social media and game practices that are already embedded in everyday-life routines and habitudes.

Chrissy, present during a follow-up interview, explained that her mother's surveillance was perhaps not as subtle as Margaret intended. "I know exactly what you're doing mum!" she laughed as her mother revealed her secret strategy. However, despite her knowledge of the inner workings of the practice, Chrissy acknowledged that her mother's attempts were still appreciated. She explained that it was preferable to a phone call or text as it was less "in the way", meaning it allowed her to respond when she felt like it, rather than "demanding" a response. In this negotiation, the friendly monitoring and concern Margaret employs through *Words With Friends* allows for a more lateral form of surveillance in which members of the social group are perceived as more equal, rather than hierarchical.

Other writers have identified similar phenomena, detailing how mobile media allows groups 'to keep a friendly eye' on each other (Hjorth et al., 2018, p. 1220). Hjorth et al., for example, explore this friendly watching in their work on locative media practices among same sex couples (2018). For these couples, locative media services such as geotagged Facebook posts or tracked Uber rides allowed partners to monitor the location of their significant other, deriving comfort and security through the intimate surveillance that the technology afforded (Hjorth et al., 2018). Much like the friendly eye of locative media highlighted by Hjorth et al., Margaret offers a maternal hand to her daughter; she can reach out if she needs to and a returning move lets Margaret know her daughter is ok. Marwick's interpretation of social surveillance, particularly her recognition of how it can operate at a decentralised and micro-level, is clearly visible in the subtle, friendly (and careful) surveillance that takes place between Margaret and her daughter. Similarly, despite the lack of geolocative technology, Margaret employs technology to surveil her daughter for similar reasons to Hjorth et al.'s participants, out of a desire to maintain feelings of closeness without direct interference (2018). As they write:

> The term careful surveillance describes the way we monitor and watch our intimates as cohabitants subject to our care. Yet, it also deliberately implies that surveillance should be a careful practice, one that we consider very carefully in terms of its impact on others.
>
> *(Hjorth et al., 2018, p. 1220)*

These notions of impact are particularly relevant in parent–child relationships, where duty of care intersects with a desire to promote independence and resilience. To this extent it is important to note that the mobile-oriented careful surveillance Margaret employs was possible in part because of Chrissy's age and her overt ownership of a mobile phone. Nearly an adult, Chrissy holds a certain amount of agency in how she negotiates the world, and the speed with which she responds to her mother. The next examples this chapter offers explore a different scenario, one in which the children being surveilled are of a younger age.

Chloe and Elish (both 13) live in Adelaide with their mother Vicky (45). Vicky, a single mother, recently allowed her daughters to get Instagram accounts, which they access both through their smartphones and the several iPads they have at home. Vicky was hesitant about allowing her daughters to use the social media platform. Many of these concerns revolved around the unexpected consequences of posting content online: "there's bad people out there, but even just innocent things like, you know, like if you take a photo of yourself ... inadvertent things can happen". She attempted to educate her daughters on these risks, explaining issues of privacy and exposure, but she still felt the need to monitor their usage.

Vicky achieved this monitoring in two ways. The first way was to follow her daughters on Instagram, explaining that: "I suppose that's why I'm on Instagram too so I can check what they're doing". Furthermore, she expanded this friendly surveillance into the social circles of her children, saying that "I follow a lot of their friends as well". She explained that she follows her daughters and their friends largely to keep track of her daughters' activities. Through this considered surveillance, Vicky was able to 'check in' on what Chloe and Elish were up to without explicitly making a phone call or sending a text message.

Likewise, monitoring their online activity allowed her to observe any potentially problematic posts or online behaviour – an increasing concern for many parents, as noted by Clark (2013). This 'checking in', enabled by the convergence of mobile and social media in communication practices, can be described in Mark Paterson's terms (2009) as a form of "mediated social touch" (p. 61). Similarly, for Farman (2011), 'social proprioception' refers to this embodied awareness of distant others that is intrinsic to communicative experiences on social media platforms and through mobile media. For Vicky, Instagram affords a mode of 'ambient presence' (Hjorth & Richardson, 2014) that allows her to 'be with' her daughters and simultaneously engage in a kind of soft surveillance that avoids more direct or intrusive pathways of communication.

Similar to Elish and Chloe, the way in which Brisbane children Sophie, aged 12, and Max, aged 14, are allowed to use mobile social media came with the caveat of 'being friends with Mum'. Even getting a mobile phone was predicated upon this agreement. As Sophie explained with much frustration: "she was like, 'You can only buy it if you're friends with me'". Her brother Max explained that being 'friends' with their Mum had a significant impact on how they used their phones while online and out of the house: "it means you can't like inappropriate stuff". Interestingly, Sophie felt that some of her friends did not adjust their practices to parental surveillance. She exasperatedly remarked:

> I see some pretty inappropriate things that my friends have liked. I'm just like, 'You want everyone to see that you've liked that?' Just like, wow. I'm like, 'Are you actually that stupid? Everyone can see it, and you can get into trouble'. Well, you can't really get into trouble for liking it I guess, but if you shared it or something.

The experiences of Sophie, Max, Elish, and Chloe all highlight a phenomenon common across the GoBM research in which parents, alongside using mobile devices to monitor their children's physical presence, carefully surveilled their children's online lives as well. In these cases, the children's mobile media practices were closely linked to social engagement with friends, a type of "messing around" (Lange & Ito, 2010) on Instagram and other social media as a mode of connection and involvement in social worlds. Parents' monitoring of these behaviours reflect the fears and risks of online behaviour Clark and other scholars have identified (Livingstone et al., 2012; Clark, 2013). However, they also highlight practices of careful surveillance through mobile technology and social media. Where direct surveillance through explicit contact was often perceived by children as obtrusive, the ambient surveillance mobile social media afford allowed parents to take a more considered and covert approach. As outlined above, such monitoring was deemed commonplace, reflecting Leaver's argument that intimate surveillance is increasingly seen as a crucial responsibility of the parent (and to not do so would be to 'fail' as a carer) (2017). By deploying careful surveillance through social media posts on mobile phones, parents are able to enact this responsibility through a lens more tolerable to their children.

Playing Together: Co-Located Surveillance

> It's not terribly strict, but there are times when we've noticed they are playing for too long. We do have to kick them off it and force sharing among them. Like, recently we changed the password so they had to come to us to get into it. So they couldn't get into it while we weren't paying attention and stay on it for hours. We kind of try to limit it a little bit.

The quote above comes from Helen, 29-year-old mother of Amy (four) and Penny (eight). Helen, her partner Charlie (also 29), and their two children live in Brisbane. A young family, they are one of the only couples within their social circle with children. They often find themselves having to watch their children's 'screen time' for fear of over-use. Such management and monitoring tactics are common among the other families she knows, with nearly all limiting children's access to devices (both mobile and static). Furthermore, these periods of time were often also spatially restricted, such as being confined to the living room or kitchen, where their engagement could be easily monitored by parents co-located within the domestic space. These examples show scenarios of use where limited mobile device access, combined with spatial limitations to particular spaces, was employed as a parental management and surveillance strategy. Techniques such as removal of the device after there has been 'enough' of a certain activity, or use within only certain rooms of the home, were frequently employed by GoBM parent participants.

The restriction of screen time has been an ongoing topic of interest in popular media and is a common method of device management for many parents (Clark, 2013). In *The Parent App*, Clark argues against the implementation of such restrictions unless a reasonable alternative is suggested, as imposed limitations without reasonable alternatives are likely to be unhelpful and contribute to feelings of obtrusive surveillance (2013). Instead, Clark suggests management strategies that "can offer an alternative that demands that [you], too, stop what [you're] doing in favour of a different activity", such that parents enact the behaviour they desire to see in their children (2013, p. 220).

More recently, Ito (2017, 2018) and other scholars such as Blum-Ross and Livingstone (2016) have maintained that screen time limitations are based on ineffective measures of whether mobile device usage is positive or negative. They claim that quantitative limits ignore the ubiquitous nature of mobile phones and call instead for management strategies that focus on context, content, and connections over quantity (Blum-Ross & Livingstone, 2016). Context concerns the situation in which the device is being used (both mediated and actual), content refers to the 'what' of mobile interaction (what is being shared, communicated, or engaged with), while connections comprise the social bonds and networks involved (Blum-Ross & Livingstone, 2016).

Charlotte (37), a mother of four children living in Sydney with her husband Oscar, explained that her two older children are now adults living out of home, but that she approached the issue of screen time a little differently with her two younger children Michael (aged ten) and Stephan (aged six), who are currently very invested in mobile videogames. In an effort to combine surveillance with 'quality time', she actively played the games her sons were interested in. As she explained:

> I helped them with their games and so I'd get to know about their games. I'd help them play, I'd learn, I'd get interested … So, I'm sort of playing with them, making

sure it is ok what they're playing and they're having fun. So a lot of my gaming has been side-by-side with my boys.

Charlotte's screen-time monitoring was therefore enacted in a more companionable and supportive manner, one that better aligns with Livingstone and Blum-Ross' advice regarding the "content, context and connections" of device usage (2016, p. 4). That is, what may be understood as a form of surveillance is closely entangled with maternal caring and 'quality time' (as Charlotte explained). What constitutes surveillance here becomes interwoven with practices of co-located intimacy and play. Charlotte deliberately avoided explicit monitoring and prohibitive rules around mobile gameplay, and through such engagement her surveillance of her children's mobile media use was more considered and careful, oriented positively around togetherness and opportunities for co-located interaction. Though similarly based on co-located management strategies, Helen and Charlie preferred explicit temporal and spatial restrictions. For both families, their considered oversight and monitoring practices are salient instances of informal, intimate, and 'domesticated' surveillance.

Implications and Conclusion

As mobile media becomes increasingly ubiquitous, parents will continue to worry about how to monitor and control their children's engagement with such technology. This chapter has explored how such monitoring is achieved through the use of 'careful surveillance' (Hjorth et al., 2018). The chapter identified two main modalities of parental watching: ambient or mediated co-presence (through social mobile media and gameplay), and co-located supervision via temporal and spatial restrictions and collaborative play. Each are managed though different modalities of presence and are partially dependent on the age of the children.

Throughout the GoBM project, ambient or mediated surveillance was most often observed in parental monitoring of older teenage children, where the fostering of independence and self-determination is deemed important by both parent and child. In contrast, co-located intimacy and spatial/temporal boundary work are far more common strategies for management of younger children, and, ideally, the specificity of content, context, and connections is recognised. In both of these manifestations of careful surveillance parents often sought to balance the wellbeing of their children alongside a desire to not appear overly determining – recalling Marwick's (2012) reframing of surveillance as potentially empowering and playful.

The implications of careful surveillance in the home and familial contexts will continue to be felt as mobile devices become thoroughly embedded in everyday life. How parents monitor and surveil their children's mobile device usage is crucial to how technology is perceived and taken up by coming generations. Surveillance through and of mobile media involves a complex interplay of power, agency, affect, and enjoyment. In the already emotionally charged parent–child relationship, such surveillance is both important and potentially risky.

As this chapter has shown, approaches deploying 'careful surveillance' appear better poised to promote ongoing considerations of the content, context, and social connections pertaining to mobile device usage. Further research into the various informal and intimate routines of watching and managing children's media engagement might explore other scenarios of use, such as school-based monitoring or the intervolved supervision of older siblings, providing further insight into the ways mobile media practices both demand and afford diverse modalities of domesticated and everyday surveillance.

Notes

1 GoBM was an Australia Research Council (ARC) discovery project.
2 All participants have been given pseudonyms to ensure anonymity.

References

Albrechtslund, A. (2008). Online social networking as participatory surveillance. *First Monday*, *13*(3). Retrieved from: www.uic.edu/htbin/cgiwrap/bin/ojs/index.php/fm/article/view/2142/1949.

Andrejevic, M. (2006). The work of watching one another: Lateral surveillance, risk, and governance. *Surveillance & Society*, *2*(4), 479–497.

Andrejevic, M. (2013). *Infoglut: How too much information is changing the way we think and know*. London, UK: Routledge.

Bakardjieva, M. (2005). *Internet society: The internet in everyday life*. London, UK: Sage.

Balmford, W., & Davies, H. (2019). Mobile Minecraft: Negotiated space and perceptions of play in Australian families. *Mobile Media & Communication*. doi:10.1177/2050157918819614.

Bellacasa Puig de la, M. (2012). Nothing comes without its world: Thinking with care. *The Sociological Review*, *60*(2), 197–216. doi:10.1111/j.1467-954X.2012.02070.

Blum-Ross, A., & Livingstone, S. (2016). Families and screen time: Current advice and emerging research. *LSE Media Policy Project, Media Policy Brief 17*. London, UK: The London School of Economics and Political Science.

Burrows, B. (2017). YouTube kids: The app economy and mobile parenting. *Social Media + Society*, *3*(2). doi:10.1177/2056305117707189.

Cincotta, K., Ashford, K., & Michael, K. (2011). The new privacy predators. *Women's Health*. Retrieved from: www.womenshealth.com.au.

Clark, L. S. (2013). *The parent app: Understanding families in the digital age*. Oxford, UK: Oxford University Press.

de Souza e Silva, A., & Frith, J. (2012). *Mobile interfaces in public spaces: Locational privacy, control, and urban sociability*. London, UK: Routledge.

Farman, J. (2011). *Mobile interface theory*. London, UK: Routledge.

Fitchard, K. (2012). *By 2016, 70M families will keep tabs on each other with GPS*. Retrieved from: https://gigaom.com/2012/09/04/by-2016-70m-families-will-keep-tabs-on-each-other-with-gps.

Gazzard, A. (2011). Location, location, location: Collecting space and place in mobile media. *Convergence*, *17*(4), 405–417.

Hjorth, L., Pink, S., & Horst, H. (2018). Being at home with privacy: Privacy and mundane intimacy through same-sex locative media practices. *International Journal of Communication*, *12*, 1209–1227.

Hjorth, L., & Richardson, I. (2014). *Gaming in social, mobile and locative media*. New York, NY: Palgrave MacMillan.

Hjorth, L., & Richardson, I. (2020). *Ambient play*. Cambridge, MA: MIT Press.

Humphreys, L. (2011). Who's watching whom? A study of interactive technology and surveillance. *Journal of Communication*, *61*(4), 575–595.

Ito, M. (2017). How dropping screen time rules can fuel extraordinary learning. *Connected Camps*. Retrieved from: https://blog.connectedcamps.com/how-dropping-screen-time-rules-can-fuel-extraordinary-learning.

Ito, M. (2018). How to shed distracted parenting guilt and transform into a digital hero. *Connected Camps*. Retrieved from: https://blog.connectedcamps.com/how-to-shed-distracted-parenting-guilt-and-transform-into-a-digital-hero.

Jakobson, R. (1960). Closing statements: Linguistics and poetics. In T. A. Sebeok (Ed.), *Style in language* (pp. 350–377). New York, NY: Wiley.

Joinson, A. (2008). Looking at, looking up or keeping up with people? Motives and use of Facebook. In *Proceeding of the Twenty-sixth Annual SIGCHI Conference on Human Factors in Computing Systems* (pp. 1027–1036).

Kirman, B., Lawson, S., & Linehan, C. (2009) Gaming on and off the social graph: The social structure of Facebook games. In *Proceedings of the 2009 International Conference on Computational Science and Engineering*, 29-31 August 2009, Vancouver, Canada: IEEE. doi:10.1109/CSE.2009.266.

Lampe, C., Ellison, N., & Steinfield, C. (2006). 'A Face (book) in the crowd: Social searching vs. social browsing. In *Proceedings of the 2006 20th Anniversary Conference on Computer Supported Cooperative Work* (pp. 167–170). New York, NY: ACM.

Lange, P. G., & Ito, M. (2010). Creative production. In M. Ito, I. Mizuko, S. Baumer, M. Bittanti, d. boyd, R. Cody, B. Herr Stephenson, H. A. Horst, P. G. Lange, D. Mahendran, K. Z. Martínez, C. J. Pascoe, D. Perkel, L. Robinson, C. Sims and L. Tripp (Eds.), *Hanging out, messing around, and geeking out: kids living and learning with new media* (pp. 243–293). Cambridge, MA: MIT Press.

Leaver, T. (2017). Intimate surveillance: Normalizing parental monitoring and mediation of infants online. *Social Media+ Society*. doi:10.1177/2056305117707192.

Livingstone, S. (2009). Half a century of television in the lives of our children and families. In: Katz, E., Scannell, P. (Eds.). *The end of television? Its impact so far. The Annals of the American Academy of Political and Social Science, 625*(1), 151–163. doi:10.1177/0002716209338572.

Livingstone, S. M., Haddon, L., & Gorzig, A. (2012). *Children, risk and safety on the internet: Research and policy challenges in comparative perspective*. Bristol, UK: Policy Press.

Lupton, D. (2016). Digital companion species and eating data: Implications for theorising digital data–human assemblages. *Big Data & Society, 3*, 1. doi:https://doi.org/2053951715619947.

Marwick, A. (2012). The public domain: Surveillance in everyday life. *Surveillance & Society, 9*(4), 378–393.

Matsuda, M. (2009). Mobile media and the transformation of family. In G. Goggin & L. Hjorth (Eds.), *Mobile technologies* (pp. 77–87). London, UK: Routledge.

Mol, A. (2008). *The logic of care: Health and the problem of patient choice*. London, UK: Routledge.

Paterson, M. (2009). *Senses of touch: Haptics, affects and technologies*. London, UK: Berg.

Shade, L. R., & Singh, R. (2016). "Honestly, we're not spying on kids": School surveillance of young people's social media. *Social Media + Society, 2*, 4. doi:10.1177/2056305116680005.

Tokunaga, R. S. (2011). Social networking site or social surveillance site? Understanding the use of interpersonal electronic surveillance in romantic relationships. *Computers in Human Behavior, 27*(2), 705–713.

Valcke, M., Bonte, S., De Wever, B., & Rots, I. (2010). Internet parenting styles and the impact on internet use of primary school children. *Computers Education, 55*(2), 454–464.

18

CHALLENGING ADOLESCENTS' AUTONOMY

An Affordances Perspective on Parental Tools

Bieke Zaman, Marije Nouwen, and Karla Van Leeuwen

Introduction

This chapter revolves around the challenging media education dynamics at home when parents seek to balance strategies of granting adolescents autonomy with respect to their media use while also protecting them from possible online harm. Adolescence is characterised by a search for autonomy, which is to be negotiated between parents and adolescents (Janssens et al., 2015). Especially for personal choices regarding media use, adolescents expect to be given significant autonomy (Cranor, Durity, Marsh, & Ur, 2014; Smetana & Asquith, 1994). It creates a challenging situation for parents. Given the increased risk profile of adolescents online, the role of parents in young people's media use remains important. However, parents are also looking for ways to give more degrees of freedom, granting opportunities for independent media use in which adolescents take responsibility for their activities (Chen & Shi, 2018; Ko, Choi, Yang, Lee, & Lee, 2015). This is at odds with the use of parental tools, i.e., apps, browsers, settings, and digital platforms that support parents with built-in technical mechanisms to guide, monitor, and control children's media use.

This chapter revolves around the affordances of parental tools. In a theoretically informed review of exemplar parental control features, their affordances are discussed in the light of parental mediation practices and parenting dimensions. It responds to a call within media and communication studies to better understand (the effects of) parental mediation by relying on insights from the domain of parenting research (Fikkers, Piotrowski, & Valkenburg, 2017). This chapter shows that the affordances of parental tools are likely to invite restrictive and monitoring practices envisioning the protection of the adolescent. However, if used in a context of parental support, they have the potential to foster adolescents' right for provision and participation in the digital world and their need to be supported in autonomy. These findings have important implications for future research on digital parenting and the design of tools that support parental mediation practices.

Parental Mediation Reconsidered from the Perspective of Parenting Dimensions

There are four common mediation practices that parents employ to guide their children's media use. These include active involvement through communication between parent and child, media co-use, restrictions, and monitoring (Valkenburg, Piotrowski, Hermanns, & de Leeuw, 2013). Parents can rely on technical tools that assist them in these practices. With technical monitoring, they can, for instance, determine in advance which websites can (not) be visited (e.g., by specifying filters about what can be downloaded or uploaded), which activities are to be automatically blocked (such as in-app purchases, multiplayer gaming, or chatting), or request weekly reports of the adolescent's online activities (Zaman & Nouwen, 2016). Only a minority of parents know how and what to install in order to technically monitor their child's media use (Pew Research Center, 2016). When parents do invest in technical monitoring, young people are often unaware of this (Livingstone & Bober, 2004), and parents tend to quickly give up because of practical problems (Cranor et al., 2014; Symons, Ponnet, Walrave, & Heirman, 2017). The perceived (mis)match between parental values can further explain why parents decide to (not) adopt parental tools (Vasalou, Oostveen, & Joinson, 2012) and what kind of effects they may have on the child and the child–parent relationship. Hence, in order to achieve this understanding, it is useful to study not only *what* parents *do* with parental tools (i.e., parental mediation behaviours) but also *why* and *how* (i.e., parenting dimensions linked to parents' underlying thoughts, feelings, and goals).

Table 18.1 provides an overview of the parallels conceptually drawn between parental mediation practices and parenting dimensions (Zaman, Nouwen, & Van Leeuwen, 2019). Parenting dimensions include different parenting practices that are related to each other in terms of content and statistics, and each dimension is considered to be a continuum: as a parent or guardian one shows to a greater or lesser extent certain parenting practices (Janssens et al., 2015; Power, 2013). Research distinguishes several dimensions, of which *behavioural control* – with subcategories *proactive behavioural* and *reactive behavioural control* – *psychological control*, and *parental support* show the most reliable empirical links with child and adolescent psychosocial development (Janssens et al., 2015; Power, 2013).

First, Table 18.1 elucidates how the practice of *monitoring* adolescents' media use can be interpreted in two ways. When parents monitor in order to prevent or reduce online risks, but without really supporting autonomy, then this is likely to be played out in a context of *proactive behavioural control*. However, if the parent's choice to monitor is based on a relationship of trust, with parents who are empathetic to the adolescent, their choice to monitor from a distance can

Table 18.1 Conceptual comparison between parental mediation practices and parenting dimensions.

Parental mediation practices	Parenting dimensions
Monitoring	Behavioural control: proactive
	Parental support
Active mediation (communication, co-use)	Parental support
	Behavioural control: proactive
Restrictions	Behavioural control: proactive
	Behavioural control: reactive
	Psychological control

Source: Zaman, B., Nouwen, M., & Van Leeuwen, K. (2019). Een interdisciplinaire kijk op mediaopvoeding: Hedendaagse praktijken van ouderkijk toezicht op mediagebruik door adolescenten. *Kind en adolescent*, *40*(2), 104–115.

be interpreted as a parenting approach based on *parental support*. In the latter situation, parents are open and respectful of the adolescent's personality, needs, and wishes (Janssens et al., 2015); they are interested in their behaviour and seek ways to promote their autonomy in a context of clear supporting rules in which the adolescents can take responsibility for their choices (Janssens et al., 2015; Joussemet, Landry, & Koestner, 2008; Timmerman, Ceulemans, De Roover, & Van Leeuwen, 2013; Wisniewski, Jia, Xu, Rosson, & Carroll, 2015).

Second, situations where parents are *actively involved* in the media use of their teenagers, whether by *talking* about it (communication) or by *using media together* (co-use), can play out in two ways (see Table 18.1). On the one hand, it can be characterised by a parenting dimension of *parental support*, when parents show a great deal of interest in initiating discussions or joint media use. Parents who follow this approach are likely to have more insight into their media use, without the adolescent experiencing this behaviour as controlling. Previous research has shown that many parents initiate discussions with their teens and monitor their online use without necessarily intervening in their online privacy, which is likely to afford autonomy and self-corrective behaviours (Wisniewski et al., 2015, p. 312). However, if the motivations to use digital media together or discuss it are an act of control and risk prevention without supporting the adolescent in their needs, then this should instead be considered as *proactive behavioural control*.

Finally, *restrictive* parental mediation practices can play out in three different ways, depending on the parenting dimension in which they are embedded. First, it can be *proactive behavioural control* as a way of preventing adverse media effects. Previous research has shown that many parents take proactive, preventive behavioural control measures that are linked to both restrictive and monitoring practices. Examples of these preventing measures are filtering or blocking content through parental software and helping set up privacy settings (Wisniewski et al., 2015). Second, restrictive parental mediation practices can also be characterised as *reactive behavioural control* when the corrective measures follow in a reaction to unwanted behaviour, which happens often without a well-considered plan of action and without paying much attention to the adolescent's needs and personality. Previous research has shown that reactive behavioural control is less effective in reducing and preventing risky behaviour than the proactive approach (Janssens et al., 2015). Third, when threats accompany restrictions, parental control takes the form of *psychological control*. Psychological control is a manipulative form of control whereby parents put their child under pressure to think, act, or feel in a certain way or make them feel guilty (Barber, 1996; Soenens & Vansteenkiste, 2010), with the expectation that they will comply and adapt to it. Psychological control affects the child's development negatively (Janssens et al., 2015; Soenens, Vansteenkiste, & Van Petegem, 2015). For adolescents, it thwarts their need for autonomy and intrinsic motivation (Joussemet et al., 2008).

Parental Control Affordances

Making an informed judgement about parental control affordances implies making sense of their potential uses, their action possibilities. Initially introduced in the domain of ecological psychology by James Gibson (1977), the notion of affordances has been picked up by scholars in media studies and design-oriented disciplines (Gillespie, Boczkowski, & Foot, 2014). It is an interesting concept to discuss the role that things, including technology, can play in people's lives; not in a deterministic way, but as something that exists as part of and not beyond the interaction between people and things. Affordances do not constitute any fixed properties, as not everyone will perceive a similar relationship between the technology's appearance and its action possibilities (Jung & Stolterman, 2012).

Affordances may 'work' in three ways, and unfold in functional, relational, and learned qualities (Lievrouw, 2014). First, *functional qualities* concern the physical and metaphysical properties that make certain actions (im)possible. As for parental tools, this would point to the buttons, settings, and functionalities as well as the language used in the commercial discourses around their promotion and sale. Second, *relational qualities* point to the way people perceive the functional qualities, give meaning to them in a particular setting, and how the interaction with the technologies result in certain adapted or emerging practices. This would elucidate how parents and adolescents perceive parental tools as (not) meaningful in the context of parental mediation practices and parenting. Third, *learned qualities* refer to the repertoire of practices and interactions shared among people from a similar community or culture and shaped by regulatory, institutional, and socio-cultural arrangements. Learned qualities, then, might put the attention on online risks and call upon parents' responsibilisation to protect their children. Alternatively, they can focus on adolescents' online opportunities and call upon parents to facilitate these as stepping stones to educational and employment achievements. The decision to (not) adopt parental tools may then be understood as serving one responsibilisation discourse more than another.

The relationship between these qualities is mutually constitutive (Lievrouw, 2014). For instance, the buttons, settings, and functionalities that are pre-defined by design, as well as the commercial 'texts' used for their promotion, reveal and shape an understanding of what is considered as 'default', 'normal', 'appropriate' (Gee, 2011). The functional design qualities, however, do not deterministically define how parental tools are used and understood, as their functions will be interpreted within the broader context of family practices and meaning-making processes. This is where the *relational qualities* come in. Understanding how family members make sense of parental tools reveals reasons for non-adoption (e.g., refusing installation because of a perceived lack of alignment with parenting values), for acceptance (e.g., when both parent and adolescent have negotiated a meaningful implementation), or refusal (e.g., when adolescents feel their autonomy is thwarted and decide to de-install or circumvent the tools). By exploring the wide variety of relational qualities, it becomes clearer why parental tools are (not) adopted and why they do not yield univocal effects.

In what follows, an illustrative reading of the affordances of parental tools is reported. The analysis took the level of functional qualities as the starting point. It then explored the potential relational qualities at the level of both parental mediation practices and parenting dimensions. Thus the aim was an informed judgement based on the conceptual framework developed earlier (see Table 18.1). The analysis considered how these functional and relational qualities could be understood against a background of learned qualities in contemporary Western 'risk societies' that circulate public discourses that tend to be fearful for and protective of children (Beck, 1992). However, this also acknowledges the increased negotiating culture in families. Before the 1970s, parents mainly exercised authority, but they have, since then, been entering into dialogue with their children in order to take account of their needs and wishes and to give children a say in the making of family agreements and rules (Chambers, 2012). The account of the parental control affordances acknowledged the possible mutual constitutive influences situated at the level of these three qualities.

The sample of parental control affordances is based on a purposeful selection. The researchers sought examples that could help us illustrate a broad spectrum of potentialities. The first and second author independently selected potential meaningful parental tools. The first author consulted the SIP-Bench III website (https://sipbench.eu) that provides a systematic benchmarking of parental control tools as the outcome of a European project within the Safer Internet Programme. She ran a search query for tools across a variety of devices and operating systems and tailored the results for relevance for families with children aged 13 and older. The outcome of the search, however, gave outdated information. In order to complement this with more recent examples, the first author approached a senior representative of the Flemish Knowledge Centre on Digital and Media Literacy in July 2018 and asked about parental tools that are popular in Flanders, Belgium. The second author relied on the findings from a previous research project ('MeToDi', n.d.) to propose a meaningful set of parental tools to consider. The intention was not to include all possible existing parental tools in the analysis; neither was the aim to reveal all possible affordances. Instead, the goal was to select convincing illustrative examples that would help us to demonstrate how parental tools might reveal and shape a broad set of affordances.

Restrictions and Monitoring 'By Design'

The findings suggest that the functional design features of parental tools are most likely to afford restrictions and monitoring as default parental mediation practices. To illustrate, the Mac Operating System's (MacOS High Sierra, 2018) built-in parental tool and the Curbi (version year 2018) provide predefined time limits and schedules, and content filters, to select blocked content, respectively. The design of the *Spyzie* parental dashboard ('Spyzie – Dashboard – Live Demo', n. d.) shows user statistics, data, and visualisations about the adolescent's activities.

Parental tools typically combine various functional qualities into one system. Most tools have *restrictive* features, inviting parents to limit time, content, or activities. Settings often allow parents to specify the *time* duration or time slots. Examples of *content* restrictions are filters of incoming content via so-called black and white lists: the first bans access to specific sites, the second allows access to only listed/pre-approved sites. Filters for outgoing content allow parents to predefine what kind of (personal) data can be revealed. An example of an *activity* restriction includes forced prevention of online purchases. In addition to risk prevention, some restrictions are put in place to promote offline activities. The *Circle* discourses frame this within a context of valuing joint family moments and parental modelling; see, for instance, its 'OffTime' feature to "get some good old fashioned family time" (Circle, n.d.-a), and the 'Pause' feature to get "everyone to the dinner table" (Circle, n.d.-b).

Many features allow the parent to *monitor and track* online activities, for example by activating the setting to receive information about browsing history, or to send a warning when the adolescent is about to be exposed to inappropriate content.

Finally, some tools come with *general safety measures* (e.g., as part of the anti-virus program) or with options to *monitor and track non-media-related activities* such as adolescents' whereabouts.

One Functional Quality, Several Potential Relational Qualities

Design functionalities that afford monitoring and restrictions can play out in diverse ways. From the literature on parenting dimensions it can be inferred that a similar feature can be interpreted differently, as more or less supporting adolescents in their autonomy. When technical measures are implemented in a relationship of trust and parental support, then their adoption might encourage adolescents to take responsibility for their choices and, as such, provide an effective means in the 'toolbox' of online and offline media education practices.

On some websites promoting parental tools, this message of building trust is made significant. For instance, on the website promoting *SafeToNet*, trust between parents and children is communicated as an important value. The home page states that "parents never get to see what their child sends and receives. This means that a child's rights to data privacy are fully maintained" (SafeToNet, n.d.-c). The company further states that 'informed safeguarding' "is about more than simply blocking devices or apps. All too often, this approach is counterproductive and results in family arguments and distrust between parents and children". As a consequence, these discourses are not only affording less risk-taking behaviours through the promoted restrictive and preventive measures but also encouraging autonomy and risk-coping behaviours by fostering a climate of trust and respecting children's privacy needs (Wisniewski et al., 2015).

Whereas these *SafeToNet* discourses build on the parental value of safety and connect it to a relationship of trust and respect for the child's privacy, the *KidGuard* discourses show how the same concern for safety is used as a motive to promote protection by 'spying' on children:

> a cell phone tracking software provided to parents to 'spy' on their kids' text messages, monitor GPS location, track phone logs, chats, allowing the parent to stay on top of issues such as cyberbullying, online predators, teen depression, and other risks to their children arising from the internet.
>
> (KidGuard, n.d.)

KidGuard considers the likelihood of 'a crisis' as a real concern that justifies revealing adolescents' media use history and their whereabouts to parents, potentially also to relatives, friends, or police. The technology is introduced as the 'solution' parents can rely on in order to guarantee children's 'protection' on a broad set of online risks (KidGuard, n.d.). Even though there are some more subtle messages on the website that warn against the secretive use of the tool, the risk-based responsibility messages are made dominant via the strategic use of online content and formatting. There is, for instance, a prominent section on the 'Resources' page (KidGuard, n.d.), entitled "5 Reasons To Spy On Your Kid's Text Messages" featuring tips on "HOW TO MONITOR & SPY ON", "LIKE A CIA AGENT".

Opposing Affordances

The affordances revolving around parental tools can be classified on a spectrum ranging from risk and safety-oriented to opportunity and rights-oriented qualities. These findings show that these opposing qualities are made salient across parental tools, and sometimes even within the affordances of one tool, as *KidGuard* exemplified.

Many of the functional qualities echo the safety and protection concerns of parents and underlie the value of its services *for* parents. However, recent tools are being launched with promotional discourses that go out from a more empowering role of the adolescent while acknowledging their digital opportunities. For instance, the *Kudos* website explicitly takes the opportunities as experienced by youth – 'empowered kids' – as a starting point, and this with a mission of engaging oneself to: "inspire kids to have the courage to express themselves, to create, to co-exist, to connect and to respect one another" (Kudos, n.d.).

There were examples where parental support is afforded by emphasising adolescents' responsibility to make their own choices. To illustrate, *OurPact* has a feature 'allowance' which grants some level of autonomy to the adolescent by inviting them to "budget screen time allowances throughout the day, independently" (OurPact, n.d.). *SafeToNet* has features that allow adolescents to report and discuss potential harmful content with their parents. The latter feature suggests that children can also initiate discussions about online safety. It sheds a bidirectional perspective on the notion of parental mediation that goes beyond the parent as the only initiator, indicating that parents and children influence one another instead (Van den Bulck & Van den Bergh, 2005; Wisniewski et al., 2015).

Discussion and Conclusion

This chapter explored and critiqued the affordances of parental tools. Its reading was theoretically informed by literature on affordances, parental mediation, and parenting dimensions.

The findings reveal a broad spectrum of affordances whereby parental tools can have qualities situated on a spectrum, with more or less of the following opposing characteristics:

- Fostering protection versus empowerment;
- Concerns about risks versus opportunities;
- Responsibilisation of parents versus responsibilisation of adolescents;
- Top-down parenting versus building a dialogue, granting the adolescent autonomy;
- One-directional versus bidirectional parent–child influences and interactions;
- Catering to the concerns of parents versus catering for adolescents' needs;
- Symbolising a means to spy on children versus a means to build trust and a dialogue.

This broad spectrum of affordances echoes the variety of discourses that run in the online public sphere (Hartikainen, Iivari, & Kinnula, 2016). The critical challenge, however, revolves around balancing children's right for protection with their needs for provision and participation in the online world (Livingstone & Third, 2017), without the risk of promoting over-controlling and over-protective parenting, which negatively affects children's development (Janssens et al., 2015; Pinter, Wisniewski, Xu, Rosson, & Caroll, 2017). In response, previous researchers have called for the participatory design of parental tools that are sensitive to the values of parents, children, and other stakeholders (such as families indirectly affected) (Czeskis et al., 2010; Nouwen & Zaman, 2018; Vasalou et al., 2012), tools that balance enabling and autonomy-supporting with restrictive and protecting parental measures (Cranor et al., 2014; Ko et al., 2015; Livingstone et al., 2017; Nouwen, JafariNaimi, & Zaman, 2017; Pinter et al., 2017), and that are flexible, dynamic, and open for renegotiation (Muñoz, Ploderer, & Brereton, 2018; Wisniewski et al., 2015).

These findings are far from conclusive, as the researchers did not engage in a systematic review of all potentialities of parental tools. However, based on an exploration of a broad spectrum of parental affordances, this chapter presents a blueprint for a taxonomy based on the following five lenses, which deserves future research to gauge its potential for social sciences analyses and as a design sensitivity:

1. *Parental tool functional qualities* including, for instance, time, content, and activity restrictions; monitoring and tracking functions;
2. *Parental mediation practices*, including parental restrictions, monitoring, active mediation, co-use as well as bi-directional influences;
3. *Parenting dimensions*, including parental support while granting the child autonomy, proactive behavioural control, reactive behavioural control, psychological control;
4. *Children's rights*, accounting for the sweet spot between avoiding and mitigating risks on the one hand and fostering opportunities on the other and acknowledging the right to protection, provision, and participation;
5. *The notion of the child*, considering the spectrum of the child as vulnerable, in need of protection versus the child as empowered, an active agent.

In sum, parental tools cannot deterministically be thought of as a homogeneous technological 'solution'. Neither can one a priori anticipate what 'effects' their uptake will have. It is hoped that in the future this taxonomy and the proposed sensitivity to account for a broad set of relational qualities at the level of both parental mediation practices (*what parents do*) and parenting dimensions (*how and why*) will foster a fruitful discussion about the role of parental tools in the lives of families with adolescents.

References

Barber, B. K. (1996). Parental psychological control: Revisiting a neglected construct. *Child Development*, *67*(6), 3296–3319. doi:10.2307/1131780.

Beck, U. (1992). *Risk society: Towards a new modernity*. London, UK: SAGE Publications.

Chambers, D. (2012). *A sociology of family life: Change and diversity in intimate relations*. Cambridge and Malden, MA: Polity Press.

Chen, L., & Shi, J. (2018). Reducing harm from media: A meta-analysis of parental mediation. *Journalism & Mass Communication Quarterly*, *96*(1), 173–193. doi:10.1177/1077699018754908.

Circle. (n.d.-a). Circle OffTime. Retrieved from *Schedule Internet-Free Times into Your Daily or Weekly Schedule*. https://meetcircle.com/offtime [URL no longer available].

Circle. (n.d.-b). Circle Pause. Retrieved from *The Internet Now Comes with a Pause Button*. https://meetcircle.com/pause [URL no longer available].

Cranor, L. F., Durity, A. L., Marsh, A., & Ur, B. (2014). Parents' and teens' perspectives on privacy in a technology-filled world. *Symposium on Usable Privacy and Security* (pp. 19–35). Menlo Park CA: USENIX Association.

Czeskis, A., Dermendjieva, I., Yapit, H., Borning, A., Friedman, B., Gill, B., & Kohno, T. (2010). *Parenting from the pocket: Value tensions and technical directions for secure and private parent-teen mobile safety*, 1–15. doi:10.1145/1837110.1837130.

Fikkers, K. M., Piotrowski, J. T., & Valkenburg, P. M. (2017). A matter of style? Exploring the effects of parental mediation styles on early adolescents' media violence exposure and aggression. *Computers in Human Behavior*, *70*, 407–415. doi:10.1016/j.chb.2017.01.029.

Gee, J. P. (2011). *An introduction to discourse analysis: Theory and method* (3rd ed.). New York, NY: Routledge.

Gibson, J. J. (1977). The theory of affordances. In R. Shaw & J. Bransford (Eds.), *Perceiving, acting, and knowing: Toward an ecological psychology* (pp. 67–82). Hillsdale, NJ: Lawrence Erlbaum Associates.

Gillespie, T., Boczkowski, P. J., & Foot, K. A. (2014). *Media technologies: Essays on communication, materiality, and society*. Cambridge, MA: MIT Press.

Hartikainen, H., Iivari, N., & Kinnula, M. (2016). Should we design for control, trust or involvement?: A discourses survey about children's online safety. *Proceedings of the 15th International Conference on Interaction Design and Children - IDC '16* (pp. 367–378). doi:10.1145/2930674.2930680.

Janssens, A., Goossens, L., Van Den Noortgate, W., Colpin, H., Verschueren, K., & Van Leeuwen, K. (2015). Parents' and adolescents' perspectives on parenting: Evaluating conceptual structure, measurement invariance, and criterion validity. *Assessment*, *22*(4), 473–489. doi:10.1177/1073191114550477.

Joussemet, M., Landry, R., & Koestner, R. (2008). A self-determination theory perspective on parenting. *Canadian Psychology/Psychologie Canadienne*, *49*(3), 194–200. doi:10.1037/a0012754.

Jung, H., & Stolterman, E. (2012). Digital form and materiality: Propositions for a new approach to interaction design research. *Proceedings of the 7th Nordic Conference on Human-Computer Interaction: Making Sense through Design* (pp. 645–654). doi:10.1145/2399016.2399115.

KidGuard. (n.d.). *#1 Call monitoring & child cell phone tracker. Track text messages, GPS, and more*. Retrieved 17 August 2018, from www.kidguard.com.

Ko, M., Choi, S., Yang, S., Lee, J., & Lee, U. (2015). FamiLync: Facilitating participatory parental mediation of adolescents' smartphone use. *Proceedings of the 2015 ACM International Joint Conference on Pervasive and Ubiquitous Computing - UbiComp '15* (pp. 867–878). doi:10.1145/2750858.2804283.

Kudos. (n.d.). *Home*. Retrieved August 17, 2018 from www.kudos.com.

Lievrouw, L. A. (2014). Materiality and media in communication and technology studies: Unfinished project. In T. Gillespie, P. J. Boczkowski, & K. A. Foot (Eds.), *Media technologies: Essays on communication, materiality, and society* (pp. 21–51). Cambridge, MA and London, UK: MIT Press.

Livingstone, S., & Bober, M. (2004). *UK children go online: Surveying the experiences of young people and their parents*. Retrieved from: http://eprints.lse.ac.uk/archive/00000395.

Livingstone, S., Ólafsson, K., Helsper, E. J., Lupiáñez-Villanueva, F., Veltri, G. A., & Folkvord, F. (2017). Maximizing opportunities and minimizing risks for children online: The role of digital skills in emerging strategies of parental mediation. *Journal of Communication*, *67*(1), 82–105. doi:10.1111/jcom.12277.

Livingstone, S., & Third, A. (2017). Children and young people's rights in the digital age: An emerging agenda. *New Media & Society*, *19*(5), 657–670. doi:10.1177/1461444816686318.

MeToDi. (n.d.). Retrieved August 30, 2018, from ResearchGate website: www.researchgate.net/project/MeToDi-Methodological-toolkit-for-publishers-and-developers-of-digital-learning-materials (last accessed 18 June 2020).

Muñoz, D., Ploderer, B., & Brereton, M. (2018). Towards design for renegotiating the parent-adult child relationship after children leave home. *Proceedings of the 30th Australian Conference on Computer-Human Interaction - OzCHI '18* (pp. 303–313). doi:10.1145/3292147.3292149.

Nouwen, M., JafariNaimi, N., & Zaman, B. (2017). Parental controls: Reimagining technologies for parent-child interaction. doi:10.18420/ecscw2017-28.

Nouwen, M., & Zaman, B. (2018). Redefining the role of parents in young children's online interactions: A value-sensitive design case study. *International Journal of Child-Computer Interaction.* doi:10.1016/j.ijcci.2018.06.001.

OurPact. (n.d.). *The #1 parental control App & family locator.* Retrieved 30 August 2018, from: https://ourpact.com.

Pew Research Center. (2016). *Parents, teens and digital monitoring.* Retrieved from: www.pewresearch.org/internet/wp-content/uploads/sites/9/2016/01/PI_2016-01-07_Parents-Teens-Digital-Monitoring_FINAL.pdf (last accessed 18 June 2020).

Pinter, A. T., Wisniewski, P. J., Xu, H., Rosson, M. B., & Caroll, J. M. (2017). Adolescent online safety: Moving beyond formative evaluations to designing solutions for the future. *Proceedings of the 2017 Conference on Interaction Design and Children - IDC '17* (pp. 352–357). doi:10.1145/3078072.3079722.

Power, T. G. (2013). Parenting dimensions and styles: A brief history and recommendations for future research. *Childhood Obesity, 9*(Suppl 1), S-14–S-21. doi:10.1089/chi.2013.0034.

SafeToNet. (n.d.). *Home.* Retrieved 30 August 2018 from: www.safetonet.com.

Smetana, J. G., & Asquith, P. (1994). Adolescents' and parents' conceptions of parental authority and personal autonomy. *Child Development, 65*(4), 1147–1162.

Soenens, B., & Vansteenkiste, M. (2010). A theoretical upgrade of the concept of parental psychological control: Proposing new insights on the basis of self-determination theory. *Developmental Review, 30*(1), 74–99. doi:10.1016/j.dr.2009.11.001.

Soenens, B., Vansteenkiste, M., & Van Petegem, S. (2015). Let us not throw out the baby with the bathwater: Applying the principle of universalism without uniformity to autonomy-supportive and controlling parenting. *Child Development Perspectives, 9*(1), 44–49. doi:10.1111/cdep.12103.

Spyzie - Dashboard - Live Demo. (n.d.). Retrieved 30 August 2018 from: https://my.spyzie.com/livedemo/dashboard.html.

Symons, K., Ponnet, K., Walrave, M., & Heirman, W. (2017). A qualitative study into parental mediation of adolescents' internet use. *Computers in Human Behavior, 73,* 423–432. doi:10.1016/j.chb.2017.04.004.

Timmerman, M. E., Ceulemans, E., De Roover, K., & Van Leeuwen, K. (2013). Subspace K-means clustering. *Behavior Research Methods, 45*(4), 1011–1023. doi:10.3758/s13428-013-0329-y.

Valkenburg, P. M., Piotrowski, J. T., Hermanns, J., & de Leeuw, R. (2013). Developing and validating the perceived parental media mediation scale: A self-determination perspective: Parental mediation scale. *Human Communication Research, 39*(4), 445–469. doi:10.1111/hcre.12010.

Van den Bulck, J., & Van den Bergh, B. R. H. (2005). The child effect in media and communication research: A call to arms and an agenda for research. In P. J. Kalbfleisch (Ed.), *Communication yearbook: An annual review* (Vol. 29, pp. 35–47). Mahwah, NJ: Lawrence Erlbaum Associates.

Vasalou, A., Oostveen, A.-M., & Joinson, A. N. (2012). A case study of non-adoption: The values of location tracking in the family. *Proceedings of the ACM 2012 Conference on Computer Supported Cooperative Work - CSCW '12* (p. 779). doi:10.1145/2145204.2145321.

Wisniewski, P., Jia, H., Xu, H., Rosson, M. B., & Carroll, J. M. (2015). Preventative vs. reactive: How parental mediation influences teens' social media privacy behaviours. *Proc. CSCW* (pp. 1258–1271). New York, NY: ACM.

Zaman, B., & Nouwen, M. (2016). *Parental controls: Advice for parents, researchers and industry.* Retrieved from: http://eprints.lse.ac.uk/65388.

Zaman, B., Nouwen, M., & Van Leeuwen, K. (2019). Een interdisciplinaire kijk op mediaopvoeding: Hedendaagse praktijken van ouderkijk toezicht op mediagebruik door adolescenten. *Kind en adolescent, 40*(2), 104–115. doi:10.1007/s12453-019-00203-w.

PART III
Complexities of Commodification

19
CHILDREN'S ENROLMENT IN ONLINE CONSUMER CULTURE

Ylva Ågren

Introduction

Contemporary Western society has become a mediatised world (Deuze, 2012; Hepp & Krotz, 2014) in which culture, lives, relationships, and social activities are affected by digital processes (Lindgren, 2017). Digital media have also become a big part of children's culture and everyday lives (Giddings, 2014). Statistical reports show how Swedish children's daily internet use is increasing, with toddlers as young as one year old participating online. Playing digital games, watching video clips on YouTube, socialising with friends, and using the internet for schoolwork are the most common activities that children engage in online (Davidsson et al., 2018; Livingstone et al., 2014). Children's digital media practices and commercial culture are also intimately intertwined. Television programmes, films, computer games, and apps are linked to merchandising and advertising. Micro-celebrities, like influencers and YouTubers who are popular among children, are monetised by integrating advertorials and product promotions into their social media posts. Companies operate across many media platforms and markets, and success is measured by visibility in a range of media (Buckingham, 2011, p. 88). This assemblage of characters, programmes, advertising, video clips, food, toys, and clothing is fuzzy and creates a complicated media ecosystem of transmedia worlds in which it can be difficult to distinguish between the role of a consumer and the role of a viewer (Cook, 2009; Giddings, 2014).

Commodification refers to the process by which goods and services become exchangeable items, called commodities (Nutter Smith, 2015). Bauman (2007) argued that, in this society of consumers, commodification has incorporated all the domains of social life, and individuals are connected to the social world primarily by their capacity as consumers. He wrote, "To consume ... means to invest in one's own social membership, which in a society of consumers translates as 'saleability': obtaining qualities for which there is already a market demand" (Bauman, 2007, p. 56). In this theory, people are both promoters of commodities and commodities themselves. Being a consumer and engaging in consumption is, therefore, something from which neither children nor adults can choose to abstain (Cook, 2013, p. 425).

Children unfold as persons in and through a consumer society, but they have been almost invisible in theories on the subject, and their role in consumer society is still unclear (Buckingham, 2011; Cook, 2009; Pugh, 2011). Discussions about children and consumption have long been characterised by moral panic and a dichotomised image of the child consumer as either naïve and in need of protection from a strong market or as a competent actor – a battle that has existed in the study of media consumption as well (Buckingham, 2011; Cook, 2009; Sparrman & Sandin, 2012). According to Cook (2013), this type of social debate has less to do with consumption and more to do with the different ways of interpreting, understanding, and defining children and childhood.

This chapter focusses on children's perspectives on commodification in their online activities and their enrolment in digital consumer culture. The chapter draws on consumer culture research and the concept of *situated child consumption*. Consumption is here regarded as a social and cultural practice, "inevitably embedded within everyday life and interpersonal relationships, and in wider social and cultural processes" (Buckingham, 2011, p. 37). Sparrman and Sandin (2012, p. 11) use the concept to emphasise the mixture of different practices, contexts, and social processes to which consumption (and media use) is always bound. In line with Cook (2010), the focus is on how children's knowledge of consumption is used in everyday practice.

Literature Review

Much of the work on the commodification of children's online activities has been conducted in relation to advertising in mobile or computer-based digital games. Many of these studies have used quantitative or experimental methods, focussing on advertising effects and advertising literacy. The primary assumption is that children are generally more vulnerable than adults to the effects of advertising (e.g., Rozendaal et al., 2011; van Reijmersdal et al., 2012). Studies have also investigated children's understanding of advertising and brand placement in social games and their desire for the brands and items advertised in those games (Rozendaal et al., 2013). Martínez (2019) wrote that few studies have focussed on the child's perspective on and engagement with advertising (see, for example, Marsh, 2014). Drawing on group interviews with 9- and 12-year-old children, Martínez (2019) analysed how children view and engage with advertising in free-to-play mobile games and what consequences this has for children's gaming. The study asserted that playing free-to-play mobile games with in-app advertising is demanding for children and takes the form of a struggle. During game play, advertising interrupts moments of achievement, engagement, and pleasure, leading to a sense of resignation in the child. However, the study also showed how advertising-based revenue models make it possible for children to easily explore and play many different games in the first place (Martínez, 2019, p. 32; c.f., Marsh, 2010).

Willett (2018) explored children's media literacy with a focus on commercial online game industries and related marketing, showing children are actively involved in cultures of consumption. Using a sociocultural approach, the study illustrated how a child's understanding of the gaming industry is influenced by the individual's surrounding context. According to Willett (2018), children who invest more in gaming, both in terms of time and money, demonstrated a larger awareness of the ownership of gaming companies and revenue generation.

Several previous studies have documented the role of consumption in online virtual worlds developed for children and how consumer ideologies are embedded in these sites (e.g., Lehdonvirta et al., 2009; Ruckenstein, 2011). For example, Wasko (2010) showed how online virtual worlds are a growing business area and a foundation for capitalist consumer culture. Focussing on textual analysis of the sites *Neopets* and *Webkinz*, she identified an ideology that encourages and educates children about the culture of consumption. Marsh (2010) explored children's play in the online virtual worlds of *Club Penguin* and *Barbie Girls*. She showed how children use gaming sites to experiment with identity and to share social networks with peers and how boundaries between online play and offline play are challenged. However, the study also demonstrated how children relate to consumption in online worlds and how it becomes a part of their play. In a later study on children's literacy practices in *Club Penguin*, Marsh (2011) stressed the need to explore further the complex relationship between childhood and the commercial world and to develop strategies for children's critical engagement.

Another area of concern related to commodifying children's online activities is YouTube. Some research has concerned the ethical implications that arise from the commercialisation of children's media and how children's digital footprints on sites such as YouTube are shared with companies for analytics and advertising (e.g., Montgomery et al., 2017; Smith & Shade, 2018). Other studies have focussed on how YouTubers and micro-celebrities construct themselves and their relationships to the viewer (e.g., Abidin, 2017; Hou, 2019; Lovelock, 2017). Martínez and Olsson (2019) explored how children make sense of YouTubers as a phenomenon by analysing how a group of 9- to 12-year-old children constructed and negotiated with a YouTuber called Misslissibell from a tutorial video. The results demonstrated how the children made sense of Misslissibell in different ways, irrespective of age and gender. Some of the children demonstrated a critical view, talking about the video as advertising and the selling of brands, while others saw her tutorial video mainly as tips and informal learning. Using an ethnographic approach, Marsh (2016) followed a four-year-old boy and documented the phenomenon of *unboxing* videos – unpacking of commercial products – on YouTube. The boy found great pleasure in watching these videos and was not interested in purchasing the products, so it was argued that he took the position of a *cyberflâneur*, or one who wanders the internet without purpose. Marsh (2016) conceptualised children's interest in YouTube – and in other online streaming platforms – as a growing peer-to-peer industry.

Methodology

The chapter draws on data from two different projects that focussed on sibling interaction and children's everyday media practices in their homes. The larger project was a six-month media ethnography of Swedish family life (Ågren, 2015) focussing on people's use of media rather than on the medium itself (Couldry, 2012). The aim was to examine how media both act as a resource for children's play and shape it, and to investigate the significance of consumption in young children's media use. The project included observations made by the participants with a video camera, as well as field notes and interviews, from six families in their homes. In total, the video recordings involved about 80 hours of videos from 14 children (eight boys and six girls) aged between four and nine years. The material was collected between December 2010 and December 2011 (Ågren, 2015). The smaller project investigated Swedish children's experiences of the Pokémon phenomenon. For one month in 2016, observations and interviews with three sibling pairs (six children, aged four to nine) and their parents were conducted. The children and parents were followed outdoors in playgrounds and public spaces by the researcher while they played *Pokémon GO*, and observations and interviews related to the game took place indoors.

In both studies, families were recruited through snowball selection (Bernard, 2006). Two key informants listed other families they knew as friends and through workplaces. Ethical research considerations are of central importance in research involving children (Alderson, 2005; Farrell, 2005), and the projects were conducted in accordance with the Swedish Research Council (2011) guidelines for good research practice. The participants were informed of the study's aim, the different data collection methods, the ways in which the data would be handled, and that their personal details would be anonymised. In most research parents give permission for their children to be involved in a given project, and children are then invited to contribute to the research process without further discussions of consent (Danby & Farrell, 2005). In these studies, special attention was given to informing children about the study and to getting informed consent directly from them as well, rather than from their parents only. The participants themselves chose their pseudonyms.

Both sibling interactions and interviews were transcribed in some detail to capture participants' own perspectives on specific media phenomena. Excerpts illuminate the commodification of children's online activities. The analysis was based on social interaction and meaning-making processes that took place with local media activities, but also extended to a broader societal context to show how social structure and social action are constantly interwoven in children's lives. The analysis is presented through three different themes: consumer culture in and outside virtual worlds, children using advertising principles, and making sense of a digital commercial lifestyle.

Consumer Culture In and Outside of Virtual Worlds

This section discusses the meaning of consumer culture for children engaged in moderated virtual worlds. In this type of gaming site many users participate simultaneously, everything is happening in real time, and the world is permanent, regardless of whether the user is currently participating. There is a range of different virtual worlds, but Marsh (2014, p. 181) highlighted two features as central for sites aimed at children: the user creates an avatar – an online representation of the self – and locates that avatar in the home environment, be it an igloo, a treehouse, or something else; this avatar is then able to socialise with other avatars, primarily through online chatting or by meeting them in online games.

This chapter focusses on the virtual worlds of *Club Penguin*, owned by Disney, and *Club Panfu*, owned by Goodbeans. The excerpt presented comes from the larger study in which several children spent time on gaming sites (Ågren, 2015). Such sites are free-to-play, but the possibilities for interaction in the virtual world are limited: to get access to all functions, the players of both *Club Panfu* and *Club Penguin* need to be paying members. With membership, the player gets extra benefits, such as game money, special clothes, or access to areas of the virtual world that are not accessible to non-paying players. Membership can be paid monthly or yearly or can be a lifelong commitment. These sites claim to be advertising-free, but the non-paying members see advertising regarding the advantages of membership, such as the possibility of doing more things on the site, being able buy clothing or things for your avatar, visiting special places, or playing special games.

The desire for and importance of getting a membership was something that was clearly communicated by the children, both within the relationship between siblings and in their conversations with parents. The children demonstrated the affordability of membership, the increase in the interaction possibilities, and how membership was, in itself, a marker of a certain status, since some goods, pets, or clothes were available for purchase by members only (c.f., Marsh, 2010, 2011). The children also presented the frequency with which advertising occurred as an argument for the parents to invest in membership. None of the children reflected on the fact that the sites could have an underlying commercial ideology (c.f., Willett, 2018). Matilda (age 8), for example, received a lifelong 'Gold' membership at *Club Panfu* after pestering her parents for a long time. She said:

> I can buy everything; I can do whatever I like. If you are not a Gold member ... well, then you cannot buy clothes or furniture and so on. Not everyone has the things my Panda does, and they think it is cool. That is fun of course. You feel a bit special when you can do whatever you like ... it is fun to be able to be whatever I want to be.

Featherstone (1994) argued that contemporary consumption culture is characterised by increasing options when it comes to choosing and displaying lifestyle. This is in line with *Club Penguin*'s special section for parents, which suggests that children would prefer a paid membership to have the opportunity "to explore exactly who they want to be". Matilda also illuminated how her

Gold membership gives her a social position both inside and outside the game. Her peers talk about the things and clothes that her Panda-avatar has, both in school and in the virtual world.

Similar findings came from another family in which the oldest brother, Melvin (age nine), was the only one who had a membership. He was, like Matilda, a Gold member of *Club Panfu*. His sister, Susann (age eight), had quite recently joined the virtual world. With his Gold membership, Melvin could buy clothes and furnishings reserved for members only. When the siblings were playing together, it was common for Melvin to use the virtual commodities and the number of friends he had to tease his sister and position himself higher.

It should be emphasised that the children in the study mainly mentioned the fun parts of the virtual worlds, such as the shared community with their friends and siblings and the challenging and exciting games (c.f., Marsh, 2011, 2014). However, the results demonstrate how they all expressed an awareness that the conditions in the gaming sites differ depending on whether or not one has a membership. Pugh (2011) held that access to consumer culture has become central to gaining acceptance and social belonging in children's peer groups. In her research she demonstrated how children use a form of *facework*: different strategies to avoid exclusion and to negotiate status and popularity. The virtual commodities in the game work similarly to material assets in social relations, indicating distinction and status between the players and making the owner of a membership exclusive and selected (c.f., Lehdonvirta et al., 2009; Wasko, 2010).

Children Using Advertising Principles

The next section presents examples of how children use advertising principles as a way of negotiating in their play and relationships. Data was analysed from the smaller project. During the summer of 2016, the phenomenon of *Pokémon GO* exploded in Sweden, as it did in several other countries (Hjorth & Richardson, 2017). Both parents and children downloaded the *Pokémon GO* app, wandering around in public spaces looking for Pokémons to catch. Three families were observed for a month, with the intent of understanding the transmediated universe of which the Pokémon phenomenon is a part. The siblings in this study did not just play the *Pokémon GO* app, they watched "Let's Play" videos[1] from other players on YouTube and followed the cartoon *Pokémon XY*. They also invented new songs from the YouTube hit *I play Pokémon GO every day*, drew Pokémon, explored the different elements of the overall Pokémon culture, made up new games and played with the characters (c.f., Buckingham, 2011; Giddings, 2014). The siblings also used the media worlds of Pokémon in their social interactions, both as a way to create community and as a way to mark their status and position within hierarchies.

In the first excerpt, Hugo (age four) is playing with his older brother Oskar (age seven). The boys have been outdoors, playing the *Pokémon GO* app with their mother, and when they arrive inside, they start to role-play with the Pokémon characters, playing different characters that battle with each other. This is like a form of wrestling and, since Oskar is older and stronger than his brother, Hugo soon suggests that they should play a different game. The new game proposed by Hugo is similar to the one they have been playing but, instead of being Pokémon, they will make plastic animals battle with each other.

Hugo: (in a complaining voice) I want to play Pokémon with the animals now!
Oskar: Nooo . . .
Hugo: YES! You told me we would do it later!
Oskar: Ok, but I know! We say that this [wrestling-game] is the commercial. If you look at it, you will get much more CP [combat power] later! Then you can fight much better later!
Hugo: No! I want to play [with animals] now! You said so!
Oskar: Yes, but now it is a commercial, and you cannot click it away. You have to look at it.

Lindgren (2017, p. 19) believed that, when we learn skills or attitudes connected to a certain medium, we are at the same time "socialised and acculturated into the symbolic environment of the medium". To understand how different media are constituted, there can be an analysis of how language or culture are used to make sense of the world. Many free-to-play mobile games use revenue models based on advertising and in-app purchases that the gamer cannot avoid. Advertising is also often a way to offer new opportunities in the games, such as game currency or the possibility of moving to a higher level (Martínez, 2019). In the excerpt, Oskar uses advertising principles as a commodity – a resource for negotiating in his play fight with his younger brother Hugo. By claiming that the play is advertising, he establishes a condition – a trump card – that defeats all arguments: "this is advertising, you cannot click it away", and his little brother just has to endure. Thus, Oskar demonstrates that he has an understanding of how advertising works and how things are imbued with monetary value. The excerpt also demonstrates how the line between online and offline are blurred in children's media worlds (c.f., Marsh, 2010).

In the following example, Max (age eight) is also talking about advertising as a form of commodity. He plays a free-to-play game app on his smartphone and his younger brother William (age six) sits next to him, watching. Max has not been playing long before the game breaks for advertising.

Max: Ah no! Advertising! So annoying!
William: Yes! Shit!
Researcher: You don't like it?
William: Sometimes I think it is fun. You can find new games that way.
Max: Yes, sometimes. But it interrupts … The best thing with it is that you can say to mum that it is a lot of advertising and make her buy a new game (*laughter*).

Buckingham (2011) stated that parents' roles in children's consumption are complex and hold ideas about childhood and concerns about their own statuses as consumers and parents. Within dominant discourses, it is argued that children are influenced by advertising and its marketising role is highlighted. Many parents expressed a preference for games that are free from advertising and considered them to be of better quality, thereby presenting themselves as caring parents (Ågren, 2015). In the excerpt, Max expresses an awareness of these discourses. He states that he can use the advertising as a commodity or a resource by emphasising its negative value and thereby getting his mother to buy a game that he would rather have, which may have less advertising.

Taken together, the excerpts in this section illustrate not only that children are familiar with the arguments about advertisements' negative effects, but also that they can elaborate critically on the topic. The children are not just aware of the commercial logic of advertising, but also its positive potential for the user. The examples highlight how consumption is not separate from a child's world but is a part of how society and its norms and values work (c.f., Buckingham, 2011; Cook, 2009; Sparrman & Sandin, 2012).

Making Sense of Digital Commercial Lifestyles

This final section discusses findings that derive from both studies and addresses how children relate to online activities, such as watching YouTube clips or following influencers – two very common activities among Swedish children.

YouTube is a social media platform, owned by Google, with user-generated content consisting of video clips. The largest revenue resource for individual users, as well as for Google, is advertising in the form of a commercial preceding a video clip or as a banner that appears during the video (Hess, 2015, p. 576). Frequent users who have become well known through their production of videos on YouTube can be described as micro-celebrities. These so-called YouTubers, or *influencers*, have gained a relatively large number of followers by uploading videos on a plethora of subjects, such as gaming (Let's Play videos) or their lifestyles. Influencers have become a branch of marketing, and companies compete for collaborations with the people who have the most subscribers (Abidin, 2017). In such cases, it is obvious that celebrities do not just sell the products but are themselves the commodities (Martínez & Olsson, 2019).

Within the study with siblings, participants often looked at different video clips and Let's Play videos on YouTube. It became clear that children's play was a re-enactment of not only the games, such as *Pokémon*, but also of the video clips they saw on YouTube, which quickly rose in popularity and then disappeared to be replaced by the next internet sensation (Ågren, 2015). Children were not allowed to upload content on YouTube themselves, but they made many Let's Play videos with their devices, and they also played at making videos. When out playing *Pokémon GO*, the brothers Max (age eight) and William (age 6) would meta-communicate what they were doing, as if someone was filming them. On one occasion, Max's phone battery ran out. The hunt for Pokémons instantly switched to a role-play of the making of a Let's Play video. Max said, "Let's play that we are making a film instead. Because I do this Let's Play video now, and then we can put it on YouTube, and I will become really famous and very rich (*laughter*)".

What is demonstrated here by Max is something of which older children in the dataset were well aware: that videos on YouTube can provide a way to become well known and make money. In various situations, such as among friends or with a parent, they talked about different YouTubers and discussed their celebrity status and numbers of subscribers (c.f., Martínez & Olsson, 2019). Several children in both studies expressed a desire to become part of the industry and produce videos themselves. In the next excerpt, two sisters, Livia (age nine) and Rebecka (age seven), sit on the sofa watching the Swedish YouTuber Misslissibell as she makes a *haul* after a shopping spree.[2]

Livia: This is so good! I also want to be a YouTuber. My absolute favourite is Therese Lindgren.
Researcher: Really? Do you want to tell me?
Livia: Yes! But then it's important to look good and to work really hard. I look a lot at others, to get ideas about how to look and so on. You need to have the right angle of the camera.
Rebecka: (*interrupts*) But mum doesn't like it when you look at her. Because it is too sexy when she makes a haul and shows her underwear (*laugh*).
Livia: (*in an irritated voice*) Ah, shut up! You're so embarrassing!

Being a micro-celebrity or an influencer is something Livia has considered as a future occupation. However, she is also well aware of the requirements and conditions that come with the task. Through her observation of the importance of looking good, working hard, and keeping the camera at the right angle, she talks about herself as a commodity and demonstrates that she understands the importance of visibility and saleability of not just commercial products, but also of herself and her lifestyle. Buckingham (2011, p. 169) wrote that children's peer talk, tastes, and preferences regarding different media simultaneously function as a way to perform identities. In the excerpt, Livia asserts how videos on YouTube are an informal learning environment for her and expresses an interest in taste and style (c.f., Martínez & Olsson, 2019). Willett (2011) argued that children have a good understanding of the discourses, norms, and values that surround them;

they are aware of the concerns around popular culture and media consumption and actively relate to these discourses in their play (see also Dyson, 2003). Buckingham (2011) further stated that childhood identities are performed in different ways in different contexts. Livia's attempt to express herself in a more grown up way is negated by Rebecka reminding her of their mother, who is not fond of Therese Lindgren's sexy approach when she is demonstrating underwear, believing that it is not appropriate for children to see.

The key argument in this section is that YouTube is a natural arena for today's children, one they consider as a future profession in a way that many of their parents, who were born before the breakthrough of the internet, do not. The children demonstrate an awareness that a good video can generate new subscribers, and possibly celebrity, but that hard work is required.

Conclusions

The aim of this chapter has been to discuss children's enrolment in digital consumer culture. The starting point was a consideration of children's interactions and perspectives to illuminate how consumption becomes important and meaningful for children in their everyday lives. Deuze (2012) suggested that contemporary society has gone from a life with media to a life *in* media. For children, the world of media consists of constant movement: an assemblage of texts, games, social relationships, commodities, pictures, and music that are recycled and deployed as material for new activities, since what is popular today may change tomorrow (c.f., Marsh, 2016). The analysis demonstrates how consumption and consumer culture does not exist outside of everyday life or in specific areas; rather, it is a pervasive part of a child's everyday life and something that exists both online and offline.

Children are consuming agents; they use the principles and rules that characterise different online activities as a resource for their own games and play and, in negotiations with parents or siblings, as a way to demonstrate their position in relation to other children or to construct and reconstruct performed identities. Their understanding of commercial intent in different online activities varies, with older children expressing greater insight into these questions (c.f., Willett, 2018). The studies further demonstrate how children are consumers of commodities, such as micro-celebrities, and also understand themselves to be commodities in terms of the conditions existing in a consumer society, such as visibility and saleability. The results show how children are well aware of the opinions of adults concerning advertising, consuming, and what is regarded as appropriate for children.

Taken together, such findings question the validity of describing a child as being either naïve or fully competent in relation to consuming. With the term *situated child consumption* (Sparrman & Sandin, 2012), the chapter brings attention to the inevitable aspects of childhood: the different practices, contexts, and social processes to which children's consumption is always bound. Consequently, to understand children's enrolment in digital consumer culture, the analysis must include their perspectives – how they relate to both the discourses that underpin cultural and social practices with media and those relating to childhood, and how they interpret and use related narratives and symbols in their everyday lives.

Finally, it is important to emphasise that consumption does not include everyone equally (Cook, 2009, p. 343). All families in the present studies can, in a broad sense, be considered part of the Swedish middle class. Buckingham (2011) stated that, since most media costs money, there are considerably more technical devices in middle-class homes than in working-class homes, which leads to different social groups living in different cultural worlds. Bauman (2007) used the concept of the *flawed consumer* and argued that the significance of being poor is, in a consumer society, no longer defined by a person's work status but by their ability to consume. Children often use consumer culture to belong to a peer group (Pugh, 2011). An increased commodification of both online and offline activities in children's everyday culture can lead to an exclusion of those children whose parents do not possesses the financial means.

Notes

1 A Let's Play video documents the play of a video or computer game, usually including commentary and/or a camera view of the face of the gamer.
2 A haul is a video in which a person discusses items, such as make-up or clothing, that they have recently purchased; it is important to note that many micro-celebrities have entered sponsorship deals and advertising programmes from major brands that are featured in these videos (Jeffries, 2011). To make a haul is similar to the phenomenon of unboxing videos, in which commercial goods are unwrapped (Marsh, 2016). Unboxing videos existed before haul videos became a trend.

References

Abidin, C. (2017). #familygoals: Family Influencers, calibrating amateurism, and justifying young digital labor. *Social Media + Society*, April–June, 1–15.
Ågren, Y. (2015). *Barns medierade värld: Syskonsamspel, lek och konsumtion*. [Children's mediated world: Sibling interaction, play and consumption] PhD diss, Stockholm University.
Alderson, P. (2005). Designing ethical research with children. In A. Farrell (Ed.), *Ethical research with children* (pp. 27–36). Maidenhead: Open University Press.
Bauman, Z. (2007). *Consuming life*. Cambridge: Polity Press.
Bernard, H.R. (2006). *Research methods in anthropology*. New York: Altamira Press.
Buckingham, D. (2011). *The material child: Growing up in consumer culture*. London: Palgrave Macmillan.
Cook, D.T. (2009). Children as consumers. In J. Qvortrop, W.A. Corsaro & M.-S. Honig (Eds.), *The Palgrave handbook of childhood studies* (pp. 332–346). Basingstoke: Palgrave Macmillan.
Cook, D.T. (2010). Commercial enculturation. Moving beyond consumer socialization. In D. Buckingham & V. Tingstad (Eds.), *Childhood and consumer culture* (pp. 63–79). Basingstoke: Palgrave Macmillan.
Cook, D.T. (2013). Taking exception with the child consumer. *Childhood*, 20(4), 423–428.
Couldry, N. (2012). *Media, society, world: Social theory and digital media practice*. Cambridge: Polity Press.
Danby, S. & Farrell, A. (2005). Opening the research conversation. In A. Farell (Ed.), *Ethical research with children* (pp. 49–67). Maidenhead: Open University Press.
Davidsson, P., Palm, M. & Melin Mandre, Å. (2018). *Svenskarna och internet 2018*. Stockholm: IIS, Internetstiftelsen i Sverige.
Deuze, M. (2012). *Media life*. Cambridge: Polity Press.
Dyson, A.H. (2003). Welcome to the Jam. *Harvard Educational Review*, 73(1), 328–361.
Farrell, A. (2005). Ethics and research with children. In A. Farrell (Ed.), *Ethical research with children* (pp. 1–14). Maidenhead: Open University Press.
Featherstone, M. (1994). *Kultur, kropp och konsumtion*. Stockholm, Sweden: Brutus Östlings bokförlag.
Giddings, S. (2014). *Gameworlds. Virtual media and children's everyday play*. New York: Bloomsbury.
Hepp, A. & Krotz, F. (2014). Mediatized worlds – Understanding everyday mediatization. In A. Hepp & F. Krotz (Eds.), *Mediatized worlds* (pp. 1–15). London: Palgrave Macmillan.
Hess, A. (2015). YouTube. In D.T. Cook & J.M. Ryan (Eds.), *The Wiley Blackwell encyclopedia of consumption and consumer studies* (pp. 576–578). London: Wiley Blackwell.
Hjorth, L. & Richardson, I. (2017). Pokémon GO: Mobile media play, place-making, and the digital wayfarer. *Mobile Media & Communication*, 5(1), 3–14.
Hou, M. (2019). Social media celebrity and the institutionalization of YouTube. *Convergence: The International Journal of Research into New Media Technologies*, 25(3), 534–553.
Jeffries, L. (2011). The revolution will be soooo cute: YouTube "hauls" and the voice of young female consumers. *Studies in Popular Culture*, 33(2), 59–75.
Lehdonvirta, V., Wilska, T.A. & Johnson, M. (2009). Virtual consumerism: Case of Habbo Hotel. *Information, Communication & Society*, 12(7), 1059–1079.
Lindgren, S. (2017). *Digital media & society*. London: Sage.
Livingstone, S., Mascheroni, G., Ólafsson, K. & Haddon, L. (2014). *Children's online risks and opportunities: Comparative findings from EU Kids Online and Net children go mobile*. London: London School of Economics and Political Science. Available at: www.eukidsonline.net and www.netchildrengomobile.eu.
Lovelock, M. (2017). "Is every YouTuber going to make a coming out video eventually?": YouTube celebrity video bloggers and lesbian and gay identity. *Celebrity Studies*, 8(1), 87–103.
Marsh, J. (2010). Young children's play in online virtual worlds. *Journal of Early Childhood*, 8(1), 23–39.
Marsh, J. (2011). Young children's literacy practices in a virtual world: Establishing an online interaction order. *Reading Research Quarterly*, 46(2), 101–118.

Marsh, J. (2014). Purposes for literacy in children's use of the online virtual world *Club Penguin*. *Journal of Research in Reading*, *37*(2), 179–195.

Marsh, J. (2016). Unboxing videos: Co-construction of the child as cyberflâneur. *Discourse: Studies in the Cultural Politics of Education*, *37*(3), 369–380.

Martínez, C. (2019). The struggles of everyday life: How children view and engage with advertising in mobile games. *Convergence: The International Journal of Research into New Media Technologies*, *25*(5–6), 848–867.

Martínez, C. & Olsson, T. (2019). Making sense of YouTubers: How Swedish children construct and negotiate the YouTuber Misslisibell as a girl celebrity. *Journal of Children and Media*, *13*(1), 36–52.

Montgomery, K.C., Chester, J. & Milosevic, T. (2017). Ensuring young people's digital privacy as a fundamental right. In S.B. De Abreu, P. Mihailidis, A.Y.L. Lee, B.S. De Abreu, P. Mihailidis, A.Y. Lee, J. Melki, & J. McDougall (Eds.), *International handbook of media literacy education* (pp. 85–102). New York: Routledge.

Nutter Smith, A. (2015). Commodification. In D.T. Cook & J.M. Ryan (Eds.), *The Wiley Blackwell encyclopedia of consumption and consumer studies* (pp. 90–93). London: Wiley Blackwell.

Pugh, A.J. (2011). Distinction, boundaries or bridges? Children, inequality and the uses of consumer culture. *Poetics*, *39*, 1–18.

Rozendaal, E., Lapierre, M.A., van Reijmersdal, E.A. & Buijzen, M. (2011). Reconsidering advertising literacy as a defense against advertising effects. *Media Psychology*, *14*(4), 333–354.

Rozendaal, E., Slot, N. & van Reijmersdal, E.A. (2013). Children's responses to advertising in social games. *Journal of Advertising*, *42*(2/3), 142–154.

Ruckenstein, M. (2011). Children in creationist capitalism. *Information, Communication & Society*, *14*(7), 1060–1076.

Smith, K.L. & Shade, L.R. (2018). Children's digital playgrounds as data assemblages: Problematics of privacy, personalization, and promotional culture. *Big Data & Society*, *5*(2), 1–12.

Sparrman, A. & Sandin, B. (2012). Situated child consumption, An introduction. In A. Sparrman, B. Sandin & J. Sjöberg (Eds.), *Situating child consumption: Rethinking values and notions of children, childhood and consumption* (pp. 9–32). Lund: Nordic Academic Press.

The Swedish Research Council. (2011). *Good research practice*. Stockholm, Sweden: The Swedish Research Council.

van Reijmersdal, E.A., Rozendaal, E. & Buijzen, M. (2012). Effects of prominence, involvement, and persuasion knowledge on children's cognitive and affective responses to advergames. *Journal of Interactive Marketing*, *26*, 33–42.

Wasko, J. (2010). Children's virtual worlds: The latest commercialization of children's culture. In D. Buckingham & V. Tingstad (Eds.), *Childhood and consumer culture* (pp. 113–129). London, UK: Palgrave Macmillan.

Willett, R. (2011). An ethnographic study of preteen girls' play with popular music on a school playground in the UK. *Journal of Children and Media*, *5*, 341–357.

Willett, R. (2018). "Microsoft bought Minecraft ... who knows what's going to happen?!": A sociocultural analysis of 8–9-year-olds' understanding of commercial online gaming industries. *Learning, Media and Technology*, *43*(1), 101–116.

20

THE EMERGENCE AND ETHICS OF CHILD-CREATED CONTENT AS MEDIA INDUSTRIES

Benjamin Burroughs and Gavin Feller

Introduction

This chapter seeks to unpack/unbox the evolving relationship between media industries and child-created content from a critical perspective. The profitability of content created for and by children on social media platforms such as YouTube has sparked an entire sector of content catering to young children. This chapter first looks at the cultivation of child 'influencers' as a part of the emergent digital media landscape and children's media industries, including the emergence of entire genres such as 'unboxing' and the family vlogging phenomenon. The chapter, ultimately, delves into the conjoining of upstart digital child-created content with traditional, legacy media industries in the example of Ryan Toys Review and Pocket Watch. Following a media industries approach (Havens & Lotz, 2012), this research tracks how child-created content is part of an emergent digital economy.

Corporations have long viewed children as a target demographic, but with the success of child-created content, large companies are also investing heavily in marketing and content through mobile phones and connected viewing practices through and by children. This chapter aims to provide a broad overview and mapping of the current landscape of child-created children's entertainment and media, including the rise of very young children as influencers. Child-created content is part of current and future media industries authorship, labour, and media consumption practices. Attention is paid to the political economy implications of a children's media industry as well as the critical and social influences on conceptions of aspirational purchasing and marketing melding with the affordances of digital technology and platform design. Child-created content is also the site for discursively codifying particular articulations of concepts such as family or gender to reinforce purchasing and marketing norms within these sites.

The confluence of ubiquitous smartphone/mobile penetration, tactile user interfaces for accessing content, and parents using phones and screens as surrogate parenting tools have all resulted in platforms such as YouTube amassing hundreds of millions of views for child-created content and content targeted toward young children (Nicoll & Nansen, 2018). This surge in young viewers, a previously untapped market for digital platforms, led to investments in attempting to enclose and capture this perceived growth area for digital media companies and legacy companies operating in the kids' media space. YouTube, in particular, aggressively pursued this demographic by developing its own YouTube Kids app to assuage parental fears of children mixing with adult content.

> Part of the work the YouTube Kids app performs is to corral young children into a controlled space without unexpected participation and play, where a more monolithic category of "child" or "kid" viewership can be codified and marketed to within the constraints of the app.
>
> *(Burroughs, 2017)*

YouTube continues to use the app as a space for building a relationship with young users that involves the consumption of YouTube content, often child-created content, and the calcifying of media practices within young children. These media practices and habits are expected to yield retention of children as platform-specific YouTube consumers in the long run.

In addition to social media channels and platforms such as "YouTube Kids", digital streaming companies like Netflix and Amazon have invested heavily in producing targeted content. In 2016, Netflix Chief Content Officer Ted Sarandos announced the company was "doubling down on kids and families", increasing the number of original programmes from 15 to 35 (Flint, 2016). Amazon struck a deal with PBS in 2016 to stream PBS Kids programming on Amazon Prime (Koblin, 2016). HBO acquired the rights to *Sesame Street* in conjunction with the launch of their streaming service HBO Now (Owen, 2018). As Steve Youngwood, COO of Sesame Workshop, explains, "There's no ambiguity that if kids and family is not an audience you serve, there's going to be a limit to how many subscribers you're ever going to have". Youngwood asserts this claim because he believes that streaming services need to be increasingly attractive to an entire household of viewers in an on-demand media consumption culture. Disney is launching their streaming service Disney+, which will target children through Disney's extensive catalogue of content and also extend existing properties to appeal to kids. These large digital media companies are increasingly targeting children through their major programming decisions.

The impact of Netflix and YouTube's investment in children's programming and child-created content has extended globally as the BBC announced in 2017 that they would invest $44 million in children's programming and content to combat the encroachment by YouTube and Netflix into young viewership. "YouTube usage is particularly popular with younger UK children – 54% of those between five and seven and 73% of those between eight and eleven use YouTube" (Tran, 2017). Legacy toy company Mattel recognised YouTube's connection to children and monetising that engagement by investing ten million dollars in advertising on the YouTube Kids platform (Schrank, 2017). Stemming from the success of child influencers like Ryan or Ryan Toys Review or FunToyzCollector and the unboxing genre, child-specific influencers spawn an entire economy of family vlogs and kids opening toys, presents, candy, and the 'stuff' of consumer culture and capitalist consumption. This child-created content is all directed towards children and the families of children, assembling a form of 'aspirational labour' (Duffy, 2017), which feeds from creators and audiences into larger corporate structures digitally and commercially.

Labour, Learning, and Playing

Integral to the history of the children's media industries are changes in labour laws, the romanticisation of childhood, educational philosophies about learning and play, and, of course, toys. Children have long been a source of cheap labour. As early in America's history as 1791, Alexander Hamilton insisted that children should be put to work. Not only could nimble fingers and fast feet help American manufacturers compete with British textile imports, but work was also deemed good for children "who would otherwise be idle" (Rosenberg, 2013, p. 4). A Puritan notion of childhood insisted that manual labour "kept [children] from idleness and rambling, and of course from early temptations to vice, by placing them for a time in manufactories" (Coxe, 1794, p. 55). Mass immigration of the late-19th and early 20th centuries infused burgeoning labour markets with children ready to work for low wages (Rosenberg, 2013). By 1890, 20% of children under the age of 16 made up 20% of the total U.S. workforce (Rosenberg, 2013).

Early children's media occupations included 'telegraph boys' who rode bicycles around city streets to deliver messages, telegraph operators running small outposts in rural towns, Pony Express riders and other 'messenger boys', and 'newsboys' selling newspapers and magazines on street corners and trains. Girls also participated, though at a much smaller scale – many believed the exposure to seedy scenes inherent in the life of messengers would lead to prostitution, for instance (Rosenberg, 2013). Children have thus been central to American media, though their 18th- and 19th-century roles often focussed on the *distribution* rather than *production* of content. Under the banner of street trades, this type of media labour was regulated long after mining and factory work (Clopper, 1912).

Changes in labour laws in the 20th century and the rise of the middle class contributed to the romanticisation of childhood. Childhood was increasingly constructed as innocent and in need of both protection and education (Mintz, 2004). As children transformed from 'useful' to 'priceless' (Zelizer, 1994), their newfound sentimental value made them increasingly valuable on the silver screen (Addison, 2015). Child film stars grew in prominence and popularity in the 1910s and 1920s. "As children were removed from the workforce", historian Gary Cross argues, "parents increasingly saw play as the core activity of childhood" (Cross, 1997, pp. 123–4). Therefore, in order to defend children's labour in Hollywood and avoid legal complications, parents and fan magazine discourse "insisted that the efforts of child stars were a form of recreation" – in other words, work was successfully framed as play (Addison, 1252). A paradox emerged: "they were child labourers paid to represent the new sentimentalised view of children. They worked to portray the useless child" (Zelizer, 1994, p. 95). Though paradoxical, the innocence and purity of child stars were crucial to maintaining the virtue of a film industry that was, particularly in the 1920s, plagued by scandal (Addison, 2015). Keeping the at-time millions of dollars in profit out of the hands of child stars was justified on the basis that the kids were happy with a menial allowance and that paying them in full would do nothing but spoil them (Addison, 2015). The California Child Actor's Bill, aka the Coogan Act, passed in 1938, forced parents to set aside half of their child star's earnings (Zelizer, 1994).

The gradual disappearance of child labour and the rise of Hollywood birthed another industry key to understanding children's media: toys. "Play had become the 'work' of children. And work required tools", argues Cross (p. 129). The toy industry answered. In the 1930s, Shirley Temple and Mickey Mouse dolls exploded in popularity – both extended blockbuster fame into the daily lives of small children (Cross, 1997). As children's roles in physical labour continually weakened, their purchasing influence as consumers of toys and media strengthened. Toys have since remained in a symbiotic relationship with legacy media. Concerns about children obtaining the benefits of labour and participatory culture have today led to calls for child rights in a digital age. Scholars and activists are fighting for children's right to free speech, privacy, and self-identification – seeking to find the nuance between protecting the innocent from dangers online and empowering future generations (Livingstone & Third, 2017).

Alongside debates over children's media rights are renewed concerns with the child labour undergirding the production of reality television, family vlogs, and other YouTube channels based on child stars. Despite the changing nature of 'work' and the increasing profitability of young children on YouTube, laws surrounding child-created media content are noticeably absent. The Fair Labour Standards Act (FLSA) of 1938, which banned children under the age of 16 from work, remains the primary piece of legislative protection against child labour 80 years later. Included in the FLSA is the 'Shirley Temple Act' – an exemption for "any child employed as an actor or performer in motion pictures or theatrical productions, or in radio or television productions" – named after the famous child star who would otherwise have been prohibited from acting at the peak of her young career (The law, Sec. 213(c)(1)(A)(ii), p. 33). In short, Congress decided that acting is not labour because it does not constitute oppressive labour and it gives children the opportunity to develop talents and skills beneficial to their future success (Podlas, 2010).

All of this has led us to a current moment wherein children are increasingly at the centre of popular media content generating enormous amounts of money, and yet little protection against exploitation exists. Capturing someone on camera – whether for a news broadcast of a public event, a documentary, or a family YouTube channel – does not inherently qualify as 'work' under current legal definitions (Podlas, 2010). Because entertainment laws regarding children are primarily decided at the state level, 17 states have essentially zero regulation of child entertainment labour (U.S. Department of Labor 2020; Popper, 2016). Podlas argues that a focus on *child* labour excludes *parents* from needed critical attention, "enabling them to avoid responsibility and risk the welfare of their children" (Podlas, 2010, p. 73).

The romanticisation of childhood and increased legal protection against dangerous physical labour has not removed young kids from the gears of the media industry machine; moreover, it has enabled them to become integral to the popularity and profitability of digital media today. Just as newsies of the 19th century were central to the distribution of daily newspapers, children going about their daily lives on camera are crucial to the production of contemporary media content.

Unboxing and Family Vlogs

Influencers or micro-celebrities have been studied by a growing number of scholars in relation to YouTube (Cunningham & Craig, 2017; Lange, 2014; Senft, 2008). Additionally, there is a small but growing body of literature related to the monetisation of child-created content and digital parenting (Abidin, 2015; Burroughs, 2017; Smith & Shade, 2018). One specific strand of this literature relates to the emergence of unboxing videos as a specific genre of YouTube videos catering to children as an emergent demographic.

Unboxing refers to videos that show people (or just hands) opening and commenting on toys, candies, and children's entertainment in the vein of a product review. Increasingly, unboxing videos lack any critical review function and instead show very young children or adults playing with the toys themselves or playing as a family. Nicoll and Nansen (2018) suggest that unboxing videos are sites of 'mimetic participation' that encourage commercialisation and play wherein children are "both sites and subjects of imitation within affinity spaces such as YouTube". This acts as a simulation of how play could (or should) be modelled for younger viewers within digital platforms and apps. The child influencer, such as Evan on EvanTube HD, is positioned as a "cyberflâneur" (Marsh, 2016). These genres reinforce a capitalist logic of consumption articulated through the viewing of other children and families immersed in toys, games, and product placement. Unboxing can serve as a lynchpin, connecting affinity spaces with consumption practices through child-created content as "the industry views these children as conduits through which they can condition purchasing habits from birth. Unboxing videos act as a kind of mini-infomercial spurring aspirational purchasing" (Burroughs, 2017). And while Craig and Cunningham (2017) rightly point out that this form of 'entrepreneurial labour' by children and families is not necessarily "beholden to the commercial interests of the toy manufacturers or the platforms", accounting for the increased agency provided by the affordances of social media, unboxing still serves to enmesh audiences within this emergent child-created media industry of digital labour.

Through these videos of consumption, the mobile phone and app technologies are the space of 'sharenting', defined as "sharing representations of one's parenting or children online" (Blum-Ross & Livingstone, 2017). The entire family is wrapped in the production of these unboxing videos. This perpetuates a media environment targeted at children, where consumption is idealised and families are projected as constantly having an abundance of free products from their digital 'labour'. Social media influencers are enabled to quit their 'regular' jobs and begin to fully rely on apps and social media accounts for their livelihood. Users compete for unique content and followers with the goal to receive paid partnerships. They manufacture this digital persona of posting approachable pictures and interacting with their fans, making it appear like they are carefree, without ever showing the audience the hard, laborious work that happens behind the scenes. Abidin (2017) labels this practice as 'calibrated amateurism' where families work to convince users "that these performers are 'family' before 'influencers'" and cultivate "followers envy and pine after their craft, unity, and family spirit to the extent of wanting to emulate after them as #familygoals". No worries, no family drama, and always already fun activities no matter where they are – a 'perfect' social media life and performance through the family vlog. The expertise and trust that is generated by the endorser has altered much of the modern consumer society, growing the perceived power of the influencer and the consumer's brand attitudes. In turn, the relationship and proximity of children to unfiltered advertising continues to shrivel.

Ryan Toys Review and Pocket Watch

The ongoing maturation of YouTube and increasing trust in the platform among advertisers, along with the emergence of new video genres explicitly aimed at children and families – such as unboxing videos and family vlogs – is opening new avenues for old media power to increase both corporate profits and ideological influence on younger and younger children. This has resulted in an industry built out of child-created content, now layered onto and integrated with traditional media industry logics. Ryan Toys Review is a site for understanding this emergent digital ecosystem, the importance of influencers catering to children, and the ethical dilemmas which arise from this shift in media industries. The rise of micro-celebrities and family influencers through platforms such as YouTube and Instagram is attracting the attention and money of traditional media and a variety of retailers. For decades television, film, and toy and clothing retailers have coordinated efforts to profit from children (Banet-Weiser, 2007; Cross, 1997). Toy companies and media producers mutually benefit from carefully calculated cross-promotional strategies. Child-created content – specifically YouTube kid stars – is the next iteration of brand integration.

At the time of this writing, the YouTube channel generating the highest number of views is not a Vevo-owned pop music star. It is Ryan Toys Review: a channel featuring a six-year-old boy unboxing new toys in his family living room from the view of his mom's iPhone. While Ryan's parents innocently describe the channel as "a little project that mommy and daddy do", it has amassed over 16.5 million subscribers in less than four years, generated over 25 billion total video views, and produced $11 million dollars of revenue in one year (Schmidt, 2017). The focus is "Toys review for kids by a kid!" and the videos are relatively simple with regards to content, narrative, and production value (channel About page, 2018). Ryan receives a box of new toys, he opens them, plays with them, and then waves goodbye to his virtual fans – all with extreme excitement, sanguine smiles, and the token YouTube calls for viewers to like, subscribe, and keep watching. In the videos, Ryan is often playing with his parents and family with the toys, as the videos generally run between 10 and 15 minutes. Ryan Toys Review generally produces a video every couple of days, so subscribers get to watch Ryan and his family open a new toy and play with a new toy as a family almost every day. While the family donates the excess to charity, the family is engaged in the formation of aspirational labour reinforced within Ryan's audience. Ideologically, the channel represents the idyllic life for millions of distant toddlers on tablets and calcifies an orientation towards constant capitalist consumption through the family and through play – who wouldn't want to open a box of brand new toys every day?

Parent reviews of the channel on the popular Common Sense Media website range from critiques of child manipulation to one commenter calling it a "plastic worshipping revenue machine kids creator". Many use terms like 'garbage', 'consumerism', and 'spoiled' while another claims, more pointedly, "it's not mindless, it's insidious". A somewhat unsettling theme emerges across review sites and video comment threads: thousands apparently loathe the channel for no other reason than the "super annoying voice" of Ryan's mom (all quotes from www.commonsensemedia.org/youtube-reviews/ryan-toys-review/user-reviews/adult).

Critiques aside, Ryan's innocuous influence is extending beyond YouTube. In the summer of 2018, Walmart launched a new toy line based on the Ryan Toys Review channel (the video of Ryan visiting the store with his parents to find the new toys for the first time has already been watched 10.5 million times). Within a highly gendered retail space, the dinosaurs, trucks, space guns, and surprise eggs are, of course, aimed primarily at boys. Importantly, the toys prominently feature Ryan as a character: wide-eyed, wide-mouthed, giving his soon-to-be iconic thumbs up. Walmart owns over 20% of the retail toy market share and is expected to reach $8 billion in toy sales soon (Fernandez, 2019). The line started as an exclusive deal with 2,500 Walmart locations but, by September, Target, another massive retail outlet with over 3% of the toy market, had also signed on to carry Ryan's new merchandise. Retailers are increasingly partnering with social media influencers, but Ryan is the first YouTube child star to have his own toy line (Jones, 2018). Of course, the six-year old and his stay-at-home mom are not doing it alone. They are backed by a new digital marketing firm with deep roots in the children's media industry, deep pockets, and decades of marketing and sales experience.

Pocket Watch launched in March of 2017, is based in Culver City, California, and currently has 40 full-time employees who are "paid to think and act like kids" (About page). The company is partnering with the biggest producers of child-created content on YouTube. Its line-up includes Ryan Toys Review, Captain Sparklez, Hobby Kids TV, and brother and sister channels EvanTube HD and JillianTube HD (each with myriad spinoff channels). The "new kind of entertainment company" ambiguously states it is "planting a flag for kids" in "today's ever-expanding, shape-shifting entertainment universe" (About page). The company's leadership includes CEO Chris M. Williams (former head of Disney Originals Online), Chief Content Creator Albie Hecht (former head of Nickelodeon) and Chief Strategy Officer Jon Moonves (entertainment representative) – some of whom have grandkids apparently well-suited for exploitation. Moonves' bio, for instance, states that "Jon is the father of two great young women and pop to two amazing grandkids/target audience members".

Pocket Watch is the latest iteration of aspirations to extend young YouTube micro-celebrity fame into traditional media structures. Many of the current Pocket Watch team first attempted to build a multi-channel network (MCN) with the launch of Maker Studios. An "uneasy collision between new and old media players" (Weiss, 2015), Maker Studios partnered with first generation YouTube stars (e.g., Pewdiepie and Shaytards) to tap into a subscriber base of nearly 400 million spread across over 50,000 YouTube channels (Barnes, 2014). Initially, the future was bright as Disney purchased Maker Studios in 2014 for $500 million (with a promise to pay another $450 million if certain milestones were met). However, the company flopped shortly thereafter due to 'internal dysfunction' and a problem symptomatic of MCNs – without owning video content MCNs can only collect advertising revenue when content plays on their channels (Patel, 2017). Pocket Watch emerged from the rubble of the crumbling Maker Studios acquisition with a tightened focus: child-created content. Nearly two-thirds of the company is made up of former Maker Studios/Disney staff – that is, television and film executives bent on leveraging their industry relationships and sales and marketing prowess to capitalise on fresh opportunities like Ryan Toys Review.

To avoid repeating the mistakes of Maker Studios, Pocket Watch is teaming up with the traditional media giant Viacom, who has invested several million dollars into forging a partnership. The aim of the partnership is to produce original content by children, for children – across various media platforms (Spangler, 2018). Pocket Watch and Viacom will, for instance, release a printed book featuring Ryan and other YouTube kid stars; and a contract with Paramount for the production of a feature-length unboxing film has been signed (Spangler, 2018).

The deals effectively cash in on the cultural cache of young YouTube stars by leveraging their authority across traditional media and further collapsing the perpetually diminishing distance between education and entertainment. The book, titled "Watch this Book!", harnesses the neoliberal logics of YouTube, encouraging kids to watch and consume rather than read, engage, and question. Perhaps most important for the financial viability of the joint venture and more worrisome for parents is the agreement for Viacom to be the exclusive third-party advertising agent on Pocket Watch YouTube partner videos. The move gives the vast and varied brands under the Viacom umbrella (Nickelodeon being one key example) direct and unfiltered advertising access to young children.

Taken together, the emergence of companies like Pocket Watch means a heightened focus on character-based development – using children, living their lives, as characters, of course. Six-year-old Ryan is, again, illustrative. The excitable and charismatic Asian-American boy can, under Pocket Watch's model, be developed as a 'character' adaptable to short-form video, a feature-length film, broadcast/streaming television, printed children's books, and toy and clothing retail. Ryan (and others who will inevitably follow in his footsteps) is on his way to becoming an icon of the new children's media sphere, both inescapable and aspirational, well before he reaches adolescence.

Conclusion

A multitude of questions involving the ethics of child-created content and media industries remain. New communicative technologies and their accompanying media industries have long served as a flashpoint for competing cultural values, hopes, and fears with regards to children. As Lynn Spigel (1992) notes, "More than any other group children [are] singled out as the victims of the new pied piper" (p. 50). Nansen, Chakraborty, Gibbs, MacDougall, and Vetere (2012) assert the need to "equip children with the knowledge and skills to be active, ethical and critical participants online" (p. 237). Ultimately, the question of safeguarding "children's rights in relation to dataveillance" (Lupton & Williamson, 2017) remains of paramount importance, especially as the boundaries between children, brands, and influencers continually shrink.

The initial promise of YouTube as a discourse of "empowerment", where anyone could make, share, and even become a "YouTube Star" or "influencer", is reified through child-created content. YouTube's Kids, like Ryan, engage in productive practices of production and disseminate that production to audiences, but YouTube's Kids, like Ryan, also open new toys seemingly every day. They remain intertwined in a system where watching and witnessing perpetuates capitalist consumption. But potentially more worrisome is that an entire generation growing up watching this mode of consumption reinforces the pernicious promise of YouTube that anyone can be like Ryan through consumption and play. Anyone can find fulfilment and joy through *constant* consumption. Child-created content is not just a potential future for digital media industries, it is the present of children and media. After all, who doesn't want to be Ryan and why can't my family be more like his?

References

Abidin, C. (2015). Micromicrocelebrity: branding babies on the internet. *M/C Journal, 18*(5).
Abidin, C. (2017). #familygoals: Family influencers, calibrated amateurism, and justifying young digital labor. *Social Media + Society, 3*(2), 1–15.
Addison, H. (2015). "Holding our heartstrings in their rosey hands": Child stars in early Hollywood. *The Journal of Popular Culture, 48*(6), 1250–1269.
Banet-Weiser, S. (2007). *Kids rule! Nickelodeon and consumer citizenship.* Durham, NC: Duke University Press.
Barnes, B. (2014). Disney buys Maker Studios, video supplier for YouTube. *New York Times.* March 24. www.nytimes.com/2014/03/25/business/media/disney-buys-maker-studios-video-supplier-for-youtube.html.
Blum-Ross, A., & Livingstone, S. (2017). "Sharenting", parent blogging, and the boundaries of the digital self. *Popular Communication, 15*(2), 110–125. doi:10.1080/15405702.2016.1223300.
Burroughs, B. (2017). YouTube kids: The app economy and mobile parenting. *Social Media + Society, 3*(2). doi:2056305117707189.
Clopper, E. (1912). *Child labor in city streets.* New York, NY: McMillan Company.
Coxe, T. (1794). *A View of the United States of America.* Philadelphia, PA: Hall.
Craig, D., & Cunningham, S. (2017). Toy unboxing: Living in a (n unregulated) material world. *Media International Australia, 163*(1), 77–86.
Cross, G. (1997). *Kids' stuff: Toys and the changing world of American childhood.* Cambridge, MA: Harvard University Press.
Cunningham, S., & Craig, D. (2017). Being "really real" on YouTube: Authenticity, community and brand culture in social media entertainment. *Media International Australia, 164*(1), 71–81.
Duffy, B. E. (2017). *(Not) getting paid to do what you love: Gender, social media, and aspirational work.* New Haven, CT: Yale University Press.
Fernandez, C. (2019). The retail market for toys. U.S. Specialized Report OD6117. IBISWorld. Retrieved from: https://my-ibisworld-com.ezproxy.lib.utah.edu/us/en/industry-specialized/od6117/about.
Flint, J. (2016). Netflix to ramp up originals targeting kids. *Wall Street Journal.* January 17. www.wsj.com/articles/netflix-to-ramp-up-originals-targeting-kids-1453058812.
Havens, T., & Lotz, A. D. (2012). *Understanding media industries.* Oxford: Oxford University Press.
Jones, C. (2018). Walmart, Nordstrom and others look to YouTube stars to woo millennials and Gen Z. *USA Today.* August 6. www.usatoday.com/story/money/2018/08/06/social-media-influencers-ocial-media-influencers/725842002.
Koblin, J. (2016). Amazon Prime strikes deal for most PBS children's shows. *New York Times.* July 1. www.nytimes.com/2016/07/02/business/media/amazon-prime-strikes-deal-for-most-pbs-childrens-shows.html.
Lange, P. (2014). *Kids on YouTube: Technical identities and digital literacies.* Walnut Creek, CA: Left Coast Press.
Livingstone, S., & Third, A. (2017). Children and young people's right in the digital age. *New Media and Society, 19*(5), 657–670.
Lupton, D., & Williamson, B. (2017). The datafied child: The dataveillance of children and implications for their rights. *New Media & Society, 19*(5), 780–794.
Marsh, J. (2016). Unboxing' videos: Co-construction of the child as cyberflâneur, discourse. *Studies in the Cultural Politics of Education, 37*(3), 369–380. doi:10.1080/01596306.2015.1041457.
Mintz, S. (2004). *Huck's raft: A history of American childhood.* Cambridge, MA: Harvard University Press.
Nansen, B., Chakraborty, K., Gibbs, L., MacDougall, C., & Vetere, F. (2012). Children and digital wellbeing in Australia: Online regulation, conduct and competence. *Journal of Children and Media, 6,* 237–254.
Nicoll, B., & Nansen, B. (2018). Mimetic production in YouTube toy unboxing videos. *Social Media+ Society, 4*(3), 1–12.
Owen, R. (2018). Cornucopia of children's content comes to streaming services. *Variety.* August 2. https://variety.com/2018/tv/features/sesame-workshop-pbs-kids-hulu-amazon-netflix-childrens-content-1202891363.
Patel, S. (2017). Inside Disney's troubled $675 mil Maker Studios acquisition. *DigiDay.* February 22. https://digiday.com/media/disney-maker-studios.

Podlas, K. (2010). Does exploiting a child amount to employing a child: The FLSA's child labor provision and children on reality television. *UCLA Entertainment Law Review*, 17(1), 39–73.

Popper, B. (2016). YouTube's biggest star is a 5-year old that makes millions opening toys: Blurring the line between playtime and business. *Verge*. December 22, 2016. www.theverge.com/2016/12/22/14031288/ryan-toys-review-biggest-youngest-youtube-star-millions.

Rosenberg, C. M. (2013). *Child Labor in America: A history*. New York, NY: McFarland and Company.

Schmidt, S. (2017, 11 December). Six-year-old made $11 million in one year reviewing toys on YouTube. Washington Post. Retrieved from: www.washingtonpost.com/news/morning-mix/wp/2017/12/11/6-year-old-made-11-million-in-one-year-reviewing-toys-on-you-tube.

Schrank, A. (2017). Goodbye cable, hello YouTube: As kids move online, so do Mattel's ad dollars. *Marketplace*. August 3. www.marketplace.org/2017/08/03/business/goodbye-cable-hello-youtube-kids-move-online-so-does-mattel-s-ad-dollars.

Senft, T. M. (2008). *Camgirls: Celebrity & community in the age of social networks*. New York, NY: Peter Lang.

Smith, K. L. and Shade, L.R. (2018). Children's digital playgrounds as data assemblages: Problematics of privacy, personalization, and promotional culture. *Big Data & Society*, 5(2), 1–12.

Spangler, T. (2018). Viacom leads $15 million round in Pocket.watch, sets content and ad pact with Startup. *Variety*. https://variety.com/2018/digital/news/viacom-pocket-watch-funding-15-million-1202875467.

Spigel, L. (1992). *Make room for TV: Television and the family ideal in postwar America*. Chicago, IL: University of Chicago Press.

Tran, K. (2017). BBC is investing heavily in children's content to combat Netflix and YouTube. *Business Insider*. July 6. www.businessinsider.com/bbc-invests-childrens-content-combat-netflix-youtube-2017-7.

U.S. Department of Labor (2020). Child Entertainment Laws as of January 1, 2020. Retrieved from: www.dol.gov/agencies/whd/state/child-labor/entertainment.

Weiss, G. (2015). Why Disney's $500 million acquisition of Maker Studios is proving less than picture perfect. *Entrepreneur*. August 17. www.entrepreneur.com/article/249659.

Zelizer, V. A. (1994). *Pricing the priceless child: The changing social value of children*. Princeton, NJ: Princeton University Press.

21
PRE-SCHOOL STARS ON YOUTUBE

Child Microcelebrities, Commercially Viable Biographies, and Interactions with Technology

Crystal Abidin

Introduction

Some of the most watched pre-schoolers today are young children of viral video fame, family influencer units, and micro-microcelebrities. While children of viral video fame may stumble into public popularity by accident or chance (Abidin, 2018a), children in family influencer units gain fame from being consistently exposed to the public as part of their parents' production of content that heavily centres on domestic life (Abidin, 2017), and children who are micro-microcelebrities are intentionally groomed by their microcelebrity mothers to become commodities and human billboards from birth (Abidin, 2015). As social-media-famous children whose public visibility in digital spaces is not only intentionally prolific but deliberately commercial, such pre-schoolers are unwittingly subject to having their biographies video-recorded and textually documented for hundreds of thousands of followers. Often, their digital estates also portray the children interacting with different devices and technology, with varying degrees of digital literacy and self-awareness. Although most of this production is managed and curated by parents of such young semi-public figures, other factors in the ecology shape parental choices, such as corporate pressures from influencer management agencies and sponsoring clients, and audience pressures from followers who request or demand specific content.

At present, contract stipulations and guidelines between child influencers and agencies or clients are guarded under legal confidentiality or obscured to preempt cultural backlash and scrutiny. Existing child labour laws in the entertainment industry, such as the Entertainment Work Permit (Department of Industrial Relations, 2013) and the Californian Coogan Law (Screen Actors Guild, 2015), stipulate protection of under-12s in the mainstream media industries such as film, television, and music. National guidelines, such as Singapore's Protection of Underaged Workers governed by the Ministry of Manpower, seem to focus on industrial work taken up outside the domestic space of the home (Ministry of Manpower, 2014). As such, despite their high visibility on social media and lucrative biographies that are archived to accumulate brand longevity on YouTube, the actual working conditions and contractual obligations of such child microcelebrities are relatively obscured.

This chapter aims to open a conversation regarding children's rights in the influencer industry by scrutinising how a group of such pre-schoolers, originating from different fame histories, interact with the camera as a stand-in for an audience. Through a content analysis of their audio-visual content on YouTube, this chapter will observe how the pre-schoolers handle devices, address the camera, and interact with their parents on film as modes of emoting and exercising their willingness to participate in filming and technology use.

Commercially Viable Biographies on YouTube

YouTube is a celebrated space of 'vernacular creativity', where users create and share content "as a means of social networking" and as an everyday culture (Burgess & Green, 2013, pp. 25–6). However, the rise of social media influencers has meant that many YouTubers are now intentionally generating content as a commercial practice, with the intention of pursuing remuneration. Even though beginners and aspirants often engage in the 'aspirational labour' of producing content without compensation, in the belief that they will experience their 'big break' and be able to monetise their content in the foreseeable future (Duffy, 2015), this route from obscurity to fame to commerce is not always readily available to everyone. Aspirants often work hard to transit from being a mere public 'face' into becoming a sustained persona that is recognisable on the internet, and later an internet celebrity who can monetise their fame (Abidin, 2018a, pp. 44–52).

For many pre-school stars on YouTube, accumulating monetisable fame often involves parent-managers who conscientiously monitor, groom, and curate a biographical narrative that can later be monetised. This requires parents to engage in 'sharenting', or the sharing of "information about themselves and their children online" (Blum-Ross & Livingston, 2017, p. 110), albeit with a higher commercial agenda. Although everyday parents have been known to use wearable devices to track their children, as an act of 'intimate surveillance' that is usually a "purposeful and routinely well-intentioned surveillance of young people by parents" (Leaver, 2015, p. 153), such young children have "no direct self-representational agency" (Leaver, 2017, p. 2). As such, unlike other child-centred parenting blogs which are useful feminist interventions to value domestic labour or resist the societal pressures and ideal constructions of 'good' motherhood (Lopez, 2009; Orton-Johnson, 2017), constructing commercially viable biographies of children on YouTube can potentially be exploitative as children are framed "to maximize advertorial potential" (Abidin, 2017). This chapter conceptualises the construction of such pre-school internet celebrities' 'commercially viable biographies' as the calculated public documentation of young children's everyday lives and especially developmental milestones, whether staged or in situ, solicited through a sustained agenda of practices to simulate situations and stimulate their reactions, with the intention to cultivate a monetisable profile.

Despite the range of social media on which child microcelebrities proliferate, this chapter focusses on YouTube as it has emerged as a central site of concern regarding children's wellbeing online, given a growing number of children who turn to the platform over television (Shnuel, 2018).

First, since 2017, there has been an explosion of age-inappropriate disturbing content tagged with child-oriented search terms that can even be viewed with YouTube's "family-friendly restricted mode enabled" (Orphanides, 2018). These include popular children's cartoons remixed into knock-off editions to contain violence, pornography, sexualisation, and suicide (Bridle, 2017; Buzzi, 2011). Although YouTube has made some efforts to moderate such content and restrict their monetisation (Hern, 2017), progress has been slow as the platform largely depends on "flagging by viewers to drive official review" (Bridle, 2018).

Second, YouTube influencers and YouTube targeted ads have been marketing contentious messages to children. One of YouTube's top stars, Jake Paul, who claims his target audience is "children between the ages of 8 and 16", has promoted digital betting company Mystery Brand's online gambling service to young viewers (Jennings, 2019). YouTube has also been accused of violating the Children's Online Privacy Protection Act by collecting the personal data of child users without parental consent and serving them targeted commercials for child products and services alongside 'kid-oriented videos' (*Washington Post*, 2018).

Third, YouTube influencers have been exploiting children in their content production. Family influencer units on YouTube have come under fire for child abuse, as they subject their children to 'pranks' as fodder for viewers, such as US YouTube channel DaddyOFive which was profiting between USD$200,000–350,000 annually from the emotional distress of their children filmed on camera (Leaver & Abidin, 2017). Viral kid reaction videos are becoming more lucrative and may drive up the demand for more staged set-ups, but such child microcelebrities are not covered by traditional workplace standards that historically protected child stars in the mainstream media industries from exploitation (Abidin, 2015).

Finally, the rise of child influencers on YouTube evidence the importance of paying close attention to such young YouTubers online. Child influencers are quickly rising through the ranks, especially in the genre of 'unboxing' videos (Marsh, 2015), with the likes of seven-year-old Ryan Toys Review topping the Forbes list of the highest paid YouTubers of 2018 (Robehmed & Berg, 2018). Since launching in March 2015, Ryan has accumulated over 17 million followers and 26 billion views (Berg, 2018) via videos in which he unboxes and plays with toys or tries out food products with "earnest and enthusiastic commentary" guided by his parents off-screen (Lynch, 2018). Ryan now owns "40 international licensing deals to use his image" and has his own toy line and TV show (Shamsian, 2019).

Against this backdrop of the variety of child microcelebrities on YouTube, this chapter focusses on three case studies of internet-famous children on YouTube who are derived from different fame origins (i.e., viral video fame, family influencer units, and micro-microcelebrities) and hail from different cultural ecologies (i.e., South Korea, USA, Singapore), to survey the landscape of pre-schoolers with commercially viable biographies on YouTube.

Context and Methodology

The case studies were selected from three different projects looking at internet-famous children in the South Korean popular culture industry (Abidin, 2018b), influencer mothers and the proximate microcelebrification of their children (Abidin, 2015), and family influencer units and their ethical practices (Abidin, 2017). Based on existing data from long-term digital ethnography projects, a sample of six videos was purposively selected for content analysis. Specifically, they were analysed for interactions between the child and the parent, the child and the object of focus (i.e., a toy, a craft paper, a mobile phone), and the child and the camera. These video snippets were studied in relation to the spoken dialogue and closed captions or textual narration if applicable, and contextualised alongside reactions from the comments section of the YouTube posts. Readings of these interactions were also cross-referenced with more extensive discussions of these children's wellbeing on various social media platforms and online forums. The specific snippets discussed in this chapter were chosen to demonstrate the wide variety of practices among child stars on YouTube. As such, the interpretations here are informed by a deeper and longer awareness of where and how these YouTube channels are situated in the internet celebrity economy.

Ye Bin (born in 2011), of the channel 'Baby Yebin', is from South Korea and has been on YouTube since 2014. She is a viral internet celebrity who eventually parlayed her fame into a sustained influencer presence. Ye Bin rose to fame after her 'stranger danger' video – in which her mother queries her reactions on various scenarios (for instance, accepting ice cream from a stranger or going out with a stranger) – went viral internationally (Ye Bin, 2014). Since then, the videos feature Ye Bin's developmental milestones and recreational activities.

Eliana (born in 2008), of the channel 'realitychangers', is from the USA and has been on YouTube since 2010. She is a member of a family influencer unit that initially began with her father Jorge and older sister Alexia. The family produces weekly vlogs of their domestic life and videos of their home-made covers of popular songs. Although Eliana initially began with cameos and was included in a handful of videos, she formally took part in the channel's cover song in 2013 (realitychangers, 2013) and became a staple in their family influencer unit after that.

Dash (born in 2013), of the channels 'Clicknetwork' and 'Xiaxue', is from Singapore and has been on YouTube since 2013. He is a second-generation microcelebrity born to a prominent influencer Xiaxue, who has been on several social media blogs since the mid-2000s. Although Xiaxue originally began as a lifestyle influencer and helmed her own YouTube series 'Xiaxue's Guide to Life' on the aggregate content channel Clicknetwork, she began to expand into the parenting genre after giving birth to Dash by intensively curating his social media presence from conception.

As a result of their different genealogies to YouTube fame, the pre-schoolers exhibit varying digital literacies in their engagement with the camera, varying awareness of audiences in their conversations on camera, and changing interactions with their parents in front of the camera, which will be summarised and analysed in the next section. This chapter builds on recent research on how content featuring social media child stars in commercial YouTube activities can be better regulated (Craig & Cunningham, 2017), how they merge play and commerce via mimetic production (Nicoll & Nansen, 2018), and how they expand their brand as they grow up online (Ramos-Serrano & Herrero-Diz, 2016). Unlike prior studies on how young children are learning to use devices such as tablets (Hourcade et al., 2015), how young children are engaged in digital literacy practices when they watch YouTube videos (Marsh, 2015), and how children develop technical identities from engaging on YouTube (Lange, 2014), this chapter focusses on pre-school-aged child YouTube celebrities, and how their different fame origins must be contextualised, to understand the varying degrees to which their parent-managers engage with them and acknowledge their agency on camera.

Child Microcelebrities' Interactions with Technology

Ye Bin

Ye Bin's videos are filmed by her mother, but there is often very little parental dialogue apart from Q&A videos in which Ye Bin is being quizzed. The videos usually begin with Ye Bin in situ, without any introduction or orientation for the viewer, and the clip usually records the moment she becomes aware of the camera filming her, before she decides whether to change her composure and engage with the lens or ignore the lens to resume her activity as if unwatched.

In one compilation of videos (Ye Bin, 2015), Ye Bin is filmed getting out of bed. She pushes her fringe away from her eyes and notices the camera. Immediately, she throws her arms onto the cushion on her bed, then reaches towards her mother to bat the camera out of her hands. The camera falls onto the bed as her mother asks, "Stop filming?" As the mother moves the camera back onto Ye Bin and awaits her response, Ye Bin pauses for a moment, then looks to her mother and pushes her palm on the lens, forcing the camera back down onto the bed again. In this brief struggle, the camera catches another glimpse of Ye Bin looking displeased and waving her palms in front of the lens. The clip then ends abruptly, to signify that the mother has honoured Ye Bin's decision to refuse being filmed. Another clip in this compilation featured Ye Bin singing a nursery rhyme when she notices that her mother is filming her. Ye Bin then turns her head slightly to face the camera, looks directly into the lens, and she completes the rest of the song with dance moves, in agreement with the filming. These two examples showcase the range of Ye Bin's gestural decisions when choosing how to respond to the camera, which are peppered throughout the videos on her channel.

In a second video (Ye Bin, 2016), Ye Bin is seen interacting with a variety of selfie filters, such as blowing digital bubbles or shifting her face in the frame so that a machine can 'apply' makeup on her. Ye Bin reacts enthusiastically to the filter's interactive displays through smiles, giggles, and repeated gestures and facial movements to solicit the same stimulations. It is evident that the video is a screen recording of the smartphone, and Ye Bin's mother is partially seen and sometimes in the shadows right beside her, presumably holding up the smartphone in front of Ye Bin since both of the latter's arms are in the frame. Such videos show Ye Bin taking the initiative to interact with technology, and demonstrating some independence as she learns to navigate the selfie filters through trial and error.

Across the videos on her channel, Ye Bin can be seen expressing on camera her desire to continue or refuse being filmed, and her mother correspondingly honours her agency. In one video, her mother had uploaded a video she apparently found on her smartphone in which Ye Bin had unknowingly recorded herself, presumably without parental supervision. Comments in the (now deleted) video praised Ye Bin for being able to pick up technical skills so quickly and at such a young age, in all likelihood from modelling her mother. The videos in which she is seen interacting with selfie filters, various smartphone apps, and the phone, evidence the processes through which she is figuring out and learning to navigate new technology. In general, the parental involvement in Ye Bin's videos is low and only to the extent of managing the technical aspects of filming behind the scenes; otherwise, Ye Bin is recorded primarily in her 'own habitat', exhibiting her own personality, and the camera is often positioned as a 'fly on the wall'.

Eliana

Eliana is usually filmed with her father and sister, via a handheld camera mostly managed by her father, or via a camera on a tripod. In their cover videos, there is usually no introduction, and the trio go straight into a song. However, often appended at the end of such 'formal' covers is a blooper reel of behind-the-scenes snippets where Eliana is seen goofing around. In their lifestyle vlogs, Eliana's father usually begins with a quick introduction situating where they are, what activity the family is engaging in, and what they would like to chat about in the clip. Eliana and her sister are usually in the background and interjecting their father's vlogs with their own opinions and thoughts without prompt, or are occasionally introduced to the audience and invited to record on camera together.

In Eliana's debut cover video (realitychangers, 2013), she joins her father and older sister to sing the choruses and bridge of the song. Throughout the song her father strums the guitar while giving her affirmation when she sings by nodding, smiling, and flashing a thumbs-up at her. At one point when she appeared to be too serious and nervous while singing, her father sticks out his tongue to humour her and Eliana smiles in acknowledgement. At the end of the song, before the father finishes strumming the outro, Eliana exclaims: "we're done! Yay! But I did a good job. I singed …", then points out that she made a mistake while singing. Her father responds: "you guys did a great job. It's not supposed to be perfect. It's just … plain fun". Towards the end of the video a two-minute clip features Eliana goofing around, dancing, and singing a children's song, and her demeanour is markedly more casual and relaxed having completed the 'formal' cover. At the very end the father prompts everyone to wave goodbye to the camera, but Eliana has run outside of the frame. He calls out to her and points to a spot in front of the tripod where she has to stand, explaining that the camera films in a single direction and that she cannot be seen even though she is waving to the camera off-screen. Eliana is successfully coaxed and comes on screen to say goodbye.

In a second video (realitychangers, 2014), Eliana, her sister, and her father are lying on a bed recording via handheld camera. Her father initially focusses the lens on himself, but Eliana spots her partial face in the frame (possibly via the camera display screen) and cheekily makes funny faces to the camera lens. When her father notices this a few seconds later, he shifts the camera to include more of Eliana in the frame. Realising this, Eliana breaks out into more exaggerated funny faces. At one point she playfully obscures the camera lens with a piece of paper, to which her father says, "baby, stop. Don't cover the camera". Eliana turns her head to look at her father, as if in acknowledgement, then returns to making goofy faces on camera. Towards the end of the video, Eliana play-wrestles with her dad and accidentally kicks the camera out of her father's hand. As the camera rolls onto the bed and then the floor, her father is heard exclaiming "Ah! Dropped the camera!". He swiftly picks it up to wrap up the video, and Eliana wrestles to get into the camera frame again to bid her imagined audience goodbye.

Across the videos on her channel, Eliana engages in a mixture of 'staged' videos where she must behave and sing cover songs, and 'casual' videos where she is given the liberty to goof off on camera. The latter snippets have become known as 'Eli cam' to her viewers, as Eliana often dominates the camera lens and, in some instances, even handles the camera herself by 'taking over' the filming. In other videos, when she is in the background and is called to film, Eliana has opted out verbally or gesturally, choosing instead to continue the activity she is focussed on. Her father almost always obliges and leaves her be. Eliana displays a learned camera presence as 'technical' instructions (i.e., how to face the camera, where to point to the camera so as not to obscure the lens) given by her father in earlier videos are always elegantly displayed in her body language in later videos. In general, the parental involvement in Eliana's videos is moderate as she is free to come and go into her father's vlogs as she wishes, but there are many instances where her behaviour is clearly rehearsed for the more 'formal' song covers. Her experiences of growing up on camera include a host of technical (i.e., how to use the camera) and social (i.e., who her audience possibly is) literacies as instructed to her by her father and unassumingly caught on video in their casual conversations, and she appears to have absorbed such tacit knowledge by exhibiting confidence on screen.

Dash

Dash is usually incorporated into his influencer mother's mostly sponsored videos. By way of advertising the sponsored message, his mother interacts with him on camera while engaging in an activity using the sponsored product or service. When Dash was younger and needed assistance sitting in a single spot to be filmed, he was often seen being coaxed by the disembodied arms of his domestic helper from off-screen, or seemingly being bribed or distracted with food to stay in the frame. When Dash was slightly older, these gestural negotiations were managed by his mother, or he would be strapped into a baby highchair in order to stay in the frame. When he was learning to be verbal, his mother would occasionally further engage him in the content by prompting him to respond to their interactions with the product they are testing on camera (i.e., is this nice? Do you want?). He would reply meekly but rarely addresses the camera directly. At times, Dash would exclaim words and short phrases (i.e., Chocolate! Nice!), to which his mother usually swiftly acknowledges him, then attempts to weave this 'intrusion' back into the narrative script for the vlog.

In a video sponsored by printer brand Epson (Xiaxue, 2018), Dash's mother attempts to bridge her promotional spiel with updates on her child's growth milestones, explaining how their recreational activities have changed now that Dash is four and a half years old. They engage in handicrafts with paper cutouts printed by the printer featured on screen; then the scene cuts to another clip where the influencer mother promotes the product in detail. Dash returns later in the video and is seen completing spelling exercise sheets, presumably printed with the sponsored product, with the help of his mother. His mother is seen guiding his hand to retrieve the paper from the printer and, when he fidgets, she places him front and centre of the camera by having him stand between her knees while she sits and 'clenches' him in place with her thighs. Subsequently, Dash is seen going off-camera, pressing his face against the lens in a close-up blurred image, and prancing around the couch behind his mother, uninterested in the activity.

In a second video on Xiaxue's dedicated YouTube series (Clicknetwork, 2017), she works through a try-out/tutorial of novelty Japanese miniature home cooking by herself. After the 8-minute mark, she transits to include Dash in her video: "so now that everything is done, I've got Dash here with me, and to see whether I can trick him into eating it … now we're going to see his reaction to the tiny little food". Dash's mother introduces him to the various foods she has made, asking which one he wants to try. He makes his selection and slowly reaches towards an item, but his arms are repeatedly held back or pushed back by his mother, who also shushes him when he interjects with verbal responses. Instead, Dash's mother quizzes him on the names of the foods, and only after he correctly guesses them for the camera is he rewarded with the items he had selected. During the outro, Dash is noticeably uninterested in filming as he leans away from his mother, nears the edge of the frame, appears visibly restless, looks out of frame, and fidgets around. However, he is unable to extract himself this time as he is sat in a baby highchair. As his mother gives her closing words, she wraps her arms around Dash, brings him into the centre of the frame and closer to her, then waves her audience goodbye while Dash's eyes are still focussed off-screen.

Across the videos featuring Dash on both channels, he is often seen being enticed by rewards for compliance to stay in the frame and continue filming. In some videos he is front and centre of the screen but not engaged with the filming despite his mother's cajoling, choosing instead to fixate on his own activities. Dash very rarely makes eye contact with the camera or acknowledges it, perhaps because of his young age, but appears to be thrust in front of it nonetheless. In general, the parental involvement in Dash's videos is extremely high, especially in front of the camera, where he is positioned to be in specific postures and prompted to respond in specific ways (e.g., verbally, gesturally, etc.). As many of these videos are sponsored collaborations, Dash's appearances are often used to promote content even though it is not clear to audiences if he is formally or contractually engaged in the filming of the product.

Pre-School Stars on YouTube

The videos discussed in this chapter feature three internet-native stars on YouTube when they are preschool-aged, between three and five. The children are seen interacting with technology *on* screen and technology *as* screen, through guidance from and negotiations with their parents. They exhibit different degrees of self-awareness with the camera, various levels of digital literacies as to how such devices and apps work, and a range of capacities to exert and emote their willingness to participate in filming and technology use, regardless of whether their parents honour it. Each case study features a child who is embedded in distinct YouTube ecologies. Ye Bin is of viral video fame and continues to be filmed in daily vlogs very casually; on YouTube her fame is primarily monetised through her channel's embedded advertisements. Eliana is a child in a family influencer unit and engages in both staged videos displaying her talents as a singer and casual daily vlogs where she appears to be a regular kindergartener; on YouTube her fame is primarily monetised through her family's influencer endorsements and advertisements. Dash is a micro-microcelebrity and features heavily in his influencer mother's various sponsored contents; on YouTube his fame is primarily monetised through his mother's extensive array of advertorials and partnerships with brands who use his likeness as their ambassador and model.

Taken as archetypes of their respective genres, these preschool stars demonstrate the nuance across the various models of child microcelebrities on YouTube, which contextualise and explain the different levels of parental intrusion into their children's lives with (techniques of) filming, and different intensities of parental acknowledgement of their children's exertion of agency regarding acceptance or refusal of technology: as Ye Bin sprang into fame from a viral video where she was known for her childlike innocence, she is still usually filmed in situ as an ordinary preschooler, and her videos often contain cues where she rejects being filmed through gestural responses; as Eliana was gradually introduced as a new member of a family influencer unit with musical talents, her videos comprise interactions with her father, with whom she actively negotiates the extent of her interest in being filmed through verbal and gestural responses; as Dash was groomed as a micro-microcelebrity from birth, his videos feature him at times positioned as a 'prop' to showcase various sponsored products, whether or not he seems to be interested in them.

This study of the front stage of child microcelebrity labour on YouTube serves as a foray into understanding the backstage operations of these prolific preschoolers. As access to contracts and the backstage of such labour is currently restricted, it is hoped that a focus on the end product and output will provide a better appreciation of how such preschool stars on YouTube are being performed, postured, and profited from online.

References

Abidin, C. (2015). Micromicrocelebrity: Branding babies on the internet. *M/C Journal*, *18*(5). Retrieved from: http://journal.media-culture.org.au/index.php/mcjournal/article/viewArticle/1022.

Abidin, C. (2017). #familygoals: Family influencers, calibrated amateurism, and justifying young digital labour. *Social Media + Society*, *3*(2), 1–15.

Abidin, C. (2018a). *Internet celebrity: Understanding fame online*. Bingley, UK: Emerald Publishing.

Abidin, C. (2018b, December). Squishy babies, soft dads, and exploding ovaries: Brand biographies and 'fan mothering' practices around celebrity babies. Paper presented at *Digital Intimacies*, Curtin University, Perth, Australia.

Berg, M. (2018, December). How this 7-year-old made $22 million playing with toys. *Forbes*. Retrieved from: www.forbes.com/sites/maddieberg/2018/12/03/how-this-seven-year-old-made-22-million-playing-with-toys-2/#5fbf262d4459.

Blum-Ross, A., & Livingston, S. (2017). "Sharenting", parent blogging, and the boundaries of the digital self. *Popular Communication*, *15*(2), 110–125.

Bridle, J. (2017). Something is wrong on the internet. *Medium*. Retrieved from: https://medium.com/@james bridle/something-is-wrong-on-the-internet-c39c471271d2.

Bridle, J. (2018). How Peppa Pig became a video nightmare for children. *The Guardian*. Retrieved from: www.theguardian.com/technology/2018/jun/17/peppa-pig-youtube-weird-algorithms-automated-content.

Burgess, J., & Green, J. (2013). *YouTube: Online video and participatory culture*. Cambridge, UK: Polity Press.

Buzzi, M. (2011). What are your children watching on YouTube? In *Proceedings of the ADNTIIC 2011: Advances in New Technologies, Interactive Interfaces and Communicability* (pp. 243–252). doi:10.1007/978-3-642-34010-9_23.

Clicknetwork. (2017, July 14). *New Popin' Cookin' - Xiaxue's Guide To Life: EP202*. [Video File]. Retrieved from: www.youtube.com/watch?v=sFQxOV54xNk&feature=youtu.be.

Craig, D., & Cunningham, S. (2017). Toy unboxing: Living in a(n unregulated) material world. *Media International Australia*, *163*(1), 77–86.

Department of Industrial Relations. (2013). *California child labor laws*. Retrieved from: www.dir.ca.gov/DLSE/ChildLaborLawPamphlet.pdf.

Duffy, B.E. (2015). The romance of work: Gender and aspirational labour in the digital culture industries. *International Journal of Cultural Studies*, *19*(4), 441–457.

Hern, A. (2017, November 10). YouTube to clamp down on disturbing kids' videos such as dark Peppa Pig. *The Guardian*. Retrieved from: www.theguardian.com/technology/2017/nov/10/youtube-disturbing-kids-videos-dark-peppa-pig-children.

Hourcade, J.P., Mascher, S.L., Wu, D., & Pantoja, L. (2015). Look, my baby is using an iPad! An analysis of YouTube videos of infants and toddlers using tablets. In *Proceedings of The CHI'15: 33rd annual ACM conference on human factors in computing systems* (pp. 1915–1924).

Jennings, R. (2019, January 4). YouTube stars promoted gambling to kids. Now they have to answer to their peers. *Vox*. Retrieved from: www.vox.com/the-goods/2019/1/4/18167341/youtube-jake-paul-ricegum-mystery-brand.

Lange, P.G. (2014). *Kids on YouTube: Technical identities and digital literacies*. New York: Routledge.

Leaver, T. (2015). Born digital? Presence, privacy, and intimate surveillance. In J. Hartley & W. Qu (Eds.), *Re-orientation: Translingual transcultural transmedia. Studies in narrative, language, identity, and knowledge* (pp. 149–160). Shanghai: Fudan University Press.

Leaver, T. (2017). Intimate surveillance: Normalising parental monitoring and mediation of infants online. *Social Media + Society*, 3(2), 1–10.

Leaver, T., & Abidin, C. (2017, May 2). When exploiting kids for cash goes wrong on YouTube: The lessons of DaddyOFive. *The Conversation*. Retrieved from: https://theconversation.com/when-exploiting-kids-for-cash-goes-wrong-on-youtube-the-lessons-of-daddyofive-76932.

Lopez, L.K. (2009). The radical act of "mommy blogging": Redefining motherhood through the blogosphere. *New Media & Society*, 11(5), 729–747.

Lynch, J. (2018, July 19). A 7-year-old boy is making $11 million a year on YouTube reviewing toys. *Business Insider*. Retrieved from: www.businessinsider.com.au/ryan-toysreview-6-year-old-makes-11-million-per-year-youtube-2017-12?r=US&IR=T.

Marsh, J. (2015). "Unboxing" videos: Co-construction of the child as cyberflaneur. *Discourse: Studies in the Cultural Politics of Education*, 37(3), 369–380.

Ministry of Manpower. (2014). Employing young persons and children. Retrieved from: www.mom.gov.sg/employment-practices/young-persons-and-children.

Nicoll, B., & Nansen, B. (2018). Mimetic production in YouTube toy unboxing videos. *Social Media + Society*, 4(3), 1–12.

Orphanides, K.G. (2018, March 23). Children's YouTube is still churning out blood, suicide and cannibalism. *Wired*. Retrieved from: www.wired.co.uk/article/youtube-for-kids-videos-problems-algorithm-recommend.

Orton-Johnson, K. (2017). Mummy blogs and representations of motherhood: "Bad mummies" and their readers. *Social Media + Society*, 3(2), 1–10.

Ramos-Serrano, M., & Herrero-Diz, P. (2016). Unboxing and brands: YouTubers phenomenon through the case study of EvantubeHD. *Prisma Social*, 1, 90–120.

realitychangers. (2013, March 13). *A thousand years - Christina Perri cover by Jorge, Alexa and Eliana Narvaez*. [Video File]. Retrieved from: www.youtube.com/watch?v=YAafNm-on50.

realitychangers. (2014, June 27) *WE WILL SEE YOU AT VIDCON! | The Family Vlog | Reality changers*. [Video File]. Retrieved from: www.youtube.com/watch?v=UIdA7NZRqKM.

Robehmed, N., & Berg, M. (2018, December 3). Highest-paid YouTube stars 2018: Markiplier, Jake Paul, PewDiePie and more. *Forbes*. Retrieved from: www.forbes.com/sites/natalierobehmed/2018/12/03/highest-paid-youtube-stars-2018-markiplier-jake-paul-pewdiepie-and-more/#7415f25a909a.

Screen Actors Guild. (2015). *Coogan Law. SAGAFTRA 2015*. Retrieved from: www.sagaftra.org/content/coogan-law.

Shamsian, J. (2019, February 15). A 7-year-old YouTuber who makes $22 million a year reviewing toys is getting a TV show. *Insider*. Retrieved from: www.insider.com/ryan-toysreview-youtube-tv-show-nickelodeon-2019-2.

Shmuel, N. (2018, October 22). The challenges with advertising safely to kids on YouTube. *The Drum*. Retrieved from: www.thedrum.com/industryinsights/2018/10/22/the-challenges-with-advertising-safely-kids-youtube.

Washington Post. (2018, April 9). YouTube under fire for allegedly targeting kids with ads. *Washington Post*. Retrieved from: www.washingtonpost.com/lifestyle/kidspost/youtube-under-fire-for-allegedly-targeting-kids-with-ads/2018/04/09/dfdaa48e-39e9-11e8-8fd2-49fe3c675a89_story.html?noredirect=on&utm_term=.6faf9b3c7fd8.

Xiaxue. (2018, March 5). *Vlog with Dash - Fun activities to do with your toddler at home!* [Video File]. Retrieved from: www.youtube.com/watch?v=9RmYRD05Vfk.

Ye Bin. (2014, July 2). *[Official] Mom teaches cute Korean baby Yebin a life lesson*. [Video File]. Retrieved from: www.youtube.com/watch?v=kN29b1-hhZ0.

Ye Bin. (2015, March 16). *Baby Yebin February Instagram compilation 예빈이 2월 인스타그램 영상 모음*. [Video File]. Retrieved from: www.youtube.com/watch?v=-Xf4uCXGIYY.

Ye Bin. (2016, May 13). *A day in the life of Yebin 예빈이의 하루*. [Video File]. Retrieved from: www.youtube.com/watch?v=V1TM0JTUmNw.

22
BALANCING PRIVACY
Sharenting, Intimate Surveillance, and the Right to Be Forgotten

Tama Leaver

Introduction

In early 2020, the daughter of a prominent Instagram influencer used an anonymous account to post to the Reddit forum 'Am I the Asshole?' where posters describe a personal situation and ask other users to judge whether they were in the right or wrong. In her message, the original poster (OP) described how she had ordered custom-made hoodies with various messages printed on them, including "no photos", "I do not consent to be photographed", "respect my privacy", and "no means no" (FinallyAnonymous6, 2020). The OP describes wearing this hoodie, and providing her younger sister with one for the same reason, to prevent her influencer mother taking photos of her and sharing them on social media. The OP made it clear that she had requested her mother stop sharing photos of her a number of times, and made it explicitly clear that she did not consent to any images being posted online. As her mother did not respect the OP's request, she had begun wearing the hoodie in her home, to family events, and anywhere her mother might be taking photos, to deliberately interrupt her mother's photography and online sharing. This upset her mother, who argued that featuring her daughters on Instagram was part of the way the family made their income. The post struck a chord on Reddit, attracting more than 3,500 responses before comments were locked. The vast majority of responses commended this as a very effective and justified tactic, and many agreed that the OP's mother urgently needed to respect her desire for privacy. Beyond this anecdote, which demonstrates a very satisfying display of children's digital literacy in negotiating their privacy boundaries, this story also points to a number of related questions. Should parental influencers share photos of their children, within what boundaries, and how might influencers model behaviour for other parents? More broadly, while 'sharenting' – parents sharing images of their children online – is incredibly widespread, what are the ongoing privacy implications of this practise? Beyond the level of images and immediate public visibility, what happens to the underlying data generated when images and media featuring young people is shared on various platforms? Moreover, do children today have a right to be forgotten online, as their digital footprints potentially last forever? Ultimately, this chapter pursues these questions to ask how exactly the digital communication and sharing of and by parents about their children can be balanced with children's rights to privacy both in the present and, more challengingly, in the future.

Child and Parent Influencers: Inadvertent Role Models?

Ryan's ToysReview, which has subsequently rebranded as Ryan's World, is the most profitable YouTube channel in the world, featuring a nine-year-old boy, making an estimated $US26 million in 2019 from sponsored posts (Spangler, 2019). Since March 2015, Ryan Kaji has been featured in toy unboxing videos in which he euphorically unwraps and examines new toys, all shared on YouTube; he was an instant hit, so much so that within two years his parents left their own jobs to focus exclusively on managing Ryan's YouTube channel and the commercial opportunities it led to. While Ryan's parents keep some details of his life private (his exact birthday, for example), he has nevertheless grown up on YouTube and his immense profitability highlights just how successful child influencers can be if a certain level of intimacy and familiarity is built with audiences, usually at the cost of a child influencer's privacy.

In the Australian context, one of the most well-known child influencers is Pixie Curtis, who is on Instagram as Pixie's Bows. Pixie is the daughter of CEO and PR executive Roxy Jacenko who, herself, is an influencer of considerable impact, with over 250,000 followers. Pixie has a more modest 95,000 followers, but commands huge reach with parents and young girls. Jacenko has been criticised publicly and in many comments for over-exposure of Pixie who has been online since she was very young (Fitch, 2017). Pixie now has a successful brand of hair products – Pixie's Bows – and has begun a modelling career at the age of seven. While Jacenko's approach to Pixie has been critiqued publicly, Jacenko has, at least, articulated a clear vision of Pixie's presence online, including ensuring that any profits made go directly into a fund for Pixie's future and education. Even if others disagree, it is certainly the case that Jacenko has considered and articulated a clear position on her daughter's online presence and the trade being made in exchanging privacy for public visibility (Archer, 2019). Pixie is an example of what Abidin (2015) calls a 'micro-microcelebrity', that is, a second generation influencer whose parents are already in the social media spotlight and whose childhood is shaped, in part at least, as part of their parents' online presence, and then fairly swiftly as an influencer in their own right. As Abidin notes, micro-microcelebrities provoke some of the most difficult questions around child influencers, including whether parents are effectively exploiting the free labour of their children, as well as more immediate questions of what privacy is really available to a child whose life and lifestyle is documented on social media for profit from birth, if not before.

While children are almost always a core part of what any parental influencer talks about, there are many different approaches to balancing the visibility and privacy of children on social media (Blum-Ross & Livingstone, 2017). Anna Whitehouse is a long-time parental influencer and flexible working advocate who blogs, and is on Instagram, as Mother Pukka; Whitehouse is one example of someone explicitly modelling best practice in terms of sharing images and information about her children. In a long blog post (also pointed to from her other social media presences), Whitehouse collates information from experts and scholarship, and reveals her own practices including: initially using pet names, and eventually just emoji, to refer to her children, protecting their real names; not revealing a host of specific information including their schools; and only photographing them, if at all, from behind or in a way that obscures their faces (Whitehouse, 2018). Moreover, on Instagram and elsewhere, Whitehouse has publicly engaged in extensive dialogue with her followers and other parental influencers about children's privacy, inviting her followers to consider and perhaps update their own practices.

Parental and child influencers are on the front lines of social media. The practices deployed by influencers are often adopted as norms by other users. Ryan Kaji and Pixie Curtis represent one end of a spectrum where their presence online is substantial and privacy has been deliberately traded for commercial success. Anna Whitehouse and her children are toward the other end of the spectrum, participating in parenting discussions while modelling a more privacy-centred approach in including, but not explicitly depicting, her children.

Sharenting: Ultrasounds and Beyond

Increasingly, a child's first image online precedes their actual birth. Sharing ultrasound images has become a rite of passage; posting the 12- or 20-week prenatal ultrasound images on Facebook or Instagram is now a very common way to reveal a pregnancy across the Western world (Lupton, 2013). Sharenting – a portmanteau of the words share and parenting, conventionally referring to parents sharing images and videos of their kids online – is thus a practice that new parents often start enacting even as they attempt to prepare for all the other new challenges parenthood can entail. Moreover, as actors, sportspeople, and other celebrities share their prenatal ultrasounds with descriptions such as 'his first photo!', they normalise a process of sharing and naming visualisations of the unborn on social media (Seko & Tiidenberg, 2016). The choice to not share increasingly seems at odds with the norms and social expectations of pregnancy and (preparing for) parenthood in the era of social media platforms.

In examining over 10,000 images and videos publicly shared on Instagram using the #ultrasound hashtag over a period of three months in 2014, Leaver and Highfield (2018) surfaced a range of practices in which ultrasounds where shared, from photos and scans of the ultrasounds themselves to excited selfies of mothers and couples heading to their first ultrasound scan, through to printed ultrasound images held in stylised poses to announce a pregnancy. In a qualitative coding, the authors found that of the prenatal ultrasounds publicly shared on Instagram, 34% of them had personally identifiable data and metadata such as the mother's full name, the hospital or facility doing the scan, the mother's date of birth, the estimated due date of the foetus, and so forth. While this metadata was usually visible as part of the image, not separate text in the image's textual description, it is nevertheless a fairly trivial task for an algorithm to 'read' the visual text and incorporate it into Instagram's metadata about that person. Moreover, as Facebook harnesses, connects, and indexes millions of data points and sources to better map their users, and better target advertising to them, it is entirely likely that such metadata not only informs advertising aimed at the expecting parents, but also that Facebook would start a proto-profile for the foetus in question. Indeed, making the process even more seamless, commercial ultrasound machines today often come bundled with the Tricefy software that delivers all the images collected during an ultrasound scan and sends these as online links that can be shared directly with family or friends, or posted directly to Facebook or Instagram. It is notable, though, that when Leaver and Highfield (2018) collected their data, Instagram had relatively simple privacy options (accounts were either fully public or fully private). Since then, direct messaging and Stories (which disappear after 24 hours) have given parents more nuanced tools to share with specific audiences rather than the whole of Instagram's userbase (Leaver et al., 2020). Yet, in February 2020, searching Instagram for #ultrasound still found 660,941 public posts, while the related hashtag #pregnancyannouncement also returned 574,633 public posts. Not all of these are ultrasound images, but a significant proportion are, as well as other visual devices to announce a pregnancy from a positive result on a pregnancy test to a pink or blue coloured cake purportedly revealing the sex of the foetus. If, as Kumar and Schoenebeck (2015) argue, new parents, and mothers especially, have to negotiate the desire other people have to see shared baby photos, this has to be weighed against a new parent's own responsibilities to the child; the first ultrasound is thus not just the beginning of sharenting, but also when a parent's 'privacy stewardship' of their child's presence and data begins.

For parents, the question of whether or not to share images of their children online is not (just) based on the present and future privacy of their child, but is often also driven by a number of other factors, including the expectation of other parents, friends, and family members who express clear desires to see newborn, baby, and growing up photos and, indeed, who may criticise new parents for any failure to share on social media (Damkjaer, 2018). For new parents, navigating the challenges of protecting their child's privacy whilst also utilising the support and community Facebook can bring, for example, can be particularly paradoxical. In a study of new Australian mothers, for example, Chalklen and Anderson (2017) found that many were acutely aware of issues with children's privacy online, but also found Facebook to be an extremely important source of support and networking with other new parents. These tensions were sometimes productive, leading to techniques for sharing but not identifying children, such as photos taken always from behind, being developed as norms within these support groups. Similarly, while some laws have come in to place to protect children's data online, these laws often rely on parents as informed champions of their children's privacy, which is not a role they are always able or willing to perform (Fox & Hoy, 2019; Steinberg, 2017). As children grow older, parents transition from being the exclusive decision-maker about sharing photos of their children online to a situation where children start exercising their voice and opinion about what should, and should not, be shared online. At times this can lead to 'boundary turbulence' in that the privacy expectations of children and their parents may not align, and difficult but important conversations can ensue (Lipu & Siibak, 2019). As children grow and usually start using their own social media accounts, their desire to shape their own identities and personality online can conflict with parental sharing, although in some contexts these conversations, too, can often be very productive with new boundaries and expectations emerging (Ouvrein & Verswijvel, 2019). However, young people's experiences of sharenting can often be predominantly negative. A study of 817 Flemish adolescents with a roughly balanced gender split, for example, found that the vast majority found their parents' sharenting practices 'embarrassing and useless' with only a small minority seeing any value in what their parents shared about them online (Verswijvel et al., 2019).

While negotiating different expectations of privacy on social media can be a confronting process, it is especially important as contemporary parents are often of an age where their own parents did not have to manage children's social media and data traces in a networked world. Moreover, rather than parents just creating their children's social media identities, as children become more active online they, too, may start posting about, and thus shaping, their parents as well. In the anecdote that began this chapter, the OP was not just resisting parental sharing, but in posting about her grievances she was also potentially shaping the online identity of her mother. These two-way streets serve as fruitful reminders that social media is actually almost always 'co-creative', in that, in so many instances when people post, they are contributing to the online presence of other people, a situation so readily visible in the realm of sharenting, but also inverted as children post about themselves and, over time, their families (Leaver, 2019). As co-creators, parents and children are thus in a dialogue about their own and others' privacy online every time they post. Making that dialogue explicit, purposeful, and, ideally, agreed upon, will be part of family (and broader) negotiations in a world where most relations take place in complex intersecting combinations of physical and digital spaces.

Wearables, Apps, and Sharable Data?

While the debates and discussions about sharenting revolve around specific objects that can be relatively easily seen and located – this is, specific images and videos – the underlying level of data and metadata can be a lot harder to define, locate, or easily understand where it is generated, what is captured, what is stored, for how long, where, and under what control, including the big question of who owns that data. While data, and big data in particular, is surrounded by a mythology that big data leads to big answers, the processes and circumstances by which this might happen are often, at best, deeply unclear (boyd & Crawford, 2012). Moreover, the generation of data about children may, in fact, be a by-product of an app, device, platform, or tool that is being used with the best of intentions to benefit children.

The Owlet 'Smart Sock' is an infant wearable device – that is, a device worn by an infant that collects certain health and metabolic information and transmits that to a device or platform – that provides parents with information about the blood oxygen levels, heart rate, and movement of a sleeping infant. This information is relayed to the cloud via a Bluetooth base station, and then the resulting data is made available to parents as a series of indicators on a smart phone app, which uses a traffic light system of indicators (green all is okay, yellow action is needed, red immediate intervention needed) to either reassure parents or indicate something is wrong. The motto in most of the Owlet sales material is that it offers weary parents 'peace of mind' in being able to be aware of their infant's health without having to physically enter the room to check (Leaver, 2017). Indeed, while many parents infer that the Owlet is a device to prevent Sudden Infant Death Syndrome (SIDS), the Owlet is not certified as a medical device, and in the fine print it warns that it, in fact, cannot prevent SIDS. The device has been the subject of warnings from the American Academy of Pediatrics (Bonafide et al., 2017; King, 2014), which notes that the Owlet and similarly wearables can both provide false warnings, needlessly distressing parents, but also falsely reassure at times when it should not, and in both cases this impacts negatively on a child and parents' health. However, despite these limitations, the company behind the Owlet continually imply that their smart sock is a viable safety measure for infants, and have enlisted a large number of parental influencers, including celebrity parent influencers such as Katherine Heigl, to promote the Owlet on their social media presences (Leaver, 2017). The Owlet is an example of what Leaver (2015, p. 153) describes as "intimate surveillance", that is, "the purposeful and routinely well-intentioned surveillance of young people by parents, guardians, friends, and so forth". While the term intimate surveillance serves as a useful reminder that surveillance practices can often be motivated by care, the term is also unsettling since surveillance is often associated with more sinister uses. In terms of the Owlet, what is perhaps less clear, and possibly more sinister depending on your perspective, is the amount of data the company collects, stores, analyses, and then *owns* about each child who uses the infant wearable. Not only does Owlet Baby Care state that they own all data generated by the smart socks – that is, measurements of every heartbeat, breath, movement, and blood-oxygen level, all linked to an exact time, place, and name – but it is clear that the company see their future success in being able to aggregate all the data from various babies and extrapolate new knowledge from that data. In this respect, the Owlet is typical of new heath apps and devices which ostensibly have two real products; one is the device or app itself, but the other is the data they collect, which can be stored and analysed as a big data set and potentially generate new forms of knowledge, but also new forms of income for the Owlet Baby Care company (van Dijck & Poell, 2016). Indeed, in its promotional videos the Owlet company is quite transparent and seemingly excited about its big dataset of baby data, claiming it has "the largest data set about infant health and sleep and wellness and safety that's ever been collected" (Owlet Baby Care, 2015). Yet, for parents who have purchased the Owlet smart sock for 'peace of mind', the amount of personal information and data about their child they have signed away is unlikely to be clear since this transaction is shrouded in Terms of Use and legal terminology that tired parents are unlikely to have the patience or time to read when they are searching for anything that might help with a baby's often very disruptive early sleep routine. These are far from ideal circumstances in which to have, effectively, made quite an important decision about the privacy of children's data.

Indeed, having enough information to judge which apps, platforms, and companies to trust is one of the biggest challenges for parents in managing their children's images and data. Peekaboo Moments is one example of a bespoke app that seemingly offers a solution for families wary of using bigger advertising-driven platforms. Instead, the Peekaboo Moments app ostensibly offers a secure way to share images and videos of children with a specific, private group in a fashion that is consistent with the ease of Facebook, but without the larger privacy questions. However, despite their sales pitch of being a safer and more secure way to share children's media and data, this was, for a period of time at least, far from true. In early 2020 security researchers discovered that over 100 gigabytes of user data from the Peekaboo Moments app was publicly accessible on an unsecured website, exposing images and videos of babies and various forms of identifiable information, from email addresses to changes in a baby's weight over time (Kirk, 2020). Security researchers report reaching out to the people running Peekaboo Moments with information about the breach, but did not hear anything back until stories ran in the media about the breach, which did then lead to Peekaboo Moments securing their data to prevent future unsecured access. However, security researchers noted that the data was likely to have been visible online for eight or nine months before the security problem was fixed. For parents trying to make informed privacy choices, the Peekaboo Moments app ostensibly appears to be a safer choice than Facebook or Instagram, but, as the breach reveals, the company's actual security did not match the rhetoric of security they were selling parents. Trying to weigh the security and privacy credentials of the plethora of apps, services, and platforms out there is extremely difficult, while app designers are often more focussed on growth and profit, and the resources put into privacy and security often do not match the sales pitch to parents.

The Right To Be Forgotten?

For almost as long as social media has existed, questions have arisen about the challenges posed by every online utterance simultaneously being a piece of media that does not, by default, ever disappear. More than a decade ago Mayer-Schonberger (2009) warned that the ability to be forgotten was being eroded and may disappear altogether, or become something of a luxury product only available to those rich enough to pay to purge their digital traces. For children, and parents trying to look after children's digital traces, the challenge of social media permanence is even more problematic. As Eichhorn argues, being able to forget, and be forgotten, matters: "Despite its bad reputation, forgetting has a function. Forgetting can help one take risks, explore new identities, embrace new ideas; it can help one grow up" (Eichhorn, 2019, p. 142). In an era of digital communication and datafied childhoods, there is no guarantee that commercial platforms and networks will ever 'forget' anything (Lupton & Williamson, 2017; Mascheroni, 2018).

In 1989 The United Nations Convention on the Rights of the Child enshrined a number of rights for children, including a specific right to privacy:

1   No child shall be subjected to arbitrary or unlawful interference with his or her privacy, family, home or correspondence, nor to unlawful attacks on his or her honour and reputation;
2   The child has the right to the protection of the law against such interference or attacks.
    (UNICEF, 1989)

While this right might have been clear 30 years ago, it is more important than ever today, but it is also less clear than ever exactly how this right should be interpreted and respected in a digital, networked society (Livingstone & Third, 2017). As children age, they clearly understand the value of their reputation, and how that reputation is visible online, but many often lack the tools and competencies to maintain control of their own reputation. While Google and many other platforms organise content by impact and interest rather than chronology, as Eichhorn (2019, p. 141) notes,

Stupid or embarrassing moments, which are simply part of growing up, hold consequences they did not hold in the past. The psychosocial moratorium – that once granted at least some adolescents a temporary pass on suffering the consequences of their actions – has eroded.

Childhood moments resurfacing and communicating different meanings, often many years after being shared, is an example of 'context collapse' in that the context for sharing stories, photos, and other information may be very different to the context in which these pieces are viewed and scrutinised (Davis & Jurgenson, 2014; Marwick & boyd, 2011). For young people, their entire futures are an unknown context where their digital traces may reappear in searches and other ways that were never envisaged when these seemingly harmless photos, videos, or anecdotes were initially posted online. In the era of Google, a right to privacy, or to be forgotten, is thus very difficult to achieve.

The prospect of children's privacy becomes even more complicated when their data is considered; the data collected by the Owlet smart sock or Peekaboo Moments, as discussed above, reveals how little control or ownership children, or their parents, have when using certain devices and apps, even if they are specifically designed for children. While data might be 'anonymised' before being collated, stored, or analysed, re-identifying individuals is relatively easy for rich data sources given there are so many ways to cross-reference various stored data. Names are only one data point. In many cases, though, the question of harm or risk is important, and sometimes very few risks are obvious. Yet one of the real challenges in thinking about children's right to privacy is that it is not just how their media or data is used today, but also in the future. If the Owlet company was purchased by a large health or insurance company in a decade or two, could the data from an infant smart sock actually reveal some sort of heart defect or weakness that would lead to that child being denied health insurance as an adult? This might seem fantastical, but it is exactly these sort of inferences that might be made from big data that gives this data its value. For OP, the daughter of an influencer parent who no longer wants to have her photographs shared as part of her mother's social media output, a right to be forgotten might entail erasing every photo OP is featured in, but the practicalities of this are hard to fathom, and, as is obvious from this example, children's images and data are deeply intertwined with the data and media of other people, from their family and friends, and beyond. Untangling one person's media and data would be a daunting and complex challenge, but a challenge that is one of the few clear paths to actually respecting children's right to privacy in a digital world.

Conclusion

Most adults struggle to find the time to pay attention to the Terms and Conditions of every app they download, and often feel ill-equipped to manage their own data and own privacy online (Leaver & Lloyd, 2015; Plunkett, 2019). When people become parents and are suddenly responsible for a vast array of things to do with their children, managing their newborn's digital footprints, social media presence, and personal data pose challenges that often the generations before them did not have to wrestle with. Without precedents to draw from, moral panics in the media about screen time and online predators may potentially drown out the seemingly more banal but equally important information about helping young people manage their online presence and privacy (Green et al., 2019). Increasingly, everything from child welfare services to interactive toys harness, generate, store, and potentially share personal data about children (Holloway & Green, 2016; Redden et al., 2020), without necessarily providing any transparency around the use, storage, or ownership of that data. While privacy itself can be conceptualised quite differently (Quinn et al., 2019), it is clear that from sharenting on social media to the data gathered by a host of apps across the fields of health, entertainment, and education, privacy is seen as a barrier, not a right, to the operation and profitability of apps, platforms, and the companies that own them. For parents today, attempting to ensure children have a right to privacy can be a time-consuming, exhausting, and confusing task, wading through Terms and Conditions on one hand, while, on the other hand, negotiating the desires of different groups from friends and family and over time children themselves, all with different opinions, about what photos, videos, information, and data should be shared, where, and with whom. Returning to the anecdote about OP and her 'no photos' hoodie, that particular tale has specific value in that it points to the deep tactical literacy of a young person who managed to intervene creatively to achieve privacy for herself and her sister, at odds with her mother's wishes. If young people are going to have a right to privacy today or in the future, it is exactly this digital literacy and bold tenacity that is needed in the face of a system of platforms, digital media, and big data which currently consume and keep as much personal data and information as possible. Moreover, it is important that researchers and educators work to provide new avenues for personal and parental literacies in understanding and managing personal data, ideally beginning before parenthood altogether, equipping new parents with the tools to curate and then help educate their children in terms of their digital traces. For parents, balancing the current and future privacy of their children is no small task, but one that matters more than ever and will likely be most successful with children as partners in the process.

References

Abidin, C. (2015). Micro-microcelebrity: Branding babies on the internet. *M/C Journal*, *18*(5). Retrieved from: http://journal.media-culture.org.au/index.php/mcjournal/article/viewArticle/1022.

Archer, C. (2019). Pre-schooler as brand extension: A tale of Pixie's bows and birthdays. In L. Green, D. Holloway, K. Stevenson, & K. Jaunzems (Eds.), *Digitising early childhood* (pp. 58–73). Newcastle upon Tyne, UK: Cambridge Scholars Publishing.

Blum-Ross, A., & Livingstone, S. (2017). "Sharenting," parent blogging, and the boundaries of the digital self. *Popular Communication*, *15*(2), 110–125. doi:10.1080/15405702.2016.1223300.

Bonafide, C. P., Jamison, D. T., & Foglia, E. E. (2017). The emerging market of smartphone-integrated infant physiologic monitors. *JAMA*, *317*(4), 353–354. doi:10.1001/jama.2016.19137.

boyd, d., & Crawford, K. (2012). Critical questions for big data. *Information, Communication & Society*, *15*(5), 662–679. doi:10.1080/1369118X.2012.678878.

Chalklen, C., & Anderson, H. (2017). Mothering on Facebook: Exploring the privacy/openness paradox. *Social Media + Society*, *3*, 2. doi:10.1177/2056305117707187.

Damkjaer, M. S. (2018). Sharenting = good parenting? Four parental approaches to sharenting on Facebook. In G. Mascheroni, C. Ponte, & A. Jorge (Eds.), *Digital parenting: The challenges for families in the digital age* (pp. 209–218). Göteborg: Nordicom.

Davis, J. L., & Jurgenson, N. (2014). Context collapse: Theorizing context collusions and collisions. *Information, Communication & Society*, *17*(4), 476–485. doi:10.1080/1369118X.2014.888458.

Eichhorn, K. (2019). *The end of forgetting: Growing up with social media*. Cambridge, MA: Harvard University Press.

FinallyAnonymous6. (2020, January 30). *AITA? My mom is an influencer. I am sick of being a part of it, I had "NO PHOTOS" hoodies printed for me and my little sister. : AmItheAsshole*. Reddit: AmItheAsshole. Retrieved from: www.reddit.com/r/AmItheAsshole/comments/evqd8/aita_my_mom_is_an_influencer_i_am_sick_of_being_a.

Fitch, K. (2017). Seeing 'the unseen hand': Celebrity, promotion and public relations. *Public Relations Inquiry*, *6*(2), 157–169. doi:10.1177/2046147X17709064.

Fox, A. K., & Hoy, M. G. (2019). Smart devices, smart decisions? Implications of parents' sharenting for children's online privacy: An investigation of mothers. *Journal of Public Policy & Marketing*, *38*(4), 414–432. doi:10.1177/0743915619858290.

Green, L., Haddon, L., Livingstone, S., Holloway, D., Jaunzems, K., Stevenson, K., & O'Neill, B. (2019). *Parents' failure to plan for their children's digital futures* (Media@LSE Working Paper Series, p. 21). LSE. Retrieved from: www.lse.ac.uk/media-and-communications/assets/documents/research/working-paper-series/WP61.pdf.

Holloway, D., & Green, L. (2016). The internet of toys. *Communication Research and Practice*, *2*(4), 506–519. doi:10.1080/22041451.2016.1266124.

King, D. (2014). Marketing wearable home baby monitors: Real peace of mind? *BMJ*, *349*, g6639. doi:10.1136/bmj.g6639.

Kirk, J. (2020, January 14). Baby's first data breach: App exposes baby photos, videos. *Data Breach Today*. Retrieved from: www.databreachtoday.com/babys-first-data-breach-app-exposes-baby-photos-videos-a-13603.

Kumar, P., & Schoenebeck, S. (2015). The modern day baby book: Enacting good mothering and stewarding privacy on Facebook. *Proceedings of the 18th ACM Conference on Computer Supported Cooperative Work & Social Computing*, 1302–1312.

Leaver, T. (2015). Born digital? Presence, privacy, and intimate surveillance. In J. Hartley & W. Qu (Eds.), *Re-orientation: Translingual transcultural transmedia. Studies in narrative, language, identity, and knowledge* (pp. 149–160). Shanghai, China: Fudan University Press.

Leaver, T. (2017). Intimate surveillance: Normalizing parental monitoring and mediation of infants online. *Social Media + Society*, *3*(2). doi:10.1177/2056305117707192.

Leaver, T. (2019). Co-creating birth and death on social media. In Z. Papacharissi (Ed.), *A networked self and birth, life, death* (pp. 35–49). Abingdon, UK: Routledge. doi:10.4324/9781315202129-3.

Leaver, T., & Highfield, T. (2018). Visualising the ends of identity: Pre-birth and post-death on Instagram. *Information, Communication & Society*, *21*(1), 30–45. doi:10.1080/1369118X.2016.1259343.

Leaver, T., Highfield, T., & Abidin, C. (2020). *Instagram: Visual social media cultures*. Medford, MA: Polity.

Leaver, T., & Lloyd, C. (2015). Seeking transparency in locative media. In R. Wilken & G. Goggin (Eds.), *Locative media* (pp. 162–174). London & New York, NY: Routledge.

Lipu, M., & Siibak, A. (2019). 'Take it down!': Estonian parents' and pre-teens' opinions and experiences with sharenting. *Media International Australia*, *170*(1), 57–67. doi:10.1177/1329878X19828366.

Livingstone, S., & Third, A. (2017). Children and young people's rights in the digital age: An emerging agenda. *New Media & Society*, *19*(5), 657–670. doi:10.1177/1461444816686318.

Lupton, D. (2013). *The social worlds of the unborn*. New York, NY: Palgrave MacMillan. doi:10.1057/9781137310729.

Lupton, D., & Williamson, B. (2017). The datafied child: The dataveillance of children and implications for their rights. *New Media & Society*, *19*(5), 780–794. doi:10.1177/1461444816686328.

Marwick, A. E., & boyd, d. (2011). I tweet honestly, I tweet passionately: Twitter users, context collapse, and the imagined audience. *New Media & Society*, *13*(1), 114–133. doi:10.1177/1461444810365313.

Mascheroni, G. (2018). Datafied childhoods: Contextualising datafication in everyday life. *Current Sociology*. doi:10.1177/0011392118807534.

Mayer-Schonberger, V. (2009). *Delete: The virtue of forgetting in the digital age*. Princeton, NJ: Princeton University Press.

Ouvrein, G., & Verswijvel, K. (2019). Sharenting: Parental adoration or public humiliation? A focus group study on adolescents' experiences with sharenting against the background of their own impression management. *Children and Youth Services Review*, *99*, 319–327. doi:10.1016/j.childyouth.2019.02.011.

Owlet Baby Care. (2015, March 2). *More than just a gadget - the Owlet vision*. Retrieved from: www.youtube.com/watch?v=fT9Vc68BfTI.

Plunkett, L. A. (2019). *Sharenthood: Why we should think before we talk about our kids online*. Cambridge, MA: The MIT Press.

Quinn, K., Epstein, D., & Moon, B. (2019). We care about different things: Non-elite conceptualizations of social media privacy. *Social Media + Society*, *5*(3). doi:10.1177/2056305119866008.

Redden, J., Dencik, L., & Warne, H. (2020). Datafied child welfare services: Unpacking politics, economics and power. *Policy Studies*, 1–20. doi:10.1080/01442872.2020.1724928.

Seko, Y., & Tiidenberg, K. (2016). Birth through the digital womb: Visualizing prenatal life online. In P. G. Nixon, R. Rawal, & A. Funk (Eds.), *Digital media usage across the lifecourse* (pp. 50–66). London & New York, NY: Routledge.

Spangler, T. (2019, December 18). YouTube Kid Channel Ryan's World pulled in estimated $26 million in 2019, Double PewDiePie's Haul. *Variety*. Retrieved from: https://variety.com/2019/digital/news/youtube-highest-earning-creators-ryans-world-pewdiepie-1203447625.

Steinberg, S. B. 1. (2017). Sharenting: Children's privacy in the age of social media. *Emory Law Journal*, *66*(4), 839–884.

UNICEF. (1989). UN Convention on the Rights of the Child (UNCRC). *UNICEF*. Retrieved from: www.unicef.org.uk/what-we-do/un-convention-child-rights.

van Dijck, J., & Poell, T. (2016). Understanding the promises and premises of online health platforms. *Big Data & Society*, *3*(1), 1–11. doi:10.1177/2053951716654173.

Verswijvel, K., Walrave, M., Hardies, K., & Heirman, W. (2019). Sharenting, is it a good or a bad thing? Understanding how adolescents think and feel about sharenting on social network sites. *Children and Youth Services Review, 104*, 104401. doi:10.1016/j.childyouth.2019.104401.

Whitehouse, A. (2018, April 27). Private: No access. *Mother pukka: for people who happen to be parents*. Retrieved from: www.motherpukka.co.uk/private-no-access.

23
PARENTING PEDAGOGIES IN THE MARKETING OF CHILDREN'S APPS

Donell Holloway, Giovanna Mascheroni, and Ashley Donkin

Introduction

Neoliberal modes of governance extend free-market enterprise to many parts of our private and public worlds, including learning and education. While all governments strive to shape the training and education of their future workforce, neoliberal societies do so in new market-based ways (Holloway & Pimlott-Wilson, 2014; Marandet & Wainwright, 2015). This chapter focusses on the use of marketing discourses as a means by which free-market economies not only shape individual citizens' education or learning but also shape the environment in which future workforce citizens are raised through the responsibilisation and mobilisation of their parents (Holloway & Pimlott-Wilson, 2014). Responsibilisation refers to indirect mechanisms through which the individual is held accountable for social risks such as poverty, illness, and unemployment. These social risks are transformed into a problem of the self and of consumption (Lemke, 2001).

The chapter also examines the way in which parental responsibilisation discourses encourage early literacy and numeracy interventions by parents. More specifically, the chapter analyses app download pages on Google Play to highlight how the app descriptions rely primarily upon an educational responsibilisation discourse aimed at parents. Implicit within this discourse is that it is good parenting practice to provide even very young children with computer-mediated educational opportunities that will help children's learning and, over time, lead to more success in the workforce when they get older (O'Connor & Fotakopoulou, 2016). Parents are constructed as pedagogues responsible for "ensuring that their children acquire skills they will need for educational success" (Buckingham & Scanlon, 2001, p. 282). At the same time, however, the specialist vocabulary and didactic educational focus of the download pages position parents as being in need of the expert help provided through these educational apps.

With more than one million early learning apps accessible through IOS or android devices (Barr & Nichols Linebarger, 2016), early childhood education is transitioning into digital spaces with commercial media, in particular, playing an ever-increasing role in very young children's educational journey. Notwithstanding questions around the educational quality of these apps in general, this new and ever-expanding market effectively positions parents and children as subjects of a specific form of educational discourse, a neoliberal, market-based discourse in which parental responsibilisation about their children's educational attainment and subsequent anxiety around this is exploited, and children's enjoyment and pleasure are leveraged.

Schoolification of Early Childhood Education

The schoolification or formalisation of early years' education, grounded in an emphasis on accountability and standardisation, and a push-down curriculum, introduces a formal literacy and numeracy pedagogy into the pre-school curriculum (Bradbury, 2018; Sims, 2014). Bradbury explains that formal education for younger children is gaining international attention and, according to England's school inspection service Ofsted, early education classes are considered a "'missed' opportunity and should involve more formal structured learning" (p. 3). Thus, what was once a child-centred and play-based education has now become a formalised pedagogy that incorporates standardised testing of children's skills (Moss, 2012; Sims, 2017).

In Australia, for instance, the federal government's emphasis on education now extends to the adoption of the Early Years Learning Framework (EYLF). This framework, which has become a national priority, has been developed for children aged 0–5 years and provides teachers with five learning goals that encompass the development of children's literacy, numeracy, social and emotional skills (Belonging, Being …., 2009). According to the framework, it is expected that digital technology will also be used in early childhood classrooms to facilitate children's learning.

In addition, the UK has its own Early Years Foundation Stage framework (EYFS), which involves the collection of data from 0–5-year-olds (Bradbury, 2018, p. 1). This framework involves the assessment of 17 Early Learning Goals every six weeks (Bradbury, 2018). These assessments require teachers to observe and take notes and photographs of children's activities within the classroom throughout the year, to determine whether children's skills are "'emerging', 'expected', or 'exceeding'" (p. 2). Likewise, the OECD has launched the International Early Learning and Child Well-Being Study (IELS) – namely, a pre-school PISA that will measure cognitive (emerging literacy, emerging numeracy) as well as socio-emotional skills (self-regulation, empathy, and trust).

The schoolification of early childhood education has been criticised as it usually results in a decline in play and the implementation of structured and more sedentary curricula for children. This schoolification is also not limited to academic settings. Digital media companies are commercialising early years' curricula through educational games and activities (educational apps in particular) that adopt literacy and numeracy pedagogies aimed at teaching pre-school children new skills.

The Business of Children's Learning

While education itself cannot be turned into a commodity, access to it can be. Hence the existence of education markets that are enhanced by the establishment of hierarchies and mechanisms of competition between individuals, schools, and states within neoliberal market-based economies. For instance, the commercialisation of education has resulted in the large-scale adoption of educational technologies and platforms (van Dijck & Poell, 2018). Educational platforms – like ClassDojo, currently used in over 180 countries (www.classdojo.com/it-it/about/), and Silicon Valley start-up schools such as AltSchool and, recently, Amazon's primary schools – incorporate a data-driven and market-oriented approach to learning and teaching that prioritises individualised learning schemes and education contracts with parents based on learning analytics (Knox, 2017; Williamson, 2017, 2018). Such an approach is sustained by policy documents – such as the 2015 OECD report "Skills for Social Progress: The Power of Social and Emotional Skills" – that emphasise the role of parents, co-responsible for ensuring data-driven learning environments which would encourage the child's development of the socio-emotional skills that maximise learning (Williamson, 2017).

Similarly, pre-school education apps are part of this movement towards "policy and broader commercial discourses [that] call for the increased responsibilisation and intensification of parenting" (Vincent & Maxwell, 2016, p. 269). The download pages of children's pre-school apps speak directly to parents, suggesting that their apps give children an advantage in the early learning years – an early foot up on the education ladder. In speaking directly to parents, these advertisements construct parents as responsible for their children's educational future and digital inclusion and mark the provision of extra-curricular activities such as these learning apps as constituting good parenting.

The download pages for pre-school children's educational apps (Google Play and Apple App Store) are spaces where corporate and independent developers compete to sell educational apps for pre-school children. In a highly competitive space, where apps are ranked and compared with each other in terms of reviews and downloads, developers often offer their apps for free "in an attempt to generate enough downloads to climb these sales tables" (*Wired*, 2012). This freemium pricing strategy relies on small, more frequent payments that are often referred to as micropayments, as it is the belief that consumers tend to be less concerned about small purchases than large ones (Krcmar et al., 2012). The use of a freemium pricing strategy enables start-ups and individual designers to secure the attention they require to generate profits – usually through in-app purchases, optional subscription fees, and sometimes advertising – and is a constituent of the evolution of neoliberal marketisation strategies for online digital products.

Previous analysis of educational apps has found that there is a marked difference between the information presented on the download pages of full-price versus freemium-priced educational apps. Vaala and colleagues (2015) found that the top 50 paid apps were more detailed compared with the top 50 freemium apps, respectively. These top 50 paid apps identified pre-school children as their target audience, which the authors noted is helpful for parents who want a specific age range. With regards to the language and literacy skills mentioned in the download page descriptions, the top paid and the top free apps mentioned three to five skills, whereas the award-winning apps only mentioned one skill being taught (pp. 21–2). The authors noted that the apps had a limited range of language and literacy skills and excluded more complex skills, such as reading fluency and self-expression (Vaala et al., 2015).

Method

A critical discourse analysis approach (CDA) was employed to analyse ten download pages of pre-school children's learning apps. Based on Fairclough and Wodak (1997), CDA deems discourse as "a form of social practice" that needs to take into account the context in which any discourse is produced, distributed, and interpreted, as well as the social and historic environment involved. Fairclough's Three-Dimensional Model was used to frame this analysis. This three-level model/framework involves: 'text analysis' where the analysis involves description of the text, which includes all semiotic indicators such as images, sounds, animations, and music (i.e., multi-modal text); 'processing analysis', which identifies the motives or objectives of the producers of these texts; and 'social analysis', where the wider social or historical context is taken into consideration in order to understand the kinds of social practices or discourses taking place and how they are interconnected (Fairclough, 1995).

Selection of Download Pages

The app download page case studies were chosen from the Google Play website, which contains over 100 apps for young children (GooglePlay, n.d.). The authors used search options to filter the gaming apps to find the top free educational apps for pre-school children. From these options, the authors chose the top apps according to their user rating (4+ stars), as well as the inclusion of a video advertisement. The ten apps discussed in this chapter (although only one example is included) claim to teach and further develop children's literacy and numeracy skills, and to prepare children for pre-school, using various pedagogical techniques and an education-approved curriculum.

Limitations

One major limitation of this analysis is the interpretive scope of media texts. There can be more than one interpretation of media texts, and these can co-occur in any one text (Jensen, 1995, p. 75). This means that there is not only one correct meaning or interpretation of any media text, with the meaning interpreted or constructed by audience members or readers of the text who read the text in a way that is compatible with their own worldview (Ritson, 2003). Nonetheless, for the purposes of this study, it is assumed that advertisers of children's apps ascribe a principal meaning to the goods or services they are promoting and anticipate "the grasping or extracting of prespecifiable meanings from the message" (Mick et al., 1999, p. 11). These prespecifiable (or main) meanings are the meanings analysed within the download pages.

A second limitation may be traced in the sample size used in this analysis. The aim was not to be exhaustive in the sample size. Rather, a case-study design was adopted that focussed on the most popular download pages available on the Google Play website. While the sample size should not be considered representative of the whole app market – where new apps are continuously being launched on the market – the pattern of discourses identified in the samples selected (and in the following case studies) is sufficiently consistent and recurrent to be assumed as indicative of the strategies in which parents are positioned as responsible for their children's educational attainment in a neoliberal ideology.

Findings and Discussion

The ten download pages were analysed and all were found to have a 'pedagogical responsibilisation' discourse firmly embedded within the texts. One of these download pages has been chosen to highlight the variety of ways in which the pedagogical responsibilisation of parents is presented. Four main discourses were embedded in the texts. The first was a pedagogical responsibilisation discourse where parents are positioned as actively responsible for their children's educational attainment. The second was an educational expertise discourse where educational expertise, knowledge, and authority is referred to which positions parents as being in need of the expertise provided within the app. The third was an edutainment discourse that assures parents that the app activities are fun and engaging and thus more likely to be used by children while fulfilling their parents' pedagogical responsibilities. And the last was a gendered discourse within the promotional videos on the app download pages which depicts the occupational stereotype of women belonging to the caring professions – specifically early childhood teaching. A less dominant risk and responsibilisation discourse which assures parents that the apps are safe and secure in terms of children's privacy and data security is also present (see Table 23.1).

Pedagogical Responsibilisation Discourse

In a post-industrial society, education is positioned as a key element in the drive for global economic competitiveness (Ball, 2008). Therefore, the care and education of even the smallest children is now seen as essential in forging a "highly skilled, competitive, and innovative future workforce, fundamental in determining the future economic wealth of a particular nation-state

Table 23.1 Case study analysis of download pages (example).

Text Analysis-Description	Processing and Social Analysis
Preschool Learning Games Kids is a free app rated 4.3 stars on GooglePlay. The app does contain advertising and offers in-app purchases. The app can be found here: https://play.google.com/store/apps/details?id=com.greysprings.games.	

Written Text

"Focuses on the motor skills and hand–eye coordination enhancements for kids"; "based on the kinaesthetic learning process"; "help your kids learn ABCs, colours, numbers, and many other basic lessons"; "experts have explained the importance of fun and interactive learning activities"; "Children enter kindergarten as kinaesthetic and tactual learners, moving and touching everything as they learn. By second or third grade, some students have become visual learners. During the late elementary years some students, primarily females, become auditory learners"; A web address (no link) for the app's Privacy Policy states "You can feel safe using our app because we don't collect your kids' personal information".

Screenshots

There are eight screenshots on the website.

Words/Phrases

"Find differences to improve observatory skills"; "colour your canvas with beautiful images"; "know house chores and manners"; "15+ games for endless learning and fun"; "count objects with beautiful animation"; "play and win beautiful stickers".

Images

Screenshot images include: a bird picture with a paintbox next to it to allow children to colour the image; a window with an alien on the other side (scratch the window to reveal the alien); a table setting with plates, cups, and cutlery; a chameleon on a lilypad in a pond about to catch a fly. The various scenes use colourful images of animals, nature, and objects to explain concepts being taught.

Video Text

The video shows various games containing cartoon animals that children need to manipulate or identify. The first game contains images of pigs that need to be matched to their correct shadow; in another game, ducklings have to be identified. The games are short and simple. The animals and scenes are colourful and varied. Stickers are shown as a reward for completing activities.

Written

Various instructions are given to players: "Match the pictures to their shadows"; "Count all the

Pedagogical Responsibilisation Discourse:

Written text is aimed at parents and defines the educational features of the app. The written text encourages parents to use the app to assist their children's educational development. "Help your kids learn ABCs, colours, numbers, and many other basic lessons".

The *video* demonstrates the game from the child's point of view. The video is slower-paced; it is longer than most other app videos. Based on the in-game instructions (e.g., "Count all the ducklings") parents are indirectly informed about the educational benefits of the game.

Expert Educational Discourse:

The *written text* contains information regarding the expert educational discourse used to promote the app, especially information about VAK (visual, auditory, and kinetic) learning styles and relationship to age range. This is also used to legitimise the educational claims of the app.

"Experts have explained the importance of fun and interactive learning activities";

"Children enter kindergarten as kinaesthetic and tactual learners, moving and touching everything as they learn. By second or third grade, some students have become visual learners. During the late elementary years some students, primarily females, become auditory learners".

This background is aimed at providing reassurance to parents that this app is based on proven educational principles.

Gendered Discourse

The adult female voice over, which instructs players in each game, is an authoritative voice similar to that of a pre-school teacher who gently instructs each activity and then provides praise for a job well done. "Spot the difference between the two pictures"; "phenomenal".

Risk and Responsibilisation Discourse

The *written text* mentions the safety of children's information, although this is at the bottom of the page. While there is a statement "Privacy Policy: You can feel safe using our app because we don't collect your kids' personal information" – no live link is given to the full policy.

(*Continued*)

Table 23.1 (Cont.)

Text Analysis-Description	Processing and Social Analysis
Preschool Learning Games Kids is a free app rated 4.3 stars on GooglePlay. The app does contain advertising and offers in-app purchases. The app can be found here: https://play.google.com/store/apps/details?id=com.greysprings.games.	

ducklings"; "Solve the puzzle by navigating the maze". Child players are praised for completing activities: "bravo"; "phenomenal"; "brilliant"; "excellent".

Oral

In-app voices. Female adult (teacher-like), and child voices give the instructions for each game. Children's voices shout "hurray" at the end of each completed activity.

Voice-Over

No voice-over narration.

Imagery

No other imagery apart from screenshots in the slideshow.

Editing Style

Montage, but slightly longer scenes.

Point of View

From the perspective of the player.

Pace

Slow.

Duration

1 minute and 56 seconds.

Target Audience

Parents and children.

Music

Xylophone-type sound whenever game images were clicked on.

So, while the app download page reassures parents that their child's personal information will not be collected, it is unclear what counts as personal information. It does provide a URL to their privacy policy. Parents would need to read the document to learn more about the app's data collection practices.

Edutainment/Gamification Discourse

The edutainment aspects of the game include scenes showing lessons such as literacy, numeracy, and recall (memory game), as fun games.

"15+ games for endless learning and fun".

The gamification of education manifests in the *video* through the use of animation to show fun, colourful images, and scenes containing various animals and shapes.

Lessons are followed by a reward. For example, matching pictures of pigs to their shadows is followed by three gold stars appearing on the screen, with the word "phenomenal" underneath as well as "120" to show how many points they scored. There is also cheering in the background (sounds like young children), which provides praise for each completed task. Rewards also include stickers of cartoon animals that children can choose.

Source: Donell Holloway, Giovanna Mascheroni, and Ashley Donkin.

on the world stage" (Brown & Lauder, 2006, p. 27 cited in Albon & Rosen, 2013 p. 32). Thus, even very young children are positioned as learners and economic units.

Commercial initiatives aimed at parents and their children's education are embedded within a responsibilisation discourse that calls for parental pedagogicalisation (Baez & Talburt, 2008; Popkewitz, 2003), where parents are expected to be increasingly responsible for educating their young children as well as forming effective partnerships with their children's schools. "They are called upon to change their parenting so as to provide their children with appropriate educational activities that have them up and running long before they enter the classroom" (Vanobbergen et al., 2009, p. 286). This pedagogical responsibilisation is not isolated to the ideology of the marketplace. Educational policy development has also taken an ideological change that positions parents and educational institutions as co-responsible for children's education (Mascheroni & Holloway, 2017). This development, to hold parents co-responsible, also hypothetically reduces the cost of government intervention (Smeyers, 2010).

Consequently, pre-school children's learning apps can be construed as part of this ongoing pedagogicalisation move. Within an entrepreneurial framework, the marketing of learning apps for pre-school children homes in on the educational benefits of the apps. These discursive texts regarding educational benefits are also a reflection on how digital technology is increasingly implicated in discourses regarding the responsibilisation of parents for their children's educational attainment.

Expert Knowledge Discourse

Parents are often constructed as in need of expert advice and help in order to be capable and responsible parents (Furedi, 2008). This 'expert knowledge' discourse emphasises that a good parent is a responsible parent who is keen to enhance their parenting skills (Widding, 2015). There is, therefore, a variety of expert advice about parenting in the form of books, magazines, television shows, and websites. This 'expert advice' discourse is also embedded in advertising material selling products that help parents maintain and support their children's health and safety, as well as their social and educational development.

These discourses, involving educational or developmental expertise within the download pages analysed, tend to problematise early childhood development and recommend that parents act on this problem. This expert knowledge discourse engenders market-based parental practices (consumption practices) that ensure children's school readiness and the long-term benefits and costs of good parental care by associating early childhood development "with (adult) traits and skills that have direct workplace and economic relevance" (Nadesan, 2002, p. 421).

The download pages analysed use the authoritative power of educational or developmental expertise (educational theory, learning styles, and curriculum objectives) as selling points to encourage parents to buy and use their products. They construct a moral imperative so that parents will wish to acquire and absorb this knowledge through consumption so that parents will be empowered to carry out their responsibilities. They also contribute to the normalisation of formal learning within early childhood. They standardise and validate supposed 'expert knowledge' about early childhood education.

Edutainment Discourse

At the same time that parents are called upon to provide extra-curricular material and activities for their children's educational benefit, children's apps need to target a dual market – the parent and the child. The apps need to meet parent expectations about what is educational and, at the same time, be enjoyable or entertaining for the child. The edutainment discourse embedded in these download pages assures parents that the app they are choosing is pleasurable and engaging, thereby more likely to be used by children and fulfil their parents' pedagogical responsibilities.

The term edutainment is simply the meshing of education and entertainment. For instance, the television show *Sesame Street* epitomises what was an early and very successful attempt to link entertainment and education on screen. However, edutainment is now a relatively stigmatised term as it is associated with lower-order thinking skills. This is because early computer-based instruction focussed more on learning and memorising facts than on analysing or engaging in other higher-level cognitive processing in Bloom's taxonomy (Jarvin, 2015, p. 35). The term gamification, on the other hand, refers to the use of game design elements in contexts without games. In the field of education, it is used to describe digital game-based learning; "game-based mechanics, aesthetics and game thinking to engage people, motivate action, promote learning, and solve problems" (Kapp, 2012, p. 10).

Thus, despite the differing emphases within the terms edutainment and gamification, preschool children's apps are, generally speaking, both a form of edutainment, in that they often comprise basic rote learnings, and a form of gamified learning, given that they contain game elements such as rewards, badges, and clapping sounds to motivate children to move along within the game and learn. Thus, alongside an education discourse within the download pages, parents are presented with texts, graphics, videos, and sounds that allude to rewards, feedback, fun, and entertainment for their children – further ensuring sustained engagement and learning for their children.

Gendered Discourse

The app download pages analysed in all but one case exclusively used female voices as narrators and in-app teachers who guide children through the app activities. These voices give the impression of a kindly female teacher and, as such, maintain a long-held stereotype regarding gender and occupation. Generally, this stereotype maintains and conveys women's occupation as belonging in the caring professions such as teaching, nursing, social work, and childcare. More specifically, and within the apps analysed, this stereotyping related to the gendered representation of early childhood educators or the 'kindy teacher'. These stereotypes, when presented to preschool-aged children, are of significance because the gender-stereotyped beliefs of children at this age are likely to become more rigid and less flexible (Ward & Aubrey, 2017).

Conventionally, women carry out the role of caring for young children whether they be mothers, nannies, childcare workers, or early childhood educators. And despite changing (more positive) attitudes toward the role of males in early childhood settings, "there is still some uncomfortableness around the idea of men in ECCE [Early Childhood Care and Education]" (King, 2018). By not evoking this uncomfortableness within the download pages app developers and promoters maintain a wider market base. The strongly gendered discourse evident in the download pages continues and validates existing responsibilisation discourses which place women in charge of children's care and development. It also reproduces an archetype of the early childhood teacher and maintains a discursive practice that excludes or ignores certain bodies (men) in early childhood education settings.

Risk and Responsiblisation Discourse

The neoliberal construction of the parents as morally responsible for the successful achievements of their children as adults-in-the-making is also pursued through a discourse of risks and responsibilities (Thomas & Lupton, 2016). Constructed around the assumption that children are powerless victims of the dangers of an adults' world, this discourse builds on and amplifies parental anxieties to ensure children's health, well-being, and a successful future.

The case studies discussed in this chapter provide an example of how a risk and responsibilisation framework can be embedded in the advertising of educational apps. In the first case study, parental anxieties over screen time are built upon and parents are encouraged to take responsibility for their children's safety through the use of parental controls. Privacy issues are also mentioned and parents are called on to familiarise themselves with the privacy policy of the app.

What is interesting here is that the discourse of risk and responsibilisation is fully functional to the neoliberal prioritisation of individual responsibilisation in the field of education. Any potential tension between providing children's access to educational opportunities while exposing them to risks (whether excessive screen time or commercial dataveillance, that is, data-based surveillance and profiling) is minimised. Parents can simultaneously ensure easier access to literacy and numeracy skills, and master children's screen time or protect them from privacy risks. Thus, the discourse of risks and responsibilisation and the discourse of the educational responsibility of parents can be better understood as complementary rather than competing (Mascheroni & Holloway, 2017).

Conclusion

This chapter has analysed the discursive regulation of parenthood that emerges from the various commercial discourses embedded in the download pages of pre-school children's learning apps. The educational focus of these download pages and the apps they describe mobilise neoliberal parenting subjectivities in the context of what was once considered a time in childhood free from over-prescriptive educational objectives.

The case studies combine and remix four contemporary normative discourses and show a range of contexts in which a 'pedagogical responsibilisation' discourse can be couched. An 'expert knowledge' discourse is embedded in the texts to varying degrees as a way to maximise the apparent educational quality of the apps and reinforce the pedagogical responsibilisation discourse. In addition, there is a noticeable emphasis on the edutainment value of these apps within the download pages. Some of the download pages briefly mention the tight privacy and security aspects of the app to be downloaded and, as such, assuage parents' concerns about their children's online safety. This speaks to the many 'risk and responsibilisation' discourses that parents are presented with where they are called to protect their children from the harms of the internet (Mascheroni & Holloway, 2017). Typical also within these download pages is a gendered discourse in which women are represented as teachers of pre-school children who guide the children through the apps' activities.

Despite possible contradictions between some of the discourses embedded in the download pages (for instance between the pedagogical responsibilisation discourse and the risk and responsibilisation discourse), the varying discourses tend to combine well to further shape and support normative understandings about responsible parenting. They extend the manner and mode of responsible parenting into new digital spaces and practices for the pre-school-aged child. Such discourses contribute to naturalise technologies, data, and analytics as an inherent component of the educational process (Couldry & Yu, 2018), and parents' responsible involvement as a required, ethical condition of its success.

References

Albon, D., & Rosen, R. (2013). *Negotiating adult-child relationships in early childhood research*. London: Routledge.
Baez, B., & Talburt, S. (2008). Governing for responsibility and with love: Parents and children between home and school. *Educational Theory, 58*(1), 25–43.
Ball, S. (2008). *The education debate: Politics and policy in the 21st century*. Bristol: Policy Press.
Barr, R., & Nichols Linebarger, D. (2016). *Media exposure during infancy and early childhood*. Dordrecht: Springer.
Bradbury, A. (2018). Datafied at four: The role of data in the "schoolification" of early childhood education in England. *Learning, Media and Technology, 44*(1), 7–21.
Brown, P., & Lauder, H. (2006). Globalisation, knowledge and the myth of the magnet economy. *Globalisation, Societies and Education, 4*(1), 25–57.
Buckingham, D., & Scanlon, M. (2001). Parental pedagogies: An analysis of British "edutainment" magazines for young children. *Journal of Early Childhood Literacy, 1*(3), 281–299.
Couldry, N., & Yu, J. (2018). Deconstructing datafication's brave new world. *New Media and Society, 20*(2), 4473–4491.

Department of Education. (2009). *Belonging, being & becoming: The early years learning framework for Australia*. Canberra. Retrieved from: www.education.gov.au/early-years-learning-framework-0.

Fairclough, N. (1995). *Critical discourse analysis*. Boston, MA: Addison Wesley.

Fairclough, N., & Wodak, R. (1997). Critical discourse analysis. In T. A. van Dijk (Ed.), *Discourse as structure and process* (Vol. 2; pp. 357–378). London: Sage.

Furedi, F. (2008). *Paranoid parenting: Why ignoring the experts may be best for your child*. London: Continuum.

GooglePlay. (n.d.). Children's apps. Retrieved from: https://play.google.com/store/search?q=children%27s%20apps&c=apps.

Holloway, S. L., & Pimlott-Wilson, H. (2014). "Any advice is welcome isn't it?": Neoliberal parenting education, local mothering cultures, and social class. *Environment and Planning A*, *46*(1), 94–111.

Jarvin, L. (2015). Edutainment, games, and the future of education in a digital world. *New directions for child and adolescent development*, *2015*(147), 33–40.

Jensen, K. B. (1995). *The social semiotics of mass communication*. London: Sage.

Kapp, K. M. (2012). *The gamification of learning and instruction: Game-based methods and strategies for training and education*. San Francisco, CA: John Wiley & Sons.

King, D. (2018). Exploring parental attitudes towards male early childhood educators in the Republic of Ireland today. *Children's Research Network*. Retrieved from: https://childrensresearchnetwork.org/knowledge/resources/exploring-parental-attitudes-towards-male-early-childhood-educators-in-the-republic-of-ireland-today.

Knox, J. (2017). Playing with student data: The learning analytics report card (LARC). Paper presented at the *Practitioner Track Proceedings of 7th International Learning Analytics & Knowledge Conference (LAK17)*, Vancouver, Canada.

Krcmar, H., Friesike, S., Bohm, M., & Schildhauer, T. (2012). Innovation, society and business: Internet-based business models and their implications. *1st Berlin Symposium on Internet and Society*, Oct. 25–27, 2011. Retrieved from: www.hiig.de/wp-content/uploads/2012/04/Business-Models-Paper.pdf.

Lemke, T. (2001). "The birth of bio-politics": Michel Foucault's lecture at the Collège de France on neo-liberal governmentality. *Economy and Society*, *30*(2), 190–207.

Marandet, E., & Wainwright, E. (2015). Geographies of education: Families, parenting, and schools. *Labouring and Learning*, *10*, 1–19.

Mascheroni, G., & Holloway, D. (Eds.). (2017). The internet of toys: A report on media and social discourses around young children and IoToys. *DigiLitEY*. Milan. Retrieved from: http://digilitey.eu/wp-content/uploads/2017/01/IoToys-June-2017-reduced.pdf.

Mick, D., Burroughs, J., & Hetzel, P. (1999). A global review of semiotic consumer research: Progress, problems. Unpublished working paper. Madison, WI: University of Wisconsin-Madison. School of Business.

Moss, P. (Ed.). (2012). *Early childhood and compulsory education: Reconceptualising the relationship*. London: Routledge.

Nadesan, M. H. (2002). Engineering the entrepreneurial infant: Brain science, infant development toys, and governmentality. *Cultural Studies*, *16*(3), 401–432.

O'Connor, J., & Fotakopoulou, O. (2016). A threat to childhood innocence or the future of learning? Parents' perspectives on the use of touch-screen technology by 0-3 year-olds in the UK. *Contemporary Issues in Early Childhood*, *17*(2), 235–247.

Popkewitz, T. S. (2003). Governing the child and pedagogicalization of the parent. In M. N. Bloch, K. Holmlund, I. Moqvist, & T. S. Popkewitz (Eds.), *Governing children, families, and education* (pp. 35–61). New York: Palgrave Macmillan.

Ritson, M. (2003). Special session summary polysemy: The multiple meanings of advertising. *Paper presented at the European Advances in Consumer Research*, Provo, UT.

Sims, M. (2014). Is the care-education dichotomy behind us? Should it be? *Australasian Journal of Early Childhood*, *39*(4), 4–11.

Sims, M. (2017). Neoliberalism and early childhood. *Cogent Education*, *4*(1), 1–10.

Smeyers, P. (2010). Child rearing in the "risk" society: On the discourse of rights and the "Best interests of a child". *Educational Theory*, *60*(3), 271–284.

The changing nature of app design and development for kids. (2012, January 16). *Wired*. Retrieved from: www.wired.com/2012/01/kids-app-design.

Thomas, G. M., & Lupton, D. (2016). Threats and thrills: Pregnancy apps, risk and consumption. *Health, Risk & Society*, *17*(7–8), 495–509.

Vaala, S., Ly, A., & Levine, M. H. (2015). *Getting a read on the app stores: A market scan and analysis of children's literacy apps*. Retrieved from: https://files.eric.ed.gov/fulltext/ED574396.pdf.

van Dijck, J., & Poell, T. (2018). Social media platforms and education. In J. Burgess, A. Marwick, & T. Poell (Eds.), *The Sage handbook of social media* (pp. 579–591). Los Angeles, CA: Sage.

Vanobbergen, B., Daems, M., & Van Tilburg, S. (2009). Bookbabies, their parents and the library: An evaluation of a Flemish reading programme in families with young children. *Educational Review, 61*(3), 277–287.

Vincent, C., & Maxwell, C. (2016). Parenting priorities and pressures: Furthering understanding of "concerted cultivation". *Discourse: Studies in the Cultural Politics of Education, 37*(2), 269–281.

Ward, L. M., & Aubrey, J. S. (2017). *Watching gender: How stereotypes in movies and on TV impact kids' development*. San Francisco, CA: Common Sense.

Widding, U. (2015). Parenting ideals and (un-) troubled parent positions. *Pedagogy, Culture & Society, 23*(1), 45–64.

Williamson, B. (2017). Decoding ClassDojo: Psycho-policy, social-emotional learning and persuasive educational technologies. *Learning, Media and Technology, 42*(4), 440–453.

Williamson, B. (2018). Silicon startup schools: Technocracy, algorithmic imaginaries and venture philanthropy in corporate education reform and venture philanthropy in corporate education reform. *Critical Studies in Education, 59*(2), 218–236.

24

DIGITAL LITERACY/'DYNAMIC LITERACIES'

Formal and Informal Learning Now and in the Emergent Future

John Potter

Thinking About Literacy and the Push and Pull of Pedagogy

Whilst many younger learners, across all levels of income and social class in the UK and elsewhere in the developed and parts of the majority world, are immersed in various media- and technology-related games and activities outside of formal learning (OFCOM, 2018), the institutional situation is often different. It is not especially surprising that this is so; earlier research in the UK found that children of primary school age hardly expected anything else when crossing the boundary between home and school (Selwyn, Potter, & Cranmer, 2010). After all, many routine aspects of life in the home are not replicated in school, which is, of course, bound by different rules and norms and generates a different learned way of being. In fact, the children participating in this research cast doubt on the proposition that formal educational settings could learn anything from informal uses of media and technology in the home.

All-pervasive use of technology, its ease of access across social and broadcast media, its various screens and various modalities of use, from passive interaction to touchscreen dragging and dropping, from consumption to production and sharing of meanings, raises the possibility of a greater disjuncture between the spaces of home and school. Pervasiveness has shifted the goalposts and media technologies are integral to, and embedded in, material culture and lived experience. In some education systems, a failure to recognise and build on this vast untapped well of skill and knowledge about media outside the school unnecessarily reduces the experience of what it is to be literate inside the school. Children being educated therein lack a critical engagement with media forms, never mind the experience to be creative and produce digital media. Of course, concerns about safety rightly drive many initiatives but, even with this agenda, digital literacy projects are still very unevenly spread in the developed and developing world, in spite of the efforts of international organisations to provide blueprints for formal engagement (UNESCO, 2016) and the way in which children experience digital media in the world outside is, like that of adults, not necessarily always on a simple risk–benefit continuum.

At the same time, education systems are increasingly dependent on an unseen but vast commercially enabled and profitable data collection project on aspects of children's learning and, increasingly, dispositions and behaviours across a range of metrics (Bradbury, 2019; Bradbury &

Roberts-Holmes, 2017; Williamson, 2017). Whilst qualitative researchers, both inside and outside formal institutions, need to provide evidence of ethical management of any data collected, including gaining informed consent from the subjects, it is not always clear that the same permissions are agentively given in respect of the compilation of league tables of achievement, and other less well understood datapoints by large corporations. Additionally, of course, by reducing literacy to simple, measurable targets and collecting data in this way, it is possible to reduce education to a functional process, disconnected from the world, its messy issues and political concerns, its inequity and lack of social justice.

Before continuing, it is necessary to think, therefore, about what it really *means* to be literate in the digital age, since how this is defined exerts a forceful push and pull on pedagogy. This suggests considering the formal development of 'literacy' as an object of study, which, in turn, means working with theoretical positions and definitions which locate literacy in its wider cultural context; a positioning which focusses attention on different phenomena than versions which arise from information science or communication studies. Arguably the most useful starting point, when considering questions of context, is Brian Street's version of the "new literacy studies", in which literacy has two overarching forms: the *autonomous* and the *ideological* (Street, 2003). In the former case, literacy *by itself* acts autonomously and confers status and success in the world; acquiring the functional codes and conventions is all that is required. It is, of course, inarguable that children who learn to read and write print are massively advantaged over those who do not. But literacy in the 'ideological' sense is a far closer definition of how literacy works in the world, because meaning-making is, ultimately, contingent and contested. It is located in literacy events and speech acts which are constructed out of particular sets of specific rules of engagement and communicative modes and its design across these many modes, in particular those other than print, now hold sway in the digital age. It is an unambitious literacy curriculum which does not consider enlarging itself better to encompass media. Note that this is not about replacing print or subverting its importance in formal and informal learning – far from it. Children and adults are arguably reading more than ever before and these skills are still vitally important for functioning in the world. It is, however, about being more ambitious with what the curriculum offers for all ages, encouraging children to become more engaged with the many modes of meaning-making in the digital age. It is about engaging in teaching and learning which recognises that meaning-making is in a more or less constant state of change and churn; it is dynamic and not static, and it is multimodal, dependent on knowledge and skills of intertextuality and of how different modes work with each other to produce meaning.

Digital Literacy and Media Literacy

The word 'literacy' confers status on everything that comes before it. Its position as inarguable and a static force for good in the autonomous definition of the word signifies a serious and structured discipline. So, '*digital* literacy' as a term promises a structured and instrumentalist version of the 'digital', one which fixes its sights on skills and technical operations, the awareness of codes and conventions. It does not catch the lived experience of the digital, the pervasive use of media devices, the cultural experience of sharing, critiquing, collecting and distributing, remediating and remixing. It fails to capture the messy reality of everyday life in the first quarter of the 21st century, with its attendant baggage from previous times and its insistence on an endlessly deferred future in which things inevitably get better, thanks mainly to technology. One thing is certain, things get more complex, because 'things' are in a constant state of flux in which the changing artefacts of new media are inextricably bound up with the different social arrangements which arise in the light of these and the subsequent altered social practices around them (Lievrouw & Livingstone, 2006).

If digital literacy is perhaps perceived as too reductive, will media literacy help as a term around which to frame thinking about learning in the digital age? Certainly, it has a longer history and there are traditions of media literacy education in countries such as Canada and the United States, and parts of Europe, which go back decades. But even with media literacy there is significant dissonance between programmes which seek to develop skillsets and those which require deeper analytical and political readings of media literacy texts, artefacts, and institutions. If digital literacy promotes safety through the understanding of codes and conventions, including some technical knowledge of the digital world, perhaps media literacy is its sibling which touches in part on citizen safety but takes its positioning from understanding the political manipulation of information, its role in hegemony. In some initiatives, and to some degree with accuracy, media literacy is portrayed as the solution to the problem of 'fake news'. But media literacy is more than this and is centrally concerned with skillsets of media analysis and production every bit as much as it is with distribution, with issues of interpretation, with economic and societal change.

'Dynamic Literacies' and Pedagogy

Digital literacy and *media* literacy are only two of the literacy labels which are part of the past, present, and children's emergent future. Could one see them, and other related labels such as '*multimodal* literacy', '*information* literacy', as subsets of an "overarching set of 'dynamic literacies' with distinct traditions which, nevertheless, frame a genuine attempt to account for the changes to the ways in which meaning is made in the world" (Potter & McDougall, 2017, p. 33)? 'Dynamic' used as a signifier in this way allows us to pay attention more closely, more responsively, to the lived experience of digital media. It does not privilege the textual over the sociocultural or even *affective* nature of meaning-making; it is an inclusive term which resists the residual definition of literacy as it relates to screens and media (which can lead to media being seen as everything else that gets done when the *real* business of working with print is finished). It brings theories together in a broader collection of concepts.

In what way might this be a useful way to think about children and their learning, now and in the emergent future? Well, it was noted in the opening section that the way in which a system defines literacy exerts a powerful push and pull on pedagogy in that system. If a narrow definition of literacy is employed, a narrow pedagogical response is generated, particularly if, as in the case of the UK, you have an assessment-dominated curriculum backed by punitive database-driven inspection. On the other hand, if you employ a *dynamic* definition of literacy, you potentially generate a more responsive pedagogy, attuned to the lived experience of children as they grow up in a media-pervasive world.

For researchers working in the field of digital media, culture, and education, approaching the world with particular frames of reference derived from the various literacies above, the important questions are around how to account for what is encountered. What is the best way to research the messy reality (Law, 2004) of the world as it relates to the texts, practices, and social arrangements of the digital media age? Researchers of children's emergent literacies should arguably aim to represent something from these messy realities in their narratives: the situated nature of classroom technologies and interactions with media texts and artefacts. This is work which is increasingly captured and theorised as the 'messy' and 'baroque complexity' of the interaction between objects, bodies, technologies, curriculum arrangements, and more in recent writing and research (see, for example, Burnett, Davies, Merchant, & Rowsell, 2014; Burnett & Merchant, 2014).

There are further large-scale efforts to focus research and dissemination in the field in the context of even younger children's engagement with these issues within an overarching frame of curiosity about the lived experience of the digital for those aged from birth to eight years. The "DigiLitEY European COST action brings researchers together to share research into digital literacy in homes and communities, settings of formal and informal learning, reading and writing onscreen, online and offline practices and new methodologies" (DigiLitEY, 2018). It runs in parallel with another multinational project which explores much of the same territory with a focus on digital 'making' in the early years (MakEY, 2018). This inclusive definition which embraces making alongside the digital and media arts is a marker of the ways in which the understanding of what it means to be literate is currently shifting some of the research agenda in new literacy studies and beyond. Certainly, it provides a more holistic and tempered view than commentary which seeks to generate panic about the 'effects' of screen media on children and young people, positioning them instead as agentive and active users of new technologies. From some of the same authors and researchers, parallel reports and opinion pieces have created nuanced accounts of what it means to be a parent or carer in this context, moving the debates beyond the risk–safety continuum and driven by three key questions: "how do parents seek to bring up their children in the digital age?" "what is parents' vision of their children's future and that of wider society?" and "what risks and opportunities will characterise the digital future?" (LSE, 2018). In all these cases, the enlarged definition of literacy prevails, moving beyond the functional, reductive codes and conventions which might be connoted by the term 'digital literacy'. Similarly, the engagement with the changing nature of meaning-making which has been captured in recent years by the various researchers and writers in the new literacies domain has moved the debate into a more dynamic engagement with the digital in this context and several writers and researchers have led the way in this (Burnett, 2016; Gee, 2015; Gillen, 2014; Marsh, 2004; Pahl, 2006; Rowsell, 2013). They have developed further the work of the earliest scholars of the new literacy studies and 'multiliteracies', the work of the New London group, introducing to the world the notion of a plethora of literacy forms and functions in a changing world, rooted in an engagement with the turn to the visual, social semiotics, multimodality, and more (Cope & Kalantzis, 2000; Kress, 2003), recently updated and remixed in new configurations (Serafini & Gee, 2017).

Researching Third Spaces

What does this multiply-placed vision of literacy as a *dynamic* force imply for teachers, researchers, and academics on the ground at this point, in many parts of the world, in many situations, attempting to operationalise some of these concepts in their broader engagement with the world, in their attempt to work with 'digital literacy' as an idea, or even to introduce new terms, concepts, and even policies appropriate to the dynamic state of literacy(ies)? It implies having frameworks for research which are responsive at a deep level to the changing nature of meaning-making and also of hierarchies in the context of digital literacy. In so doing it becomes important to think about the spaces and locations of the digital. Where is this engagement possible within and between formal/informal boundaries of learning? Some have invoked the 'third space' as a useful concept for this (Gutierrez, 2008), though it generates misunderstandings and misapplications of the term. Nevertheless, it can work in the context of children now and in the emergent digital future, if it is understood as not always an actual, physical space, but more as a space in which hierarchies are flattened and practices adapted beyond the original conception in culture (Bhabha, 1994) into educational space in the context of the all-pervasive uses of digital technologies (Potter & McDougall, 2017, see especially pp. 37–60).

For those of us working and researching in the spaces between formal and informal education these third spaces are potential locations for observing a dynamic conception of literacy in action. It becomes something more than a discursive account of digital literacy practices. It is realisable and acted out in the world in such activities as filmmaking, animation, gaming, augmented and virtual reality in a range of settings. But it depends fundamentally on a working relationship between two key aspects of pedagogy: the roles of the various social actors in the setting and the negotiation into the space of popular culture or vernacular literacies, the welcoming into the space of children's funds of knowledge, their skills and dispositions from outside across the semi-permeable membrane between home and school (Marsh, 2004; Moll, Amanti, Neff, & Gonzalez, 1992; Pahl, 2003; Parry, 2013; Potter, 2011).

Three exemplar projects might be useful at this point. The first examines the impacts of the use of culturally familiar devices such as touch screens in the teaching of filmmaking and moving image grammar. This work comprised a series of observations, interviews, and focus groups over the course of a project which lasted for one school term, with a group of 20 children aged 9 and 10, as well as a similar number of 14-year-olds. In the participating schools, the data showed clear impact on practices around filmmaking and editing, with the affordances of immediate review and iterative filmmaking by the children a real possibility, without the encumbrances of other kinds of technical filmmaking equipment. In this case the "culturally familiar artefact represented an opportunity for boundary crossing between formal and informal settings of education" (Potter & Bryer, 2016, p. 124). The artefact itself was part of the process, the descriptions of its use and those of the children playing a part in describing what has been referred to elsewhere as the 'Baroque complexity' of interactions in educational settings in and around social actors and technology (Burnett & Merchant, 2014). The research noted also its centrality in the creative process, a key component of digital media education (Cannon, 2018), and its findings were broadly in line with how touchscreen devices had previously been found to be potentially useful in many early literacy activities (see, for example, Flewitt, Kucirkova, & Messer, 2014), though the study reported here was working in the expanded and inclusive definition of literacy, beyond print and into meaning-making with digital moving-image production.

The second project, in an out-of-school setting, employing similar methods to those described above, worked with similar-aged groups of children in different project locations (see Flewitt et al., 2017). In this research the interest was in finding out how children's experiences of material disadvantage could be represented by the child co-researchers, using digital artefacts, voice recorders, media production, audio recordings, alongside pencil and paper methods. These were embedded within discussions of lived experience and ideas of representation drawn from popular culture as well as personal accounts. Across the range of documentary-style productions, in the child-produced videos (in one setting a horror film and also a dance movie), there were flattened hierarchies of adults and children in the setting, the positioning of children as expert reporters of their own experience, and the emergence of thinking and working in a 'third space' (Gutierrez, 2008; Potter & McDougall, 2017), the connection between texts, artefacts, and practices adding up to an emergent negotiation with existing skills and dispositions which the children employed in a fresh, revelatory context.

Finally, a current project is working with children in two primary schools to find out more about their playground games (Playing the Archive, 2018). The project, like an earlier iteration (Burn & Richards, 2014), has its origins in the games collected by folklorists Peter and Iona Opie over a period of some 30 years (Opie & Opie, 1954). In this version, children have been recruited as co-researchers of their playground experiences of play with a view to casting new light on the collection and, ultimately, helping to represent it to new audiences in digitally enhanced museum exhibits and play trails. This research is using innovative research methods, including thinking about embodied literacy and movement through space enabled by new thinking on multimodal transcription (Cowan & Kress, 2017). In the early stages of the project it became clear how much YouTube takes centre stage in the playground as the main media space to be represented and remediated. Children profess admiration for YouTubers and a desire to have their own followers; one ten-year-old who was interviewed already has her own. This active engagement with the vast swathes of content on YouTube results in playground games becoming inflected with the performance of their idols among the YouTubers. Dances from current crazes are performed and enacted within the template of earlier games from times gone by. Just as the Opies found in their work and just as colleagues on the earlier project found, popular culture is remixed into play (Willett, 2014). In this most recent case, the provisional world of social media is the anchor for play which finds roots and echoes in much earlier rhyming patterns and clapping games. This research is at the beginning stages of understanding and theorising these phenomena but there are parallels with the earlier projects which reported on the ways in which dynamic literacies are operating.

YouTube is inevitably at the heart of the viewing experience of children who have access to tablets and smartphones which are present in a variety of forms and different levels of use in many homes in the UK. The point here, again, is to state that adults, like children, are in thrall to a platform which reaches into most aspects of their lives, viewing YouTubers, TV shows, recorded gameplay, self-help clips, and more. From a video-sharing platform, it has grown into a central, first port-of-call for many searches for media, entertainment, and information. In terms of lived experience, it acts as a kind of ecosystem in its relationship to both playful engagements with media and an interaction with the dynamic of digital life. Dances from Instagram have moved across into online video gameplay, via the medium of YouTube, back out into the physical, offline world of the playground. Children are running around as much as they ever were during these minutes in between lessons and their play is a rich engagement with digital culture. To what extent they are agentively, actively curating their play – as in the previous project (Potter, 2014) – back into the world leads us to a wider discussion of exactly which elements might be components of 'digital literacy'.

Digital Lives, Agency, and Curation: Components of Digital Literacy

This chapter presents a mostly positive interpretation of children and young people's ability to act for themselves in the world in the digital age, whilst much contemporary discourse assumes that there are dire consequences of digital media use in terms of screen addiction, danger from strangers, and more. Many of these fears are exaggerated, some are evidently not, and there are excellent resources for educating in a nuanced and research-led way about them, including culturally sensitive, detailed, and expanded datasets and reports from across the European Union (Sonck, Livingstone, Kuiper, & de Haan, 2011).

Some of the less obvious forces which act on children's agency are arguably even more present in their lives than those traditionally associated with risk; those corporations quietly accruing information about their subjects under the guise of educational assessment and improvement. Children's attainments, and even behavioural actions in the world, are recorded digitally and stored as assets by companies and agencies, some of whom are engaged in profiting from such profiling (Williamson, 2017). However, in this, children should not necessarily be 'othered' as unknowing victims with adults positioned as their knowing guardians; adults are also prey to ignorance of the same levels of surveillance and data 'sharing' in which the notion of consent is a very loose conception of the term. Without serious time and effort, for example, it is not a simple process for adults of any age to erase purchases, browsing histories, uploaded social media files, emails, and more which accrue through (digital) life.

Children's use of social media as it grows, moves over time from perhaps being the object of other people's gaze at the behest of parents and carers sharing images, to becoming producers of their own content, curators of their own exhibitions of their achievements, likes, collected items, and more. Younger learners can add to their profile the data they give away to that which is collected without consent. In many senses this curatorial process is agentive and positive, a part of participatory culture which is playful and under the control of the end user.

Behind it, of course, lie corporations framing the ways in which the media can and should be shared and controlling both the access, storage, and ultimate purposes of the productions. Social media production is also as complex as it is 'playful' and 'agentive', framed differently across the many spaces in which the images, videos, and audio files are published and displayed. Each space has its own rules, logic, affordances, and audiences; there is a particular grammar and syntax associated with each one of them from Instagram to Twitter, WhatsApp to WeChat, Facebook to WordPress. The author has suggested elsewhere that 'curation' is in itself a new literacy practice in digital media and 'curatorship' is the ability to navigate these processes. It is way beyond the simple act of editing and conflates many different skillsets and dispositions across performance, exhibition, reflexivity, performativity, and more (Potter, 2012; Potter & McDougall, 2017). In keeping with the notion of an enlarged definition of what it means to be literate, encompassing the making and sharing of meanings in a wider form of media than print, it would be useful in years to come to think about 'curation' itself becoming part of what these children learn about. In England, where it has become important for children to know what the term 'fronted adverbial' means, it is surely as important for them to understand curation in digital media.

In conclusion, it is arguably important to consider a set of useful and usable component parts of 'digital literacy' which somehow capture the present and emergent state of play for children, young people, and their carers living with media and technology which is all pervasive and ever changing. The following could be useful, potential locations of research and thinking also about 'dynamic literacies', the knowledge domains which acknowledge four key facets of the lived experience of both children and their parents and carers in the digital age:

1   Technology as part of material culture and lived experience;
2   Digital media and learner identity as bound and contingent on one another;
3   Literacy in the digital age recognised as a dynamic phenomenon, inclusively and ideologically defined;

and, finally,

4   Curation as a new literacy practice (with all its attendant contradictions around agency and control).

Researchers might begin to do better by all social actors in the field by paying attention to the detail of people's lives in the digital age and not being fixated on static, reductive systems which miss the detail of the lived experience of children of all ages. The emergent future may well be one in which technologies such as Artificial Intelligence will have a decisive impact on all aspects of life and learning, and there is much debate and hype around this at the time of writing, but the critical considerations around the digital, around media, remain the same, even as the technology is evolving. Thinking about this and living with it is about thinking beyond the technology (Buckingham, 2007) into the processes of digital media consumption and production, examining the structures around them, holding larger education technology businesses to account and thinking about the ethical and moral considerations of this rise of a particular form of 'learning analytics'. It is important also to be very clear that more is involved than a reductive, technicist notion at the level of the individual child and their family if researchers are going to agree on using 'digital literacy' as a label, as a subject around which to focus debate. One argument elsewhere (Potter & McDougall, 2017) has been that labelling like this inevitably underlines unreal divisions in the locus of investigation and debate with other domains, such as 'media literacy'. The term 'dynamic' in relation to literacy appears to offer more in terms of keeping in play the notion of churn and change and anchoring that with the ever-constant need to make meaning in the world anchored by the use of the word 'literacies' after it. It needs to be a key component of what is understood when talking about 'digital literacy'.

References

Bhabha, H. (1994). *The location of culture*. London: Routledge.

Bradbury, A. (2019). Datafied at four: The role of data in the 'schoolification' of early childhood education in England. *Learning, Media and Technology*, 44(1), 7–21.

Bradbury, A., & Roberts-Holmes, G. (2017). Creating an Ofsted story: The role of early years assessment data in schools' narratives of progress. *British Journal of Sociology of Education*, 38(7), 943–955.

Buckingham, D. (2007). *Beyond technology: Children's learning in the age of digital culture*. London: Routledge.

Burn, A., & Richards, C. (Eds.). (2014). *Children's games in the new media age: Childlore, media and the playground*. Farnham: Ashgate.

Burnett, C. (2016). *The digital age and its implications for learning and teaching in the primary school*. York: Cambridge Primary Review Trust.

Burnett, C., Davies, J., Merchant, G., & Rowsell, J. (Eds.). (2014). *New literacies around the globe*. London: Routledge.

Burnett, C., & Merchant, G. (2014). Points of view: Reconceptualising literacies through an exploration of adult and child interactions in a virtual world. *Journal of Research in Reading*, 37(1), 36–50. doi:10.1111/jrir.12006/

Cannon, M. (2018). *Digital media in education: Teaching, learning and literacy practices with young learners*. London: Palgrave Macmillan.

Cope, B., & Kalantzis, M. (Eds.). (2000). *Multiliteracies: Literacy learning and the design of social futures*. New York: Routledge.

Cowan, K., & Kress, G. (2017). Documenting and transferring meaning in the multimodal world: Reconsidering "transcription". In F. Serafini & E. Gee (Eds.), *Remixing multiliteracies* (pp. 50–61). New York: Teachers College Press.

DigiLitEY. (2018). DigiLitEy website – "About" page. Retrieved from: http://digilitey.eu/about [Access date: Feb 1st 2019].

Flewitt, R., Kucirkova, N., & Messer, D. (2014). Touching the virtual, touching the real: IPads and enabling literacy for students experiencing disability. *Australian Journal of Language and Literacy*, 37(2), 107–117.

Flewitt, R., Jones, P., Potter, J., Domingo, M., Collins, P., Munday, E., & Stenning, K. (2017). "I enjoyed it because . . . you could do whatever you wanted and be creative": Three principles for participatory research and pedagogy. *International Journal of Research & Method in Education*, 41(4), 1–15.

Gee, J. P. (2015). *Literacy and education*. London: Routledge.

Gillen, J. (2014). *Digital literacies*. London: Routledge.

Gutierrez, K. (2008). Developing a sociocultural literacy in the third space. *Reading Research Quarterly*, 43(2), 48–164.

Kress, G. (2003). *Literacy in the new media age*. London: Routledge.

Law, J. (2004). *After method: Mess in social science research*. London: Routledge.

Lievrouw, L. H., & Livingstone, S. (Eds.). (2006). *The Handbook of new media (updated student edition)*. London: Sage.

LSE. (2018). Parenting for a digital future – About this blog. Retrieved from: http://blogs.lse.ac.uk/parenting4digitalfuture/about/about-this-blog [Access date June 1st 2018].

MakEY. (2018). Makerspaces in the early years: Enhancing digital literacy and creativity. Retrieved from: http://makeyproject.eu [Access date: Feb 1st 2019].

Marsh, J. (Ed.). (2004). *Popular culture, new media and digital literacy in early childhood*. London: Routledge.

Moll, L. C., Amanti, C., Neff, D., & Gonzalez, N. (1992). Funds of knowledge for teaching: Using a qualitative approach to connect homes and classrooms. *Theory into Practice*, 31(2), 132–141.

OFCOM. (2018). Children and parents: Media use and attitudes report. London: OFCOM Retrieved from: www.ofcom.org.uk [Access date Feb 12th 2019].

Opie, I., & Opie, P. (1954). *The lore and language of schoolchildren*. Oxford: Oxford University Press.

Pahl, K. (2003). Children's text-making at home: Transforming meaning across modes. In C. Jewitt & G. Kress (Eds.), *Multimodal literacy* (pp. 139–154). New York: Peter Lang.

Pahl, K. (2006). An inventory of traces: Children's photographs of their toys in three London homes. *Visual Communication*, 5(95), 95–114.

Parry, B. (2013). *Children, film and literacy*. London: Palgrave Macmillan.

Playing the Archive. (2018). Playing the Archive: "About the project" pages. Retrieved from: https://playingthearchive.net/about [Access date: Feb 1st 2019].

Potter, J. (2011). New literacies, new practices and learner research: Across the semi-permeable membrane between home and school. *Lifelong Learning in Europe*, XVI(3), 22–35.

Potter, J. (2012). *Digital media and learner identity: The new curatorship*. New York: Palgrave Macmillan.

Potter, J. (2014). Co-curating children's play cultures. In A. Burn & C. Richards (Eds.), *Children's games in the new media age: Childlore, media and the playground* (pp. 187–206). London: Palgrave Macmillan.

Potter, J., & Bryer, T. (2016). "Finger flowment" and moving image language: Learning film making with tablet devices. In B. Parry, C. Burnett, & G. Merchant (Eds.), *Literacy, media, technology: Past, present and future* (pp. 111–128). London: Bloomsbury.

Potter, J., & McDougall, J. (2017). *Digital media, culture and education: Theorising third space literacies*. London: Palgrave Macmillan/Springer.

Rowsell, J. (2013). *Working with multimodality: Rethinking literacy in a digital age*. Abingdon: Routledge.

Selwyn, N., Potter, J., & Cranmer, S. (2010). *Primary ICT: Learning from learner perspectives*. London: Continuum.

Serafini, F., & Gee, E. (Eds.). (2017). *Remixing multiliteracies: Theory and practice from new London to new times*. New York: Teachers College Press.

Sonck, N., Livingstone, S., Kuiper, E., & de Haan, J. (2011). *Digital literacy and safety skills*. London: EU Kids Online, London School of Economics & Political Science.

Street, B. (2003). What's 'new' in new literacy studies? Critical approaches to literacy in theory and practice. *Current Issues in Comparative Education*, 5(2), 77–91.

UNESCO. (2016). Literacy. Retrieved from: www.unesco.org/new/en/education/themes/education-building-blocks/literacy [Access Date June 1st 2018].

Willett, R. (2014). Remixing children's cultures: Media-referenced play on the playground. In A. Burn & C. Richards (Eds.), *Children's games in the new media age: Childlore, media and the playground* (pp. 132–152). Farnham: Ashgate.

Williamson, B. (2017). *Big data in education: The digital future of learning, policy and practice*. London: Sage.

25

BEING AND NOT BEING

'Digital Tweens' in a Hybrid Culture

Inês Vitorino Sampaio, Thinayna Máximo, and Cristina Ponte

Introduction

In Latin America, Brazil has the greatest number of children and adolescents aged 9–16 who access social networks (Pavez, 2014). Around 24.3 million Brazilian children (9–17) are part of the connected generation (CGI, 2017). By interacting with digital devices, they experience mobility, connectivity, and privatised access to communication, in line with international studies such as EU Kids Online (Livingstone, Haddon, Görzig & Ólafsson, 2011), Net Children Go Mobile (Mascheroni & Cuman, 2014), and Global Kids Online (Byrne, Kardefelt-Winther, Livingstone & Stoilova, 2016). Focussed on pre-teens, this chapter adopts an equivalent theoretical position as those international studies, considering children's and adolescents' rights as well as the opportunities and risks offered by Information and Communication Technologies (ICTs) for children's wellbeing.

Following a sociology of childhood perspective (Corsaro & Eder, 1990; Pasquier, 2008; Sarmento, 2004), children and adolescents are constructed as active agents in the configuration of digital culture, its dynamics and trajectories. They participate within this culture through acts of liking, disliking, posting, and sharing. They are involved through interactive processes which connect and disconnect people and groups, invigorating and/or challenging beliefs, rituals, symbols, values, preferences, etc. In their daily dialogue with adults and peers, either close or distant, entangled in online and offline relationships, children and adolescents learn how to negotiate concepts and practices, permissions and prohibitions, gains and losses. All this makes the experience of living in a digital culture both fascinating and frightening. In the words of Clarissa, aged 11: "the internet is dangerous, but it's nice" (Sampaio & Ponte, 2017).

For those who are transitioning from childhood to adolescence, often referred to as *tweens*, this online universe is especially attractive. The concept of tweens is generally applied to children aged between 8 and 12 years, and has emerged as a marketing tool, as postulated by Abiala and Hernwall (2013). It is understood as a cultural age in which identity issues are intensified, such as who a child is and/or who a child wants to be. This implies an exploratory process of children discovering who they are through their relationships with others and the world around them. The two European surveys, EU Kids Online (2010) and Net Children Go Mobile (2013–2014), confirm this trend: in comparison with the younger age group (9–10 years old), children aged 11–12 years clearly climb a 'ladder of opportunities' as defined by Livingstone and Helper (2008). According to Pruulmann-Vengerfeldt and Runnel (2012), they add communication-based activities (using messages, visiting social networking sites, playing games with others) to the content-based activities they used to do, thus enlarging their experiences of communication with peers and their sources of entertainment.

This chapter discusses how children aged 11–12 participate (or not) within this digital culture, in a country marked by high social inequality and cultural hybridity. After considering the Brazilian tweens that are digitally excluded, it explores how factors such as social inequality affect children participating within digital culture. Reflecting upon the impact of cultural context, the following sections analyse children's digital practices, focussing on their modes of access and on their main activities, especially in relation to message-based social media interactions and YouTube.

Being and Not Being a 'Digital Tween' in Brazil

In the words of poet Tom Jobim, "Brazil is not a country for beginners" (Silva, 2014). The population of Brazil is approximately 208.7 million people, while the country as a whole is divided into five geographical regions (North, Northeast, Midwest, Southeast, and South) (IBGE, 2010, 2018). More than 80% of the population live in urban areas, and the majority identify themselves as Christians (IBGE, 2010, 2018). For many, Brazil is merely associated with Carnival and soccer. However, this "tropical country, blessed by God and beautiful by nature" – words from a song by Jorge Ben Jor (1969) – is also one of the most socially unequal countries in the world. *Mestizos*, Brazilians who are part-white, part-black, and part-Indian, have in their genetic and cultural formation the mark of being mixed, reflecting the genuine encounters and/or the violence that has accompanied the colonising process. Contrary to classifications that try to define the country, Brazil and its people recreate themselves daily in order to survive amid both the advances and backwardness that have marked its history.

In recent years, Brazil has gone from celebrating being a "country for all" – the slogan of the government led by Luís Inácio da Silva – advancing towards a culture that was both inclusive and plural, including in ICT use to a country that was impelled to maintain "order and progress" – the slogan of Michel Temer, who took over the presidency after the coup of 2016; to being seduced by the 2018 presidential campaign slogan of "Brazil above everything, God above all", used by the current president, Jair Messias Bolsonaro. This political change has occurred at the expense of constitutional rights and social protection policies, such as public investments in education and in the *Bolsa Família* Program – two measures that have directly impacted the daily life of Brazilian children and adolescents.

In such an unequal, culturally diverse, and politically unstable country, it is worth noting that 5.2 million children and adolescents are not internet users (CGI, 2017). Of these, the 2.9 million children who have never accessed the web are especially drawn from rural areas in the North and Northeast regions, as well as being of low socioeconomic status (SES). Among this group, 18% of children aged 11–12 are disconnected, and 29% of these have never accessed the web.

Before experiencing the condition of digital exclusion, these children and adolescents were first and foremost excluded from citizenship. Many have been exposed to child labour and/or sexual exploitation, being deprived of access not only to school but also to safe living conditions with basic sanitation and electricity. Some were already living in the streets of the country's cities, as reported by CONANDA (2018), the National Council for Children and Adolescents' Rights. If the 'tween times' are understood as a search for autonomy, in which children still rely on parents to secure survival (Abiala & Hernwall, 2013), being a 'tween' becomes an abstract idea which does not translate to the lived experiences of children who, alone and fending for themselves, have to be accountable for their own survival. With these critical issues in mind, this chapter now considers digitally connected children and adolescents in Brazil.

The adult gaze categorises contemporary children as 'digital natives', in consonance with global marketing discourses that reverberate in Brazilian media, which celebrate children's positioning as 'experts' in technology. Research has suggested, though, that the relation of children and adolescents to digital culture is much more complex, being also contingent on factors such as SES, gender, religion, region, interest groups and/or belonging (Livingstone & Haddon, 2009). Such factors engender different forms of access and appropriation of ICTs by children, challenging the notion that 'digital natives' know how to use them competently and critically in an intuitive way. By highlighting social inequalities and cultural trends, this chapter explores and analyses how these disparities are present in Brazilian adolescents' online practices concerning both digital access and use.

Methodological Procedures

Since 2012, the ICT historical series *ICT Kids Online Brazil*, overseen by the Brazilian Internet Steering Committee (CGI.Br), has offered a robust statistical database. The depth and breadth of this resource allows a longitudinal analysis of ICT access by children aged 9 to 17 years. The quantitative research follows the conceptual and methodological models of the European network EU Kids Online (Livingstone, Mascheroni, & Staksrud, 2015), which has the goal of identifying the risks and opportunities represented by the relationship between children and the internet. As with other CGI studies, the *ICT Kids Online Brazil* reports are available online.

The analysis presented here is based on two kinds of data:

1. Statistical data from the historical series of *ICT Kids Online Brazil*, particularly the results collected in 2016, which involved 2,999 children. According to the data collection procedures, children's answers were collected through two structured questionnaires; one was interviewer-administered and the other, which included sensitive questions, was self-completed. The five economic strata classifications (classes A, B, C, D, and E) were here combined into high SES (A and B), middle SES (C), and low SES (D and E) for data analysis and cross-country comparability.
2. Recent qualitative studies that investigate Brazilian pre-teens and digital culture (Ferreira, 2018; Máximo, 2017; Monteiro, 2018; Rezende, 2017; Sampaio & Ponte, 2017; Tomaz, 2017). These studies use and combine distinct approaches: ethnographic observation of children's environments of media use, focus groups and interviews. The authors of this chapter conducted some of these studies, while others were identified through databases of Brazilian academic research. Qualitative data were explored through thematic axes that considered children's practices and reports on their digital experience. Children's testimonials were extracted from these studies.

This dialogue between two different kinds of data is productive: the qualitative approach not only contributes to identifying contextual issues that affect children's access to and use of the internet; it is also important to account for process and cultural aspects hidden in the quantitative results produced through the historical series and statistically controlled procedures.

Ways of Accessing the Internet

This section demonstrates what quantitative data can show, and also what it can hide. More issues regarding internet access are visible than the ones revealed in statistics. In addition, qualitative data also show children' strategies for participating in and shaping digital culture in the context of inequality.

As the historical series of *ICT Kids Online* reveal, the smartphone has become the main device used by children and adolescents to access the internet, increasing from 21% in 2012 to 91% in 2016. In contrast, use of other devices for accessing the internet decreases as a child's age increases. Among the age group ranging from 11 to 12 years, 87% use the smartphone to access the internet, compared with 83% of children aged 9 and 10. When considering the use of smartphones by children aged 11 to 12, the data associated with family income do not suggest significant differences: 91% of high SES, 86% of medium SES, and 86% of low SES children use this digital device. The income variable negatively impacted children's and adolescents' access to other devices such as tablets and desktop computers, however.

While quantitative data reveals little difference in children's access to smartphones, qualitative research suggests singularities in such access. Shared use of smartphones is associated with low SES children in this age group. Given that mobility trends identified in European studies such as Net Children Go Mobile (2014) suggest a more individualised use of the smartphone and greater autonomy by children and adolescents (Vincent, 2015), Brazilian studies from Monteiro (2018), Ferreira (2018), Rezende (2017), and Máximo (2017) indicate a shared use of devices by children living in marginalised contexts. Reflecting the low purchasing power of families who are unable to provide individual devices for their children, children aged 11–12 from low SES families share smartphones with their parents or siblings. This aspect has not been adequately investigated in quantitative research.

The shared use of smartphones has implications for children's digital access and use. One is the reduction of privacy, since parents can access the content shared by their children. To deal with this situation, some children use strategies like deleting messages. Monalisa, aged 12, reported: "I delete the conversations so she [the mother] can't see". This situation may also have implications for parental mediation practices. Since parents can easily access children's digital content, they may engage in more direct mediation. Melody, aged 11, shares the smartphone with her mother and reported: "sometimes she tells me to take down some pictures" (Máximo, 2017).

Just as parents can access the content generated by their children, children can also view content exchanged by parents or older siblings, at times leading to situations in which they have viewed inappropriate content. A seven-year-old boy, for example, saw pornography when he accessed his mother's smartphone since she had an account designated for adults over 18 years (Ferreira, 2018). Children's limited access to and use of smartphones was also reported. Lis, aged 11, stated that she shares her smartphone and Facebook account with her 15-year-old sister. However, Lis is not allowed to post online, she can only see her sister's profile (Máximo, 2017).

Mobility trends associated with the use of smartphones are also representative of SES in Brazil. Although the smartphone is the main device used by children aged 11 and 12, their mobile access to the internet (24%) is significantly lower than access from other people's places (79%) and from their own homes (77%). Indeed, children's access to the internet is predominantly via wi-fi (80%), which demands a broadband connection, something still inaccessible to many poorer families. Access to the internet at home is common for those from high SES (98%), while those from low SES typically access the internet from other people's places (82%). Mirela, from the outskirts of Fortaleza (a Northeast region), aged 12, said "Sometimes I use my uncle's wi-fi" (Máximo, 2017).

Since access to a high-bandwidth connection is not a reality for many Brazilian households and public schools, children report a particular strategy for accessing the network: they discover other people's wi-fi passwords. In the words of Emilia, aged 11: "my cousin spent all day trying to figure out the password from our neighbour. He discovered it and gave it to us. But the neighbour didn't know" (Sampaio & Ponte, 2017). This conduct, in which the child circumvents adult rules and may experience risky situations, reflects contextual conditions of social inequality affecting children. It also reveals how children of this age may feel pressured to achieve connectivity, a phenomenon increasingly reported by children and adolescents around the world (Mascheroni & Ólafsson, 2014).

In an environment where 'connectivity imperative' is increasingly important, 62% of Brazilians aged 11 to 12 access the internet more than once per day. Some children mentioned their difficulty in controlling the time they spend online, signalling the risk of excessive use. Mateus, a middle-class boy aged 11, says: "you spend too much time on your cell phone, then you can't have control between cell phone and study" (Sampaio & Ponte, 2017). In this regard, when analysed in terms of SES, results indicate a greater proportion of tweens from high SES accessing the internet more than once a day (77%) in comparison with tweens from low SES (42%).

Considering the balance between opportunity and risk, children from low-income families are theoretically less exposed to the risk of internet overuse but may have fewer opportunities due to their limited access. Neymar, aged 11, reports:

> I have to work with my father to make money for me. If I do not win, there's no way I can see YouTube. I did not pay the guy there when I played [at the LAN (local area network) house], but I'm going to pay. I owe [him].
>
> *(Monteiro, 2018)*

However, some lower SES children may also be at risk of internet overuse, as factors other than income influence this process: "I spend 90% of my time on the internet", said a boy from a low SES family (Sampaio & Cavalcante, 2016).

While it is difficult to measure accurately how much time children and adolescents spend on the internet, it is possible to identify the main online activities, as discussed in the following section.

Children's Digital Experiences

Contacting and Curating

According to *ICT Kids Online* 2016, the most frequent online activities of Brazilian children aged 11 to 12 were instant messaging (39%), using social media (35%), and watching videos (27%), followed by researching topics of their interest (18%), playing games (15%), and doing school activities (10%). Activities related to content creation and civic participation are present in low or even residual values. Thus, communication stands out as the most prevalent daily online practice for Brazilian children, surpassing activities related to entertainment which is the trend in other countries, as shown by Haddon and Vincent (2014).

Six out of ten Brazilian children aged 11 to 12 use instant messaging applications such as WhatsApp, one of the most popular applications used in the country. With this app, children can usually interact more freely with peers and keep the messages exchanged private, i.e., away from adults' surveillance: "because those are my conversations with my friends, I don't like her [mother] to see them", says Melody, aged 12 (Máximo, 2017). As considered previously, this is not always possible for children from low SES families who have to share their phone use.

Connected with their peers through WhatsApp, children collaborate on processes of self-discovery and of finding out about the world, negotiating identities and belongings. The application can be integrated with social networking sites, thus facilitating content sharing, especially of visual material. For tweens, the impacts of body changes of adolescence are intensified with media use, with significant implications for identity processes. The act of sharing self-images in peer groups becomes a recurring practice in this age group (Abiala & Hernwall, 2013). The exposition of the 'perfect body' is reinforced by both colonial and patriarchal traditions in Brazil, which are actualised in the objectification of the feminine body through advertising or Carnival pictures that circulate around the world.

Tween girls especially report the practice of digitally curating their appearance through media representations. That is, they use strategies such as sharing, evaluating, and selecting previous photos through WhatsApp. Those images are then exposed in wider groups and on social media such as Facebook. "Sometimes I show it to my friends, then they tell me to post that one", says Mirela, aged 12 (Máximo, 2017). Thus, WhatsApp is used for the performance of being digitally curated by peers, aimed at achieving peer recognition – that is, receiving *likes* in Facebook.

Since being accepted by friends is a key part of peer culture (Corsaro, 2011; Pasquier, 2008), the process of curating their appearance, especially for tween-aged girls, is in line with the centrality of body culture in Brazil. From a contextual point of view, it also reveals the unequal pressure experienced by Brazilian girls to conform to certain body models that do not reflect their *mestizo* and diverse constitutions. In some situations, body exposure becomes a bargaining chip to get likes on posts and followers on channels such as Gemeas.com where, for example, teenagers dance and sing funk music with appealing lyrics (Monteiro, 2018). Mirela, aged 11, indicates the type of photos that are most appreciated: "it is the ones with bikini because people give more likes and enjoy them more" (Máximo, 2017).

In line with Brazilian digital users in general, children at this age are active users of social media (76%). Their participation on platforms such as Facebook and Instagram is performed mainly through photos and/or videos posted about daily situations. While some are curated, others are often published instantly. Such continuous exposition tends to contribute to the maintenance of peer relationships (boyd, 2014).

As previously considered, while sharing online content through their profiles on social media, young people are not always aware of who is watching their online performances. Depending on the privacy configuration selected, their self-presentation may be accessible to the broader public. Many times, tweens deal with what is, effectively, an invisible audience, since not all users are visible when they post their online information. In this type of self-exposition, malicious comments posted on the network may cause harm and embarrassment, due to harassment, regardless of any physical contact with strangers. Gabi, 11 years old, says: "once a guy posted it like this ... I'm ashamed to say [it] ... he said so 'this one should be very good in bed'" (Máximo, 2017). Malicious comments are prevalent on public profiles, which is the largest group of profiles used by Brazilian children aged 11–12 (42%). Even when configuring their profiles to be private (33%) or partially private (6%), tweens still connect with a high number of friends on social media. National data indicates that one out of five children in this age group has between 101 and 300 friends on their contact lists on social media, a high amount when compared with other countries (CGI, 2017; Sozio et al., 2015).

Generalised narratives about Brazilian people are multiplied through numerous binomials: 'feminist and antifeminist', 'catholics and protestants', 'southern and north-eastern', 'white and black', 'fascist and revolutionary', among many others. In dialogue with such terms, collectivities, communities, and movements are formed, either conforming to the established order or promoting resistance. On the internet, social networking sites, particularly WhatsApp, are active vehicles for circulating such information. These general tensions and conflicting messages become manifest in children's experience of the digital world. As such, having access to the internet, Brazilian children also have access to hate speech and intolerance. In 2016 41% of Brazilian children reported having seen, at some point in the previous twelve months, someone suffering discrimination as a result of skin colour and race (24%), physical appearance (16%), or sexual orientation (13%). Body image and homophobia stand out as important cultural elements around which othering and discrimination processes take place.

By contrast, it is worth highlighting that Brazilian children use social networks within 'communities of belonging', 'movements' and/or 'collectivities' which are structured not only in terms of personal interests and affinities, but also around shared projects. The experiences of boys and girls from *Fundação Casa Grande*, in Ceara (Barbalho, 2010), and *Movimento Sem Terrinha*, affiliated with *Movimento Sem Terra* (Ravena, 2015), are examples of these communities. To a lesser extent, these forms of social media have also allowed the emergence of a counterpoint to the hegemonic discourses of mainstream media.

Producing Popularity and Audiences around Consumption

Besides accessing social networking sites, many Brazilian children aged 11–12 mentioned watching online videos on platforms such as YouTube. Though this has not yet been explored through quantitative audience research, videos from YouTubers have stood out as important digital products in qualitative research on children's media consumption (Tomaz, 2017). Entertainment videos, such as music, movies, and YouTubers' videos, was the content most likely to be accessed (Rezende, 2017; Sampaio & Ponte, 2017). According to the mapping made by the ESPM Lab of the 100 channels most viewed on YouTube in Brazil, 48 offered content for children (Corrêa, 2016). The data also revealed that in 2016 230 national channels targeting children had more than 52 billion views.

In a country of *mestizos*, the most popular YouTuber children are white, southeastern pre-adolescents (8–14 years old) from middle-income families (Tomaz, 2017). Often, the production of their videos is sophisticated, with the use of editing, lighting, and other professional techniques contributing to their channels' popularity and dissemination (Marôpo, Sampaio & Miranda, 2017). Famous YouTubers are usually managed by specialised agencies and maintain a close – but not always transparent – connection with the brands they advertise. In their videos, some child YouTubers display expensive products, trips abroad, glamorous and luxurious rooms, and, in a number of cases, the celebration of ostentation (Rezende, 2017). For the millions of Brazilian children living in poverty (61% of this age group, according to the UNICEF report, 2018), engaging with such videos is to face the evidence of social inequality and disparity. Yet YouTubers' products also provide a platform for the possibility of ascending to a higher social position in the symbolic sphere. While some poor children entertain themselves by consuming videos of countless products, others are amused by watching others' consumption of such products (Monteiro, 2018). Thus, disadvantaged tweens virtually exploit a world that is, in fact, inaccessible to them.

There is a contrast between the more homely productions of children from the periphery and the glamorous productions of more privileged children who have already achieved celebrity status (Miranda, 2017). Celebrities offer guidance to their followers on 'How to become a successful YouTuber', encouraging them not to give up on that dream through the courses, books, and videos that celebrities package and sell. The most common recipe for success that guides the performance of children in these two different worlds is, however, the same: the construction of narratives around consumption.

By watching these videos, children and young people are exposed to a form of marketing communication, which is present both in the advertising that precedes the video and in the video itself, disguised in the YouTubers' testimonies, unboxings, reviews, and so on. In 2016, 69% of the *ICT Kids Online* respondents aged 11 to 17 reported having seen advertising on video-sharing websites. This figure is 63% for children aged 11 and 12 (CGI, 2017). As a young boy from São Paulo said, advertising is everywhere on the internet, "on every website; on almost all of them, [advertising] appears" (Sampaio & Cavalcante, 2016). This situation happens despite the Brazilian legal framework which defines marketing communication directed at children as abusive and, in effect, illegal (Nunes Junior & Souza, 2016).

Finally, it is worth noting that some videos presented on child YouTuber channels promote and justify widespread discrimination as being merely a 'joke'. This is the case of the *Rich versus*

Poor YouTuber Kid playlists cited by Monteiro (2018), in which children are encouraged to trivialise social inequality and even laugh at the differences it creates.

Conclusion

As evidenced by quantitative data, many findings from the Global North, such as the trends towards connectivity, mobility, and privacy (Mascheroni & Cuman, 2014), are also confirmed in the Brazilian context. However, this superficial equivalence is challenged by the nuance offered in qualitative studies and it is further complicated by factors associated with social inequality. Although the majority of the 11–12 age group is connected, as in the Global North, children from low SES families are more likely to suffer precarious connections, via smartphone use without data support, dependence on wi-fi, and through sharing devices with family members. For many children, intermittent connection is the only option. Such restrictions have implications for children's experiences of mobility and for their right to privacy. Brazilian children's access to the internet is often impacted by restricted connectivity within their own household, while their use of a smartphone is frequently shared with others. This type of shared use, associated with social inequality, may provide opportunities for direct parental mediation. Even so, it also increases the likelihood of children's access to inappropriate content, affecting their privacy and limiting their online experiences, via time restrictions, limited access to platforms, freedom to post, etc. Undoubtedly the dynamics of shared use require further investigation.

Within the market logic of global digital culture, Brazilian children find new possibilities for self-expression in digital space, and these opportunities are evident in studies that discuss the digital participation of child YouTubers. Despite a legal prohibition on marketing to children, Brazilian tweens – including those from very low SES families – watch videos that celebrate the consumption of brands, products, and lifestyles produced by rich middle-class children.

Framed as entertainment and treated as jokes, class and gender biases are also disseminated through digital content. Children are exposed to hate speech which targets, above all, body characteristics (colour and race), and appearance. In this context, digitally curating one's self-representation, especially among girls, reveals the unequal social pressures manifest by girls when compared with boys. These imperatives to conform to certain body types do not reflect the *mestizo* reality. Instead, they are aligned with the emphasis upon the body within Brazilian culture, and tweens risk using their bodies as bargaining chips to get likes in posts and to attract followers on YouTuber channels.

In sum, apart from the high number of Brazilian children that are still digitally excluded, preteens with internet access in different conditions experiment, play, circumvent rules, and trust each other to deal with market and societal pressures, such as the imperative to be beautiful, rich, famous, intelligent, and competitive. While these values conform to the dominant market logic, pressures to live up to these unrealistic expectations are exacerbated by the high levels of inequality characterising Brazil as a South-American country that identifies with the Global South. The challenges faced by Brazilian children in terms of digital risks and opportunities highlight the relevance of specific cultural processes associated with reducing the impact of social inequality in promoting children's rights in digital contexts.

References

Abiala, K., & Hernwall, P. (2013). Tweens negotiating identity online – Swedish girls' and boys' reflections on online experiences. *Journal of Youth Studies, 16*(8), 951–969. doi:10.1080/13676261.2013.780124.

Barbalho, A. (2010). Meninas, meninos e suas políticas: Ideias e práticas midiáticas da Fundação Casa Grande [Girls, boys and their policies: Ideas and media practices from the Casa Grande Foundation]. *Intercom – Revista Brasileira de Ciências da Comunicação [Brazilian Journal of Communication Sciences], 33*(2), 87–102. doi:10.1590/rbcc.v33i2.594.

boyd, d. (2014). *It's Complicated: The social lives of networked teens*. New Haven: Yale University Press.

Byrne, J., Kardefelt-Winther, D., Livingstone, S., & Stoilova, M. (2016). *Global kids online research synthesis, 2015–2016*. UNICEF Office of Research Innocenti and LSE. Retrieved from: https://unicef-irc.org/research/270.

CGI, Brazilian Internet Steering Committee. (2017). *Survey on internet use by children in Brazil – ICT kids online*. São Paulo. Retrieved from: https://cetic.br/tics/kidsonline/2016/criancas.

Co-nanda. National Council for the Rights of Children and Adolescents. (2018). *Migrados: Pesquisa do Conanda revela as condições de vida de crianças e adolescentes em situação de rua* [Migrants: Conanda research reveals the live conditions of street children and adolescents]. Retrieved from: www.direitosdacrianca.gov.br.

Corrêa, L. (2016) *Geração YouTube: Um mapeamento sobre o consumo e a produção infantil de vídeos para crianças de zero a 12 anos* [YouTube Generation: Mapping video production and consumption for children from 0 to 12 years old]. Retrieved from: https://criancaeconsumo.org.br/biblioteca/geracao-youtube-um-mapeamento-sobre-o-consumo-e-a-producao-de-videos-por-criancas.

Corsaro, W. A. (2011). *The sociology of childhood*. Los Angeles: Pine Forge Press.

Corsaro, W. A., & Eder, D. (1990). Children's peer cultures. *Annual Review of Sociology, 16*, 197–220. doi:10.1146/annurev.so.16.080190.001213.

Ferreira, M. (2018). *Infância (n)ativa: Potencialidades de participação e cidadania às crianças na mídia digital* [(N) active childhood: Potentialities of participation and citizenship to children on digital media] (Doctoral dissertation, Universidade Estadual Paulista, São Paulo, Brazil). Retrieved from: https://repositorio.unesp.br/handle/11449/157357.

Haddon, L., & Vincent, J. (Eds.). (2014). *Net children go mobile: European children and their carers' understanding of use, risks and safety issues relating to convergent mobile media* (Report No. D4.1). Milan, Italy: Unicatt. Retrieved from: http://eprints.lse.ac.uk/id/eprint/60147.

IBGE, Brazilian Institute of Geography and Statistics. (2010). *Atlas of the demographic census 2010*. Retrieved from: https://ww2.ibge.gov.br/home/estatistica/populacao/censo2010/default_atlas.shtm.

IBGE, Brazilian Institute of Geography and Statistics. (2018). *Population projection of Brazil and of the Federation units*. Retrieved from: www.ibge.gov.br/apps/populacao/projecao.

Jor, J. (1969). País Tropical. On *País Tropical*. Retrieved from: https://open.spotify.com/album/3V3XJ3Sh62jPUYUMSQ1Tsf?highlight=spotify:track:4877bJ149OUJZHTiU5Jg8P.

Livingstone, S., & Haddon, L. (Eds.). (2009). *Kids online: Opportunities and risks for children*. Bristol, UK: Policy Press.

Livingstone, S., Haddon, L., Görzig, A., & Ólafsson, K. (2011). *Risks and safety on the internet: The perspective of European children. Full findings*. London, UK: EU Kids Online. Retrieved from: http://eprints.lse.ac.uk/33731.

Livingstone, S., & Helsper, E. J. (2008). Parental mediation of children's internet use. *Journal of Broadcasting & Electronic Media, 52*(4), 581–599. doi:10.1080/08838150802437396.

Livingstone, S., Mascheroni, G., & Staksrud, E. (2015). *Developing a framework for researching children's online risks and opportunities in Europe*. London, UK: EU Kids Online. Retrieved from: http://eprints.lse.ac.uk/64470.

Marôpo, L., Sampaio, I. V., & Miranda, N. P. D. (2017). Top girls on YouTube: Identity, participation, and consumption. In I. Eleá & L. Mikos (Eds.), *Young & creative: Digital technologies empowering children in everyday life* (pp. 65–76). Gothenburg: Nordicom.

Mascheroni, G., & Cuman, A. (2014). *Net children go mobile: Final report: Deliverables D6.4 and D5.2*. Milan, Italy: Educatt. Retrieved from: http://eprints.lse.ac.uk/60231.

Mascheroni, G., & Ólafsson, K. (2014). *Net children go mobile: Risks and opportunities*. Milan, Italy: Educatt. Retrieved from: http://eprints.lse.ac.uk/60231.

Máximo, T. M. (2017). *Público ou privado?: A compreensão de crianças cearenses sobre privacidade online*. [Public or private? How children from Ceará understand online privacy] (Master's thesis, Universidade Federal do Ceara, Brazil). Retrieved from: www.repositorio.ufc.br/handle/riufc/31440.

Miranda, N. P. D. (2017). *Beijos monstruosos e eletrizantes: Os direitos à provisão, à proteção e à participação no canal de Julia Silva no YouTube* [Monstrous and electrifying kisses: The rights to provision, protection and participation in Julia Silva's YouTube channel] (Master's thesis, Universidade Federal do Ceará, Brazil). Retrieved from: www.repositorio.ufc.br/handle/riufc/34463.

Monteiro, M. C. (2018). *Apropriação por crianças da publicidade em canais de YouTubers brasileiros: A promoção do consumo no YouTube através da publicidade de experiência* [Children's appropriation of advertising in Brazilian YouTubers channels: Promoting consumption on YouTube through experience advertising] (Doctoral dissertation, Universidade Federal do Rio Grande do Sul, Brazil). Retrieved from: https://lume.ufrgs.br/bitstream/handle/10183/189071/001087498.pdf?sequence=1&isAllowed=y.

Nunes Junior, V. S., & Souza, A. C. de (2016). A discussão legal da publicidade comercial dirigida ao público infantil [The legal discussion of commercial advertising aimed at children]. In L. Fontenelle (Ed.), *Criança e consumo: 10 anos de transformação [Children and consumption: 10 years of transformation]* (pp. 342–352). São Paulo, Brazil: Instituto Alana.

Pasquier, D. (2008). From parental control to peer pressure: Cultural transmission and conformism. In K. Drotner & S. Livingstone (Eds.), *The International Handbook of Children, Media and Culture* (pp. 448–459). London, UK: Sage.

Pavez, M. I. (2014). *Los derechos de la Infancia en la era de internet: América Latina y las nuevas tecnologías [Children's rights in the internet era: Latin America and new technologies]*. Santiago, Chile: United Nations – CEPAL.

Pruulmann-Vengerfeldt, P., & Runnel, P. (2012). Online opportunities. In S. Livingstone, L. Haddon, & A. Gorzig (Eds.), *Children, risk and safety on the Internet* (pp. 73–85). Bristol, UK: Policy Press.

Ravena, M. (2015, July). Os Sem-terrinha: Uma história da luta social no Brasil [The landless children: A history of social struggle in Brazil]. The XXVII Simpósio Nacional de História, Florianópolis: ANPUH. Retrieved from: www.repositorio.ufc.br/handle/riufc/7096.

Rezende, A. S. B. (2017). *Entre o olhar da pobreza e o som da ostentação: Os imaginários do consumo na construção midiática da infância na cena musical do funk ostentação [Between the poverty look and the ostentation sound: Imaginary of consumption in the media construction of childhood by the funk music]* (Master's thesis, Escola Superior de Propaganda e Marketing, São Paulo, Brazil). Retrieved from: http://tede2.espm.br/handle/tede/260#preview-link0.

Sampaio, I. V., & Cavalcante, A. P. (2016). *Publicidade infantil em tempos de convergência* [Children advertising in times of convergence]. Retrieved from: www.defesadoconsumidor.gov.br/portal/biblioteca/93-conteudos-diversos/190-relatorio-grim-pesquisa-sobre-publicidade-infantil-ines-vitorino.

Sampaio, I. V., & Ponte, C. (2017). *Relatório técnico da pesquisa TIC Kids Online Brasil-Portugal* [Technical report of the ICT Kids Online Brazil-Portugal Research]. Retrieved from Research Gate: www.researchgate.net/publication/328963769.

Sarmento, M. J. (2004). As culturas da infância nas encruzilhadas da 2ª modernidade [Childhood cultures in the crossroads of second modernity]. In M. J. Sarmento & A. B. Cerisara (Eds.), *Crianças e miúdos: Perspectivas sociopedagógicas da infância e educação [Children and the little ones: Socio-pedagogical perspectives of childhood and education]* (pp. 9–34). Porto, Portugal: Asa Editores.

Silva, D. da (2014). *De onde vêm as palavras: Origens e curiosidades da língua portuguesa [Where the words come from: Origins and curiosities of the Portuguese language]*. Rio de Janeiro, Brazil: Lexikon Editora Digital.

Sozio, M. E., Ponte, C., Sampaio, I. V., Senne, F., Ólafsson, K., Alves, S. J., & Garroux, C. (2015). *Children and internet use: A comparative analysis of Brazil and seven European countries*. London, UK: EU Kids Online. Retrieved from: www.lse.ac.uk/media@lse/research/EUKidsOnline/EU%20Kids%20III/Reports/FullReportBrazilNCGM.pdf?fbclid=IwAR0xLxqbDVVQa8WpK99Zo6fuS0Hj0fhHXjuwOCuC2mnSBgj65giFUozdA0I.

Tomaz, R. (2017). *O que você vai ser antes de crescer: Youtubers, infância e celebridade* [What you will be before you grow up: Youtubers, childhood and celebrity] (Doctoral dissertation, Universidade Federal do Rio de Janeiro, Brazil). Retrieved from: www.compos.org.br/data/arquivos_premio_anual/trabalhos_arquivo_4ZYHAXG1IPTLCLUWYHZY_627__29_01_2018_09_15_17.pdf.

UNICEF United Nations Children's Fund. (2018). *Pobreza na infância e na adolescência* [Childhood and adolescent poverty]. Retrieved from: www.unicef.org/brazil/media/156/file/Pobreza_na_Infancia_e_na_Adolescencia.pdf.

Vincent, J. (2015). *Mobile opportunities: Exploring positive mobile opportunities for European children*. London, UK: LSE-Polis Journalism and Society. Retrieved from: http://eprints.lse.ac.uk/61015.

26

"TECHNICALLY THEY'RE YOUR CREATIONS, BUT..."

Children Making, Playing, and Negotiating User-Generated Content Games

Sara M. Grimes and Vinca Merriman

Introduction

From creating house rules for *Monopoly*, to constructing elaborate make-believe play scenarios, making (and modifying) games has long been a core part of children's cultural experience, as well as a key site for children's learning, socialisation, and development (Evaldsson & Corsaro, 1998; Gussin Paley, 2004). The emergence of child-friendly digital games centred around user-generated content (UGC) and do-it-yourself game design (herein referred to as 'UGC games') introduces important new forums for children to shape their *digital* play in much the same way (Fields & Grimes, 2017; Willet et al., 2009). Like other forms of making, children's game design (i.e., game design activities undertaken *by* children) is currently a popular topic among educators, child advocates, and policymakers (Kafai & Burke, 2015). It is also the focus of a burgeoning market niche. UGC games extend traditional practices into the digital world, but they are also unique, in that they enable children to publish their game ideas at a mass level (e.g., Comunello & Mulargia, 2015). They are thus part of an unprecedented cultural development, in which children are increasingly assuming the roles of producers, authors, and designers of their own media and popular culture.

While UGC games offer promising opportunities, they also introduce new challenges. As commercial products, many UGC games resituate children's creativity within a quasi-public context that is corporately controlled and market-driven (Grimes, 2014). This raises complex questions about children's cultural rights (including fair use and freedom of expression), access (who is included/excluded in the games' designs and marketing), and the responsibilities of the game companies providing these new participatory spaces for children. To date, however, most of the research on children's UGC games has focussed on educational applications and outcomes (e.g., Niemeyer & Gerber, 2015). There are notable gaps in the literature when it comes to the frequency with which different groups of children engage in UGC game design, how children's participation is shaped by the companies who publish UGC games, and what types of games children are creating and sharing with them.

This chapter discusses findings of a recent study aimed at uncovering children's thoughts and experiences of UGC game tools, their opinions about the potential and limitations of these tools, as well as their motivations for creating game content. This chapter focusses on children's understanding of the legal implications of making content in a commercially owned UGC game, and highlights the depth, diversity, and occasional contradictions found within children's knowledge of complex legal concepts like copyright. It argues that there is a need for a deeper integration of legal issues within digital literacy curricula for children, as well as a broader inclusion of children within public discussions of authorship, ownership, and other rights in the digital age.

Literature Review

Easy-to-use customisation tools are now found in a wide range of digital games – from sports titles featuring intricate character creation tools, to first-person shooters containing map and level editors. As in other areas of the digital realm, web 2.0 and participatory culture are prevalent in gaming culture and integral to many game companies' business models and promotional strategies (Banks & Potts, 2010; Young, 2017). Concurrently, several game design programs and engines aimed at non-specialist (or non-professional) users, including children, are now available. This has fuelled a surge in amateur game development and renewed interest in using game design to teach children how to code (Resnick et al., 2009).

The titles referred to here as 'UGC games' lie at the intersection of these two trends – games in which the central focus of activity consists of game making and/or customisation. The games in this category feature 'what you see is what you get' tools and templates that do not require coding or other sophisticated technical skills to use. Instead, players select menu options, click and drag, move and modify, combine and restyle a wide range of objects, features, and mechanics to make original or derivative creations. While many of the titles in this category do include some officially produced content or storylines, they are, for the most part, unstructured and prioritise *player creativity* as the main mode of play. Most contain copyrighted assets – such as characters, set designs, or theme songs – associated with well-known media brands that players can incorporate into their creations for a fee (as purchasable downloadable content, or DLC). The UGC games market is dominated by a handful of high-profile titles, most of which are either targeted to or are inclusive of children. They largely carry ratings that classify them as appropriate for children and feature media brands that are popular among children. Key examples include *Little Big Planet*, *Minecraft*, *Disney Infinity*, *Super Mario Maker*, and *Roblox*.

The rise of UGC games has motivated the formation of vibrant new cultures of practice. It has also attracted a growing body of scholarship, a significant portion of which focusses on the highly popular sandbox game *Minecraft* and its potential benefits for children's learning. For example, Niemeyer and Gerber (2015) propose that *Minecraft* fosters participatory learning. Other scholars emphasise the creative dimensions of *Minecraft*, arguing that its unique combination of 'limitless' tools and building materials, emergent design, and social aspects function as a catalyst for invention (Cipollone et al., 2014; Nguyen, 2016). Absent from much of this literature is a consideration of the commercial and legal relationships that children enter into when they make and share content in *Minecraft* (and other corporately owned titles), and how this might shape their creative process and experience.

Notable exceptions include Willett's (2016) study of the socio-economic contexts of children's literacy relating to *Minecraft*'s business model, in which children were asked how the game makes money, who owns it, and why it contained in-game advertising. Another is Bak's (2016) analysis of *Disney Infinity*'s promotion and adherence to the official 'versions' of well-known Disney characters, and how this emphasis puts discernible constraints on players' creative freedom. Similarly, Grimes (2015) argues that *Little Big Planet*'s closed technical infrastructures 'tether' players and their creations to the game's proprietary system and its associated brand identity. Together, these works cover important ground, providing crucial insight into the educational and political economic dimensions of UGC games. What is missing from the literature to date, however, is a focussed exploration of how these aspects of UGC games overlap, or how they both shape and are shaped by the activities and experiences of the games' players. How do children understand the terms and conditions that are placed on their creativity within commercial UGC games? Does this limit or extend their creative process? What are children's thoughts on who owns and controls the content they make within UGC games, and how do the games in turn contribute to their emerging understandings of authorship?

While very little is known about how children experience these aspects of UGC game making, there *is* a wealth of relevant research to draw upon on the topics of children's creativity (Marsh, 2010), evolving notions of ownership over things and ideas (Shaw et al., 2012), and the benefits of 'remix'-type practices for children's media and digital literacy (Jenkins, 2008). For example, research by Olson and Shaw (2011) challenges the assumption that younger children are unable to grasp complex concepts like intellectual property. Their study found that children as young as six years old made "negative moral evaluations about those who plagiarise as compared to those who produce unique work" (p. 438). Overall, the literature suggests that even young children can have nuanced opinions about key facets of intellectual property, from the ownership of ideas to what makes a work 'original' or derivative. Contrary to traditional child development models, many children develop a very early awareness, and at least a burgeoning understanding, of these concepts. While products aimed at children tend to downplay such processes in their packaging and promotional materials, children are clearly impacted by the business mechanisms and legal rules that shape commercially owned game titles and platforms.

The Current Study

This study builds on the emerging body of academic work examining the political economic dimensions of UGC games and contributes important new insight into the perspectives and experiences of child game makers. Previous research on children's learning and playing in *Minecraft* and other UGC games supports the idea that children engage in important forms of creativity when they make or modify game content in these contexts. Yet, still very little is known about how children experience this form of creative expression, or what feelings of ownership they have over their creations. To fill some of these gaps, the researchers conducted a series of focus groups and interviews with elementary-school-aged children who regularly participate in UGC game making. Data collection was done in the form of a 'game jam'.[1] The children were invited to participate in an afternoon session that interspersed game making with semi-structured interviews, followed by a group-wide show-and-tell, and finally a small group discussion. The methodology was inspired by Gauntlett's (2007) 'creative explorations' approach, which seeks to engage participants in hands-on creative activities through which complex questions can be explored in a participatory and reflexive way. It also drew on child-centric participatory research traditions advanced by new sociology of childhood scholars such as Jenks (2005).

Recruitment

The call for participants aged six to 12 years who "like to make things in *Minecraft*, *Little Big Planet*, *Super Mario Maker* or another video game" was posted to various social media networks, email lists, and blogs, and shared with an intentionally diverse range of children's organisations. A screening survey was conducted over the phone with the parent or caregiver to establish eligibility. Although the researchers strived to include a diverse group of children, most of the participants were recruited through university-related networks and reflected demographic trends common to Canadian university communities, but not to the general population. For instance, all the participants came from households in which at least one parent had (at minimum) an undergraduate education. Despite prolonging the recruitment stage by several weeks in the hopes of reaching gender parity, the researchers failed to recruit an even number of boys (15) and girls (six). Participants did include children of varying ages and several children (7) who were identified by their parent as members of a visible minority/person of colour.

Participants

Participants consisted of 21 children between the ages of six and 12 years.[2] Each participant self-identified as someone who liked making game content. The majority (18) mostly made content in *Minecraft*. However, more than half (13) had also made content in at least one other game. Only three of the participants 'mostly' played a UGC game that was not *Minecraft* (*Super Mario Maker*, *Project Spark*, and *Roblox*, respectively). Experience levels varied, from those who had only 'recently' (i.e., less than one year) started making content in one specific game, to those who had been making content in games for several years, to those who had received formal training in game design. Participants had varying levels of access to digital games in the home: some had strict 'screen time' limits (e.g., one pair of siblings was only allowed two hours per week), while others engaged in 15–18 hours (or more) of UGC game-making on a weekly basis. Some participants rarely shared their creations with anyone, while others frequently shared their work with family and friends. Still others uploaded their creations to online communities or posted videos about them on YouTube. Despite these differences, participants had a shared enthusiasm for game-making that was evident in their responses to researchers' questions, as well as in the regular expressions of excitement and joy displayed during the game jams.

The Game Jams

A total of three standalone game jams were conducted between August and September 2016. Each had seven child participants.[3] Upon arrival, participants were divided into pre-selected teams – three teams of two participants and one researcher, and one team composed of one participant and one researcher.[4] Each participant attended one game-jam session and each session lasted three hours. The game jams were held at the authors' home university, in a spacious multi-purpose room set up in the style of an open concept 'design studio', with a 'design station' assigned to each team.

For the game jams, children were tasked with working together to make (or modify) a game, while the researcher asked questions, took notes, and observed their actions. Each design station included console systems 'pre-loaded' with the UCG games that parents had identified as the ones their child(ren) used most for making games. When the children arrived, the gaming systems were already on, with their 'preferred' game open and ready to play at their assigned stations. Although *Minecraft* was by far the most popular, three design teams began with a different title.[5] The *Roblox* team elected to switch to *Minecraft* almost immediately, while another switched back and forth between *Minecraft* and *Little Big Planet*. The predominance of *Minecraft* among the other design teams appeared to be a contributing factor in these teams' decision to switch to *Minecraft* as well, as they each expressed excitement to try some of the texture packs the other teams were building with.

Each design team included a researcher as participant-observer. Researchers were instructed to let the children take the lead in all design decisions. Instead, they focussed on incorporating interview questions into the conversation, keeping the participants focussed on the task at hand, and mediating any minor conflicts that arose (e.g., one participant not letting the other have a turn). If participants ran into technical problems, the researchers served as knowledgeable but 'hands off' helpers, prioritising the children's own knowledge of the games and design processes. In the three teams comprised of one researcher and one participant, researchers assumed a more active role in the design process, but always deferred to the children and supported their choices. Three additional researchers ensured that the recording equipment functioned without interruption,[6] and a fourth served as the 'reference librarian', available to look up information on the internet for the children at their request.[7]

Toward the end of the session, researchers held a show-and-tell that consisted of a tour of all four design stations. The children each presented or co-presented their creations. Overall, the participants seemed very excited about the show-and-tell. They were engaged and enthusiastic about the other teams' designs, and many of them provided each other with praise, suggestions, and constructive criticism. In the final group discussion, the research team shared some preliminary observations, workshopped themes to explore at the data analysis stage, and gave the participants an early opportunity to correct, clarify, or add to the record.

Discussion of Findings

During the game jams, participants made an assortment of highly creative and sophisticated game 'builds'.[8] While they designed, and negotiated, these creations they also discussed a range of topics related to their experiences and knowledge of how UGC games work. In response to the interview questions, in dialogue with the games and with each other, participants talked about gaming, popular culture, creativity, where ideas and inspiration come from, family dynamics and the key role of siblings and parents in collaborative creation, thoughts on why games contain advertisements and in-game purchases, licensed game content, and a range of issues relating to the corporate ownership of games and whether this extends to player-made content. A wealth of data was generated out of these sessions. As a comprehensive analysis of the patterns that emerged among participants of different ages, genders, previous gameplay experience, and other variables is still underway, the findings presented herein are partial and preliminary. They include some overall trends, but largely centre on examples and outliers that have been identified as compelling potential themes of inquiry. Below, the focus is exclusively on the participants' thoughts about who owns UGC games and player-made content, who *controls* player-made content, and the role of copyright within these dynamics.

Who Owns UGC Games?

Participants varied in terms of the precision of their knowledge about what company (or companies) 'owned' the games they played. Most participants had some understanding that a company, person, or entity had created the game software, that someone owned it, and that these two things were not necessarily the same. Nearly all the players knew at least one of the companies associated with *Minecraft* – either Mojang, the game's original developer, or Microsoft, the company that acquired Mojang in 2014. Some participants said that "Not" owned *Minecraft*, referring to the game's original creator, Markus Persson.

Participants had mixed ideas about whether they owned the content *they* created. Though one participant said confidently that she owned the content she made, most had more ambivalent opinions about their ownership of in-game creations. Many participants seemed to be grappling with ambiguous and somewhat contradictory ideas about ownership and control. In keeping with previous work on people's perceptions of what constitutes an original creation, several of the participants expressed a perceived linkage between effort and ownership. The more effort one put into making something, the stronger one's ownership claim over the result. Nonetheless, many participants described that there were restrictions on what they could *do* with their creations. The youngest participants expressed a relatively fluid understanding about the ownership of player-made and in-game content, viewing it all as a shared resource or as a sort of 'commons'. Conversely, many of the older participants reported that another entity (companies, other players, server hosts, etc.) had some claim and power over their work.

In response to questions about ownership, 'Simber'[9] (age 9) stated, "I own my build, but Mojang technically owns *Minecraft*". As such, the company could come to her house and take away her build, by taking back her copy of *their* game. When researchers asked if she owned a picture that she drew on paper, she said the same rule applied. The person who had invented paper could come take her picture from her (no matter "how much you've drawn on it"), just as the inventor of bricks could come and take back the bricks that made up her house. This applied to all commodities, Simber explained, "Everything isn't *owned* by you, you just bought it". Her description revealed a sophisticated understanding of the closed, proprietary software licensing model, which indeed underlies *Minecraft* and most other digital games, apps, and media 'purchases'. Her expansion of this model to all areas of market exchange, however, raises questions about its spread and, ultimately, normalisation. Simber's responses both confirm and problematise findings uncovered in previous research on children's understanding of *transfer of ownership*, which suggest that this concept can be particularly challenging for children to grasp (e.g., Berti & Bombi, 1988). On the one hand, her description suggests some important gaps in her comprehension of this aspect of market exchange. On the other hand, as more businesses move toward license and subscription models, her assertion that creators (or companies) maintain ownership rights over their products – and can take them back 'anytime in the world' – is becoming increasingly accurate.

Who Controls UGC?

When asked about the game companies' authority and control over the game, player creations, and saved files (i.e., copies of builds stored on the child's own gaming device), responses were often tentative and conditional. Very few participants had experienced a clear or direct form of *interference*, a term used here to describe any form of official reprimand, warning, or disciplinary action (such as having one's content removed or account suspended) taken by a game's corporate owner or distributor. Most of the participants were unsure about what type of content or activity could invite such a response. Several of them questioned whether Microsoft even had the ability to delete or alter player-made worlds. Others suggested that perhaps their content *had* previously been deleted 'by the game', though these participants were unclear as to how or even if that had occurred. Nonetheless, most participants insisted that the potential for interference did exist. Notably, most of them also described that corporate interference was always justifiable. At the very least, it could not be challenged or overturned by a player. Many participants were furthermore uncertain about what happened to player-made builds once they were deleted. For instance, Trixie (age 8) agreed that, once deleted, a world was "gone forever, you can never see it again", but also replied that she didn't know if Microsoft kept a copy of it for themselves.

The younger brother on the one team that contained a sibling pair,[10] 'Cloudy' (age 8), became agitated when researchers asked if the makers of Minecraft could change or delete his world without notice. He did not overtly question their ability to do so, but insisted that they would not because "Mojang is nice and that would be mean". His older brother, 'Mr. Minecraft' (age 10), agreed that the worlds could be deleted, but had a different view of the risk. He explained that it was no different than a competition server he played on in which the culture was that players destroyed each other's creations soon after they were built. He said that once he knew this was the culture of the server and understood that it was not personal, he no longer minded when his creations were destroyed. He thought he would feel similarly if he found out that a world he had created was removed.

Some participants pointed out that interference was not the only way players could lose access to their creations. For example, 'Nicholas' (age 10) told us that he lost access to a world he had created when he accidentally left the phone it was 'on' in the pocket of a pair of pants that went through the washing machine. When the phone came out of the wash it was no longer usable, and he believed that the world he had created on it was lost forever. Another participant mentioned that if a player forgets their password, their builds would still exist but would become inaccessible to them. These players put the deletion of player-made content by Microsoft in the same category as other random acts of fate, and justified it in similar terms. While frustrating, ultimately no one was to blame and no recourse was available.

Navigating Copyright

Issues pertaining to corporate copyright and copyright infringement surfaced quite frequently during discussions about ownership, as well as in response to the questions asked about licensed content, in-game purchases, and advertising. Notably, many of these issues were raised by the participants themselves. Although several of the research questions related to intellectual property, transfer of ownership, copyright and fair use/dealing, the researchers rarely, if ever, used the legal terminology when broaching these topics with the participants. Instead, participants were asked if they owned the content they created, who they considered to be the owner(s) of the game itself, and who (if anyone) could delete or change player-made content. However, several participants' responses included legal terms like 'copyright' to describe licensed content, or 'infringement' to talk about derivative player-made content. The older participants were most likely to utilise such terms. Interestingly, the older children were also more likely to think that their UGC creations were owned by someone other than themselves – either by the game owner, or by a corporate copyright holder.

One of the participants, 'Bob!' (age 10), a self-described 'professional' *Super Mario Maker* designer, had an especially deep understanding of copyright and authorship. Unlike most of the other children in the study, he reported that he himself had directly experienced interference related to copyright, although not exactly within the context of a UGC game. He explained that he regularly posted 'Let's Play' videos of levels he had made in *Super Mario Maker* and *Minecraft* to his YouTube channel, and had received one or more cease and desist notices. Some of his videos had also been 'taken down' by YouTube. With the help of his parents, he reposted the videos with the sound removed, which 'solved the problem'. He was not sure why the sound made a difference, but he knew that was the way to ensure his content remained posted. As he later replied to the researcher's question about who owned his player-made levels, "Technically they're your creations, but ... I can't put a copyright on it or anything". This led to a longer conversation about the nature of copyright. Neither he nor any of the participants described copyright as something *they* could claim. For the children in this study, ownership may be fluid, variable, and complex, but copyright belongs solely to corporations.

Notably, many children, including some of the participants, learn about copyright in the classroom, as part of a digital literacy curriculum. While an analysis of these curriculum materials was beyond the scope of the current study, previous work in this area has flagged multiple problems with the information contained in child-targeted copyright lesson plans. As Gillespie (2009) describes, when children are taught about copyright, the emphasis is often placed on delineating *corporate* copyrights. Meanwhile user rights, such as fair use, are downplayed or omitted altogether. The digital literacy materials included in his study largely positioned children as (potential) copyright infringers – not as content creators or as possible copyright holders themselves. While copyright law is indeed highly complex and beyond the full comprehension of many adults, let alone children, Moore's (2018) research demonstrates that even kindergartners can grasp the underlying principles of authorship, attribution, and fair use that guide intellectual property rights. He advocates for a more comprehensive approach to teaching copyright at every grade level, one that encourages children "to confidently and thoughtfully claim their rights as both creators and users of copyrighted material" (p. 272). These findings support the argument that there is a clear need for a firmer delineation of children's rights as authors, creators, and emerging digital citizens, within digital literacy curriculum.

Conclusion

A preliminary review of the findings from the game-jam study yields a compelling snapshot of the complex relationships that children of various ages have with ownership and copyright in UGC games. Even the youngest participants had strong opinions about who owns and controls the content they create in these games, as they navigated the complex terrains of corporate sovereignty and user rights embedded in corporately controlled UGC game titles. Previous studies of UGC games largely focus on educational applications, emphasising their potential to contribute to children's learning and creativity. Other works highlight how the commercial priorities of many UGC games introduce unexpected political economic relationships into children's creative processes. The current study builds a bridge between these disparate bodies of research by revealing some of the ways in which the political economic dimensions of UGC games are experienced, understood, and negotiated by the children who play them.

These findings support the conclusions drawn in recent studies conducted by Shaw et al. (2012), Olson and Shaw (2011), and Moore (2018). Although the concepts of idea ownership and fair use are abstract, variable, and traditionally considered to be beyond children's (especially younger children's) grasp, young game makers are clearly engaging with these concepts. They have situated knowledge about various legal terms, and formulate judgements about the meanings and implications of these complex processes for themselves and other players. At the same time, in reviewing the children's descriptions of their ownership rights, and those of the companies who make and manage UGC game titles, there was evidence of important gaps in children's understanding of both the scope and specificities involved in creating original and derivative content within corporately controlled forums. This supports Moore's conclusions that there is a clear need for a deeper and more concerted integration of legal issues within children's digital literacy curricula.

More than this, however, there is a growing need to include children, their needs and vulnerabilities, within copyright discourses and policy development. The expansion of children's access to digital creation tools brings with it a wide range of exciting possibilities for supporting children's cultural rights, fostering their sense of agency, and increasing their participation in shaping shared digital culture. Previous research on UGC games and the broader children's consumer culture makes it clear that the responsibility for realising this potential cannot be delegated to the tools alone. Nor should the onus be offloaded onto children, teachers, and their caregivers through a narrow focus on digital literacy strategies. Fully supporting children's newfound roles as game makers and mass media creators will also require a disruption and shift in the industry standards, regulatory policies, and social conceptualisations that continue to configure the child as first and foremost a consumer or passive user – rather than the active, engaged *producers* of content so many of them already are.

Notes

1 The term 'game jam' refers to a popular activity in digital game culture in which teams of people come together over a short period of time, either a day, a night, or a weekend, etc., to collaboratively create one or more games.

2 Our participants included two six-year-olds (one girl, one boy), one seven-year-old boy, four eight-year-olds (two girls, two boys), two nine-year-olds (one girl, one boy), eight ten-year-olds (one girl, seven boys), and four 12-year-olds (one girl, three boys).

3 For each session, eight participants had been confirmed to attend. However, in all three instances, one participant cancelled at the last minute.

4 As much as possible, participants were paired with another child close in age and with similar gaming habits.

5 On teams made up of children with different 'preferred' UGC games, we pre-loaded a game that both children had previously made content with instead. Before starting the game jam, these teams were consulted about their game selection and given the chance to switch.

6 Recording equipment was set up at each design station, and an additional camera was positioned to capture the room in its entirety. Pictures were taken throughout the day. All but one of the design teams' game levels or 'builds' were preserved for later analysis and reference (one was deleted by a participant, as per an option outlined in our ethics protocol).

7 Children were prohibited from directly accessing the internet during the game jam, as per our ethics protocol.

8 The term 'build' is commonly used by *Minecraft* and other game makers to describe their creations.

9 All the participants were asked to suggest a 'code name' or pseudonym for themselves that the researchers could use in any reports or writings about the study.

10 All but one of our teams comprised participants and researchers who did not know each other prior to the game jam. The sole exception was a pair of brothers who insisted on joining the same team. Three other sibling pairs participated in our study, including one set of twins, all of whom happily agreed to be on different teams.

References

Bak, M. (2016). Building blocks of the imagination: Children, creativity, and the limits of *Disney Infinity*. *The Velvet Light Trap* (78), 53–64.

Banks, J., & Potts, J. (2010). Co-creating games: A co-evolutionary analysis. *New Media & Society*, 12(2), 253–270.

Berti, A. E., & Bombi, A. S. (1988). *The child's construction of economics*. Cambridge, UK: Cambridge University Press.

Cipollone, M., Schifter, C. C., & Moffat, R. A. (2014). Minecraft as a creative tool: A case study. *International Journal of Game-Based Learning*, 4(2), 1–14.

Comunello, F., & Mulargia, S. (2015). User-generated video gaming. *Games and Culture*, 10(1), 57–80.

Evaldsson, A.-C., & Corsaro, W.A. (1998). Play and games in the peer cultures of preschool and preadolescent children: An interpretive approach. *Childhood*, 5(4), 377–402.

Fields, D. A., & Grimes, S. M. (2017). Pockets of freedom, but mostly constraints: Emerging trends in children's DIY media platforms. In I. Elea & L. Mikos (Eds.), *Young & creative: Digital technologies empowering children in everyday life* (pp. 159–171). Goteborg, Sweden: International Clearinghouse on Children, Youth & Media/UNESCO.

Gauntlett, D. (2007). *Creative explorations: New approaches to identities and audiences*. New York: Routledge.

Gillespie, T. (2009). Characterizing copyright in the classroom: The cultural work of anti-piracy campaigns. *Communication, Culture, & Critique*, 2(3), 274–318.

Grimes, S. M. (2014). Child-generated content: Children's authorship and interpretive practices in digital gaming cultures. In R. J. Coombe & D. Wershler (Eds.), *Dynamic fair dealing: Creating Canadian culture online* (pp. 336–345). Toronto: University of Toronto Press.

Grimes, S. M. (2015). Little big scene: Making and playing culture in media molecule's. *LittleBigPlanet*. *Cultural Studies*, 29(3), 379–400.

Gussin Paley, V. (2004). *A child's work: The importance of fantasy play*. Chicago, IL: University of Chicago Press.

Jenkins, H. (2008). *Confronting the challenges of participatory culture: Media education for the 21st Century*. Chicago, IL: The John D. and Catherine T. MacArthur Foundation.

Jenks, C. (2005). *Childhood*. London, UK: Routledge.

Kafai, Y. B., & Burke, Q. (2015). Constructionist gaming: Understanding the benefits of making games for learning. *Educational Psychology*, 50(4), 313–334.

Marsh, J. (2010). *Childhood, culture and creativity: A literature review*. Newcastle upon Tyne, UK: Creativity, Culture and Education.

Moore, D. C. (2018). I got it from Google. In R. Hobbs (Ed.), *The Routledge companion to media education, copyright, and fair use* (pp. 258–273). New York: Routledge.
Nguyen, J. (2016). *Minecraft* and the building blocks of creative individuality. *Configurations, 24*(4), 471–500.
Niemeyer, D. J., & Gerber, H. R. (2015). Maker culture and *Minecraft*: Implications for the future of learning. *Educational Media International, 52*(3), 216–226.
Olson, K. R., & Shaw, A. (2011). "No fair, copycat!": What children's response to plagiarism tells us about their understanding of ideas. *Developmental Science, 14*(2), 431–439.
Resnick, M., Maloney, J., Monroy-Hernández, A., Rusk, N., Eastmond, E. N., Brennan, K., . . . Kafai, Y. (2009). Scratch: Programming for all. *Communications of the ACM, 52*(11), 60–67.
Shaw, A., Li, V., & Olson, K. R. (2012). Children apply principles of physical ownership to ideas. *Cognitive Science: A Multidisciplinary Journal, 36*, 1383–1403.
Willet, R., Robinson, M., & Marsh, J. (Eds.). (2009). *Play, creativity, and digital cultures*. New York: Routledge.
Willett, R. (2016). "Microsoft bought Minecraft . . . who knows what's going to happen?!": A sociocultural analysis of 8–9-year-olds' understanding of commercial online gaming industries. *Learning, Media and Technology*. doi:10.1080/17439884.2016.1194296.
Young, C. J. (2017). Game changers: Everyday gamemakers and the development of the video game industry. (Doctoral dissertation). Retrieved from TSpace database: http://hdl.handle.net/1807/89734.

27
MARKETING TO CHILDREN THROUGH DIGITAL MEDIA
Trends and Issues

Wonsun Shin

Introduction

Digital media have become an integral part of children's lives. Marketers recognise the access that digital media offer in terms of reaching young consumers, and they actively harness digital platforms to appeal to this market. While digital media offer unprecedented opportunities for marketers to target children, however, some of the current youth-directed digital marketing practices have raised concerns. For instance, branded environments provided by online, social, and mobile media often blend commercial and non-commercial content, making children susceptible to the persuasive intentions of marketers. The interactive nature of digital media also increases the possibility that children will disclose personal information to unknown others, including marketers. Overall, the new generation of consumers and media users faces unique challenges that previous generations have not seen or experienced.

Defining 'children' as anyone under the age of 18, this chapter considers children as consumers in the changing media environment and examines how digital media pose new challenges to this consumer segment. It begins with an overview of what is known about children as consumers and media users and the theoretical perspectives underpinning the knowledge. It then explores how children are constructed as marketing targets in the digital age and addresses growing concerns associated with current marketing practices. The chapter concludes by identifying gaps in the current understanding of marketing to children through digital media and highlighting areas for future research.

Children as Consumers

Children constitute a lucrative market in several respects. First, although children may not be the final decision-makers for household purchases, they substantially affect their caregivers' buying decisions. Three out of four parents in the US report that their children influence family purchase decisions (Viacom, 2018). According to a survey conducted with children aged 6–13 in Australia, about 4 out of 10 children 'help their parents decide' clothes for themselves (38.1%), DVDs (37.8%), toys (35.5%), and fast food (35.3%) (Roy Morgan, 2016). Another reason that children are an important consumer segment is that they represent future consumers. Marketers promoting adult products often reach out to children, with the hope that children will develop their brand preference at an earlier age and become lifetime consumers for their brands. Toyota's ToyToyota mobile app ('Backseat Driver') and McDonald's Happy Meal are good examples of such marketing practices, also known as *cradle-to-grave marketing*.

With an increase in dual-income households, smaller families, and more permissive parenting practices among the younger generations of parents, today's children learn to be active and competent consumers who are proactive about what they want and persistent in pursuit of their needs, using various persuasion techniques – from begging and pestering to bargaining and negotiating with their parents (Hawkins, 2016). Children on average make approximately 3,000 requests to their parents for products or services per year (Schor, 2004). Their persuasion tactics, often referred to as 'pestering power', are known to have substantial influence on the spending decisions of parents at a global scale (Calvert, 2008).

However, children are also viewed as vulnerable victims of commercialisation who are easily persuaded or 'manipulated' by marketers to pursue products that they do not need or which may have detrimental effects on their physical and psychological wellbeing (Lapierre, Fleming-Milici, Rozendaal, McAlister, & Castonguay, 2017). Extensive research has demonstrated positive links between children's exposure to fast food, alcohol, and tobacco ads and their favourable attitudes toward the consumption of those products (Wilcox et al., 2004). Excessive commercialism through marketing messages is also associated with materialism in young people, leading them to ascribe greater importance to the acquisition and ownership of material goods (Buijzen & Valkenburg, 2003).

The answer to the question of 'whether children are active agents or victims in the commercialised world' is not straightforward, as children's consumption-related attitudes, skills, and behaviours are shaped by various developmental and social factors (Hawkins, 2016). Regarding the role of cognitive development in children's responses to marketing, a general consensus has been that children's age (maturity) matters. It is more difficult for younger children to understand the commercial intentions behind marketing messages, as compared with older children, due to their limited cognitive capability. For example, according to the American Psychological Association (Wilcox et al., 2004), children under the age of seven tend to have difficulty comprehending the true purpose of advertising. As they grow older, they become more critical about marketing practices and no longer believe that advertising always represents the truth. This line of thought has been influenced by age-based developmental-stage models, including Piaget's *four stages of cognitive development* (1970), Selman's *theory of perspective taking* (1980), and Roedder-John's *model of consumer socialisation* (1999).

Aside from the level of cognitive development, the social environment in which children grow up and learn social norms and proper conduct plays a crucial role in their responses to marketing practices (Roedder-John, 1999). The theory of *consumer socialisation* (Moschis, 1978) has long been applied to examine and explain the process by which children acquire and develop consumption-related knowledge, skills, and behaviours through their interactions with socialisation agents, which include parents, friends, schools, and media. According to the consumer socialisation perspective, children's interactions with socialisation agents result in an array of outcomes. For instance, the degree to which children and parents engage in critical discussions about advertising practices can reduce children's vulnerability to advertising (Buijzen, 2009). On the other hand, children's frequent interactions with peers and excessive use of media can make them less critical about marketing practices (Moschis & Churchill, 1978).

Children as Media Users

These unique and influential young consumers are also avid media users; they spend considerable time on diverse types of media. In addition, the amount of time spent on media tends to increase as children grow older. According to the Australian Institute of Family Studies (2015), children aged 4–5 spend 2.2 hours per day on screen media. This increases to 3.3 hours when children reach the age of 12–13. Another important trend in children's media use is that they rely heavily on digital media, and this trend is steadily increasing. Eight out of ten teenagers aged 14–17 in Australia think that the internet is extremely/very important to them (Australian Communications and Media Authority, 2013). Ofcom's survey with children in the UK (2017) found that children aged 5–15 spent 15 hours and 18 minutes per week on the internet in 2017, which represents a dramatic increase from 2007 (9 hours and 42 minutes). Pew Research Center (2018) shows that 45% of teens in the US are online almost constantly, which is almost double the rate from the 2014–2015 survey (24%).

Social media in particular represent important parts of young people's digital media routine. In Australia, almost all online teenagers aged 14–17 use social media, engaging in such activities as posting status updates, sending messages, tagging others, and joining groups (Australian Communications and Media Authority, 2013). Children are also increasingly mobile. Teens' access to smartphones increased from 73% in 2014–2015 to 95% in 2018 in the US (Pew Internet Research, 2018). Across eight different countries (Belgium, Denmark, Ireland, Italy, Japan, Portugal, Romania, and UK), 71% of children aged 9–16 use their mobile phones to access the internet and 81% of these kids use social networking services on mobile phones (GSMA, 2014).

Digital Marketing to Children: Issues and Concerns

Inspired by the mounting potential of digital media to reach this younger consumer group, marketers have employed various strategies to appeal to digital youth. Well-known examples of marketing strategies directed to young consumers include brand websites with interactive features, advertising displayed on those websites, brand placement embedded in digital content, advergames (i.e., online or mobile games created by a marketer to promote a specific brand), social media advertising, and branded mobile applications. Given that children spend excessive amounts of time on social media and mobile devices, this chapter focusses on marketing practices utilising social and mobile media.

Social Media Advertising

A key characteristic of social media as a marketing communication platform is that they allow marketers to 'target' specific consumer groups using the demographic characteristics, interests, and online activities of the users. These pieces of user information enable marketers to offer personalised promotional content to different consumer segments. Users' personal information is collected through their voluntary disclosure to social media (e.g., information they provide to join a social networking site), as well as through their digital footprints (e.g., what users see and do on their social media profiles and other websites). *Social media retargeting* (i.e., exposing a social media user to an advertisement promoting a product or service that was shown on a previously visited website) is thus a widely used marketing strategy to target both adult and teen social media users (Zarouali, Ponnet, Walrave, & Poels, 2017). Let's say that a teen Instagram user visits an apparel brand's website, browses, and clicks on a few items there. If the apparel brand is a client or 'partner' of Instagram, the user's behaviours on this apparel website will be known to Instagram through a cookie. When the same user later visits Instagram, he or she will be 'retargeted' by advertisements promoting the products shown on the apparel website. In other words, marketing messages are personalised based on consumers' individual online behaviours.

From the marketers' perspective, personalised marketing content is a logical choice, as it results in more positive outcomes as compared with non-personalised content, including more favourable attitudes toward the marketers and greater purchase intentions for the advertised brands (Zarouali et al., 2017). Consumers are more likely to perceive personalised content to be relevant and useful as compared with non-personalised content, as the former is in closer keeping with their current lifestyle, context, and interests (Tucker, 2014). However, more precisely targeted personalisation requires a greater degree of personal information from social media users. In other words, users may have to sacrifice their privacy in exchange for personalised offerings. A problem is that young consumers often underestimate the risks associated with information disclosure and tend to share a wide range of personal information on social media (Madden et al., 2013). The fact that they often have difficulty understanding how their information is collected and used by social media platforms and other third-party marketers puts young social media users at greater risk.

Another concern associated with social media marketing targeted at youth is that many of the promotional messages, including personalised advertising, are blended into the users' social media profiles, blurring the line between commercial and non-commercial content. This is known as *social media newsfeed ads*, referring to advertising messages that appear within users' personal feeds. Social media newsfeed advertising is a type of *native advertising* – paid advertising that matches the look, feel, and function of its surrounding editorial content. According to eMarketer (2018), native advertising like newsfeed advertising constitutes the main source of revenue for social media companies.

Another type of native advertising popular among marketers targeting digital youth is *influencer marketing* (De Jans, 2018). Influencer marketing refers to a marketing practice in which marketers work with social media influencers (i.e., individuals with access to a substantial social network of people following them and the power to influence the followers' opinions and behaviours) to promote their brands (Folkvord, Bevelander, Rozendaal, & Hermans, 2019). It is considered native advertising because it allows marketers to blend their promotional messages into the content created by the influencer (van Dam & van Raimersdal, 2019). When social media influencers work for (or are 'sponsored by') marketers, they endorse the marketers' brands by featuring the brands as part of their social media stories (Coates, Hardman, Halford, Christiansen, & Boyland, 2019). Because the brand stories are seamlessly integrated into the influencers' social media posts, young consumers are less likely to view the stories as marketing messages (Coates et al., 2019). Furthermore, social media influencers are often viewed as friends or friendly experts (Folkword et al., 2019). Given that young consumers tend to be vulnerable to peer influence, brand messages endorsed by 'peer' influencers are more likely to be considered authentic and credible as compared with the overt forms of advertising (De Jans, 2018).

Consumers are more likely to view, share, and click native advertising compared with more overt forms of advertising like banner ads (Folkword et al., 2019; Marketing Land, 2016). However, because native advertising, such as social media newsfeed ads and influencer marketing, obscures the distinction between advertising and non-advertising content, it is also considered a misleading and deceptive practice (Taylor, 2017). The organic form of native advertising on social media is less likely to activate young consumers' cognitive defences to cope with persuasion, possibly leading them to be less critical about such marketing practices (Zarouali et al., 2017).

Lastly, most of the established social media platforms (e.g., Facebook, Instagram, Snapchat, Twitter, etc.) require their users to be 13 or older to join, in order to comply with the Children's Online Privacy Protection Act of 1998 (COPPA) (Office of eSafety Commissioner, 2016). However, Ofcom's (2017) survey indicates that about half of children aged 11–12 have social media profiles. This means that many young children who are not supposed to use social media can be exposed to age-inappropriate content, including marketing messages targeting older consumers, through their social media use.

Mobile Marketing

Mobile devices offer a variety of tools for marketing, including SMS (short message service), push notifications, mobile applications (apps), in-app advertising (ads that appear on mobile webpages or in apps), QR (quick response) codes, and location-based advertising. As an increasing number of children and teenagers own mobile devices and rely heavily on those devices to undertake a wide range of activities, marketers actively utilise mobile technology to reach young consumers (Common Sense Media, 2014).

Advanced tracking technologies, as well as the prevalence of GPS- and wi-fi-enabled mobile devices, have empowered marketers to identify and monitor the locations of their target consumers and to deliver customised advertising messages based on their current locations. Using geo-location data from young consumers, marketers deliver location-specific promotions – for example, sending ads or coupons when children are around particular stores or restaurants (Common Sense Media, 2014). Marketers also encourage children to 'check in' at fast food restaurants and to share that information via social media (World Health Organization, 2016). These tactics are about targeting children at the right time in the right context.

However, location-based marketing targeted at children raises two important concerns. First, it targets children when they are most vulnerable to marketing messages (World Health Organization, 2016). This is likely to make children less analytical about promotional messages and more likely to lower their guard. Given that location-based marketing is often used by fast food brands to target kids (World Health Organization, 2016), its impact on children cannot be underestimated. Second, location-based marketing involves personal data, including the users' current location. In short, users' privacy is at risk. Wang, Yang, and Zhang (2015) note that many advertisers that utilise location-based advertising collect extensive personal information from mobile users without providing clear explanations for how the data will be used.

The collection of personal data and the intrusions into consumer privacy that are commonplace among marketers are particularly pressing issues regarding mobile apps targeting children. Apps often collect an array of personal information and seek 'permission' to access the user's ID, contact list, address book, calendar, network connections, camera, and storage associated with the mobile device. For example, the *Minecraft* mobile app, a popular mobile game for children and teenagers, requests access to users' contacts, phone, storage, and full network connections to other users (Google Play's *Minecraft* page, n.d.). The Instagram mobile app, one of the most popular social networking sites among teenagers, demands access to users' camera, contacts, location, microphone, phone, SMS, storage, Bluetooth setting, and network connections on their phones. Many other widely used apps have similar requirements and yet the Federal Trade Commission's (FTC) survey of mobile apps targeted at children in 2012 showed that only 20% of these apps provided a link to a privacy policy available to parents (FTC, 2015). This improved three years later, with more than 45% of kids' apps including links to their privacy policies on their app store pages in 2015 (FTC, 2015). Nevertheless, according to the FTC (2015), those apps do not provide easy enough access for parents or young users themselves to learn about how user data are collected and used. That is, while mobile marketers collect extensive personal information from young mobile users, they are not diligent in protecting the privacy of those consumers.

Another concern related to mobile marketing targeted at children is that it often forces children to view advertisements and nudges them to spend money on virtual goods. When children use free-to-play mobile apps to play games, for example, they are often required to watch or click in-app ads to earn game money or skip to the next level. They are also prodded to make in-app purchases for a variety of reasons – to access extra functions, unlock the game's full features, get new accessories or abilities for their game characters, buy rare items, speed up the game's progress, or enjoy the game without advertisements. These kinds of marketing practices may induce materialistic attitudes in children, leading them to associate money with solutions (Opree, Buijzen, & van Reijmersdal, 2013). While in-app purchases represent the primary revenue source for mobile marketers (Business of Apps, 2018), they can also result in parent–child conflict. Numerous news reports have covered accidental and expensive unauthorised purchases made by children across the world, like a seven-year-old child who spent £4,000 on a *Jurassic World* in-app purchase (*Daily Mail*, 2015).

What Is Known: a Summary of the Current Knowledge

Overall, the literature shows that children are many-sided consumers. They are influential consumers with great indirect buying power. They are also active agents, persistent about what they want and strategic about the manner in which they fulfil their consumption needs. Children are also ardent media users, and digital media constitute a substantial part of their lives. In response to these characteristics, marketers aggressively target young consumers using numerous digital marketing tools. However, the literature also suggests that children, especially younger ones, are susceptible to marketing influences due to their limited developmental capacity and consumption experience. Current digital marketing practices appear to put children in a more vulnerable position, as outlined below.

- *Privacy intrusion*: Just as adult consumers are targeted through data-driven marketing, young consumers are also targeted through online tracking, location-based and behavioural targeting, and retargeting strategies. Zarouali et al. (2017) show that retargeted Facebook ads lead to greater purchase intention among adolescents compared with non-retargeted Facebook ads. That is, content personalisation through online tracking 'works' to attract young consumers. However, children often input various types of personal information when they join social networking sites or download and use mobile apps without understanding how their personal information is collected and used by marketers. This raises important concerns regarding privacy.
- *Covert advertising*: Young consumers who spend extensive amounts of time on social media are exposed to various forms of covert advertising such as social media newsfeed advertising and influential marketing (Lapierre et al., 2017). These forms of advertising integrate commercial messages into non-commercial content and obscure the line between advertising and neutral messages. Research suggests that covert advertising can be effective when it is considered nonintrusive by viewers (Lee, Kim, & Ham, 2016). However, the subtle nature of covert advertising makes it difficult for young consumers to understand that they are being targeted by marketers (Lapierre et al., 2017). It can also lower consumers' persuasion knowledge, making them less critical about marketing practices (Taylor, 2017).
- *Ad-induced materialism*: When engaging with digital media such as app-based mobile games, children are exposed to ongoing pressure to spend money to enjoy better digital experiences (Kelion, 2013). This can foster a materialistic orientation in children and cause parent–child conflicts. Unauthorised spending on in-app purchases can also result in a significant financial loss for children and parents.
- *Exposure to inappropriate content*: The prevalence of underage social media use is also concerning in that it can expose young children to commercial content that is not appropriate for their age.

What Needs to be Known: Gaps in Current Understanding

Despite the importance of children as consumers and media users, as well as various concerns associated with digital marketing directed at children, there are many gaps in the research literature.

Gap 1. The Lack of Understanding Regarding Age Differences in Children's Recognition and Understanding of Digital Marketing Strategies

The aforementioned age-based cognitive developmental models, as well as the conventional views regarding children's understanding of advertising (e.g., children aged five can distinguish advertising from television programmes) emerged in the pre-digital era, when digital media was largely foreign to children. Given the dramatic changes in the consumer and digital marketplaces over the past few decades, the existing theories and models may not adequately explain today's children.

Currently, little is known regarding the relationship between children's age and their ability to recognise and understand digital marketing practices (Common Sense Media, 2014). A deeper understanding of those issues, such as "when children recognise native advertising as a form of marketing communication" and "when they understand how personalised advertising works" will help policy-makers assess the fairness of different forms of marketing communications targeted at different ages of children (Common Sense Media, 2014). It will also help parents and media educators to develop age-appropriate educational programmes to enhance children's digital marketing literacy.

Future research needs to shed light on age-related differences in children's recognition and understanding of various forms of overt and covert advertising across different platforms (e.g., websites, social media, and mobile apps) and their interactions with marketing content (e.g., liking or sharing social media newsfeed advertising with peers). Important insights will emerge if researchers carefully consider the role of social environmental factors (e.g., children's interactions with parents, peers, and media) as mediating or moderating factors that possibly affect the relationship between children's age and their understanding of and responses to digital marketing.

Gap 2. The Lack of Empirical Evidence Regarding the Impact of Digital Marketing on Children

This chapter has addressed a number of concerns associated with digital marketing targeted at children, including content personalisation and privacy intrusion, unclear distinctions between commercial and non-commercial content, and materialistic attitudes induced by in-app advertising. However, little research has been carried out to investigate the impact of these marketing practices on children. Although many studies address teenagers' online information disclosure or protection behaviours (e.g., Shin & Kang, 2016; Walrave & Heirman, 2013), not much is known regarding children and teenagers' responses to personalised and targeted digital marketing content and the implications of those choices for their privacy, with a few notable exceptions (e.g., Youn & Shin, 2019; Zarouali, Poels, Pottet, & Walrave, 2018; Zarouali et al., 2017). Likewise, research on young consumers' responses to covert social media advertising and mobile marketing is currently underdeveloped (De Jans, Van de Sompel, Hudders, & Cauberghe, 2017). Thus, little is known regarding how covert advertising presented across different digital platforms affects children's buying intentions, whether children's awareness of the data collection practices of mobile apps influences their use of those apps, and to what extent children's in-app purchases have adverse effects on their wellbeing and that of their parents.

Future research will generate new breakthroughs by exploring a broader range of digital marketing practices, especially covert, targeted, and personalised ones that may lower young consumers' cognitive defences and invade their privacy. While a few studies focus on teenagers' responses to personalised social media advertising (Youn & Shin, 2019; Zarouali et al., 2017, 2018), pre-adolescent children's responses to and interactions with digital marketing are largely unknown. Given that children under the age of 13 often engage in social media activities and can be targeted by covert and personalised marketing messages on social media, greater attention needs to be given to this younger target segment.

Gap 3. Need for Reconceptualisation of Persuasion Knowledge

In the advertising and marketing literature, persuasion knowledge refers to consumers' ability to recognise and evaluate advertisers' persuasive motivations, which is a critical skill for young consumers to obtain and develop in order to cope with persuasive efforts by marketers (Friestad & Wright, 1994). When a consumer recognises the persuasive intentions of a marketer, his/her knowledge of persuasion is activated. This activated persuasive knowledge helps the consumer counter the marketer's persuasive attempts and critically assess marketing communication messages (Boerman, van Reijmersdal, Rozendaal, & Dima, 2018).

Wojdynski (2016) argues that an advertisement that blends itself to the surrounding content, like native advertising on social media, "imposes a high bar to the activation of persuasion knowledge" (p. 1478). This implies that the covert advertising prevalent in digital marketing is less likely to activate children's persuasion knowledge, leading them to be less critical about, and more susceptible to, promotional messages.

However, it is also possible that extensive social media use and frequent exposure to social media newsfeed advertising may familiarise children with these advertising formats and practices, making them more knowledgeable about covert advertising. Such persuasion knowledge developed through repeated exposure and experience will help children cope with advertising blended with non-commercial social media content, and thus to become more resilient to covert advertising. However, this persuasion knowledge may not be useful when they encounter different forms of digital advertising like retargeted advertising or location-based advertising. They may have to develop different types of persuasion knowledge to deal with these variations.

The current digital marketing environment, crowded with diverse tools and platforms for reaching young consumers, requires children to have multiple sets of persuasion knowledge to cope with diverse and constantly changing marketing strategies. This requires researchers to reconceptualise persuasion knowledge and reconsider how it works in digital contexts. In the context of fast-changing marketing practices especially well-suited to target children, important questions to ask are as follows:

- What constitutes persuasion knowledge in the digital media environment?
- How do young digital consumers acquire and cultivate persuasion knowledge?
- How can one's persuasion knowledge be measured in digital marketing contexts?

Recently, Boerman et al. (2018) developed scales for measurement of adult consumers' persuasion knowledge of sponsored content (i.e., promotional messages integrated into television programmes, video games, and blog posts) and demonstrated that persuasion knowledge of sponsored content comprises nine different components. Future research can examine whether Boerman et al.'s scales are applicable to assess young consumers' persuasion knowledge of covert advertising.

Conclusion

This chapter has described children as multifaceted consumers who live in a fast-changing digital environment and are heavily targeted by various digital marketing strategies. Current marketing practices directed to youth raise numerous concerns. However, the existing research literature has significant gaps in understanding how children recognise, process, and are affected by diverse marketing practices. Identifying the gaps in current knowledge, this chapter offers concrete suggestions for future research. A deeper understanding of children as consumers, and of their responses to the transforming digital and social media marketing environments, will enable media educators and policy-makers to assess the fairness of digital marketing practices and develop effective guidelines to raise more digitally resilient consumers.

References

Australian Communications and Media Authority. (2013). Like, post, share: Young Australians' experience of social media: Quantitative research report. Retrieved from: https://apo.org.au/sites/default/files/resource-files/2013-08/apo-nid35223.pdf.

Australian Institute of Family Studies. (2015). The longitudinal study of Australian children – Annual statistical report 2015. Retrieved from: https://growingupinaustralia.gov.au/sites/default/files/asr2015.pdf.

Boerman, S. C., van Reijmersdal, E. A., Rozendaal, E., & Dima, A. L. (2018). Development of the persuasion knowledge scales of sponsored content. *International Journal of Advertising*, 37(5), 671–697.

Buijzen, M. (2009). The effectiveness of parental communication in modifying the relation between food advertising and children's consumption behavior. *British Journal of Developmental Psychology*, 27, 105–121.

Buijzen, M., & Valkenburg, P. (2003). The effects of television advertising on materialism, parent–child conflict, and unhappiness: A review of research. *Journal of Applied Developmental Psychology*, 24(4), 437–456.

Business of Apps. (2018, 11 May). App Revenue (2017). Retrieved from: www.businessofapps.com/data/app-revenues.

Calvert, S. L. (2008). Children as consumers: Advertising and marketing. *Future Child*, 18(1), 205–234. Retrieved from: https://pdfs.semanticscholar.org/afad/423524b4d080b2ae1bfbf4073fae5a37924b.pdf.

Coates, A. E., Hardman, C. A., Halford, J. C. G., Christiansen, P., & Boyland, E. J. (2019). Social media influencer marketing and children's food intake: A randomized trial. *Pediatrics*, 143(4), 2018–2554.

Common Sense Media. (2014). Advertising to children and teens: Current practices. Retrieved from: www.commonsensemedia.org/research/advertising-to-children-and-teens-current-practices.

Daily Mail. (2015, 31 December). Boy, 7, racks up massive £4,000 bill playing dinosaur video game on his father's iPad - including £1,500 in just one hour. Retrieved from: www.dailymail.co.uk/news/article-3378667/Boy-charges-4-000-father-s-Apple-account-game-purchases.html.

De Jans, S. (2018). How an advertising disclosure alerts young adolescents to sponsored vlogs: The moderating role of a peer-based advertising literacy intervention through an informational vlog. *Journal of Advertising*, 47(4), 309–325.

De Jans, S., Van de Sompel, D., Hudders, L., & Cauberghe, V. (2017). Advertising targeting young children: An overview of 10 Years of Research (2006–2016). *International Journal of Advertising*, 38(2), 173–206.

eMarketer. (2018, 11 April). Native ad spend will make up nearly 60% of display spending in 2018. Retrieved from: www.emarketer.com/content/native-ad-spend-will-make-up-nearly-60-of-display-spending-in-2018.

Federal Trade Commission. (2015, 3 September). Kids' apps disclosure revisited. Retrieved from: www.ftc.gov/news-events/blogs/business-blog/2015/09/kids-apps-disclosures-revisited.

Folkword, F., Bevelander, K. E., Rozebdaal, E., & Hermans, R. (2019). Children's bonding with popular YouTube vloggers and their attitudes toward brand and product endorsements in vlogs: An explorative study. *Young Consumers*, 20(2), 77–90.

Friestad, M., & Wright, P. (1994). The persuasion knowledge model: How people cope with persuasion attempts. *Journal of Consumer Research*, 21(1), 1–31.

Google Play. *Minecraft*. Retrieved from: https://play.google.com/store/apps/details?id=com.mojang.minecraftpe&hl=en_AU.

GSMA. (2014). Children's use of mobile phones: A special report 2014. Retrieved from: www.gsma.com/publicpolicy/wp-content/uploads/2012/03/GSMA_Childrens_use_of_mobile_phones_2014.pdf.

Hawkins, C. (2016). Brand consumers. In C. Hawkins (Ed.), *Rethinking children as consumers: The changing status of childhood and young adulthood* (pp. 86–105). London: Routledge.

Kelion, L. (2013). In-game app fees face OFT consumer protection crackdown. BBC News. (25 September 2013). Retrieved from: www.bbc.com/news/technology–24272010.

Lapierre, M. A., Fleming-Milici, F., Rozendaal, E., McAlister, A. R., & Castonguay, J. (2017). The effect of advertising on children and adolescents. *Pediatrics*, 140(2), S152–S156.

Lee, J., Kim, S., & Ham, C.-D. (2016). A double-edged sword? Predicting consumers' attitudes toward and sharing intention of native advertising on social media. *American Behavioral Scientists, 60*(12), 1425–1441.

Madden, M., Lenhart, A., Cortesi, S., Gasser, U., Duggan, M., Smith, A., & Beaton, M. (2013). Teens, social media, and privacy. *Pew Research Center*. Retrieved from: www.pewinternet.org/2013/05/21/teens-social-media-and-privacy.

Marketing Land. (2016). Native advertising, the new marketing workhorse. Retrieved from: http://marketingland.com/native-advertising-new-marketing-workhorse-197856.

Moschis, G. P. (1978). *Acquisition of consumer role by adolescents*. Atlanta, GA: Georgia State University Publishing Services Division.

Moschis, G. P., & Churchill, A. (1978). Consumer socialization: A theoretical and empirical analysis. *Journal of Marketing Research, 15*, 599–609.

Ofcom. (2017). *Children and parents: Media use and attitude report*. Retrieved from: www.ofcom.org.uk/__data/assets/pdf_file/0020/108182/children-parents-media-use-attitudes-2017.pdf.

Office of eSafety Commissioner. (2016). Is there an age limit for kids on social media? Retrieved from: www.esafety.gov.au/education-resources/iparent/staying-safe/social-networking/is-there-an-age-limit-for-kids-on-social-media.

Opree, S., Buijzen, M., & van Reijmersdal, E. A. (2013). Children's advertising exposure, advertised product desire, and materialism: A longitudinal study. *Communication Research, 41*(5), 717–735.

Pew Research Center. (2018). Teens, social media & technology 2018. Retrieved from: www.pewinternet.org/2018/05/31/teens-social-media-technology-2018.

Piaget, J. (1970). *Science of education and the psychology of the child*. New York, NY: Viking.

Roedder-John, D. (1999). Consumer socialization of children: A retrospective look at twenty-five years of research. *Journal of Consumer Research, 26*(3), 183–213.

Roy Morgan. (2016). Pester power and household purchasing decisions. Retrieved from: www.roymorgan.com/findings/6698-pester-power-purchasing-decisions-201602292247.

Schor, J. B. (2004). *Born to buy: The commercialized child and the new consumer culture*. New York, NY: Scribner.

Selman, R. L. (1980). *The growth of international understanding*. New York, NY: Academic Press.

Shin, W., & Kang, H. (2016). Adolescents' privacy concerns and information disclosure online: The role of parents and the internet. *Computers in Human Behavior, 54*, 114–123.

Taylor, C. R. (2017). Native advertising: The black sheep of the marketing family. *International Journal of Advertising, 36*, 207–209.

Tucker, C. E. (2014). Social networks, personalized advertising, and privacy controls. *Journal of Marketing Research, 51*(5), 546–562.

van Dam, S., & van Raimersdal, E. A. (2019). Insights in adolescents' advertising literacy, perceptions and responses regarding sponsored influencer videos and disclosures. *Cyberpsychology: Journal of Psychological Research on Cyberspace, 13*(2). doi:10.5817/CP2019-2-2.

Viacom. (2018). Kidfluence: How kids influence buying behavior. Retrieved from: https://v.viacom.com/kidfluence-kids-influence-buying-behavior.

Walrave, M., & Heirman, W. (2013). Adolescents, online marketing and privacy: Predicting adolescents' willingness to disclose personal information for marketing purpose. *Children & Society, 27*(6), 434–447.

Wang, W., Yang, L., & Zhang, Q. (2015). Privacy preservation in location-based advertising: A contract-based approach. *Computer Networks, 93*, 213–224.

Wilcox, B. L., Kunkel, D., Cantor, J., Dowrick, P., Linn, S., & Palmer, E. (2004). Report of the APA task force of advertising and children. *American Psychological Association*. Retrieved from: www.apa.org/pi/families/resources/advertising-children.pdf.

Wojdynski, B. W. (2016). The deceptiveness of sponsored news articles: How readers recognize and perceive native advertising. *American Behavioral Scientist, 60*(12), 1475–1491.

World Health Organization. (2016). Tracking food marketing to children in a digital world: Trans-disciplinary perspectives. Retrieved from: www.euro.who.int/__data/assets/pdf_file/0017/322226/Tackling-food-marketing-children-digital-world-trans-disciplinary-perspectives-en.pdf.

Youn, S., & Shin, W. (2019). Teens' responses to Facebook newsfeed advertising: The effects of cognitive appraisal and social influence on privacy concerns and coping strategies. *Telematics and Informatics, 38*, 30–45.

Zarouali, B., Poels, K., Pottet, K., & Walrave, M. (2018). "Everything under control?": Privacy control salience influence both critical processing and perceived persuasiveness of targeted advertising among adolescents. *Cyberpsychology, 12*(1), 77–95.

Zarouali, B., Pottet, K., Walrave, M., & Poels, K. (2017). "Do you like cookies?" Adolescents' skeptical processing of retargeted Facebook-ads and the moderating role of privacy concern and a textual debriefing. *Computers in Human Behavior, 69*, 157–165.

PART IV
Children's Rights

28
CHILD-CENTRED POLICY
Enfranchising Children as Digital Policy-Makers

Brian O'Neill

Introduction

The need for child-centred policies in the digital domain is now recognised as an important priority for governments and the wider policy community. Landmark publications such as UNICEF's *State of the World's Children 2017: Children in a Digital World* have provided evidence of the global nature of the pervasive presence of digital culture in 21st-century childhood. Much policy attention understandably focusses on issues of online harms, reflecting concerns from an adult perspective for child safeguarding and welfare. A child-centred approach to digital policy is one that would similarly recognise the importance of children's safety in their use of digital technologies while formulating policy that seeks to advance the quality of children's digital engagements. That such an approach should be grounded in children's own experiences – in the form of both evidence and testimony from children themselves – would appear to be self-evident. Yet, despite the central role digital technologies play in the lives of children, progress in the area of advancing children's active participation in digital policy-making is still at an early stage.

This chapter reviews the case for children as digital policy-makers and examines the challenges as well as the potential benefits of involving children in the process of formulating and implementing policy initiatives relating to digital practice. Policy-making in the digital environment comprises a complex multi-stakeholder space where the diverse interests of governments, industry, and civil society compete to achieve equilibrium in one of the most dynamic and fast-moving sectors. Even in multi-stakeholder platforms such as the Internet Governance Forum, which advocates open and inclusive dialogue and where principles of democratic participation are strongest, it can be challenging for end users, especially children, to have their voice heard (Epstein & Nonnecke, 2016). Yet, with one third of the total global population of internet users estimated to be under the age of 18 (Livingstone, Carr, & Byrne, 2015), the missed opportunity and the gap in terms of policy-making is a significant one. Building on the emerging discourse on children's rights in the digital age (Gasser & Cortesi, 2016), the chapter highlights conceptual, policy-based, and practical issues related to children as digital policy-makers, arguing that children's participation enhances public decision-making and contributes to better policy-making overall.

Participation in the Policy Process

Public policies lie at the heart of the relationship between citizens and the state. A range of opportunities may be available to citizens to be involved in decision-making regarding the formation of laws, regulatory measures, strategies, or funding decisions that make up the policy process (Kilpatrick, 2000). Such involvement may take the form of *consultation* whereby the public's views are sought and listened to by policy-makers, or, more actively, *participation*, which provides some level of public responsibility, power, and influence in the formation of decisions (Partridge, 2005). A further dimension may include actual involvement in *policy governance*, which implies participation in the organisation and management of policies as well as the coordination of the interactions between different sectors of society in the policy process (Althaus, Bridgman, & Davis, 2013).

Children's participation in policy-making stems from a recognition of their rights as citizens to be involved in matters that affect them. This has been recognised most notably in the UN Convention of the Rights of the Child (UNCRC) (2009), specifically Article 12 (the 'Right to be Heard'). Article 12 ascribes to children the right to be heard in all matters affecting them and to participate in decision-making processes that have a bearing on their lives in accordance with their age and maturity. Article 12 is something of a touchstone for international efforts to reinforce governments' responsibilities to facilitate consultation with children through representative authorities such as children's ombudspersons and children's commissioners, advocating on behalf of children's *participation* rights alongside rights to *protection* and indeed rights of *provision* – the so-called three 'Ps' of the UNCRC.

Elaborating on what Article 12 may mean in practice, the UN Committee on the Rights of the Child has argued:

> The views expressed by children may add relevant perspectives and experience and should be considered in decision-making, policy-making and preparation of laws and/or measures as well as their evaluation … The concept of participation emphasises that including children should not only be a momentary act, but the starting point for an intense exchange between children and adults on the development of policies, programmes and measures in all relevant contexts of children's lives.
>
> *(CRC, 2009, p. 7 at para. 12)*

What could this mean in a digital policy context? Digital policy refers to the process of developing and implementing various forms of policies, procedures, and standards for the proper use, management, and development of digitalisation (Floridi, 2018). This may include, for instance, regulation of digital and electronic communications, network and information security, issues concerning broadband access and digital infrastructure, as well as online safety and civic participation. Public policy invariably impacts on some aspect of children's everyday lives and experiences, all the more so in the case of the digital world where children and young people are most often to the fore in early adoption (Fortunati, Taipale, & de Luca, 2017). Yet the issues that dominate the digital policy agenda which most explicitly refer to children are often about protecting young people from harmful content or contact through restricting their access. Prominent examples of digital policy initiatives that are ostensibly child-focussed include, therefore, the European Union's Audiovisual Media Services Directive with its specific requirements for the protection of minors (ERGA, 2017); measures introduced in the UK to restrict access by under-18s to online pornography (Blake, 2019); or the introduction of a digital age of consent as part of the EU General Data Protection Regulation (GDPR) whereby an age limit is set between 13 and

16 years below which children require parental consent to register for many social media services (Macenaite & Kosta, 2017; Milkaite & Lievens, 2018). Key drivers in this respect are growing public and political concern about the lack of regulation of digital platforms, the perceived scant regard such operations have for children's safety or welfare, and the pressure for a more urgent political response to curb the power of global digital undertakings.

In each of these areas of significant policy debate and development, consultation with children has been limited or entirely absent (Livingstone, 2018). The concerns that children themselves raise receive relatively little attention when it comes to: providing better online tools to deal with nasty comments, hate speech, or cyberbullying on social media platforms (Livingstone, Kirwil, Ponte, & Staksrud, 2013); their concerns about having to confront disturbing online content or being pestered with unwanted sexual messaging (European Institute for Gender Equality, 2018); and, importantly, their need for more support in developing their own media and digital literacy skills as well as positive content relevant to their lives, language, and culture.

Children also receive many conflicting and confusing messages about their use of digital technologies. On the one hand, they are encouraged to acquire digital skills and use ICT in their learning. On the other, they face restrictions – often stoked by parental fears about the harmful impact of digital technologies – despite its pervasive presence in the home. For this reason, a more considered incorporation of and reflection on children's perspectives on digital policy matters has been taken up as a rights-based issue. This includes the fundamental principle that children have a right to be heard and that their input merits meaningful attention as a contribution to the policy debate (Byrne & Burton, 2017; Perez Vallejos et al., 2016).

Empowering Children as Digital Policy Actors

While the UNCRC was developed before the digital age, its drafting in 1989 anticipated the media and communications sphere as an important context in which to exercise and fulfil children's rights. Article 13 ('Freedom of Expression') states: "this right shall include freedom to seek, receive and impart information and ideas of all kinds, regardless of frontiers, either orally, in writing or in print, in the form of art, or through any other media of the child's choice". Article 17 recognises "the important function performed by the mass media and shall ensure that the child has access to information and material from a diversity of national and international sources" (UNCRC, 1989). Combined, this formulation of the rights of children places a spotlight on the role of media – which inescapably is now a digital phenomenon – emphasising the importance of access to high-quality media content, opportunities for young people's voices to be heard, and advocating for responsible and ethical media representation of children (Livingstone, 2007; Tobin, 2004; Von Feilitzen, Carlsson, & Bucht, 2010).

Scholarly attention has more recently highlighted the digital environment as an important and relevant context for the elaboration of children's rights and specifically to advance children's participation (Lievens, Livingstone, McLaughlin, O'Neill, & Verdoodt, 2018; Livingstone & O'Neill, 2014). Consideration of children's rights in a digital context has, to date, centred around three interconnecting issues (Livingstone, Lansdown, & Third, 2017):

1 *Digital use*, in particular the right to access content and services;
2 *Digital environment* including rights within online and networked spaces; and
3 *Digital citizenship*, for instance, how such media impacts upon wider rights in society (Livingstone & Third, 2017; Third & Collin, 2016).

The UN Committee on the Rights of the Child, for its part, devoted a Day of General Discussion on 'Digital Media and Children's Rights' (2014) and has undertaken to publish a General

Comment on the subject (Livingstone et al., 2017). Addressing both *risks* and *opportunities* in the digital sphere, the Committee has argued for effective and immediate implementation of human rights-based laws and policies which integrate children's access to digital media and ICTs (UN Committee of the Rights of the Child, 2014, pp. 18–19). Addressing children's participation, it recommended that:

> States should recognise the importance of access to, and use of, digital media and ICTs for children and their potential to promote all children's rights, in particular the rights to freedom of expression, access to appropriate information, participation, education, as well as rest, leisure, play, recreational activities, cultural life and the arts.
>
> *(CRC Committee, 2014, p. 18)*

In a report prepared for the UK Children's Commissioner, it is also argued that engaging with children in the development of legislation and policy on such topics as digital participation and protection is vital and that "digital means of consulting and collaborating with children in the wider policy domains" and "enabling and empowering children to participate in wider political citizenship online and through social media" is a crucial development of the practical application of Article 12 (Livingstone, Lansdown, and Third, 2017, p. 42).

The Council of Europe has added its voice to empowering children as digital policymakers in a number of key policy statements. Its 2018 Recommendation to member states, *Guidelines to respect, protect and fulfil the rights of the child in the digital environment*, is the most comprehensive statement to date on the articulation of children's rights within a digital context. The Recommendation sets out detailed policy guidance regarding children's right to be heard, their right to access to the digital environment, rights to freedom of expression and information, and empowerment through digital literacy, while considering the importance of safety, security, and data protection and privacy (Council of Europe, 2018). It recommends that governments review their legislation, policies, and practice to ensure children's rights are promoted within a digital context, that appropriate oversight is developed to ensure that business enterprises meet their responsibilities, and all relevant stakeholders ensure concerted action and cooperation at the national and international level to uphold and respect children's rights.

The Recommendation's guidance on the right to be heard, encapsulated in the statement "Children have the right to express themselves freely in all matters affecting them, and their views should be given due weight in accordance with their age and maturity" (2.4) encompasses specific recommendations on the development of practical opportunities for children to be actively and meaningfully involved in the policy-making process:

6. States and other relevant stakeholders should *provide children with information on their rights*, including their participation rights, in a way they can understand, and which is appropriate to their maturity and circumstances. They should *enhance opportunities for them to express themselves through ICTs* as a complement to face-to-face participation. Children should be informed of mechanisms and services providing adequate support, and of procedures for complaints, remedies or redress should their rights be violated. Such information should also be made available to their parents or carers to enable them to support children in exercising their rights.
7. Furthermore, States and other relevant stakeholders should actively engage children to participate meaningfully in devising, implementing and evaluating legislation, policies, mechanisms, practices, technologies and resources that aim to respect, protect and fulfil the rights of the child in the digital environment.

(emphasis added) (Council of Europe, 2018)

Notably, digital literacy and support for children to acquire the necessary skills to exercise their rights to participation is further identified as an important pre-condition. Children should receive adequate support through digital literacy education to ensure they have the skills and digital competence to engage in online communication and should not be disadvantaged by socio-geographical or socio-economic factors (paras 41–46).

Furthermore, states should introduce greater coordination and policy coherence across the full range of children's rights in the digital environment. A comprehensive strategic national approach is advocated, engaging all relevant stakeholders, "such as ombudspersons for children and other independent human rights institutions, education stakeholders, data-protection authorities, business enterprises and civil society, including child and youth-led organisations" and ensuring adequate resources for children's meaningful participation (para 84). This should also be supported by investment in "research and knowledge development, including child and youth participation in the field of the rights of the child in the digital environment" (para 110).

Building on the concept of the right to be heard in a digital context, Vromen (2008) has identified three key aspects of the digital sphere, specifically the internet, that are of particular relevance to its participatory potential.

First, the digital sphere represents an immense gateway to *information* that empowers through its open dissemination of knowledge about campaigns and issues of importance to young people. One of the most popular and basic things that children do when they first go online is to seek out information and use the internet as a vast encyclopaedia (Livingstone, Mascheroni, Ólafsson, & Haddon, 2014). Vromen (2008) argues that engaging and empowering young people through information about topical and political issues is key to more active participation. In the policy domain, this has been especially significant in terms of informing young people of their rights, making information available in accessible ways and providing them with trustworthy and authoritative sources of information.

Second, the internet is by its nature an *interactive communication* medium that facilitates a variety of different types of online conversations, from one to one, to online platforms, chat rooms, and discussion forums. The importance of interactivity from a policy-making point of view is its potential to facilitate communication and feedback from large numbers of people to government and other agencies and institutions, of which online petitions and online voting are the most prominent examples. Young people are often critical of internet resources that simply provide information and do not provide opportunities for interaction and engagement, and they seek out those resources that do (Coleman & Rowe, 2005).

Third, the internet may be seen as a vast *virtual public sphere*, thus "providing a platform for rational critical debate rather than simple registration of individual views through information aggregation tools, such as polls or surveys" (in Vromen, 2008, p. 81). Coleman (2008) advances the argument that for governments wishing to promote more active involvement of youth, such initiatives themselves have to be democratic in character. To avoid being more than a top-down exercise in bureaucratic management, terms of engagement should "be determined in partnership between official policy-makers and young people themselves, using wikis and other forms of collaborative decision-making software" (Coleman, 2008, p. 204). Openness and transparency in how conversations are initiated and structured, or how topics are prioritised, is also essential.

The respective *informational*, *interactive*, and *participatory* dimensions of the digital sphere, as presented by Vromen, may be said to represent an idealised space for digital participation. As Third and Collin argue (2016), digital citizenship is a concept "*brimming with promise for rethinking citizenship through the digital*" (p. 42, emphasis in original). However, as they also note, the reality of children's experiences and the attendant policy responses is such that such potential is overwhelmed by the many challenges that children – as much as adults – face, such as being confronted with manipulation of information or 'fake' (political) news, the filter bubble, hate speech, and even radicalisation through, among other means, digital media (Third, Livingstone, & Lansdown, 2019).

It is also the case that just as the existence of digital divides underscores the fact that digital opportunities are not equally available to all, there is also a notable participation gap when it comes to those children and young people who have the digital skills and the opportunity to access its participatory potential and those who do not (Helsper, 2012).

Methodological and Other Challenges

While there has been something of a shift within policy circles towards accentuating positive opportunities – notwithstanding the urgent imperative to respond to online harms – giving effect to children's participation in policy-making is also a subject of considerable methodological debate. A number of theoretical models have been developed to conceptualise and support effective and meaningful participation of children and young people. Hart's eight-rung hierarchal ladder of participation (1992), for instance, building on Arnstein (1989), proposes that only mechanisms which facilitate *actual* decision-making, whether shared with adults or child-initiated, can be considered truly participatory in nature.

Persistent systemic challenges or barriers to making children's participation effective, i.e., involving *active* participation and *actual* decision-making, have been identified. Tisdall (2015) summarises the following six key areas of concern:

1. *Tokenism*: children may be consulted but with little discernible impact on decisions or outcomes (see also Arnstein, 1969; Partridge, 2005; Sinclair, 2004);
2. *Lack of feedback*: children are given insufficient information on what happens to their contributions (see also Gerison Lansdown, 2016; Lister, 2007);
3. *Who is included or excluded?* The 'over-consultation' of some children and not enough representation from seldom-heard or hard-to-reach groups (see also Kelleher, Seymour, & Halpenny, 2014; Kirby, Lanyon, Cronin, & Sinclair, 2003);
4. *Consultation but not dialogue*: children and young people are frequently consulted in one-off activities but are not involved over time in on-going, respectful dialogue (see also Collin, 2008);
5. *Adult processes and structures exclude children and young people*: a lack of integration of children's participation into formal established policy-making processes, in effect making children's participation a specialisation and risking that it will be side-lined (see also Cockburn, 2005; Kilkelly et al., 2007);
6. *Lack of sustainability*: with inadequate long-term support, participation initiatives risk being one-off and short term in nature and will not become embedded in the policy process (see also Asthana, 2006; Jochum, Pratten, & Wilding, 2005).

Models developed by Treseder (1997) and Kirby et al. (2003) address some of the contextual factors that can impact on the form of children's and young people's participation. Lundy's model (2007) aims for a more comprehensive approach in drawing attention to four integrated elements – each related to Article 12 of the UNCRC. These are *space, voice, audience,* and *influence*, which act as chronological stages in the development of an effective model of child participation.

Lundy's first element, *space*, refers to the provision of opportunities for children to express their views. These opportunities should be safe, inclusive, and voluntary. In addition to the decision to take part, children should also be allowed to choose which matters they wish to discuss and what methods of participation they would like to use. Following on from this, the second element, *voice*, highlights that children and young people should be able to express their views. Once children are capable of forming views, they are entitled to communicate them. In line with Article 5 of the UNCRC, Lundy (2007) emphasises that parental assistance can be called upon to help formulate views if required. Further to this, the third element, *audience*, focusses on the importance of children's views being listened to by decision-makers. Finally, the fourth element, *influence*, states that children's views should be appropriately acted upon. The level of competence children possess for decision-making should be viewed according to their evolving capacities and within a child-empowering perspective (Lundy, 2007).

From a practice-based perspective, the literature on the use of digital technologies in youth work similarly provides important insights into the factors that are likely to make participation more effective (Grönlund & Åström, 2009; Panopoulou, Tambouris, & Tarabanis, 2014; Zimmermann, 2016). Drawing on the use of e-participation tools for involving youth in decision-making, the International Youth Service of the Federal Republic of Germany (IJAB, 2014) has outlined five key principles to underpin successful engagement.

First, *alignment with young people's realities*: to encourage active participation requires consultation and structured dialogue to relate closely with young people's lives and to address issues of concern to them. Processes should be designed to interest, stimulate, and motivate young people using diverse methods and creative applications. Social and digital media have intrinsic interest for many young people; yet design and technical implementation have to be carefully adapted to their needs and requirements.

Second, the adequate *resourcing of effective participation is crucial*. While the use of social and digital media can be a cost-effective way of reaching larger audiences and involving more young people who might not otherwise participate, it is not a cost-saving tool and needs to be adequately resourced to be successful. Sufficient resources for expertise, the time required to achieve the outcomes, and for appropriate technology development and support are needed.

Third, to be effective participation must have *defined outcomes* with a structural link to public decision-making processes defined in advance. A formal linkage to the policy-making cycle is an essential element. Delivering concrete results quickly, sharing them in an accessible fashion and broadcasting them across wider social media has positive benefits in reinforcing effectiveness.

Fourth, the issue of *transparency* is crucial, particularly given public concerns about the role of digital technologies in democratic processes. Social and digital media platforms can be opaque in terms of processing. Success factors include making the process of consultation or participation transparent for everyone, including the tools and software used with clear demonstration of information flows, input, and outcomes.

Finally, it is vital that *involvement is inclusive*. In order to promote an inclusive, participatory culture, young people should be involved at all stages, including feedback opportunities through successive phases. Young people's input at the concept and piloting stage has been found to be particularly important and can positively impact on its design effectiveness (García-Peñalvo & Kearney, 2016).

Models of successful participation, whether technology-based or not, will always require close matching of the objectives set for the particular consultation or dialogue process, and engagement with as well as comprehensive feedback to the populations concerned (Peixoto, Fall, & Sjoberg, 2016). Experience from the field shows that selecting the appropriate methodologies and choosing the right digital tools is always a delicate balancing act between wider engagement and a more focussed deliberative process designed to achieve a specific outcome (Edelmann, Krimmer, & Parycek, 2008). For children and youth, those methodologies, while showing promise, are still in development – especially in the case of digital methodologies – and necessarily require higher levels of safeguarding and oversight if they are to achieve the objectives of fostering better participation.

Conclusion

Despite its evident promise and the underlying policy imperatives that have attracted increasing international attention, the mobilisation of children as digital policy-makers remains at an early stage of development. The nature of participation itself remains complex and if effective mechanisms such as that mapped out by Lundy (2007) are to be realised in and through digital media, the barriers to participation, both contextual and systemic, need to be addressed.

Active participation may be defined as a process where citizens are engaged in policy-making and have a role in defining the issues, structuring the consultation process and where they can have an impact on the policy outcomes (OECD, 2003). Here, digital technologies can provide a range of supporting interactive communication tools that can bring policy-makers and end users closer together by sharing information and channels for feedback on an unprecedented level. However, as argued by Vromen (2008), participation in this context is a deliberative process which means that citizens have the opportunity to be actively involved in the decision-making process and its outcome. Applying digital technologies to this process suggests "a new framework for decision-making and legislation formation" that is more inclusive and more wide-ranging than what has gone before (Ergazakis, Metaxiotis, & Tsitsanis, 2011, p. 5).

Ultimately, to be successful, children's involvement in policy-making – digital and otherwise – needs to be addressed both at the level of the individual child, with appropriate supports to foster a democratic ethos in the child's immediate environment, as well as at the systemic level to include supportive professional attitudes and resources dedicated to fostering children's participation, an enabling regulatory regime as well as a willingness and acceptance at the socio-political level of children's legitimate role in policy-making. That digital policy itself can benefit from greater inclusion of youth perspectives is a key contributory consideration. But the underlying rationale remains that mobilising children's digital participation is not just a more sophisticated application of digital literacy but also a higher order of citizen engagement, something that is central to digital citizenship, the positive use of digital media technology, and active participation in democratic culture (Council of Europe, 2017).

References

Althaus, C., Bridgman, P., & Davis, G. (2013). *The Australian policy handbook, 5th edition*. Crows Nest, NSW: Allen & Unwin.

Arnstein, S. R. (1969). A ladder of citizen participation. *Journal of the American Planning Association*, 35(4), 216–224.

Arnstein, S. R. (1989). A ladder of citizen participation. *Journal of the American Planning Association*, 35(4), 216–224. doi.org/10.1080/01944366908977225.

Asthana, S. (2006). *Innovative practices of youth participation in media: A research study on twelve initiatives from around the developing and underdeveloped regions of the world; 2006*. Retrieved from: http://unesdoc.unesco.org/images/0014/001492/149279e.pdf.

Blake, P. (2019). Age verification for online porn: More harm than good? *Porn Studies*, 6(2), 228–237.

Byrne, J., & Burton, P. (2017).Children as internet users : How can evidence better inform policy debate? *Journal of Cyber Policy*, 8871(August), 39–52.

Cockburn, T. (2005). Children's participation in social policy: Inclusion, chimera or authenticity? *Social Policy and Society*, 4(2), 109–119.

Coleman, S. (2008). Doing IT for themselves: Management versus autonomy in youth E-citizenship. In W. Lance Bennett (Ed.), *The John D. and Catherine T. MacArthur foundation series on digital media and learning* (pp. 189–206). Cambridge, MA: The MIT Press.

Coleman, S., & Rowe, C. (2005). *Remixing citizenship: Democracy and young people's use of the internet*. London: The Carnegie Trust.

Collin, P. (2008). The internet, youth participation policies, and the development of young people's political identities in Australia. *Journal of Youth Studies*, 11(5), 527–542.

Council of Europe. (2017). *Digital citizenship education. Vol. 1: Overview and new perspectives*. Strasbourg: Council of Europe.

Council of Europe. (2018). *Recommendation CM/Rec(2018)7 of the Committee of Ministers to member States on guidelines to respect, protect and fulfil the rights of the child in the digital environment*. Strasbourg: Author. Retrieved from: https://search.coe.int/cm/Pages/result_details.aspx?ObjectID=09000016808b79f7.

Edelmann, N., Krimmer, R., & Parycek, P. (2008). Engaging youth through deliberative e-participation: A case study. *International Journal of Electronic Governance, 1*(4), 385–399.

Epstein, D., & Nonnecke, B. M. (2016). Multistakeholderism in praxis: The case of the regional and national Internet Governance Forum (IGF) initiatives. *Policy & Internet, 8*(2), 148–173.

ERGA. (2017). *Protection of minors in the audiovisual media services: Trends & practices*. Brussels. Retrieved from: http://ec.europa.eu/newsroom/document.cfm?doc_id=44167.

Ergazakis, K., Metaxiotis, K., & Tsitsanis, T. (2011). A state-of-the-art review of applied forms and areas, tools and technologies for e-participation. *International Journal of Electronic Government Research, 7*(1), 1–19.

European Institute for Gender Equality. (2018). *Gender equality and youth: The opportunities and risks of digitalisation*. Luxembourg: Publications Office of the European Union.

Floridi, L. (2018). Soft ethics and the governance of the digital. *Philosophy and Technology, 31*(1), 1–8. Retrieved from: https://theoccasionalinformationist.com/2017/02/02/why-lis-doesnt-have-a-quick-fix-for-the-post-factual-society-and-why-thats-ok.

Fortunati, L., Taipale, S., & de Luca, F. (2017). Digital generations, but not as we know them. *Convergence, 25*(1), 95–112.

García-Peñalvo, F. J., & Kearney, N. A. (2016). Networked youth research for empowerment in digital society. In *Proceedings of the Fourth International Conference on Technological Ecosystems for Enhancing Multiculturality – TEEM '16* (pp. 3–9). New York, NY: ACM Press.

Gasser, U., & Cortesi, S. (2016). Children's rights and digital technologies: Introduction to the discourse and some meta-observations. In M. D. Ruck, M. Peterson-Badali, & M. Freeman (Eds.), *Handbook of children's rights: Global and multidisciplinary perspectives* (pp. 417–436). London: Routledge.

Grönlund, Å., & Åström, J. (2009). DoIT right: Measuring effectiveness of different eConsultation designs. In A. Macintosh & E. Tambouris (Eds.), *Electronic participation. ePart 2009. Lecture notes in computer science, Vol. 5694* (pp. 90–100). Berlin, Heidelberg: Springer.

Hart, R. A. (1992). *Children's participation: From tokenism to citizenship. UNICEF: Innocenti Essays (No. 4)*. Florence: UNICEF International Child Development Centre.

Helsper, E. (2012). Which children are fully online? In S. Livingstone, L. Haddon, & A. Görzig (Eds.), *Children, risk and safety on the internet* (pp. 45–58). Bristol: Policy Press.

IJAB. (2014). Guidelines for successful e-participation by young people in decision-making at local, regional, national and European levels. Retrieved from: www.ijab.de/uploads/tx_ttproducts/datasheet/Guidelines_eParticipation_engl.pdf.

Jochum, V., Pratten, B., & Wilding, K. (2005). *Civil renewal and active citizenship*. London: NCVO. Retrieved from: www.ncvo.org.uk/images/documents/policy_and_research/participation/civil_renewal_active_citizenship.pdf.

Kelleher, C., Seymour, M., & Halpenny, A. M. (2014). *Promoting the participation of seldom heard young people: A review of the literature on best practice principles*. Dublin: Dublin Institute of Technology. Retrieved from: http://arrow.dit.ie/aaschsslrep.

Kilkelly, U., Whyte, J., Buckley, H., Fitzgerald, F., Mark McCafferty, J., & Kilkelly, U. (2007). Barriers to the realisation of children's rights in Ireland. *Senior Clinical Psychologist North Kildare Child and Adolescent Mental Health Service*. Dublin: Office of the Ombudsman for Children. Retrieved from: www.oco.ie/library/barriers-realisation-childrens-rights-ireland/content/uploads/2014/03/Barrierstorealisationofchildren_x0027_s rights.pdf.

Kilpatrick, D. G. (2000). *Definitions of public policy and the law*. Washington, DC: National Violence Against Women Prevention Research Center. Retrieved August 27, 2017, from: https://mainweb-v.musc.edu/vawprevention/policy/definition.shtml.

Kirby, P., Lanyon, C., Cronin, K., & Sinclair, R. (2003). *Building a culture of participation: Involving children and young people in policy, service planning, development and evaluation: A handbook*. London: National Children's Bureau. Retrieved from: www.ncb.org.uk.

Lansdown, G. (2016). The right to be heard: Taking child participation to a new level. *Reaching the heights for the rights of the child* (pp. 1–3), Sofia, 5–6 April 2016.

Lievens, E., Livingstone, S. M., McLaughlin, S., O'Neill, B., & Verdoodt, V. (2018). Children's rights and digital technologies. In T. Liefaard & U. Kilkelly (Eds.), *International children's rights law* (pp. 487–513). Singapore: Springer.

Lister, R. (2007). From object to subject: Including marginalised citizens in policy making. *Policy and Politics, 35*(3), 437–455.
Livingstone, S. (2007). Children's television charter. In J. J. Arnett (Ed.), *Encyclopedia of children, adolescents, and the media* (pp. 164–165). London: Sage. Retrieved from: www.wsmcf.com/charters/charter.htm.
Livingstone, S. (2018). Children: A special case for privacy? *InterMedia, 46*(2), 18–23.
Livingstone, S., Carr, J., & Byrne, J. (2015). *One in three: Internet governance and children's rights*. London: Centre for International Governance Innovation and the Royal Institute of International Affairs.
Livingstone, S., Kirwil, L., Ponte, C., & Staksrud, E. (2013). *In their own words: What bothers children online?* London: LSE. Retrieved from: http://eprints.lse.ac.uk/48357.
Livingstone, S., Lansdown, G., & Third, A. (2017). *The case for a UNCRC general comment on children's rights and digital media*. London: The Children's Commissioner. Retrieved from: www.childrenscommissioner.gov.uk/wp-content/uploads/2017/06/Case-for-general-comment-on-digital-media.pdf.
Livingstone, S., Mascheroni, G., Ólafsson, K., & Haddon, L. (2014). *Children's online risks and opportunities: Comparative findings from EU Kids Online and Net Children Go Mobile*. London: LSE, EU Kids Online, LSE. Retrieved from: http://eprints.lse.ac.uk/60513.
Livingstone, S., & O'Neill, B. (2014). Children's rights online : Challenges, dilemmas and emerging directions. In S. van der Hof, B. van den Berg, & B. Schermer (Eds.), *Minding minors wandering the web: Regulating online child safety* (Vol. 24, pp. 19–39). The Hague: T.M.C. Asser Press.
Livingstone, S., & Third, A. (2017). Children and young people's rights in the digital age: An emerging agenda. *New Media & Society, 19*(5), 657–670.
Lundy, L. (2007). "Voice" is not enough: Conceptualising Article 12 of the United Nations Convention on the Rights of the Child. *British Educational Research Journal, 33*(6), 927–942.
Macenaite, M., & Kosta, E. (2017). Consent for processing children's personal data in the EU: Following in US footsteps? *Information and Communications Technology Law, 26*(2), 146–197.
Milkaite, I., & Lievens, E. (2018). *Counting down to 25 May 2018: Mapping the GDPR age of consent across the EU*. Ghent: University of Ghent.
OECD. (2003). *Promise and problems of E-democracy: Challenges of online citizen engagement*. Paris. Retrieved from: www.oecd.org/gov/digital-government/35176328.pdf.
Panopoulou, E., Tambouris, E., & Tarabanis, K. (2014). Success factors in designing eParticipation initiatives. *Information and Organization, 24*(4), 195–213.
Partridge, A. (2005). Children and young people's inclusion in public decision-making. *Support for Learning, 20*(4), 181–190.
Peixoto, T., Fall, M., & Sjoberg, F. (2016). *Evaluating digital citizen engagement: A practical guide*. Washington, DC: Governance and Social Development Resource Centre. Retrieved from: https://openknowledge.worldbank.org/bitstream/handle/10986/23752/deef-book.pdf?sequence=1&isAllowed=y.
Perez Vallejos, E., Koene, A., Carter, C. J., Statache, R., Rodden, T., McAuley, D., . . . Coleman, S. (2016). Juries: Acting out digital dilemmas to promote digital reflections. *ACM SIGCAS Computers and Society, 45*(3), 84–90.
Sinclair, R. (2004). Participation in practice: Making it meaningful, effective and sustainable. *Children and Society, 18*(2), 106–118.
Third, A., & Collin, P. (2016). Rethinking citizenship through dialogues on digital practice. In A. McCosker, S. Vivienne, & A. Johns (Eds.), *Negotiating digital citizenship: Control, contest and culture* (pp. 41–59). London: Rowman and Littlefield.
Third, A., Livingstone, S., & Lansdown, G. (2019). Recognizing children's rights in relation to digital technologies: Challenges of voice and evidence, principle and practice. In B. Wagner, M. C. Kettemann, & K. Vieth (Eds.), *Research handbook on human rights and digital technology* (pp. 376–410). London: Elgar. Retrieved from: www.elgaronline.com/view/edcoll/9781785367717/9781785367717.00029.xml.
Tisdall, K. (2015). Promoting the participation of children and youth across the globe: From social exclusion to child-inclusive policies. In T. Gal & B. F. Duramy (Eds.), *International perspectives and empirical findings on child participation* (pp. 381–404). Oxford: Oxford University Press. Retrieved: from www.research.ed.ac.uk/portal/en/publications/addressing-the-challenges-of-children-and-young-peoples-participation-considering-time-and-space(f14df609-ab9a-4bbc-8296-0fa937c5837f)/export.html.
Tobin, J. (2004). Partners worth courting: The relationship between the media and the Convention on the Rights of the Child. *International Journal of Children's Rights, 12*(2), 139–167.
Treseder, P. (1997). *Empowering children & young people: Training manual : Promoting involvement in decision-making*. London: Save the Children. Retrieved from: https://books.google.ie/books/about/Empowering_Children_Young_People.html?id=SFDoAAAACAAJ.

UN Committee on the Rights of the Child (CRC). General Comment No.12. (2009). *The right of the child to be heard*. Pub. L. No. CRC/C/GC/12 (2009). Retrieved from: www2.ohchr.org/english/bodies/crc/docs/AdvanceVersions/CRC-C-GC-12.pdf.

UN Committee on the Rights of the Child (CRC). (2014). *Report of the 2014 day of general discussion "Digital Media and Children's Rights"*. Retrieved from: www.ohchr.org/Documents/HRBodies/CRC/Discussions/2014/DGD_report.pdf.

United Nations. (1989). *Convention on the Rights of the Child*. Retrieved 22 June 2020 from: www.ohchr.org/en/professionalinterest/pages/crc.aspx.

Von Feilitzen, C., Carlsson, U., & Bucht, C. (2010). *New questions, new approaches, new insights: Contributions to the research forum at the world summit on media for children and Youth 2010. Media*. Goteborg: International Clearinghouse on Children Youth and Media.

Vromen, A. (2008). Building virtual spaces: Young people, participation and the internet. *Australian Journal of Political Science, 43*(1), 79–97.

Zimmermann, H.-D. (2016). Youth e-participation: Lessons learned from an ongoing project in Switzerland. In *Proceedings of the 29th Bled eConference* (pp. 588–596). Retrieved from: https://domino.fov.uni-mb.si/proceedings.nsf/Proceedings/DABFCEF97B8EAA93C125800D004944AA/$File/1_DieterZimmermann.pdf.

29
LAW, DIGITAL MEDIA, AND THE DISCOMFORT OF CHILDREN'S RIGHTS

Brian Simpson

Introduction

This chapter seeks to bring a 'counter-narrative' to discussions about children and their use of digital media. This narrative is centred on a view of children's rights that stresses the autonomy rights of children ahead of their protection rights. In challenging more orthodox stances about the place of children and adult emphases on the need to protect children, this narrative is often highly contested by many who hold to more conservative views of family. Thus, the conceptualisation of children's rights argued for here gives rise to discomfort for some adults, but it will be explained here that this is a discomfort that is truly necessary if the meaning of childhood is to be protected while giving proper effect to the rights of children. This discussion is also of contemporary importance as it connects the transformation of children's lives by digital technology with other challenges to the authority of adults, institutions, and governments over children. The advent of social media, for example, has meant that individuals under 18 who previously had minimal media presence, if any, and thus little voice to call to account those who caused them harm, can now challenge orthodox understandings and explanations of social phenomena that affect them. In positive terms, children have become active participants in defining their identities and what they stand for through their access to digital media. This is not, of course, to argue that such participation of children is straightforward or without problems, but it is important to recognise the transformative nature of what is occurring and how children and young people use new media to explore their place in society (Chalfen, 2009; Simpson, 2005). Importantly, regarding the sole focus of the law as the need to protect children from the purported 'harmful' effects of digital media ignores the manner in which the law must also support the right to transgress norms (sometimes outdated) as part of enabling individuals to challenge narratives that seek to inhibit their potential or subordinate them (Abiala & Hernwall, 2013; boyd, 2014; Karaian, 2012; Presdee, 2000).

The role of the law in regulating or supporting this process of allowing individuals to transgress norms is muddied and confused. What is meant by this is that legal responses to the role of digital media in the lives of children often fit within what could be called a traditional understanding of the role of law. This understanding of law tends to see law as a set of 'rules' that has, as its purpose, the protection of a set of social understandings about what is 'good' and 'bad', what is 'beneficial' and what is 'harmful' about digital media, as applied to children. What this notion of law disguises, however, is that those who make the law also construct the definitions of what is 'good' and 'bad'. In history, this has usually been about supporting the definitions of the powerful who in fact manipulate the law to advance their interests while paying lip service to the notion that law is the product of a democratic process and social consensus. (See, for example, Kairys, 1998.) The messiness of the law's response to the use of digital media as a tool of identity formation, and as a challenge to established and potentially outdated norms, is that while many of the stated tenets of the law articulate the rights of individuals to dissent and, in effect, transgress, this creates a struggle for legal institutions that have tended to see their purpose historically as the preservation of the rights that underpin the status and political power of those with wealth and influence. (See, for example, Kennedy, 2004.) In this sense, law has more to do with ideology, politics, and economics than legal doctrine, which itself is often ambiguous and lacking in coherence (Carson, 1980) leading to more symbolism than sense (Freiberg, 2007, p. 81). For this reason, it is important to recognise that while a discussion of the nature of law in this context is important, it would be folly to assume that it is possible to come to a position where there is any clarity about the role of law, or what reforms are necessary to create 'better' laws. To understand 'law' does not imply any insight as to how to make it 'better'.

Debates about the role of law in regulating digital technology rarely include significant discussion about what is meant by 'law'. Such debates seem to assume that, when providing a 'legal' response to, say, children's use of social media, the role of the law is to bring to the matter some kind of neutral arbiter. It is assumed that the law is itself a result of a process that rationally considers competing views, weighs up the evidence, and then formulates appropriate legal principles to apply to the situation. This unquestioning approach to what law is, and hence the role that law does or can perform, is against a proper understanding of how law operates in relation to social events. A better understanding of law, and hence a basis for discussing how it impacts on children and digital media, is to acknowledge its primary role in preserving status, power, and privilege within society while cloaking this "in the fabric of a discourse of rights" (Williams, 1987, p. 133). This understanding of law is an important underpinning to the counter narrative discussed here about children, law, and digital media. While the law mythologises its manner of development as a rational and scientific one, in fact the law is formulated around shifts in society that direct its development rather than in any necessary coherent or formulaic manner. Many of those who operate within the law understand the extent to which ideology and politics – counter-narratives if you will – influence what law 'is'. To that extent, and to the extent that those other narratives enter legal debates from time to time somewhat haphazardly, it should be of no surprise that law can often seem more ambiguous or contradictory in its response to social problems or phenomena than its stated legal principles would suggest. (See, for example, King & Piper, 1995.) In effect, and as will be further articulated below, in the area of children and digital media, the law tends to adopt understandings of the child that both support adult romantic notions of childhood and also meet society's needs to produce citizens that are broadly economically productive and unquestioning of the existing social order. This leads to the focus on children's protection rights mentioned previously, leading the law away from rights that support challenges to the social order. Considering the conjunction of children, law, and digital media, however, offers the opportunity to embed the counter-narrative in law's role, and to add to the tension surrounding law's purpose.

The Shifting Terrain of Law, Children, and Status

An understanding of the law's approach to the regulation of digital media as it affects children also requires an understanding of how law views the status of children. The legal status of children is shifting and dynamic. It cannot be assumed that the concept of children's legal status results from some developmental and coherent process. Nor should it be assumed that the legal notion of consent – pivotal in stated legal doctrine to the capacity of the child to make life decisions – has held the same meaning through legal history. As Holly Brewer (2005) demonstrates, the way in which the law constructs the legal capacity of children reflects ideological shifts in society. She traces the development of society through the 17th and 18th centuries from an authoritarian system of government towards a democratic one. In this period, she also identifies an important shift in constructions around the legal capacity of children. Prior to the formation of democracies, the child's capacity to consent on its own behalf was attached to their status. In effect, the aristocratic child could enter into various legal relationships that relied on this status (Brewer, 2005). The advent of democratic theory, however, shifted the basis of the meaning of consent away from status and towards reason; that is, to be governed democratically required a form of consent that depended on an understanding of this nature of government. This excluded children from democratic participation. As she explains:

> 'Consent' has not had an unchanging meaning. The new principle that consent must be 'informed' and reasonable, which led to the exclusion of children, was part of what made democratic political ideology viable, acceptable, and above all, legitimate. It became the marrow of the law. The principle that responsibility was necessary for both criminal matters and voting became established as consent became more important to the law, at the same time as birth and perpetual status became less important.
>
> *(Brewer, 2005, p. 341)*

By the mid-18th century "some began to characterise teenagers, in particular, as ruled by passion, whereas adults were guided by reason" (Brewer, 2005, p. 335). It would be a mistake to understand this shift simply in terms of a greater enlightenment about the capacity and maturity of children. Instead, other contemporaneous changes provide a more credible explanation of what was occurring around this conceptualisation of the child. At that time, older power structures were being challenged by new ideas about how society should be governed. Within that context, the recasting of the child's capacity as diminished, based on children's inability to reason, had the effect of removing children's influence in those new forms of power. Other groups within society were also having their capacity to participate in democracy nullified, for example women and indigenous people, who were said to be unable to be full citizens because of their 'superior virtue' or emotional immaturity (Russell, 1950). Thus, as Brewer acknowledges, the law constructed an 'age of reason' in such a way that it portrayed children as having an almost complete inability to exercise judgement, elevating reason as important beyond all other human attributes and, in the process, putting great weight on this supposed difference between the adult and the child. The dominant narrative of the immaturity and incapacity of the child persists today (Brewer, 2005, p. 351).

Law, Digital Media, and the Protection of Children as the Dominant Paradigm

Viewed as a legal and not a psychological construct, the claimed immaturity of the child has arguably done more to harm children than protect them (Ferguson, 2007, p. 134; Simpson, 2015, p. 345). In the first instance, this state of immaturity forms the basis for removing from the child the capacity to consent in law on their own behalf in relation to how their body will be dealt with by others. Of course, children can and do consent as a matter of fact, but the law removes this as operative for the purposes of many legal decisions. The protection of children in this context thus depends on the proper and responsible behaviour of adults, usually parents or guardians, but sometimes the state, to exercise their judgement on behalf of the child. However, experience shows that this is problematic for many reasons.

One problem is that there is a legal culture created by the stated immaturity of the child that removes from the child the possibility of participation in decisions that affect them, even where some legal principles seem to support their involvement. For example, there was a time in the past when the Australian Law Reform Commission described the evidence of children as based on an "assumption of unreliability" (Australian Law Reform Commission, 1997, para. 14.15). Formally, judges are now not permitted to warn juries that children are unreliable witnesses. (See, for example, Evidence Act 1995 (NSW), ss.165A(1).) However, that does not preclude a judge warning a jury about the unreliability of a particular child's evidence for reasons "other than solely the age of the child" (Evidence Act 1995 (NSW), ss.165A(2)). The problem is that, in saying the child's age should not determine their capacity, it affirms that this may be an issue. Thus, while the law attempts to place children in the same position as adults in relation to their competence to give evidence, attention is drawn to the historical treatment of children as immature while, at the same time, trying to remove that very perception. This means that even where the law attempts to involve children in legal processes that affect them, it must confront a view of the child that is against granting them the capacity to participate meaningfully. (See, for example, *RCB and The Hon Justice Colin James Forrest* [2012] HCA 47, per Heydon, J at paras. 51–52.) Of course, there are, as stated in the example of the formal rules of evidence, shifts in legal discourse that represent other narratives of the child as capable and mature. However, this is not to say that this alternative way of understanding children's position is in any way in the ascendancy. It is still fair to say that the dominant narrative in discussions about law, children, and digital media persists, with an overriding concern with the welfare and protection of children that needs to be understood to appreciate fully the role the 'counter-narrative' plays.

Digital Media, Harm to Children, and Their 'Best Interests'

The legal test to determine whether a course of action is harmful to a child is often expressed in terms of whether or not that course of action is in the child's 'best interests'. The mechanics of this legal concept is that it rests on the assumption that a child is generally unable to make their own decisions about such matters as their body, interactions, or living arrangements, and so it becomes the standard against which other persons are expected to make those decisions for them. Thus, quite simply and some might say sensibly, parents, guardians, and the state are often expected to act in the child's best interests when substituting their decisions for those of the incapable or immature child. The problem, however, with the 'best interests' approach lies within its own internal logic. For many adults, the determination of what is in a child's best interests is regarded as self-evident, when in fact this matter is heavily value-laden. In removing from the child its capacity to make its own decisions, recourse to the best interests of the child as the justification for various courses of action can allow the interests of others – parents, guardians, or the state – to operate under the smokescreen that the legal standard creates.

The dilemmas this creates for decision-makers in the field of children and the law are illustrated by the points made by Brennan, J in his dissenting judgment in the High Court of Australia in Marion's case, about the way in which the best interests standard operates. The case is not about children and digital media, but its discussion of general principles to do with the protection of children is still relevant. The case was concerned with the sterilisation of an intellectually disabled child. The parents wished to have their child undergo the procedure, and, in the usual case (that is, where the medical procedure does not involve invasive surgery such as in sterilisation), it was accepted that parents could consent to the treatment on behalf of a child incapable of making their own decision. In Marion's case, however, the nature of the treatment being undertaken raised the question of whether parental agreement would suffice or whether the law required that court approval was required in such cases. While the majority found such approval was required, and that the determination of the matter must be based on the best interests of the child concerned, Brennan, J dissented, finding that any authorisation of such an invasive procedure would undermine any claims that a child has a right to bodily integrity. In effect, he held that the right of a child to own their own body would be rendered meaningless by others who were deciding the matter for the child based on their view of the child's best interests. In his judgment, he provided a critique of the best interests principle that many would agree with. He said:

> In ascertaining where the welfare of a child lies, the courts have sought to discover what is in the child's 'best interests'. The 'best interests' approach focusses attention on the child whose interests are in question. By asserting that the child's 'best interests' are 'the first and paramount consideration', the law is freed from the degrading doctrines of earlier times which gave priority to parental or, more particularly, paternal rights to which the interests of the child were subordinated ... But, that said, the best interests approach does no more than identify the person whose interests are in question: it does not assist in identifying the factors which are relevant to the best interests of the child ... the best interests approach offers no hierarchy of values which might guide the exercise of a discretionary power to authorise sterilisation, much less any general legal principle which might direct the difficult decisions to be made in this area by parents, guardians, the medical profession and courts ... it must be remembered that, in the absence of legal rules or a hierarchy of values, the best interests approach depends upon the value system of the decision-maker. Absent any rule or guideline, that approach simply creates an unexaminable discretion in the repository of the power. Who could then say that the repository of the power is right or wrong in deciding where the best interests of an intellectually disabled child might lie when there is no clear ethical consensus adopted by the community?
>
> (Department of Health & Community Services v. JWB & SMB ('Marion's Case') [1992] HCA 15; (1992) 175 CLR 218 (6 May 1992), pp. 139–142)

Brennan went on to state that "the power [to decide such matters] cannot be left in a state so amorphous that it can be exercised according to the idiosyncratic views of the repository as to the 'best interests' of the child" on the basis that "that approach provides an insubstantial protection of the human dignity of children" (p. 142).

What then is the place of considerations of the human dignity of children when it comes to digital media? For the most part, as has already been observed, such discussions tend to focus on matters to do with the protection of children, which is of course one aspect of human dignity. Such discussion of the protection of children in the context of digital media does require consideration of harm from which children are to be protected, and an incapacity on the part of children to protect themselves. As noted above, Brewer's work illustrates the construction of the child as incapable of judgement in law from the 18th century. However, the identification of harm from digital media also has to be established to justify the protection of the child in this context, and this has generally been achieved by identifying those parts of digital media that harm, endanger, or threaten 'childhood innocence'. (See, for example, Simpson, 2015.) Childhood innocence in this context might be broadly understood as the nature of childhood which explains the child's incapacity to make mature judgements. In other words, the counter-narrative regards discussion of the innocent child as fraught, problematic, and a social and legal construct itself.

However, both the perception of the harms that digital media contains for children and the construction of the child as innocent are highly problematic. The notion that digital media contains aspects that can harm or threaten the child, while other parts may bring benefits to that child, itself relies on a utopian versus dystopian view of digital technology which has been a common approach to all new technologies throughout history, but which also depends on the acceptance of a number of myths about that technology (Papacharissi, 2010). Clearly, what is to be regarded as 'good' or 'bad' online will be a matter of values which are often left unstated for the very reason that clear definitions are fraught, if not impossible. There may be general agreement that cyberbullying is wrong, but can any agreement be reached on how it should be defined? Beyond that common example, is the child who explores their sexual identity online engaging in the 'positive' or the 'negative' aspects of digital media? The answer here is probably not one that even begins with a universal consensus that then flounders on subsequent definitions.

A possible reason for believing that digital technology has clear positive and harmful aspects is that deciding matters in this context for the protection of children based on their best interests becomes a relatively easy exercise for adults entrusted with their care; they need simply direct the child away from the 'harmful' parts of digital media, and towards those parts of the media that are 'good'. Indeed, such a view of digital media underpins and appears in many legal systems. One such example is the Australian Enhancing Online Safety Act 2015 (Commonwealth) which creates an e-Safety Commissioner with specific functions to promote online safety for Australians and for Australian children (s.3). The legislation defines 'online safety for children' as the "capacity of Australian children to use social media services and electronic services in a safe manner and includes the protection of Australian children using those services from cyber-bullying material targeted at an Australian child" (s.4). Such provisions contain many unstated assumptions about the nature of digital media and what constitutes 'good' or 'safe' behaviour online. The explanation of cyberbullying material highlights the extent to which such definitions are value-laden as they depend on the judgement being made that an ordinary reasonable person would conclude that:

(i) It is likely that the material was intended to have an effect on a particular Australian child; and
(ii) The material would be likely to have the effect on the Australian child of seriously threatening, seriously intimidating, seriously harassing or seriously humiliating the Australian child. (s.5)

(It may well be appropriate to ask here "who is the 'ordinary reasonable person' that the judgement is to be based upon?" Certainly, it is a standard that itself could change over time.)

In addition to this ambiguity around how cyberspace and online activity is seen, there is also the matter of how the child is constructed within this context. As previously indicated, children are often constructed in one of two ways. The first way leads to a focus on their vulnerabilities and immaturity, which then leads to an obligation to protect them from harm. This approach to children is one that is well entrenched in everyday culture and that is constantly reinforced in mainstream media and, as a consequence, applied to debates about children and digital media. It forms part of a romantic notion of children that portrays them as angelic and chaste and fits nicely within many people's notion of what a child should be (Synnott, 1983). This view of childhood also draws heavily on notions of childhood innocence, which is seen most clearly in arguments that digital media, and what children can access through it, corrupts or removes children's innocence. Governments, eager to show that they are addressing parental anxieties about digital media and children, have long utilised the concept of the innocent child when explaining their policies on online regulation. For example, in 2007 in Australia, the then Howard Government mailed to all Australian households the document *NetAlert protecting Australian families online* (Australian Government, 2007), which was presented as an informative guide clearly addressed to parents about how to protect their children online. The section on 'inappropriate material' began:

> An eight-year-old boy came across offensive images when he innocently conducted an Internet search for films about boys. Devastated and afraid he would get into trouble, he initially refused to explain why he was upset when his mother discovered him in tears at bedtime. His parents contacted NetAlert for advice on how to block sites with inappropriate content.
>
> (Australian Government, 2007, p. 12)

Of course, this story is far more likely to have been manufactured in a government policy unit than in a real Australian home. The referencing to the child's age – young enough to be credibly 'innocent' (would the story have had the same resonance if the child here was 14 years old?) – his 'innocently' conducting a search resulting in 'confirmation' that "offensive materials are just a few clicks away" online (Australian Government, 2007, p. 3) leading to 'tears at bedtime' creates a narrative that draws heavily on childhood innocence being corrupted by 'bad' digital content. It also explains the role of the e-Safety Commissioner's office, mentioned above, to promote online safety. This concern with protecting the child is grounded in these notions of childhood innocence and immaturity. It could be argued that, because children may contact the Commissioner directly where they feel unsafe online, this recognises the capacity of the child to claim their right to protection. This is the 'digital resilience' notion promoted in the United Kingdom by various commentators. (See, for example, Children's Commissioner for England, 2017, p. 4.) But this fails to articulate a complete understanding of children's capacity and their digital rights. If children's capacity is to be fully recognised, then this must also embrace the right to be 'annoying' online and digitally, because this means that the child would possess the most valuable aspect of a right – to assert it against powerful interests who would otherwise define their behaviour as inappropriate (Simpson, 2018, p. 60). Thus, the granting to children the ability to claim protection disguises a subtle reinforcement of children's continuing innocence and incapacity to claim a fuller set of rights in this domain.

Yet 'childhood innocence' is as problematic a concept as is the notion of what is 'inappropriate content' online. The innocence of children is often proclaimed in a sexual context, especially in relation to children's use of social media. Yet commentators such as James Kincaid note that the child's sexual innocence can itself become eroticised, as focussing on the very notion of a child's sexual innocence necessarily raises the issue of children's sexuality (Kincaid, 1998, p. 55). Debates about children, sexuality, and innocence often become proxy debates about children's assumed incompetence more generally. Jenny Kitzinger points out that childhood innocence becomes an effective way of denying children their rights:

> The twin concepts of innocence and ignorance are vehicles for adult double standards. A child is ignorant if she doesn't know what adults want her to know, but innocent if she doesn't know what adults don't want her to know.
>
> (Kitzinger, 2015)

Judith Ennew has also argued that, in relation to the exposure of children to sexual exploitation, "the key to solving the problem lies not in denouncing repressive morality, but in denying the presence of childhood innocence" (Ennew, 1986, p. 61). Ultimately, Ennew's position seems to be that the education of children about sexuality in a manner that is age-sensitive is more likely to lead to their ability to protect themselves from sexual exploitation (Simpson, 2018, p. 107). Similarly David Archard argues that the dominant narrative around children is that they are "incompetent innocents" (Archard, 1993, p. 218), which justifies denying children rights. Yet, to the extent that innocence is equated with ignorance, Archard emphasises that "any strategy to protect children from abuse will be inadequate if it maintains children in their ignorance and powerlessness" (Archard, 1993, p. 206).

However, while the concept of the innocent child is perhaps not as clear as first thought, the related question is whether the notion also clouds the discussion of child protection where the perpetrator is also a child. In other words, children's innocence may be utilised as the rationale for protecting children from harm, but how does this model accommodate the child perpetrator, the child who causes harm to other children? What happens to the innocence of children in such cases? The short answer is that the model of innocence is dispensed with and replaced with the 'demonic' child, the child that is worthy of blame (Synnott, 1983). The notion that children can be viewed as angelic or as uncontrollable devils is embedded in law and popular culture, but this dichotomy sits uneasily with notions that children need to be protected by adults from unwanted harm. The demonic child may actually be the child who knows things that adults do not want them to know, and for that reason is more likely to be seen as more in need of punishment or control rather than protection. Clearly, such competing views of the child are not readily reconciled, and create problems for legislators and policymakers seeking to demonstrate their concern for children. They lead, as is often the case in juvenile justice policy, to often contradictory positions about the offending child that, on the one hand, they are innocent, immature, and unworthy of being blamed for their deeds, while, on the other hand, they are seen as little devils that need to be punished and controlled. But if punishment is to be justified as a deterrent, it requires a certain degree of understanding on the part of the child of their behaviour. Under this view, the child must be accorded a certain level of understanding or maturity as would justify their punishment as being knowing and responsible (for their behaviour). The logical consequence of this position is that they must also be accorded certain legal rights, such as due process.

This was acknowledged by the United States Supreme Court in its landmark decision *In re Gault* in 1967. In that case, a child in Arizona aged 15 had been accused of making an offensive telephone call. On the basis that the juvenile court proceedings were focussed more on 'helping' children rather than punishing them, the accused was accorded no due process, including notification of the complaint nor cross-examination of their accuser. Gault was, in effect, placed in state care until he was 21, while an adult convicted of the same offence would have received a maximum sentence of two months and/or a fine of up to $50. The United States Supreme Court eventually heard the case and remarked of the Arizona State law and its rationale:

> The idea of crime and punishment was to be abandoned. The child was to be 'treated' and 'rehabilitated', and the procedures, from apprehension through institutionalisation, were to be 'clinical', rather than punitive.
>
> These results were to be achieved, without coming to conceptual and constitutional grief, by insisting that the proceedings were not adversary, but that the state was proceeding as parens patriae . . .
>
> The right of the state, as parens patriae, to deny to the child procedural rights available to his elders was elaborated by the assertion that a child, unlike an adult, has a right 'not to liberty, but to custody'. He can be made to attorn to his parents, to go to school, etc. If his parents default in effectively performing their custodial functions – that is, if the child is 'delinquent' – the state may intervene. In doing so, it does not deprive the child of any rights, because he has none. It merely provides the 'custody' to which the child is entitled. On this basis, proceedings involving juveniles were described as 'civil', not 'criminal', and therefore not subject to the requirements which restrict the state when it seeks to deprive a person of his liberty.

> ... The absence of substantive standards has not necessarily meant that children receive careful, compassionate, individualised treatment. The absence of procedural rules based upon constitutional principle has not always produced fair, efficient, and effective procedures. Departures from established principles of due process have frequently resulted not in enlightened procedure, but in arbitrariness ...
>
> Failure to observe the fundamental requirements of due process has resulted in instances, which might have been avoided, of unfairness to individuals and inadequate or inaccurate findings of fact and unfortunate prescriptions of remedy. Due process of law is the primary and indispensable foundation of individual freedom. It is the basic and essential term in the social compact which defines the rights of the individual and delimits the powers which the state may exercise.
>
> *(In re Gault 387 US 15–20)*

It is difficult to envisage now but in 1967 to speak about children in terms of their due process rights was a watershed moment. It shifted the paradigm about the punishment of children away from simple notions of paternalism and gave children in effect the same rights as adults. But such change is never simple, and to think that this shift in thinking was universally accepted – then or now – would be wrong. To this day, debates in juvenile justice between 'welfarist' (paternalistic) and 'justice' models continue. In part, this is because the first approach in many ways recognises a form of childhood innocence that speaks more to the idea that children need to be nurtured and allowed to mature, thus making discussion of their rights unnecessary, while the latter approach accords children substantive and due process rights, but on the basis that children are mature enough to possess and exercise those rights. For those that adhere to the former approach to children, there is great discomfort in accepting that children have that level of maturity, even if this means denying them various rights.

Law can thus be portrayed as a pendulum that swings between various conceptions of childhood. Or it might be explained as a confused and muddled 'grab bag' of ideas about children and their capacity to make their own decisions. Either way, any notion that law relies on a consistent and coherent set of rules that applies to the treatment of children must be disavowed. The argument in this chapter has been that the need to protect children based on their immaturity often prevails as a narrative. But the chapter has also argued that a counter narrative exists that challenges the dominant one and, in doing so, identifies various flaws in the protectionist approach. There are of course various legal principles pertaining to the treatment of children that are agreed almost universally, such as the need to act in the child's 'best interests' and that children can and do possess a number of rights, as for example appear in the United Nations Convention on the Rights of the Child. But these principles set up contests over meaning and content rather than settle any understandings of the role of law in relation to children generally if the competing narratives are understood. It is in this legal context that the child in digital media can be further explored [See Chapter 30].

References

Abiala, K., & Hernwall, P. (2013). Tweens negotiating identity online – Swedish girls' and boys' reflections on online experiences. *Journal of Youth Studies 16*(8), 951–969.

Archard, D. (1993). *Rights and childhood* (2nd ed.). London: Routledge.

Australian Government. (2007). *NetAlert protecting Australian families online*.

Australian Law Reform Commission. (1997). *Seen and heard: Priority for children in the legal process* (ALRC Report 84).

boyd, d. (2014). *It's complicated: The social lives of networked teens.* New Haven and London: Yale University Press, Kindle Edition.

Brewer, H. (2005). *By birth or consent: Children, law and the Anglo-American revolution in authority*. Chapel Hill: University of North Carolina Press.
Carson, W. G. (1980). The institutionalization of ambiguity: Early British factory acts. In G. Geis & E. Stotland (Eds.), *White collar crime: Theory and research* (pp. 142–173). London: Sage.
Chalfen, R. (2009). "It's only a picture": Sexting, 'smutty' snapshots and felony charges. *Visual Studies 24*(3), 258–268.
Children's Commissioner for England. (2017). *Growing up digital*, a report from The Growing Up Digital Taskforce. London: Children's Commissioner for England.
Ennew, J. (1986). *The sexual exploitation of children*. New York: St Martin's Press.
Ferguson, H. (2007). Abused and looked after children as 'moral dirt': Child abuse and institutional care in historical perspective. *Journal of Social Policy 36*, 123–139.
Freiberg, A. (2007). Jurisprudential miscegenation: Strict liability and the ambiguity of law. In A. Brannigan & G. Pavlich (Eds.), *Governance and regulation in social life: Essays in honour of W. G. Carson* (pp. 74–90). Oxford: Routledge. Kindle edition.
Kairys, D. (Ed.). (1998). *The politics of law: A progressive critique*. New York: Basic Books.
Karaian, L. (2012). Lolita speaks: 'Sexting', teenage girls and the law. *Crime Media Culture 8*(1), 57–73.
Kennedy, D. (2004). *Legal education and the reproduction of hierarchy: A polemic against the system: A critical edition*. New York and London: New York University Press.
Kincaid, J. R. (1998). *Erotic innocence: The culture of child molesting*. Durham and London: Duke University Press.
King, M., & Piper, C. (1995). *How the law thinks about children* (2nd ed.). Aldershot: Ashgate.
Kitzinger, J. (2015). Children, power and the struggle against sexual abuse. In A. James & A. Prout (Eds.), *Constructing and reconstructing childhood: Contemporary issues in the sociological study of childhood* (Classic ed., pp. 145–166). Oxford: Routledge.
Papacharissi, Z. A. (2010). *A private sphere: Democracy in a digital age*. Cambridge: Polity Press.
Presdee, M. (2000). *Cultural criminology and the carnival of crime*. London and New York: Routledge.
Russell, B. (1950). The superior virtue of the oppressed. In Bertrand Russell, *Unpopular essays* (Chapter 5). First published 1950. London: George Allen & Unwin.
Simpson, B. (2005). Identity manipulation in cyberspace as a leisure option: Play and the exploration of self. *Information and Communications Technology Law 14*(2), 115–131.
Simpson, B. (2015). Sexting, digital dissent and narratives of innocence: Controlling the child's body. In Sampson L.B, P. N Claster & S.M. Claster (Eds.), Technology and youth: Growing up in a digital world. *Sociological Studies of Children and Youth 19*, 315–349.
Simpson, B. (2018). *Young people, social media and the law*. London and New York: Routledge.
Synnott, A. (1983). Little angels, little devils: A sociology of children. *Canadian Review of Sociology and Anthropology 20*(1), 79–95.
Williams, R. A. (1987). Taking rights aggressively: The perils and promise of critical legal theory for peoples of color. *Law & Inequality: A Journal of Theory and Practice 5*(1), 103–134.

Legislation

Enhancing Online Safety Act 2015 (Commonwealth).
Evidence Act 1995 (NSW).

Cases

Department of Health & Community Services v. JWB & SMB ('Marion's Case') [1992] HCA 15; (1992) 175 CLR 218.
Gillick and Wisbech AHA [1985] UKHL 7.
In re Gault 387 US 15.
RCB and The Hon Justice Colin James Forrest [2012] HCA 47.

Treaties

United Nations Convention on the Rights of the Child.

30

NO FIXED LIMITS?

The Uncomfortable Application of Inconsistent Law to the Lives of Children Dealing with Digital Media

Brian Simpson

Introduction

The previous chapter [Chapter 29] explored how the law's approach to children's relationship with digital media is shaped by ideological, political, economic, and romantic narratives as much as it is constructed by scientific ones. It was argued that a dominant legal narrative is one that is heavily weighted towards protecting the child rather than granting them autonomy rights. While there are strands within law that speak to children's agency, they often overlap with the dominant narrative and, as a result, law often lacks coherence and consistency. For example, the very different ways in which children's rights can be understood bears testament to that point. In this chapter, the application of those principles in a few important cases is examined to better understand the legal process, and to explore the extent to which it might be possible to better articulate 'children's rights' in the context of digital media through re-thinking what is in the best interests of the child.

While many commentators on children, law, and digital media are unlikely to have read *Gault* or considered the relevance of debates around competing conceptions of the child in juvenile justice law and policy to their area, those debates have great relevance for understanding laws which affect children and digital media today. However, it must also be noted that in the modern day there appears to have been a shift back to the paternalism of yesteryear. This regressive shift may reflect the manner in which governments pitch their efforts to regulate the digital terrain as a means to appease parents rather than to liberate children. This is evident in the existence of (for example) the e-Safety Commissioner in Australia, which was initially set up to protect children from online harm. Such offices rarely, if ever, speak to the online rights of children to act independently or autonomously. Instead, while the Office of the e-Safety Commissioner professes a concern for children, it initially spoke principally to parents. Another example of this is the General Data Protection Regulation (GDPR) of the European Union. The GDPR raises the age until which parental consent is required for data collection from 13 to 16, although it can be lowered by a member state, but not below 13 (GDPR, art 8(1)). The requirement of parental consent to access social media clearly removes children's capacity to make their own decisions in this space, and the debate over the appropriate age here underlines the extent to which this area is governed by competing notions of the child held by adults rather than the practical use, say, of social media by children which would support laws that address that reality rather than parents' fears (Simpson, 2018, p. 83).

The return to the paternalism of previous years is also evident in a central concern of much of the law today on children and digital media with its focus on cyberbullying. The narrative that now surrounds cyberbullying is mainly concerned with the protection of the child victim. Of course, those bullies are often other children. As with general debates on juvenile justice, if the innocent child is the child in need of protection and nurture, then how should the law respond to the child cyberbully? If the innocent child victim must be protected from online harm because of their immaturity to understand the risks, then how can a same-aged cyberbully be dealt with? Is the child cyberbully as immature as their victim? Should they be punished for what they do not understand? Or are they a wicked and knowing child that bullies, who should learn the consequences of their behaviour?

Casting law around 'good' and 'bad' aspects of digital media tends to embed a utopian versus dystopian view of the technology. Such an approach relies on various mythologies about digital media rather than embodying a more nuanced and sophisticated understanding of children's realities with respect to their use of the technology. Likewise, the ideology of childhood that constructs the child as both angelic and demonic also reinforces and creates various tensions and contradictions around how children are to be understood in their interactions with digital media. As a consequence, the relationship between children, law, and digital media is fuelled as much by ideology and narrative as it is by any semblance of scientific analysis of children's use of the media. It is in this context that the best interests of the child might be recast through an alternative narrative that moves away from a simple focus on the protection of children towards the articulation of their rights in digital contexts.

Re-Articulating the Best Interests of the Child in the Digital Age Through the Uncomfortable Nature of Children's Rights

A contemporary consideration of the law, children's rights, and digital media has its roots, as is often the case when formulating legal principles, in an age before the advent of digital technology and the internet. Legal principles may aim to address current problems, but the law tends to seek deeper and ongoing principles to invoke as the basis for its response. A case that is not about cyberspace, cyberbullying, or cybersex, but for law raises principles relevant to those matters, was a case about children's capacity to consent to medical treatment independent of their parents. In 1985, in the United Kingdom, the then highest court in that country, the House of Lords, decided that children had the capacity to make their own decisions regarding medical treatment provided they had sufficient maturity to do so (*Gillick and Wisbech AHA* [1985] UKHL 7). This case is relevant for the manner in which that court analysed the capacity of children to determine matters that affect them, creating a template for understanding current concerns about children and digital media. It also illustrates a central theme of this chapter: the discomfort that the case brought to discussion of the rights of children.

'Children's rights' as a juristic concept has become one of the most misrepresented, manipulated, and misunderstood concepts in legal and political discourse (Simpson, 2018, pp. 51–2). It is often mentioned as if its meaning is self-evident and it is often assumed, because of the connection with children, that the purpose of such rights is to support a wholesome and virtuous idea of childhood. Such representations of the concept of children's rights has evolved from the manner in which adults have historically controlled the meaning of childhood and employed various smokescreens, such as the paternalism of the 'best interests' of the child, to consistently oppress, harm, and endanger children while justifying such treatment for their welfare (Ferguson,

2007, p. 134; Simpson, 2015, p. 345). What is good for children has all too often been about advancing the interests of adults. For the most part this has been enabled by the difficulty children have had throughout time in finding a means to have their voice heard.

A large part of the paternalism that has always underpinned discussions of the child may be grounded in a desire to have certainty around what constitutes 'good parenting' and what is 'bad parenting'. While the notion of the best interests of the child is clearly based on normative content, it is also arguable that, for the most part, adult society can formulate some consensus about how children should be treated, often based on highly idealised notions of the child. The articulation of children's rights as granting the child independent action is both threatening and disruptive to such a consensus. However, the groundwork for children's independent rights was not based on an alternative romantic notion of what childhood should be like; it was articulated in terms of certain social realities, as challenging as that made the legal conclusion. As Lord Scarman said in *Gillick*:

> Certainty is always an advantage in the law, and in some branches of the law it is a necessity. But it brings with it an inflexibility and a rigidity which in some branches of the law can obstruct justice, impede the law's development, and stamp upon the law the mark of obsolescence where what is needed is the capacity for development. The law relating to parent and child is concerned with the problems of the growth and maturity of the human personality. If the law should impose upon the process of 'growing up' fixed limits where nature knows only a continuous process, the price would be artificiality and a lack of realism in an area where the law must be sensitive to human development and social change.
>
> *(Gillick v. Wisbech AHA, per Lord Scarman)*

In other words, legal principle about the capacity of the child should be formulated around the acceptance that the nature of childhood is changing, as is the idea that parents can always make decisions on behalf of their children. One of the Law Lords in the majority, Lord Scarman, thus concluded that

> the parental right to determine whether or not their minor child below the age of 16 will have medical treatment terminates if, and when, the child achieves a sufficient understanding and intelligence to enable him or her to understand fully what is proposed.
>
> *(Gillick v. Wisbech AHA, per Lord Scarman)*

However, the decision in *Gillick* (which is also accepted to state the law in Australia) carried with it a level of discomfort about what it meant to give children such effective control over their lives. John Eekelar famously said at the time that the decision gave children "that most dangerous but most precious of rights: the right to make their own mistakes" (Eekelar, 1986). That children had such a right caused much anxiety for both parents and judges in later cases – often involving the refusal of medical treatment by children – and it would be wrong to suggest that the adoption of such a legal principle was simple or without challenge. Even in recent cases, there continues this tension between recognising children's capacity to decide and the role of others to determine the matter based on the child's best interests. *In Re Kelvin*, for example, the Family Court of Australia decided that court authorisation was no longer required in the case of stage 2 treatment for gender dysphoria in cases involving children wishing to transition, where the child consents to the treatment, the child is *Gillick* competent, and the parents do not object to the treatment. This case is often presented as the court removing itself from people's lives and, thus, a progressive development for children. But the fact that *Gillick* competence alone is not sufficient to determine the matter (as in other countries such as the UK) indicates how the notion of children's rights is continually contested and qualified and, by extension, what is in the best interests of children.

By 1989, a view of children's rights that embraced children's independent capacity to decide matters began to appear in such documents as the United Nations Convention on the Rights of the Child (UNCROC). Article 13 of that Convention states:

> The child shall have the right to freedom of expression; this right shall include freedom to seek, receive and impart information and ideas of all kinds, regardless of frontiers, either orally, in writing or in print, in the form of art, or through any other media of the child's choice.
>
> (UNCROC, Art. 13)

While the overarching principle in the Convention is that in all areas affecting children their best interests shall be the primary consideration (UNCROC, Art. 3(1)), other articles, such as Article 13, indicate that the paternalism of bygone days and the use of the child's 'best interests' to conceal acts done according to adult's views of how children should behave, may be under siege. There is a greater sense today, at least, that children have a right to be heard and to be listened to seriously, lest their perspective on what should happen to them be ignored. This also finds expression in Article 12 of the UNCROC:

> States Parties shall assure to the child who is capable of forming his or her own views the right to express those views freely in all matters affecting the child, the views of the child being given due weight in accordance with the age and maturity of the child.
>
> (UNCROC, Art. 12(1))

This statement of the position of children clearly reflects the conclusion in *Gillick* and underscores the point that that case reaches far beyond the question of medical treatment in its reasoning. The difficulty is in the detail, as giving effect to the process of listening to children is as challenging for many adults as it is to give effect to the child's views in appropriate cases. The participation of children in deciding matters that affect them is easy to state in principle, but as a practical matter remains the cause of much anxiety to many adults.

For some adults, children are, by definition, incapable of acting maturely, and to countenance a conclusion about their welfare that is contrary to their own views is anathema. That such a position runs counter to the legal principles that inform this area may not matter to such adults whose position is usually based on particular views of the child's best interests or welfare, and thus may gain much currency. In effect the tension, as Michael Freeman has described it, is often between different notions of the rights of children, between the protection rights of children and their autonomy rights (Freeman, 1983).

In the context of children's use and access to digital technology and social media there is a tendency to stress the 'positive' aspects of the technology as something that is 'good' for children, while also pointing to those 'negative' areas of cyberspace that children need to be protected from. The extent to which this construction of children and online activity has permeated popular consciousness results in it being accepted as essentially unobjectionable. In that context, the idea that children may claim uses of digital media that challenge such views of childhood are both uncomfortable and challenging for adults. Children now create their identity and forge new connections on the internet that disrupt older views about who should guide and define what it means to be a child. In effect, digital media grants to children a higher degree of autonomy than ever before and the possibility of them participating in the construction of childhood in meaningful ways (Simpson, 2018). In this sense, law's failure to rearticulate children's best interests around greater autonomy rights risks making the law either irrelevant for children's lives, or it being applied against children because of their cultural practices.

Good Children, Bad Children: The Importance of Rights Talk for Children and Digital Media

Rights mean little if they are only asserted when others approve. Ultimately, the value of rights is in their capacity to effect change (Donnison, 1999). As argued previously, what is 'good' and what is 'bad' in relation to children is often what is subjected to challenge in children's use of digital media. To the extent that this is about the capacity of children to use digital media to create identities that upset adults or to ask questions about their treatment that challenge parental and state authority, this is in effect to ask whether children have a right to be 'really annoying'.

Much of the law in this area is geared towards supporting children so that they access the 'good' material online while being shielded from the 'bad'. But in fact, defining what is good and what is bad is difficult, because as with any attempt to articulate the best interests of the child, it eventually falls to a normative judgement that is always going to be subjective and value laden. The construction of digital media as a place with 'good' and 'bad' in it panders to similar notions about children that assume a good child will result from exposure to only the good things online. An assertion along these lines rarely if ever engages with what is meant by 'good' in this context.

These strands can be seen in high-profile examples of legal cases considering children and digital media such as that of Michelle Carter in the United States. Michelle Carter was a young woman, aged 17, who was found guilty of involuntary manslaughter on the basis that she had encouraged her 18-year-old boyfriend to commit suicide through a series of texts she had sent to him. She was sentenced to two and a half years in prison for the crime (Logan, 2018). Carter appealed her conviction to the Massachusetts Superior Judicial Court which upheld her original sentence. The various arguments advanced in support of her appeal highlight the conflicting notions around how children are perceived generally, and in relation to digital media.

Much of the case is not about digital media at all. Massachusetts has no offence of encouraging suicide, so a large part of the case involved whether the definition of involuntary manslaughter could embrace her acts. Another aspect of the case is whether her acts – the sending of texts – was causative of her boyfriend's death. However, the appeal also raised the question of whether Carter's words were protected speech under the United States Constitution protection of free speech. The point here is that while it may seem abhorrent to send texts that encourage someone to kill themselves, this is the very point of free speech, to protect a category of speech even if others find it distasteful (Carter Appellant Brief, p. 46). This goes to the purpose of such protection of free speech. In effect, although some may find the words annoying or unpleasant, this is the very reason for protecting that speech. A person encouraging suicide may present as cold and lacking in concern, but is this a basis for criminalising their behaviour? As the appellant brief remarked:

> Encouragement, even if ugly or strident, remains protected, and a law that penalises such speech (or chills related speech about suicide, including by physicians or family) is unconstitutional.
>
> *(Carter Appellant Brief, p. 49)*

The American Civil Liberties Union submitted an *amici curiae* brief in support of Carter's appeal and explained further the basis for arguing the speech was protected under the Constitution:

> Because the prohibition at issue here criminalises speech encouraging suicide, and because [the decision of the trial court] seems to draw distinctions between those encouraging suicide for reasons that are deemed compassionate and those that are not and between those who encourage suicide by people 'coping with a terminal illness' and those who encourage suicides for other reasons ... it is both content and indeed viewpoint based.
>
> *(ACLU Brief, p. 36)*

What is unstated is that Carter as a young person was also engaging in behaviour that does not fit well with the notion of the angelic child discussed above. And while part of the appeal argument focussed on the extent to which Carter should receive the same rights as adults with respect to how her speech was to be treated – no matter how distasteful it was – another part of the appeal focussed on her lack of maturity. Massachusetts law allows children to be dealt with as adults where they have inflicted 'serious bodily injury'. The Youth Advocacy Division of the Committee for Public Counsel and the Massachusetts Association of Criminal Defence Lawyers also submitted an *amici curiae* brief on the appeal. They argued that, as a juvenile, Carter's brain functioning was not that of an adult and she should not be held accountable for her actions as an adult. Their core submission was that there should have been further evidence to examine whether Carter actually understood her actions:

> All juveniles have structurally and functionally immature brains, which influence their conduct. Experts on juvenile brain development are relevant to whether a juvenile's conduct departs from that of a reasonable juvenile by defining what can be expected of juveniles.
>
> *(Youth Advocacy Division of the Committee for*
> *Public Counsel and the Massachusetts Association*
> *of Criminal Defence Lawyers, Amici Curiae brief, p. 1)*

Arguments that rely on the immature child do not challenge the nature of the behaviour. Carter was alleged to have sent many texts to her boyfriend that encouraged her boyfriend to kill himself. Those read into the evidence at trial were certainly lacking in compassion on one reading. Read as the actions of a wicked juvenile, they can support the lawyer's recourse to the immaturity of the child as a defence. On the other hand, to claim that the child has the right to free speech sits uncomfortably with many adults as it supports the proposition that children may also have the right to engage in conduct (or speech) that others find not only unpalatable but also at odds with what a child should be, innocent, naïve, but certainly not knowing and challenging of dominant views about how to behave. Yet again, in all of the briefs presented on this appeal, the competing and contradictory views of the child are in evidence.

The appeal court judgment reinforces this conclusion as to the confused messages about children that are embedded in the applicable legal principles. On the argument that Michelle Carter's actions should have been evaluated as those of a juvenile and not those of an adult, the court concluded:

> The defendant argues essentially that, when considering a juvenile's actions under the objective measure of recklessness, we should consider whether an ordinary juvenile under the same circumstances would have realised the gravity of the danger. It is clear from the judge's findings, however, that he found the defendant's actions wanton or reckless under the subjective measure, that is, based on her own knowledge of the danger to the victim and on her choice to run the risk that he would comply with her instruction to get back into the truck. That finding is amply

supported by the trial record. Because the defendant's conduct was wanton or reckless when evaluated under the subjective standard, there is no need to decide whether a different objective standard should apply to juveniles. Moreover, it is clear from the judge's sentencing memorandum that he did in fact consider the defendant's age and maturity when evaluating her actions and that he was familiar with the relevant case law and 'mindful' of the general principles regarding juvenile brain development. He noted that on the day of the victim's death, she was seventeen years and eleven months of age and at an age-appropriate level of maturity. Her ongoing contact with the victim in the days leading to his suicide, texting with him about suicide methods and his plans and demanding that he carry out his plan rather than continue to delay, as well as the lengthy cell phone conversations on the night itself, showed that her actions were not spontaneous or impulsive. And, as the judge specifically found, '[h]er age or level of maturity does not explain away her knowledge of the effects of her telling [the victim] to enter and remain in that toxic environment, leading to his death'. Where the judge found that the defendant ordered the victim back into the truck knowing the danger of doing so, he properly found that her actions were wanton or reckless, giving sufficient consideration to her age and maturity.

(Commonwealth v. Michelle Carter (2019) SJC-12502, pp. 30–32)

What is apparent here is that the court's judgment about the maturity of the child was heavily focussed on the nature of the actions rather than the individual circumstances of the child. Emphasis was placed on her age being close to 18 and that, as such, she was at 'an age-appropriate level of maturity' which is the very issue in question. There was no discussion of the role of digital technology in her life and the manner in which digital culture itself creates new cultural norms within which young people's behaviour can be understood.

Orthodox narratives about children's digital behaviour in cases such as Michelle Carter become concerned about cyberbullying, the potential of the 'bad' aspects of digital media to harm young people, and the potential for young people to get into legal difficulty across jurisdictions. However, this narrative assumes that what is 'good' and 'bad' in digital domains is self-evident. It does not consider that there are often competing values over such questions. Moreover, it fails to consider that, while there may well be negative outcomes of some behaviour, that same behaviour may also rest on important principles that need to be defended. Thus, while the right to speak in digital and other contexts may lead to speech that many find distasteful or against normal values, there will be other examples where such free speech leads to the accountability of others that do harm to children. And in the case of children, it should also be remembered that the freedom to self-expression in digital contexts contains developmental aspects. The children who become skilled in developing their own digital norms online today while still children will likely become better and more active citizens tomorrow. In this regard, the role of adults is not to deny children access to digital media 'in their best interests' but to offer guidance that enhances their rights rather than stymies them.

Conclusion: Why Uncomfortable Rights Matter for Children in Digital Media

It is important to have a clear understanding of the nature of the rights claimed in relation to children using digital media. David Donnison argues that rights are valuable commodities in the hands of the powerless that challenge the powerful and their norms (Donnison, 1999). The discomfort that the powerful feel when others claim rights is palpable. One tactic utilised to weaken such rights is to argue that the claiming of a right may be fair, but with it comes responsibilities to act in certain ways. This is simply a mechanism to weaken the right held by the right holder. As Judith Ennew remarks, quoting the work of Paul Sieghart:

> In all legal theory and practice, rights and duties are symmetrical. It is a popular fallacy that this symmetry applies within the same individual: that if I have a right, I must also have a correlative duty. This is not so: if I have a right, someone else must have a correlative duty; if I have a duty, someone else must have a corresponding right.
> *(Paul Sieghart cited in Ennew, 1986, p. 36)*

The importance of this is that what is *not* being claimed for children here is a simple right to do as they please online. It may be that their behaviour will offend or disappoint at times, but the correlative responsibility on adults – parents and others – is to ensure that children are able to fully develop their rights online, rights which embrace their right to an identity and to transgress norms as a means of improving their situation, and also quite simply the right to play. The advancement of such rights may shift the norms of behaviour online and in society in many ways, but this is not of itself a bad thing.

Christian Fuchs argues that cyberspace cannot be understood without also understanding its political economy (Fuchs, 2015). Clearly, much of the articulation of responsibility online, and of steering children towards the 'positive' and away from the 'negative' areas of digital media, has the hallmarks of ensuring that children grow up to be productive consumers and compliant workers. It is only recently, and after much public campaigning, itself often annoying to government and corporations, that debate has begun to move away from a simple concern about how much privacy people have in relation to each other online, and what large social media corporations do with personal and private information (Vaidhyanathan, 2018). A citizenry that claims the right to speak out about such behaviour will be annoying to those who benefit from the profits of data-mining. However, such rights may be the only bulwark against the erosion of civil liberties.

So far, legal discourse on children and digital media has tended to focus on the consequences of social media that relate to traditional notions of legal harm (such as bullying, identity fraud, and loss of privacy) rather than attempting to regulate it in a way that addresses the rights of others, and especially the rights of children, in their fullest sense. It is easy to see the rights of children only in terms of protection from harm and harmful online content as this has historically been the dominant discourse. But that concern relates to legal tests that were as much about denying children a voice or a place as they were about actually protecting children. Those tests also handed unaccountable power to adults to act in the child's best interests that could then be used by adults to protect and disguise their own interests. Digital technology empowers children on a practical level to articulate their own wants and needs. It allows them to transgress norms, often in spite of the law. In this new age, the challenge for the law is not to simply prevent such usage, but to frame the law in such a manner that it preserves the rights that children can now claim in relation to media as one aspect of how it is possible to protect children's interests. In that regard, young people such as Michelle Carter are neither immature nor knowingly wicked, but individuals that present the opportunity for the whole community to demand more sophisticated laws in this space, as uncomfortable as that exercise may be.

References

Donnison, D. (1999). Rethinking rights talk. In L. Orchard & R. Dore (Eds.), *Markets, morals and public policy* (pp. 219–231). Sydney: The Federation Press.

Eekelaar, J. (1986). The emergence of children's rights. *Oxford Journal of Legal Studies, 6*, 161.

Ennew, J. (1986). *The sexual exploitation of children*. New York: St Martin's Press.
Ferguson, H. (2007). Abused and looked after children as 'moral dirt': Child abuse and institutional care in historical perspective. *Journal of Social Policy, 36*, 123–139.
Freeman, M. D. A. (1983). *The rights and wrongs of children*. London: F. Pinter.
Fuchs, C. (2015). *Culture and economy in the age of social media*. New York and London: Routledge.
Logan, E. B. (2018, July 11). Michelle Carter's texts urging boyfriend to kill himself were protected speech, lawyers argue. *The Washington Post*. Retrieved from: www.washingtonpost.com/news/true-crime/wp/2018/07/10/she-urged-her-boyfriend-to-kill-himself-her-lawyers-say-it-was-free-speech.
Simpson, B. (2015). Sexting, digital dissent and narratives of innocence: Controlling the child's body. In Sampson L.B., P.N. Claster and S.M. Claster (Eds.), Technology and Youth: Growing Up in a Digital World. *Sociological Studies of Children and Youth, 19*, 315–349.
Simpson, B. (2018). *Young people, social media and the law*. London and New York: Routledge.
Vaidhyanathan, S. (2018). *Antisocial media: How Facebook disconnects us and undermines democracy*. Oxford: Oxford University Press.

Legislation

European Union General Data Protection Regulation.

Cases

Commonwealth v. *Michelle Carter* (2019) SJC-12502.
Gillick and Wisbech AHA [1985] UKHL 7.
In re Gault 387 US 15.
Re Kelvin [2017] FamFC 258.

Treaties

United Nations Convention on the Rights of the Child.

Other

Michelle Carter case: Appellant, ACLU and Youth Advocacy Division of the Committee for Public Counsel and the Massachusetts Association of Criminal Defence Lawyers Briefs (accessed at www.ma-appellatecourts.org/display_docket.php?dno=SJC-12502).

31
CHILDREN'S AGENCY IN THE MEDIA SOCIALISATION PROCESS

Claudia Riesmeyer

Introduction

Media socialisation research discusses the negotiation of norms and skills for media use and concentrates often on children and their socialisation through elders (e.g., Grusec, 2002; Riesmeyer, Abel & Großmann, 2019; Riesmeyer, Pohl & Ruf, 2019), named socialisation agents (Hurrelmann, 1990; Hurrelmann & Bauer, 2018; and as illustrated in the EU Kids Online model; EU Kids Online, 2014). While these agents are thought of as 'fundamental', other agents include the media (Beaudoin, 2014; Prot et al., 2015) and the legal system (Arnett, 1995a, 1995b, 2007). By the mid-1980s, media-pedagogical and development-psychological socialisation research began to move away from the individual's role as the object and more toward their role as the subject within the socialisation process. The concepts of self-socialisation and agency consider the active role of the individual and compare it with their socialisation through others. This recent shift in perspective has been triggered by social and media changes such as the digitalisation of educational and socialisation processes and their possible consequences for childhood (Honig, 2002; Van Dijck, 2009; Himmelbach, 2013). The ability to contribute to individual socialisation and thus to the acquisition of skills and norms is also conceded to children – they could take an active part within the media socialisation process.

With the progression of digitalisation, the spread of (mobile) communication technologies, and extensive media use by children over the last decades, a new transformation process has taken place, questioning the importance of the various external agents in the media socialisation process. Due to their intuitive, individualised, and ubiquitous use of (mobile) media technologies, some children and adolescents are now entering the limelight themselves as they acquire skills, values, and norms for sophisticated media use. What is more, they are able to communicate their skills to the socialisation agents, who should communicate their skills to them ('reverse socialisation'; Mead, 1970; Peters, 1985; Clark, 2011; Correa, 2014).

Despite these changes and challenges, however, media socialisation research in communication studies has thus far largely ignored the individual's active role in the media socialisation process. It is against this background that this chapter argues that media socialisation research should consider the individual's contribution within this process. It discusses the theoretical concepts of media socialisation, self-socialisation, and agency. This chapter also shows, based on a systematic literature review of articles published in peer-review journals and anthologies, as well as monographs, since 2000, the significance of concepts in media socialisation research to communication studies. Finally, the chapter formulates four theses for potential research perspectives on media socialisation concerning children's agency.

Media Socialisation Process

Media socialisation is part of the socialisation process, which aims to develop individuals into subjects capable of social action (Smetana, Robinson, & Rote, 2015; Pfaff-Rüdiger & Riesmeyer, 2016; Genner & Süss, 2017). Grusec (2002, p. 143) defines socialisation as a process in which "individuals are assisted in the acquisition of skills necessary to function as members of their group". In this respect, individuals (should) learn a) to regulate their emotions, thoughts, and behaviour; b) to appropriate cultural norms and values to integrate into society; and c) to resolve conflicts, to evaluate social relationships, and to assume active roles (Grusec, 2002). It is also a matter of the individual knowing and acknowledging their own abilities and limitations in everyday life (Arnett, 1995a, 1995b).

Within the framework of media socialisation, the individual acquires skills and is taught norms and standards for his or her media use (Hobbs, 2011, 2013; Mihailidis, 2014; Martens & Hobbs, 2015). Krämer (2012, p. 32) speaks of "dispositions that are (can be) socially structured in a typical and sufficiently momentous way with regard to media use, i.e. have as their object the use of the media", and which are acquired. According to Krämer's understanding, media socialisation happens through the processing of media content. This process of teaching skills, values, and norms for media use takes place within social relationships between the individual and the socialisation agent, whereby the relationship is structured by "individual and group dispositions, media offerings with their previous meanings (classifications, connotations, evaluations), and strategies of mediation between these levels acquired or to be acquired" (Krämer, 2012, p. 187). Krämer emphasises that both the group in which the individual interacts (e.g., their family or their friends) and their individual characteristics and attitudes influence media socialisation. By emphasising the individual's characteristics, Krämer moves away from concentrating on the individual as an object to considering them a subject in the process of media socialisation.

Self-Socialisation and Agency: Concepts of Media Socialisation

The concepts of self-socialisation and agency focus on the individual's status in the socialisation process and his or her influence upon this process (Abels & König, 2010; Süss, 2010; Heinzel, Kränzl-Nagl, & Mierendorff, 2012). Both concepts have in common the notions that individuals of all generations make self-regulating contributions to the socialisation process, and that people are producers of their own development by processing their needs and their environment throughout their lives (Hurrelmann & Bauer, 2018). This process does not end at adulthood, but affects the entire life cycle (and thus all generations, regardless of their age). The concepts of self-socialisation and agency thus expand the number of socialisation agents impacting the individual because the agents' influence shifts over the course of the socialisation process as a result of developmental tasks (for example, from parents to teachers to peers; Arnett, 1995a, 1995b).

The theoretical concepts of self-socialisation and agency have been discussed using various educational, sociological, or communication studies perspectives. These discussions are often driven by 'non-theoretical' research such as everyday life observations and empirical findings. Yet they are also based on theoretical assumptions. The discussion of media socialisation research as 'non-theoretical' must be evaluated carefully (Chakroff & Nathanson, 2008) however, because both concepts are based on theoretical assumptions, which are presented below.

The understanding of self-socialisation can be differentiated based on two characteristics: the independence of the individual and their scope of actions on the one hand, and whether the concept of self-socialisation is discussed in general or with a concrete reference to media socialisation on the other hand. If self-socialisation is related to the media, then, in addition to the individualisation of society, technological change is inter-related with changes in media use behaviour, an increase in the media spectrum and differentiated media content. Such developments lead to self-socialisation gaining importance (Arnett, 1995a, 1995b, 2007), because "institutions (such as family and community) have lost their binding power, and individuals have gained more control of and responsibility for the direction of their lives" (Arnett, 2007, p. 214). Because of self-socialisation processes, socialisation agents have to support individuals less; instead, individuals have to make their own decisions and independently acquire skills, values, and norms for media use.

Self-Socialisation

A characteristic of this concept is the idea that the individual always makes an independent contribution to the socialisation process (Luhmann, 1987). This contribution is carried out in three steps. Individuals socialise themselves by a) attributing a meaning of their own to things and to themselves, b) developing their own logic of action, and c) formulating their own actions that should be achieved in the future. From this individual activity, a "childhood space, a childlike environment, in contrast to the world of adults" is developed (Zinnecker, 2000, p. 279). Children's self-socialisation serves to develop and maintain identity through active and productive engagement with the child's own environment and everyday life. The individual selects, interprets, and changes their social reality over the course of their lifetime (Hurrelmann, 1983; Müller, 1999). Nelissen and van den Bulck (2017) differentiate between three forms of self-socialisation, whereby the degree of independence increases according to the classification of understandings made and the developmental tasks undertaken throughout childhood and adolescence. Children could a) act as co-creators of their socialisation, interpreting and classifying information, b) socialise themselves and develop their own strategies without the influence of others, and c) socialise others.

Finally, Arnett (1995a, 1995b, 2007) and Süss (2010) discuss the concept of self-socialisation in the process of media socialisation. Arnett (1995a, p. 622) defines self-socialisation as the ability to use media for coping with developmental tasks so that children "are free to choose materials that contribute to their socialisation". Based on the required, acquired, or the existing independence of the child (the assumption), children could make selections from the media content that "best suit[s] their individual preferences and personalities" (Arnett, 1995b, p. 527). Media content provides identity-creating identification possibilities and helps to open up the world. The characteristics of such self-socialisation are control over the social developmental tasks that need to be mastered; a selection of media according to the individual's needs; as well as the self-reliant, independent actions of the individual. Self-socialisation through media use means that individuals "control the choice of media and media content themselves, decide on media times and media locations in relative autonomy and independently construct the significance of media content in the reception process", and they do not direct other socialisation agents' media dealings "with regard to externally determined socialisation goals" (Süss, 2010, p. 110). Because the individual is actively involved in the socialisation process, there is no subordination or media control by other socialisation agents. The adaptation and application of imparted abilities, values, and norms, as well as the acquisition of new abilities, take place with the individuals themselves. These subjects exercise their reflective abilities through their media use (e.g., with regard to media literate media use). For children, this implied freedom means not only using media in accordance with their wishes and needs (Pfaff-Rüdiger & Riesmeyer, 2016) but also in dealing responsibly with media offerings and using media to reflect opportunities and minimise risks (Livingstone, 2004).

Agency

The concept of agency also assumes that individuals are competent social actors. Agency is synonymous with power, the ability to act; or is simply equated with action (Raithelhuber, 2008). Following this concept, agency focusses less on the *socialisation process* (like self-socialisation) than on the *result of socialisation*, the concrete action or non-action of the individual, and the consequences of actions. "Having a sense of agency means that one can be generative, creative, proactive, and reflective" (Levesque, 2011, p. 92).

Agency is embedded in Barnes' social theory (1995), Bandura's learning theory (2001), and Giddens' structuring theory (1984) among others, with Giddens defining agency as being linked to the individual's ability to influence actions, to intervene in events, or to affect something causally. He states, "agency refers not to the intentions people have in doing things but to their capability of doing those things" (Giddens, 1984, p. 9). Expectations are formulated, corresponding action plans are drawn up, self-regulation is implemented, and self-reflexes are evaluated (Bandura, 2001). Barnes (1995) goes further, arguing that the consequences of the action, or of the decision to act, assume that the individual is also able to think through the consequences of the action. Individuals thus contribute to the shaping of the social worlds in which they participate.

The common thread regarding the idea of agency is that the individual is not only seen as a subject capable of acting (as in the concept of self-socialisation) but that he or she is also granted power – "the power to produce an effect, to have influence, to make a difference" (Buckingham, 2017, p. 12). Individuals must ensure that others recognise their capacity to act and their sense of responsibility for the consequences of their actions. This desire to be recognised for their abilities is intrinsically motivated (Giddens, 1984, p. 80), and when applied to the process of media socialisation this means that if socialisation agents (can) trust the individual child and his/her contribution to his/her socialisation they allow greater freedom to act independently. Alternatively, the child might claim that agency, whether or not the socialisation agents permit him/her to do so, creating potential conflict.

Self-Socialisation and Agency: State of Research

Both the concept of self-socialisation and agency have in common the notion of the individual as an independently acting subject with his or her own needs, ideas, and actions. The concepts assume that children and adolescents are independent social actors with specific rights, duties, and requirements as well as abilities and limitations regarding their actions. These characteristics should also be accounted for in research. Given this, what role has the individual played thus far in media socialisation research within communication studies?

A systematic literature review was conducted to answer this question. It included all publications since 2000 including monographs, articles in anthologies, and articles in peer-reviewed journals in English and German. The year 2000 was chosen as the starting point due to changes in the media ecosystem (such as the establishment of mobile communication technologies). Publications were searched for in the *EBSCO Host* database and in the archives of peer-reviewed journals *Journal of Children and Media* (English language), *Publizistik, Medien & Kommunikationswissenschaft*, and *Merz–Medien und Erziehung* (both German language), and *SCM – Studies in Communication and Media* (with articles in both English and German). All publications that mentioned the keywords media socialisation, mediation process, socialisation agent, self-socialisation, agency, and media in the title, the abstract, and/or the keywords were included. The search terms were deliberately broad in scope because it could not be guaranteed in advance that the publications would exclusively use the terms 'self-socialisation' or 'agency'.

Both 'self-socialisation' and 'agency' can also be used, for example, when comparing the different socialisation agents or the consequences of the socialisation process. In addition, despite the different conceptualisation of each term, they are treated equally for the literature review since both concepts focus on the individual and his or her role in the socialisation process. The sample was not limited to empirical studies of children and adolescents, but included studies of all ages in order to capture phenomena relating to different groups, such as socialisation by children and socialisation as an intergenerational task. Articles that did not contain an empirical study but discussed the concepts theoretically were also included in the sample.

The sample, once cleared of duplicates, comprised 1,082 publications. The broad search strategy meant that the sample also contained articles from journalism research and from the field of organisational or political communication research. Therefore, the second stage excluded from the sample all publications that either had no focus on communication studies (e.g., articles dealing with diplomatic relations) or that did not focus on any of the search terms mentioned (e.g., as a theoretical basis or as an empirical construct). This revision led to 159 publications being included in the systematic literature review (152 publications in English, 7 in German). This sample comprised 11 monographs, 22 articles in anthologies, and 126 peer-reviewed journal articles.

In the final step the articles were read and coded as to whether they used one or both concepts or at least referred to them. Twenty-four categories were created to allow the systematic ordering of article contents. This approach was necessary in order to capture the content, to categorise it, and to ensure that the texts could be correctly encoded even if they did not use the specific terms 'self-socialisation' and/or 'agency'.

The literature review shows that, despite the relevance of the concepts of self-socialisation and agency, they have thus far only made a small contribution to media socialisation research. Only 19 of the 159 publications use the term self-socialisation or agency and/or deal with the role of the individual as a subject in the socialisation process without using either of the two terms. Second, where other socialisation agents are taken into consideration, the publications were deemed to address 'self-socialisation' and/or 'agency' where they primarily focus on the role of the media within the media socialisation process (e.g., television, books, video games, or social networks). Such articles often also deal with non-medial agents, such as parents (or the nuclear family), teachers, and peers. Very few publications that compare the influence of agents and their importance for media socialisation also observe that the influence of the agents changes over the course of childhood and adolescence.

With regard to the topics dealt with by the publications, they are primarily concerned with the role of the media; and media use or influence on the formation of identities, self-representation, and self-perception. Mediated norms for media use, the processes, and the importance of media socialisation are discussed. The sample also contains numerous fields of application of media socialisation, e.g., the connection between media socialisation and political socialisation, sexual education, consumer, and religious socialisation.

The systematic literature review not only illustrates the low importance of the individual and the concepts of self-socialisation and agency, but also the at times very broad use of these terms. On the one hand, the boundary between self-socialisation and socialisation through others is drawn inconsistently. This applies to more than the question of whether peers are to be counted as self-socialisation or socialisation agents because of a very similar living environment. Some authors also define media as self-socialisation because they are used by individuals to socialise themselves, as Arnett (1995a) proposes. Other authors separate the media from self-socialisation and thus emphasise the educational mandate of media as a socialisation agent. While the concept of self-socialisation is discussed, so too is the media content the individual uses for his or her socialisation and how other agents use media in order to be able to socialise and pass on their knowledge. Some of these aspects would have to be characterised by the concept of socialisation through others. Finally, the sample contains texts that combine agency with the possibility of the individual producing media of their own, thus emphasising the active component of the concept, focussing on the action result.

Open Up for the Future: Four Theses

The aim of this chapter is to demonstrate the relevance of self-socialisation and agency for media socialisation research relating to children in the field of communication studies. Self-socialisation is understood as the socialisation of the individual, the person themselves, and thus as a process, while agency looks at the outcome of the process. The state of research makes it clear that there are various starting points that can be considered in future research endeavours and which are summarised in four theses, as follows.

Thesis 1: Media Socialisation as Comparative Research

One basic question asked by media socialisation relates to the origin of socialisation: who learns which skills, when, and where? Up until now, media socialisation research in the field of communication studies has focussed on the media as an agent, followed by parents (or the nuclear family), teachers, or peers, and their influence at one measuring point. As a rule, the focus is on one agent; a comparison between agents is almost absent from the selected publications. This could be a starting point for further discussions.

Closely linked to this absence is one relating to the perception of the mediation process over time: how do the socialisation agent and the individual mutually assess their roles in the socialisation process? How do they perceive each other? Precisely because media socialisation is a process that begins at childhood, and because there may be different and contested ideas about its end (Hurrelmann & Bauer, 2018), it is a challenge to grasp the (mutual) comparison of all socialisation agents at different points in time. Research shows that media socialisation research in the field of communication studies has thus far largely failed to make this comparison. This may reflect methodological challenges: researchers either have to rely on self-reflection by the socialisation agents and their ability to remember, or they would have to fall back on a panel design in order to survey long-term influences and proportions. However, for reasons of research pragmatism and economics, panel designs are often only partially feasible. 'The Class' project by Sonia Livingstone and Julian Sefton-Green (2016) is an exception, during which both communication scholars accompanied a London school class for a year and conducted interviews with the students, teachers, and parents at various times.

When media socialisation as a process is investigated empirically, the role of the individual should always be considered. Children and adolescents acquire skills independently in the process of media socialisation since the acquisition of knowledge does not necessarily have to be carried out by other bodies but can also be intrinsically motivated. Initial studies indicate that children and adolescents can name their own contribution to socialisation ("Who taught you how to use and deal with the media?"); compare their own socialisation activities with those of other bodies (Pfaff-Rüdiger & Riesmeyer, 2016; Riesmeyer, Pfaff-Rüdiger, & Kümpel, 2016); and define norms and values for their media use. This freedom of children and adolescents to take part in socialisation in a self-determined way and to make decisions independently means that older socialisation agents (e.g., parents, teacher) have to support and trust them to acquire skills and knowledge in order to counter risks from the very beginning (Blum-Ross et al., 2018; Riesmeyer, Abel, & Großmann, 2019).

Which abilities can be made concrete in self-socialisation, and when children and adolescents need support from other socialisation agents, has not yet been clarified. Krämer notes, in addition to self-socialisation, in the sense of "testing along and in a variation on the practical knowledge acquired so far", that "the family is probably one of the essential sources of strategies of media use" (Krämer, 2012, p. 170). Initial research findings show that the attribution of who contributed what to children's media socialisation varies in terms of the skills learned. The majority of those surveyed acquire technical skills themselves (following the principle of trial and error); parents and school play the major role in imparting background knowledge and (self-)reflection (evaluative media literacy; self and social skills; Pfaff-Rüdiger & Riesmeyer, 2016; Riesmeyer, Pfaff-Rüdiger, & Kümpel, 2016). To promote "critical understanding" which "should also lead to action" should be the aim of media education and the media socialisation process (Buckingham, 2019).

This implies that children and adolescents need guidance in the media socialisation process; they need to be taught values and norms in order to be able to apply them and adapt them to new conditions and media environments. Only in this way are they able to make their own decisions and reflect on them (e.g., with regard to the evaluation of received media content or interactions in a chat group). This decision-making power should be recognised in future research, and not either/or but with both guidance and self-direction, and, ideally, all possible socialisation agents considered. Such an approach includes regularly reviewing the definition of socialisation agents, and, if necessary, extending it if new agents arise. Traditional concepts do not yet consider agents that operate on social media platforms: neither followers as individuals (subjects who follow an account, e.g., peers), nor followees (objects followed by an account, e.g., influencers or friends) are currently accounted for. These should be considered, however, since initial studies already emphasise the importance of social media platforms in providing a benchmark for adolescents (Riesmeyer, Abel, & Großmann, 2019; Riesmeyer, Pohl, & Ruf, 2019).

Finally, in addition to the skills taught to children and young people, the comparative perspective concerns the origin of knowledge and the way in which knowledge is imparted: what is the knowledge of the socialisation agents based on and how do they intend to impart this knowledge? The contexts of everyday life become particularly relevant here. Arnett (1995a, p. 619), for example, notes that parents always educate within the cultural context around them and adapt cultural patterns and peculiarities that their parents have taught them. Especially with regard to technological change, this observation raises the question of whether the adaptation of abilities and educational patterns can be or should be media-dependent or media-independent. Individuals may be able to apply unknown standard patterns to new media technologies, but they must define and adopt new values and standards of media use into their futures – media socialisation also means a lifelong-learning process for all socialisation agents.

Thesis 2: Media Socialisation Means Lifelong Learning

Future research should, therefore, understand media socialisation as a lifelong-learning process that does not end when early adulthood is reached ('emerging adulthood'; Arnett, 2007, p. 208). Until now, media socialisation has often been defined as a process that begins in childhood where older socialisation agents teach younger people skills, knowledge, values, and norms for media use. Here, research into media socialisation in the field of communication studies should consider the changes in media offerings. In the meantime, more intuitive media technologies have been developed, and older socialisation agents (parents, grandparents, and teachers) can and must themselves acquire the skills of applying these. Against this background, all socialisation agents are called upon to constantly check their knowledge, and, if necessary, acquire new/further skills in order to be able to set values and standards. If the concept of self-socialisation or agency is thus redirected away from children and young people toward the generation of adults' skills, this can help to explain how adults acquire new technologies and associated skills.

Thesis 3: Media Socialisation Is Not a Unidirectional Process

Closely linked to thesis two is that media socialisation should not be understood as a unidirectional process. Using the example of self-socialisation, the previous logic of the socialisation process breaks down because children and young people can also take over a socialisation function (e.g., toward their parents; Correa, 2014; and/or their followers; Riesmeyer, Pohl, & Ruf, 2019). If the basic assumption of the individual as an independently acting and responsible subject applies, then this not only emphasises the active role of the subject within the process but also implies its importance as a socialisation agent, since the self-acquired knowledge can, in turn, be passed on to others – irrespective of generational affiliation. The perception that the younger generations socialise the older generations is not a new one: Mead defined 'reverse socialisation' in 1970. Socialisation is a bidirectional process between parents and children, between generations, that imparts skills, values, and norms from each to the other. Within this concept of the socialisation process, the active role of the individual and thus self-socialisation is already in place. There is an equal agency of parents and children (Kuczynski, 2003; Clark, 2011; Van den Bulck, Custers, & Nelissen, 2016; Nelissen & van den Bulck, 2017) that is assumed. However, this concept of the socialisation process has rarely been implemented in empirical media socialisation studies in communication studies thus far.

Thesis 4: Media Socialisation as an Interdisciplinary Common Starting Point

Finally, current research indicates that media socialisation in general, but also the concepts of agency and self-socialisation in particular, are repeatedly associated with specific fields of application. These include where research deals with the connections between media socialisation and sexual education, for example, and political, religious, or consumer socialisation (e.g., how Muslims use Google to research religious practices instead of discussing them with their parents, or how young people use media offerings to make purchase decisions; e.g., Davignon, 2013; Moeller & de Vreese, 2013; Wright, 2014). Since these issues are at the interface of media socialisation, and since they deal with the role of the individual, media socialisation research in the field of communication studies should also take up these common starting points in order to grasp what part 'young people' play in the construction "of their own social lives" (Poynotz, Coulter, & Brisson, 2016, p. 51).

References

Abels, H., & König, A. (2010). *Sozialisation (Socialisation)*. Wiesbaden: VS Verlag.
Arnett, J. J. (1995a). Broad and narrow socialization: The family in the context of a cultural theory. *Journal of Marriage and the Family, 57*(3), 617–628.
Arnett, J. J. (1995b). Adolescents' use of media for self-socialization. *Journal of Youth and Adolescence, 24*(5), 519–533.
Arnett, J. J. (2007). Socialization in emerging adulthood: From the family to the wider word, from socialization to self-socialization. In J. E. Grusec & P. D. Hastings (Eds.), *Handbook of socialization: Theory and research* (pp. 208–231). New York: Guilford Press.
Bandura, A. (2001). Social cognitive theory: An agentic perspective. *Annual Review of Psychology, 52*(1), 1–26.
Barnes, B. (1995). *The elements of social theory*. Princeton: Princeton University Press.
Beaudoin, C. E. (2014). The mass media and adolescent socialization: A prospective study in the context of unhealthy food advertising. *Journalism & Mass Communication Quarterly, 91*(3), 544–561.
Blum-Ross, A., Donoso, V., Dinh, T., Mascheroni, G., O'Neill, B., Riesmeyer, C., & Stoilova, M. (2018). *Looking forward: Technological and social change in the lives of European children and young people*. Report for the ICT Coalition for Children Online. Brussels: ICT Coalition.
Buckingham, D. (2017). Media theory 101: Agency. *Journal of Media Literacy, 64*(1&2), 12–15.
Buckingham, D. (2019). *The media education manifesto*. Cambridge: Polity Press.

Chakroff, J., & Nathanson, A. I. (2008). Parent and school interventions: Mediation and media literacy. In S. L. Calvert & B. J. Wilson (Eds.), *The handbook of children, media, and development* (pp. 552–576). Malden: Blackwell.

Clark, L. S. (2011). Parental mediation theory for the digital age. *Communication Theory, 21*(4), 323–343.

Correa, T. (2014). Bottom-up technology transmission within families: Exploring how youths influence their parents' digital media use with dyadic data. *Journal of Communication, 64*(1), 103–124.

Davignon, P. (2013). The effects of R-rated movies on adolescent and young adult religiosity: Media as self-socialization. *Review of Religious Research, 55*(4), 615–628.

EU Kids Online. (2014). *EU kids online: Findings, methods, recommendations*. Retrieved from: http://eprints.lse.ac.uk/60512.

Genner, S., & Süss, D. (2017). Socialization as media effect. In P. Rössler, C. Hoffner, & L. van Zoonen (Eds.), *The international encyclopedia of media effects* (pp. 1890–1904). Chichester: Wiley Blackwell.

Giddens, A. (1984). *The constitution of society. Outline of the theory of structuration*. Berkeley: University of California Press.

Grusec, J. (2002). Parental socialization and children's acquisition of values. In M. Bornstein (Ed.), *Handbook of parenting: Practical issues in parenting* (pp. 143–168). Mahwah: Erlbaum.

Heinzel, F., Kränzl-Nagl, R., & Mierendorff, J. (2012). Sozialwissenschaftliche kindheitsforschung-Annäherungen an einen komplexen forschungsbereich (Social science childhood research—approaches to a complex research field). *Theo-Web. Zeitschrift für Religionspädagogik (Theo-Web. Academic Journal of Religious Education), 11*(1), 9–37.

Himmelbach, N. (2013). Kindheit, jugend und sozialer wandel: Gegenwärtige und zukünftige herausforderungen für die internationale kindheits- und jugendforschung (Childhood, adolescence, and social change: Current and future challenges for international children and youth research). *Diskurs Kindheits- und Jugendforschung (Discourse Childhood and Youth Research), 8*(2), 237–241.

Hobbs, R. (2011). *Digital and media literacy. Connecting culture and classroom*. Thousand Oaks: Sage.

Hobbs, R. (2013). Media literacy. In D. Lemish (Ed.), *The Routledge international handbook of children, adolescents, and media* (pp. 417–424). Abingdon: Routledge.

Honig, M.-S. (2002). Konzeptionelle emanzipation? Systematische probleme der kindheitssoziologie (Conceptual emancipation? Systematic problems of childhood sociology). In H. Uhlendorff & H. Oswald (Eds.), *Wege zum selbst: Soziale Herausforderungen für Kinder und Jugendliche (Ways to yourself: Social challenges for children and young people)* (pp. 13–35). Stuttgart: Lucius & Lucius.

Hurrelmann, K. (1983). Das modell des produktiv realitätsverarbeitenden subjekts in der sozialisationsforschung (The model of the productive reality-processing subject in socialisation research). *ZSE, 3*, 91–103.

Hurrelmann, K. (1990). Parents, peers, teachers, and other significant partners in adolescence. *International Journal of Adolescence and Youth, 2*(3), 211–236.

Hurrelmann, K., & Bauer, U. (2018). *Socialisation during the life course*. Abingdon: Routledge.

Krämer, B. (2012). *Mediensozialisation. Theorie und empirie zum erwerb medienbezogener dispositionen (Media socialisation. Theory and empiricism for the acquisition of media-related dispositions)*. Wiesbaden: Springer VS.

Kuczynski, L. (2003). Beyond bidirectionality: Bilateral conceptual frameworks for understanding dynamics in parent-child relations. In L. Kuczynski (Ed.), *Handbook of dynamics in parent-child relations* (pp. 1–24). Thousand Oaks: Sage.

Levesque, R. J. R. (2011). Agency. In R. J. R. Levesque (Ed.), *Encyclopedia of adolescence* (p. 92). Wiesbaden: Springer.

Livingstone, S. (2004). Media literacy and the challenge of new information and communication technologies. *The Communication Review, 7*(1), 3–14.

Livingstone, S., & Sefton-Green, J. (2016). *The class. Living and learning in the digital age*. New York: NYU Press.

Luhmann, N. (1987). Sozialisation und erziehung (Socialisation and education). In N. Luhmann (Ed.), *Soziologische aufklärung 4 (Sociological enlightenment)* (pp. 173–181). Opladen: Westdeutscher Verlag.

Martens, H., & Hobbs, R. (2015). How media literacy supports civic engagement in a digital age. *Atlantic Journal of Communication, 23*(2), 120–137.

Mead, M. (1970). *Culture and commitment: A study of the generation gap*. New York: Natural History Press/Doubleday & Company, Inc.

Mihailidis, P. (2014). *Media literacy and the emerging citizen: Youth, engagement and participation in digital culture*. New York: Peter Lang.

Moeller, J., & de Vreese, C. (2013). The differential role of the media as an agent of political socialization in Europe. *European Journal of Communication, 28*(3), 309–325.

Müller, R. (1999). Musikalische selbstsozialisation (Musical self-socialisation). In J. Fromme, S. Kommer, J. Mansel, & K. P. Treumann (Eds.), *Selbstsozialisation, kinderkultur und mediennutzung (Self-socialisation, children's culture, and media use)* (pp. 113–125). Opladen: Leske & Budrich.

Nelissen, S., & van den Bulck, J. (2017). *Bidirectional influences among parents and children in their digital media use and the association with Internet self-efficacy: An application of the actor-partner interdependence model in media research.* Paper presented at the 67th International Communication Association Conference, San Diego.

Peters, J. F. (1985). Adolescents as socialization agents to parents. *Adolescence, 20*(80), 921–933.

Pfaff-Rüdiger, S., & Riesmeyer, C. (2016). Moved into action. Media literacy as social process. *Journal of Children and Media, 10*(2), 164–172.

Poynotz, S. R., Coulter, N., & Brisson, G. (2016). Past tensions and future possibilities: ARCYP and children's media studies. *Journal of Children and Media, 10*(1), 47–53.

Prot, S., Anderson, C. A., Gentile, D. A., Warburton, W., Saleem, M., Groves, C. L., & Brown, S. C. (2015). Media as agents of socialization. In J. E. Grusec & P. D. Hastings (Eds.), *Handbook of socialization: Theory and research* (2nd ed., pp. 276–300). New York: Guilford Press.

Raithelhuber, E. (2008). Von akteuren und agency—eine sozialtheoretische einordnung der structure/agency-debatte (By actors and agencies—a socio-theoretical classification of the structure/agency debate). In H. G. Homfeldt, W. Schröer, & C. Schweppe (Eds.), *Vom adressaten zum akteur. Soziale arbeit und agency (From addressee to actor. Social work and agency)* (pp. 17–45). Opladen: Barbara Budrich.

Riesmeyer, C., Abel, B., & Großmann, A. (2019, in print). The family rules. The influence of parenting styles on adolescents' media literacy. *Medien Pädagogik: Zeitschrift Für Theorie Und Praxis Der Medienbildung (Mediaeducation: Journal for Theory and Practice of Media Education), 35,* 74–96.

Riesmeyer, C., Pfaff-Rüdiger, S., & Kümpel, A. S. (2016). Wenn wissen zu handeln wird: Medienkompetenz aus motivationaler perspektive (When knowledge becomes action: Media literacy from a motivational perspective). *Medien & Kommunikationswissenschaft (Media and Communication Research), 64*(1), 36–55.

Riesmeyer, C., Pohl, E., & Ruf, L. (2019). *Your best friend and influencer? Perception of and dealing with peer pressure on Instagram among adolescents.* Paper presented at the 69th Annual Meeting of the International Communication Association, Washington, DC.

Smetana, J. G., Robinson, J., & Rote, W. M. (2015). Socialization in adolescence. In J. E. Grusec & P. D. Hastings (Eds.), *Handbook of socialization: Theory and research* (2nd ed., pp. 60–84). New York: Guilford Press.

Süss, D. (2010). Mediensozialisation zwischen gesellschaftlicher entwicklung und identitätskonstruktion (Media socialisation between social development and identity construction). In D. Hoffmann & L. Mikos (Eds.), *Mediensozialisationstheorien (Media Socialisation Theories)* (pp. 109–130). Wiesbaden: VS.

Van den Bulck, J., Custers, K., & Nelissen, S. (2016). The child-effect in the new media environment: Challenges and opportunities for communication research. *Journal of Children & Media, 10*(1), 30–38.

Van Dijck, J. (2009). Users like you? Theorizing agency in user-generated content. *Media, Culture & Society, 31*(1), 41–58.

Wright, P. J. (2014). Pornography and the sexual socialization of children: Current knowledge and a theoretical future. *Journal of Children & Media, 8*(3), 305–312.

Zinnecker, J. (2000). Selbstsozialisation—Essay über ein aktuelles konzept (Self-socialisation—essay about a current concept). *ZSE, 20*(3), 272–290.

32
DIGITAL CITIZENSHIP IN DOMESTIC CONTEXTS

Lelia Green

The Evolving Policy Context around Digital Citizenship

In March 2019 the United Nations Committee on the Rights of the Child advised it was "drafting a General Comment on children's rights in relation to the digital environment" (OHCHR, n.d.). Importantly, this notification was made under the auspices of the United Nations Commission on Human Rights. The initiative aligns with an increasing policy emphasis on developing and recognising children's digital citizenship. According to a United Nations Educational, Scientific and Cultural Organization (UNESCO) report, *Digital Kids Asia-Pacific*, digital citizenship

> is about preparing children to become true digital citizens, with both the skills and the socio-emotional abilities to engage with digital technologies and other users in a critical and ethical manner while being aware of their own and others' rights and responsibilities.
>
> *(UNESCO Bangkok Office, 2019, p. 50)*

This chapter focusses on the development of i) socio-emotional abilities, ii) rights, iii) responsibilities, and iv) critical and ethical digital engagement, principally in the domestic context of the family home. Other definitions of digital citizenship call attention to how digital media offer a channel through which children may 'speak truth to power' about issues that affect them now, and which will be crucially important to the world they will inherit as adults (Green, 2020). That definition is a cogent one, but less relevant to most domestic contexts.

The current focus on digital citizenship is the most recent transformation in a journey that began by constructing children's digital engagement as a matter of provision (approximately 1995–2004), then as a matter of protection (approximately 2005–2014), and most recently as an emerging discussion around participation (2015 onwards). Participation is crucial to the enactment of citizenship. Arguing for a specific focus on children's rights in digital environments, Livingstone and Third (2017) note that the policy emphasis has tended towards protection: "over and again, efforts to protect them [children] unthinkingly curtail their participation rights in ways that they themselves are unable to contest, given the nature of Internet governance organizations" (2017, p. 661).

Recognising the zeitgeist of the time, a flurry of recent policies and pronouncements relating to children's rights in digital environments specifically reference digital citizenship. The European

Union, for example, has embarked on an EU-wide discussion of these issues (EU Council of Europe, 2019), alongside such initiatives as the General Data Protection Regulation (GDPR) ('EU data protection rules', n.d.). These generally positive regulatory advances, which include, for example, 'the right to be forgotten' (Bunn, 2019), nonetheless have a sting in their tail since they effectively increase the age of digital consent for children in some European countries from 13 to 16 (Milkaite & Lievens, 2019).

In the United States, the Center for Digital Democracy (CDD) particularly champions children's and young people's rights to privacy and seeks to protect them from online commercial exploitation, especially in terms of the commodification of their data (CDD, n.d.). Elsewhere in the world, UNESCO's *Digital Kids Asia-Pacific* reports leading-edge work on investigating children's digital citizenship in terms of a "comprehensive and holistic set of competencies" (UNESCO Bangkok Office, 2019, p. xiii). These competencies, explored via benchmark research in Bangladesh, Fiji, South Korea, and Vietnam, comprise five domains: Digital Literacy; Digital Safety and Resilience; Digital Participation and Agency; Digital Emotional Intelligence; and Digital Creativity and Innovation (2019, pp. 8–10). Extrapolating across these dimensions and relating them to the domestic context, this chapter considers the development of digital citizenship in children's domestic lives.

Children's Everyday Lives and Digital Citizenship

Although there is significant activity to promote children's digital citizenship, the impetus is arguably adult-driven and top-down, engaging with children on occasion, but not necessarily reflecting children's priorities and preoccupations. The case study that follows offers a bottom-up perspective: evidence of developing recognition of digital citizenship with specific reference to a clan of teen gamers who play Dota 2. The analysis suggests that there is an articulation between proactive parental mediation, which aligns with Livingstone, Haddon, Görzig, and Olafsson's notion of "active mediation – the parent talks about content (e.g. interpreting, critiquing) to guide the child" (2011, p. 103), and digital citizenship. These engaged parental mediation approaches, which were largely followed by the families discussed here, support the growth of key skills in children's digital activities and behaviour, and the competencies that feed into the development of digital literacies. At its best, parental mediation may induct young people into digital citizenship.

This section addresses aspects of parents' mediation activities, especially as these relate to gaming, before introducing the specific characteristics of Dota 2, the focus game. Apperley has previously argued that children have a right to digital play, including a right to play digital games, which he sees as contributing to "literacy and civic engagement" (2015, p. 193). He notes that: "the process of playing digital games and being a part of gaming communities fosters the development of skills that support civic behavior and participation" (2015, p. 200).

In their paper on parental mediation of First Person Shooter (FPS) and Massively Multiplayer Online Role Playing Games, Jiow, Lim, and Lin (2017) also suggest that family discussions around game play may themselves fuel children's awareness of digital citizenship rights. Jiow et al.'s work focusses on parents' mediation of gamer children aged between 12–17, since this is "the developmental stage where adolescents begin to exhibit individuation through negotiating and asserting their rights" (2017, p. 314). Arguably, negotiation and the assertion of their own priorities are key indicators of a realisation by adolescents that they have rights.

An awareness of rights develops over time. Willett notes, of a younger gamer age group (7 to 11), that "'big gift' items (namely gaming consoles or tablets) [are] a frequent point of negotiation between parents and children" (2016, p. 467) in relation to birthday and Christmas presents. Between them, these researchers indicate a trajectory of awareness in children that transitions from hopes regarding gifts to the claiming of rights. Children's realisation of their growing autonomy around making decisions and setting their own priorities becomes more evident as they earn or are given their own money. In the discussion to follow, when Mike purchased his own computer it became the catalyst for him to change the family rule around having the computer in a shared space. Mike located his new computer in his bedroom.

According to Nikken and Jansz, children's videogaming practices from the 1980s onwards have "produced considerable public concerns, in particular about the effects of violent game content, the stereotypical representation of women and non-white ethnic groups, and the time-consuming nature of gaming" (2006, p. 182). These researchers draw upon their survey of 536 Dutch parent–child (aged 8–18) dyads to observe that, with regard to parents' mediation of videogaming, "all three forms of parental mediation (restrictive, active and co-viewing) were more often directed towards younger children and girls than towards older children and boys" (2006, p. 185). This contrasts somewhat with Eklund and Helmersson Bergmark's view (2013, p. 63) that, in Sweden, "Boys and young adolescents are controlled more than girls and older adolescents". This latter finding might reflect Swedish parents' "quite negative views on gaming" (Eklund & Helmersson Bergmark, 2013, p. 63).

Leaving gendered aspects of mediation to one side, the general view concerning older children is that parents feel a "need to grant more decision-making authority to young people as they age" (Clark, 2011, p. 325), implicitly acknowledging that young people living in the family home have an increasing right to act autonomously. Negotiations around potential points of parent–child disagreement, such as screen time restrictions, or adherence to media classification categories, can be challenging emotional work, however. One of the parents involved in the case study indicated a strong antipathy towards violent content in video games, saying that the game his son plays, Dota 2, is "not that sort of game. It's a fun game [pauses] I know it's intense but it's a fun game they play. You know, there's no level of violence that I'd consider to be extreme" (Father B). This father was particularly keen that his son should respect the 18+ classifications of some of the popular FPS games.

While Common Sense Media suggest a rating of 13+ for the case study game, Dota 2, describing it as a "Polished, fun fantasy multiplayer game [that] stands test of time" (Chapman, 2013), others take an alternative view. The Anti-Defamation League for example, in their report *Free to play? Hate, harassment, and positive social experiences in online games* (ADL, 2019), ranked 15 games according to players' experiences of online harassment. Dota 2 tops the list, with 79% of players reporting toxic experiences in-game. "Online multiplayer gamers who experience harassment believe they were targeted because of their race/ethnicity, religion, ability, gender or sexual orientation" note ADL (2019, p. 7), subsequently observing that "A majority of players (62%) feel that companies should do more to make online games safer and more inclusive for players" (ADL, 2019, p. 28). Arguably, the public discussion around violent content in videogames may distract parents and commentators from paying attention to other aspects of children's online experiences.

With socio-emotional abilities previously identified as a component of digital citizenship, Clark notes that "Parents attempt to utilize media for positive familial and developmental goals that may not be directly related to the media" (2011, p. 324), adding that "parents and children negotiate interpersonal relationships in and through digital mobile media" (2011, p. 335). These issues will now be explored in greater depth through a case study that uses ethnographic data gathered as part of an Australian Research Council-funded project, *Parents or peers: which group most affects the experiences of young people online, and how?* (DP110100864: see Green & Haddon, 2015), with the author and Leslie Haddon as co-Investigators. Although these materials provide evidence of a discussion around digital citizenship, the initial impetus for the project was a comparison of parental influence on high school students' digital activities compared with the influence of their peers.

Method and Approach

The teens in this case study (Yin, 2009) were aged 16~17 at the time of the research in 2014. Glynn, Louden, Mike, and Rob (all pseudonyms for the purposes of de-identification) constituted the inner circle of a well-established Dota 2 clan which had played together for about two years. A fifth clan member was unable to take part because of lack of parental consent. The gamers all attended the same high school in the British Midlands, and were comparatively strong academic achievers, which may have meant their parents experienced less anxiety around their gaming practices.

The author had found it difficult to recruit a cohort of gamers who were willing to take part in the research and had parents who were similarly willing to give consent and participate themselves. This clan was eventually recruited through the author's personal networks. The four teen gamers were first interviewed individually and then gathered together for a focus group, with the same data collection strategy used with the (five) participating parents. The parents represented three of the four families, a mother and father from two families, and a mother from the third. Given the requirements of privacy and non-identifiability for all participants, mothers are numbered Mother 1 to Mother 3, while Fathers are A or B. Mother 1 does not necessarily co-parent the same child as Father A.

The nine interviews and two focus groups were recorded, and then transcribed, and the constant comparative method of analysis (Fram, 2013) was used to interrogate the resulting dataset. Constant Comparative Analysis (CCA) shares some similarities with the analytic processes of Grounded Theory but does not require that the outcome is inductive. As Hodkinson notes, however

> although highly influential, grounded theory is not very often followed to the letter and ... it is more common for researchers to adopt one or more elements associated with the approach as part of their efforts to develop theory through research.
>
> *(2008, p. 80)*

A CCA approach indicates that data are constantly analysed and compared, within and between: interviews; focus groups; interviews and focus groups; and, different groups of participants. Echoing Hodkinson, Fram notes that researchers often "pragmatically use the CCA method to support the emergence of a substantive theory from working the data" (2013, p. 4). Further details around recruitment and methodology are addressed in Green and Haddon (2015).

Dota 2

The clan's preferred game, Dota 2, is a spin-off of the Warcraft franchise and a successor to a mod (modification) of Warcraft III, Defence of the Ancients. It is a free-access real-time strategy game that pits two five-person teams against each other in a multiplayer online battle arena with the aim of one team destroying the other's Ancient. With a high global profile that rivals Fortnite, Dota 2 has a significant eSports component. In 2019, for example, the competitive prize pool for professional gamers exceeded 30 million USD (Kaser, 2019).

The international community engaged in Dota 2 both fuels and reflects the richness of the gamer experience as well as, potentially, adding to its toxicity (ADL, 2019). As Apperley (2018, p. 7) notes, "the work of 'making meaning' of ... games *does not only take place within algorithmic constraints*; rather, it is also situated in relation both to a community of players and the circumstances of the individual". Gamers have round-the-clock opportunities for competition, where one clan of gamers can take on another with the hope of establishing a relative pecking order and moving up the league tables. Dota 2 games typically take between 40 and 60 minutes to reach a result and, because of the importance of all players to the strategic outcome of each contest, there are significant penalties imposed by the competitive framework upon teams where a player or team drops out before the end of the competition. Mike explains: "you get put in a low priority, which means it takes longer to find a [good] match. The people you are with are also in low priority, so the games won't be as good" (Mike).

Given the strategy element to Dota 2, it is advantageous for an established team to play games together, since they know each other's strengths and weaknesses and can develop effective ways of collaborating. Even so, it can be challenging to get five teens online at the same time, with each having negotiated an hour's uninterrupted access within their domestic context. Glynn is the eldest in his family and his parents have strict rules around no screen time after 9.00 p.m., which he finds especially frustrating:

> Normally in the week everyone else stays on a bit later than me, so I could end up waiting the whole evening then I have to get off 'cos my brothers and sister are going to bed, then everyone else ... plays a match after I've gone.
>
> *(Glynn)*

As well as the core group of gamers within most Dota 2 clans, represented by the four teen participants, there is also a floating pool of substitutes who may be incorporated within the team if one or more of the key players is unavailable when other members want to play. In extremis, it is possible to recruit 'randoms', people unknown to the team but offered to them by a Dota 2 matching system that suggests the player on the basis of skills and a 'behaviour score', which classifies their approach to the game (Cook, 2019).

Findings

The case study data suggest that core aspects of what policy makers deem digital citizenship are developed and recognised within the daily domestic negotiations of parents and teens around young people's lives online. Examples of how this happens will be considered in relation to earlier discussions of four key aspects of digital citizenship: i) socio-emotional abilities, ii) rights, iii) responsibilities, and iv) critical and ethical dimensions.

Socio-Emotional Abilities

Looking back over their shared years in high school, and as gamers, this clan has gradually internalised the realities of the impact of their gaming on others, and particularly on their families. Louden notes how the clan works around the fixed and moving points of domesticity, while at the same time justifying his ongoing close connection with digital technology:

> Say, I have [dinner] early and Rob has it late, there's a period in between where we're both free ... [you] have to be at the point where you're on your computer for a lot of the time after school, so there's just more chance of everyone being available.
>
> *(Louden)*

The challenges of managing to find an hour or so of shared time, and the sense of time as an investment and a scarce resource, have come to be accepted as a responsibility by these clan members, who also talk about the days when they play a 'bad' game. Louden argues that "you have to remember, it's an hour of someone else's time. If you're ruining the game for them they're not going to be particularly happy". Rob offers a more sanguine perspective: "you've both probably been bad in one match or another, so it's just accepting the fact that the person you're playing with has had a bad match and they know they've had a bad match". This capacity to take a longer view and put one day in perspective against a general background of the everyday is part of digital emotional intelligence. As a socio-emotional journey, it builds resilience and a confidence in planning for longer-term horizons.

Families within this tight-knit gamer clan have different perspectives about how to respond to classification standards relating to game content. For example, Father B recalls that at 14 his son

> wanted to get Call of Duty, which is an 18+ game, and we said "no", and he said "well, so and so's playing it", and we said "well sorry, but that's up to their parents. We're not going to let you play that. It's an 18 for a reason, they're age rated for a reason".

While none of the Dota 2 clan could recall how they came to start playing the game, apart from the fact that is was free, enjoyable, and challenging, it could be the case that Father B's refusal to allow his son to play any 18+ FPS games meant that the friends sought an alternative. This would be another indicator of emotional maturity and the accommodation of a group member's specific circumstances. Given that the clan had been playing Dota 2 together for about two years at the time of the interviews, they would have started when Father B's son was about 14.

Recognising and supporting their teens' growing socio-emotional abilities, parents may also start paying greater attention to their child's perspective. Mother 3, for example, acknowledges that: "In the last year, up until probably about a year ago I was, I didn't, I was anti it, I was anti the gaming". Over time, however, she came to accommodate her son's right to be passionate about Dota 2. "You grow up yourself in recognising that, you know, there isn't just one way the family's living, or one way a boy's living in the family, there's [pauses] other ways". This mother acknowledges the influence of dominant discourses that position gaming as potentially problematic but embraces the reality of the evidence experienced in daily life.

> Rather than just accepting what you read in the paper and saying "Oh, this is bad for us", we're thinking "well, hang on a minute, our boy seems to be doing well at school, he seems to be having friends ... What are we worried about? What are our complaints?"

These vignettes show the growth of emotional intelligence and of reciprocal acceptance by parents and sons of the others' points of view. As young people become more aware of their parents' priorities, such as around family meal times in the evening, so some parents also recognise their child's growing autonomy by practising an increasingly soft-touch mediation of video gaming.

Rights

As noted above, one of the teens had changed his family's rules around only having computer access in shared spaces within the home. According to Mike's mother, he

> bought his own computer and built it, and it was up in his bedroom. I [pauses] it was a long time before I was comfortable with it ... just frequently popping in and out of his room, just to see what he was doing ... and every time I went in there he was just on the game.

The implication of Mother 2's response to Mike's new computer, and its location in Mike's bedroom, is that there was more at stake for her than increased access to computer time. The 'popping in and out' of Mike's room is part of an active mediation strategy, while Mother 2's reference to Mike's being 'just on the game' indicates some relief that this was indeed the reason for Mike's desire to have private access to his own technology. In terms of respecting her son's rights to digital privacy, however, and in response to a suggestion that she might have wanted to check Mike's browsing history, Mother 2 was clear about what she saw as acceptable limits of parental enquiry: "No, I wouldn't check it, actually ... I don't know, just teenage boys, I don't know what I'd find on there".

Mother 3 also argued that the activity of checking her son's computer would be "stalking your children". In addition to constructing her son's right to not be stalked, Mother 3 noted the lack, for her, of appropriate ways to respond to any outcome of such surveillance:

> it will just pull you into a different world you wouldn't want to know about, possibly. 'Cos if you do [find] something [then] you think "Well, now I've got to tell them that I've looked at their PC and do I want to do that?" I've got no reason to look at it. I'd rather not, so no, I don't.

Father A puts the issue of accessing inappropriate content into the context of a preparation for adulthood: "I kind of think they've got to negotiate that world [internet content] for all their life". In this respect, he sees parental prohibitions for this 16–17 age group as counterproductive. In particular, he is unable to see the value in saying "'we'll monitor everything and once they're 18 they can watch anything they like', I think that's probably more destructive".

These different negotiations around young people's rights to digital participation and agency demonstrate teens and their parents finding ways to respect the rights of other members in the family home. There is also a direct acknowledgement, by Father A, that the notional control that parents have over their child's digital activities ceases at the point at which they become 18. For that parent, the aim of mediating his son's digital engagement in domestic space was to lay the foundations for his son to conduct his own negotiations with digital content for the rest of his life.

Responsibilities

Aspects of digital citizenship associated with digital participation and agency involve self-directed activity on the part of gamers, particularly in terms of acquiring and using the high-end technological equipment and connectivity required to be an effective clan member. Father A, for example, was impressed with his son's commitment to gaming in terms of the evidence it provided of long-term planning and goal-oriented activity. "His machine's very high spec so, he chose it himself. He saved up his money and he bought it himself." One clan member's desire for bigger, better, faster, gaming tech can have a ratcheting effect on other families, however. Mother 2 identified that her son Mike was concerned about their internet connection:

> Mike said "I'm lagging behind and, yeah, can we just look for something that's faster, faster broadband speeds?" And [we ...] then researched and found an affordable [pause] well the fastest speed at an affordable price for us ... But Mike did actually say that he was prepared to contribute [money] to a faster internet 'cos it affected his gaming so much if it was slow.

(Mother 2)

It made a difference to these parents that Mike was helping take responsibility for the impact of his request for better internet access. At the same time, Mike's parents were indicating their acceptance of his desire to participate in gaming with his peers on an equal basis.

One family can chart the process by which their son gradually took responsibility for aspects of his gaming behaviour as the two-year engagement with Dota 2 progressed. Mother 3 began by voicing her frustration around

> [you] find he's suddenly gone on a game and it's going to last an hour. And you know he's got a dentist appointment or we're just about to eat, you know, and he's saying "Well, I can't come off it", and you're thinking "This is ridiculous, our life is being determined by one-person-in-the-family's game!"

But then, this mother recalled that these frustrations were mainly a thing of the past, and that her own changes in behaviour had also helped create a more reciprocal environment where both mother and son took responsibility for the smooth running of the household. These days, says Mother 3, her son will come and quickly check and say

> "Is it OK if I go on a game?" So sometimes I go, "yeah", [or] "no", [or] "that's fine". So mentally I have to allow them an hour ... We just know that we give him a warning ... and he can see, he's intelligent, he can see that obviously the meal thing is a big issue, that he can't [pauses] we can't all sit down and wait and have the food go cold.

As well as appreciating that their sons were displaying greater responsibility as their Dota 2 gaming practices developed, two parents spoke about how digital engagement had led to their boys displaying financial responsibility. Mother 1 described how her teenager buys things on Steam, the video gaming distribution service operated by Valve, Dota 2's developer and publisher.

> He has to give me the money, obviously, but he always comes and asks ... We've left the [credit card] details on there [Steam] because it just got so [pause]. It actually got to be a bit of a pain, always having to put them in, so there's a high level of trust in that respect.

Mike's family had gone one step further.

> [Mike] wanted his own debit card [so] that he could do it himself ... He does seem to know exactly what he's doing ... because before that it was our credit card that was on there. And I wasn't really comfortable with that because, you know, the sky's the limit, but with his debit card he can't go overdrawn. The only worry is fraud.
>
> (Mother 2)

Given the integration of gaming across these teens' daily lives, it is unsurprising that their gaming activities offer a range of ways in which they can develop and display an increasingly evident sense of responsibility to others, in domestic spaces and beyond.

Critical and Ethical Digital Engagement

This section considers how citizenship-like activities can encompass, and are not negated by, rule-breaking, where an in-the-moment responsibility to the peer group may trump an abstract responsibility to rules. It recognises the citizenship is an inherent attribute, it is not earned by good or bad behaviour, even when people act as good or bad citizens at different times and in different contexts.

Although there are many positive aspects to these boys' relationships with digital media, they also discussed a range of non-compliant behaviours. Two specific examples were proffered during the focus group discussion. Since the teens all attended the same school, and had privileges as a result of being in the sixth form, they had periods of free time when they were trusted to go online and behave responsibly:

Rob: They do filter games and TV sites at school, but you can get quite inventive and find ...
Mike: Dutch websites.
Rob: We've tried all sorts. It got to one point where we went and learnt the Arabic Google [all laughing] and Googled [unclear] and so ... and typed in like "play online games" and then translated it into Arabic, and then pasted it to Google. I was trying to get round the filtering system.

There is some incidental evidence that contesting established authority strengthens the bonds that link the boys. The examples of non-compliance certainly fuelled moments of hilarity in the focus group. As noted above, Mike has his own debit card and takes responsibility for buying some of his digital games. He explained the challenge encountered when a younger player likes:

Mike: ... the trailer for an 18+ game, you have to put your age in.
Louden: You can just lie.
Rob: ... and I've just got it auto set to, I was born in 1907 [all laughing]. I just click okay and then it's all fine.

Relevantly, the policy settings around access tend to be made without reference to those they are intended to protect, representing adults' views of what constitutes responsible citizenship for young people. Further, parents may model a comparatively laissez faire attitude to some of the restrictions upon this age group, although they may feel strongly that such rules should apply to younger children. Mother 1, for example, suggests that the family's internet filter is little more than an inconvenience for Louden: "I'm sure techno-savvy teenagers know what to do to get around a basic filter system in a house". Such an attitude aligns with a (teen-friendly) perception that filters are only necessary for people unable to circumvent them. The parental hope seems to be that by the time a filter can be beaten, the child is sufficiently mature to handle the material they access.

In terms of the perennial concern of parents that activities other than schoolwork may compromise their child's future, Mother 3 shared a recent development in her own philosophical approach:

> I'm just going [speaking to myself ...] "Actually, you know, he's a lovely boy, do we want to spend our lives in complete conflict? He's not going to change, he's not voluntarily going to give this up, it's not affecting his school work". Well, maybe it has, maybe he could get better marks but, you know, who knows? ... Maybe not. Maybe he'd just be depressed or something.
>
> *(Mother 3)*

Taking these four points into consideration: i) socio-emotional abilities, ii) rights, iii) responsibilities, and iv) critical and ethical digital engagement; the overall impression is that the digital citizenship project for this group of gamers is working well, with significant respect shown by parents and sons for issues of socio-emotional intelligence on the one hand and digital participation and agency on the other.

Conclusion

Willson notes that "parents want happy and healthy (and successful) children. How to understand and achieve healthy, happy and successful, however, is less clear" (2019, p. 623). This case study examines a journey towards 'healthy, happy and successful' in terms of the digital citizenship dynamics at work in four families selected for their teen sons' engagement in an online game. In many families, at a critical point of a child's educational journey, a hobby such as videogaming might be constructed as a negative, or a challenge. In the families in this study, however, the boys and their parents used gameplay as a means for learning more about what matters to each, in relation to the other. Whilst this is a small-scale study and of limited applicability to wider digital citizenship issues, it has demonstrated that these families' generally active mediation practices (Livingstone et al., 2011, p. 103) have helped foster the conditions for nurturing and refining certain aspects of digital citizenship. Given that the national and international focus on this area is placing these issues at the forefront of public debate, it is important to recognise that parents have been helping prepare their children for digital citizenship for as long as children have had domestic access to digital media.

Acknowledgements

This chapter draws upon data collected by the author that has previously informed a Media@LSE Working Paper (Green & Haddon, 2015). That material has been reanalysed in the context of digital citizenship. The Australian Research Council (ARC) Discovery Projects programme funded the author and Leslie Haddon as co-Chief Investigators of DP110100864: *Parents or Peers: Which group most affects the experiences of young people online, and how?*, which also included Donell Holloway and Kylie Stevenson as Research Associates. The ARC specifically supported an International Collaboration Award, enabling the author's collection of UK data. Finally, the author thanks the reviewers for their valuable comments and suggestions.

References

ADL. (2019). Free to play? Hate, harassment, and positive social experiences in online games. *Anti-Defamation League*. July. Retrieved from: www.adl.org/free-to-play.

Apperley, T. (2015). The right to play in the digital era. In S. Conway & J. deWinter (Eds.), *Video game policy: Production, distribution, and consumption* (pp. 193–205). New York, NY: Routledge.

Apperley, T. (2018). Counterfactual communities: Strategy games, paratexts and the player's experience of history. *Open Library of Humanities*, 4(1), 15, 1–22.

Bunn, A. (2019). Children and the 'Right to be Forgotten': What the right to erasure means for European children, and why Australian children should be afforded a similar right. *Media International Australia*, 170(1), 37–46.

Center for Digital Democracy. (n.d.). *Digital youth*. Retrieved from: www.democraticmedia.org/projects/focus/digital-youth.

Chapman, D. (2013). Dota 2 game review. *Common Sense Media*. Retrieved from: www.commonsensemedia.org/game-reviews/dota-2.

Clark, L. S. (2011). Parental mediation theory for the digital age. *Communication Theory*, 21(4), 323–343.

Cook, P. (2019, July 20). Dota 2: How important is your behavior score? *The Game Haus*. Retrieved from: https://thegamehaus.com/dota/dota-2-how-important-is-your-behavior-score/2019/07/20.

Eklund, L., & Helmersson Bergmark, K. (2013). Parental mediation of digital gaming and internet use. In *FDG 2013-The 8th International Conference on the Foundations of Digital Games* (pp. 63–70).

EU Council of Europe. (2019). *Digital citizenship education handbook: Being online, well-being online, rights online*. Council of Europe. Retrieved from: https://rm.coe.int/168093586f.

EU data protection rules. (n.d.). Retrieved from: https://ec.europa.eu/commission/priorities/justice-and-fundamental-rights/data-protection/2018-reform-eu-data-protection-rules/eu-data-protection-rules_en.

Fram, S. M. (2013). The constant comparative analysis method outside of grounded theory. *The Qualitative Report*, 18(1), 1–25. Retrieved from: www.nova.edu/ssss/QR/QR18/fram1.pdf.

Green, L. (2020). Confident, capable and world-changing: Teenagers and digital citizenship. *Communication Research and Practice*, 6(1), 6–19.

Green, L., & Haddon, L. (2015). Parents' reflections upon mediating older teens' gaming practices. In B. Cammaerts, N. Anstead, & R. Garland (Eds.), *Media@LSE Working Paper Series*. Retrieved 27 January 2020 from: www.lse.ac.uk/media@lse/research/mediaWorkingPapers/pdf/WP37-FINAL.pdf.

Hodkinson, P. (2008). Grounded Theory and inductive research. In N. Gilbert (Ed.), *Researching social life* (3rd ed., pp. 80–100). London: Sage Publishing.

Jiow, H. J., Lim, S. S., & Lin, J. (2017). Level up! Refreshing parental mediation theory for our digital media landscape. *Communication Theory*, 27(3), 309–328.

Kaser, R. (2019, July 23). Dota 2 international prize pool surpasses $30M, becomes largest in eSports history. *The Next Web*. Retrieved from: https://thenextweb.com/gaming/2019/07/22/Dota-2-international-prize-pool30m-becomes-largest-esports-history.

Livingstone, S., Haddon, L., Görzig, A., & Ólafsson, K. (2011). *Risks and safety on the internet: The perspective of European children*. London: EU Kids Online. Retrieved from: http://eprints.lse.ac.uk/33731.

Livingstone, S., & Third, A. (2017). Children and young people's rights in the digital age: An emerging agenda. *New Media & Society*, 19(5), 657–670.

Milkaite, I., & Lievens, E. (2019). *Status quo regarding the child's article 8 GDPR age of consent for data processing across the EU*. Retrieved from: www.betterinternetforkids.eu/web/portal/practice/awareness/detail?articleId=3017751.

Nikken, P., & Jansz, J. (2006). Parental mediation of children's videogame playing: A comparison of the reports by parents and children. *Learning, Media and Technology*, 31(2), 181–202.

Office of the United Nations High Commissioner for Human Rights. (n.d.). *Committee on the Rights of the Child: General Comment on children's rights in relation to the digital environment*. Retrieved from: www.ohchr.org/EN/HRBodies/CRC/Pages/GCChildrensRightsRelationDigitalEnvironment.aspx.

UNESCO Bangkok Office. (2019). *Digital Kids Asia-Pacific: Insights into children's digital citizenship*. UNESCO. Retrieved from: https://unesdoc.unesco.org/ark:/48223/pf0000367985.

Willett, R. (2016). Online gaming practices of preteens: Independent entertainment time and transmedia game play. *Children & Society*, 30(6), 467–477.

Willson, M. (2019). Raising the ideal child? Algorithms, quantification and prediction. *Media, Culture & Society*, 41(5), 620–636.

Yin, R. K. (2009). *Case study research: Design and methods* (4th ed.). Thousand Oaks, CA: Sage Publishing.

33

DIGITAL SOCIALISING IN CHILDREN ON THE AUTISM SPECTRUM

Meryl Alper and Madison Irons

Introduction

Autism is a complex cognitive, biological, and behavioural phenomenon that, in simple terms, shapes how people move, think, and perceive the world around them, though it shapes all individuals differently (Fletcher-Watson & Happé, 2019). Some autistic people are very talkative while others may be unable to reliably communicate through oral speech; some may be highly gifted while others have intellectual impairments.[1] For children on the autism spectrum, social interactions can be particularly challenging (Cresswell, Hinch, & Cage, 2019). This includes initiating social encounters, displaying emotional reciprocity, and interpreting non-verbal cues. Frustration arising from social exchanges, pressure to conform to neurotypical expectations, and peer victimisation can all lead to increased feelings of depression and anxiety (e.g., Whitehouse et al., 2009). These challenges also occur among broader conditions of contemporary childhood and adolescence, within which media and technology are increasingly central. This chapter delves into these nuances of sociality in relation to autistic youth and their uses of media and communication technologies.

The more that researchers learn about autism, the more challenging it becomes to summarise or universalise. The lived experience of autism differs across age, race, ethnicity, class, gender, sexuality, and geography (Brown, Ashkenazy, & Onaiwu, 2017). The story of autism has historically been told by non-autistic people, though autistic individuals are increasingly taking narrative ownership (e.g., Yergeau, 2017). Over the course of its long and contentious history as a medical classification (Silberman, 2015), autism has been associated with a personal preference for 'aloneness' (Kanner, 1943) and a retreat from society (i.e., Bruno Bettelheim's much-maligned book *The Empty Fortress*, 1967). The Diagnostic and Statistical Manual of Mental Disorders (DSM-5) (American Psychiatric Association, 2013), which is used by clinicians to diagnose autism, characterises it as a spectrum of closely related disorders that present as 'persistent deficits' in an individual's development of social relationships and communication, as well as repetitive patterns of behaviour, interests, or activities.

The assumption of preferred solitude among those on the autism spectrum has undergone significant challenge from psychologists, anthropologists, and autistic individuals (Biklen, 2005; Jaswal & Akhtar, 2019). Some contend that 'autistic sociality' (Ochs & Solomon, 2010) is a different, rather than less, social way of being in the world. Not looking someone in the eye, for instance, may be a reflexive avoidance of visual stimuli rather than an intentional personal slight (Robison, 2008). Moreover, the social motivations of autistic children and adults do not rest solely with the diagnosed individual but arise from dynamic interactions and relationships with people, communities, and institutions in specific contexts over time (Kapp, 2018). For example, when young people on the autism spectrum enter the complicated landscape of adolescence, research has shown that they infrequently participate in social activities and rarely hang out with friends outside of school despite expressing a desire to connect (Wagner et al., 2004).

The discussion in this chapter spans digital technologies characterised as 'social media' (e.g., websites and apps that facilitate the networked flow of ideas and communication), instructional technologies used by therapists and educators to modify the social behaviour of autistic children, and media technologies that are made social through their co-use with others. The analyses herein also touch upon general concerns that pertain to the development of all children and adolescents in the digital age: the relationship of social-emotional development to other domains (including language, physical, and physiological) and the myriad cultural, political, and historical factors shaping how children react to and interact with society and social institutions.

After reviewing relevant theoretical and conceptual framings of disability, autism, and youth, this chapter encompasses three main areas: technologies for *socialisation* (educational tools and therapeutic devices; e.g., robots), materials for *socialising* (everyday media used at home and on the go, e.g., YouTube), and media that purportedly promote *anti-social* behaviour in children and exacerbate social isolation. With added reflection from ethnographic fieldwork on this topic, this chapter highlights how digital socialising not only pertains to autism or youth but has broader implications for technology, society, and the sociotechnical writ large. The argument is made that modern media and technology practices of autistic youth reveal tensions and contradictions in how social norms are made, remade, and unmade through highly complex technologically mediated interactions and relationships occurring on both interpersonal and institutional levels.

Conceptual and Theoretical Background

Defining autism exclusively through its diagnostic criteria fits into a 'medical model' of disability, in which disability is located solely in the individual's body (Silverman, 2012). The aim of medical interventions and research underpinned by this model is to prevent, diminish, or correct for the disability. In the case of autism, this medicalisation regularly manifests in language used to describe autism as an 'epidemic' or 'crisis' (Eyal et al., 2010; Sinclair, 1993). As mentioned above, the DSM-5 diagnostic criteria for autism incorporates multiple mentions of sociality. This includes "deficits in social-emotional reciprocity" such as "reduced sharing of interests, emotions, or affect"; "deficits in nonverbal communicative behaviours used for social interaction"; and "deficits in developing, maintaining, and understanding relationships". There are numerous ways to understand how autistic people might or might not be 'social', with the DSM-5 framing focussed on lack and deficit serving as only one possible guidepost.

Therapeutic efforts tend to proceed with the goal of changing the child in some manner but may do this by altering the behaviour of others (e.g., parent- and peer-mediated interventions) or the environment (e.g., visual supports). Other interventions seek to accommodate the child by modifying others' behaviour or the environment but are less concerned with whether this results in long-term changes within the child. Recognition that interpersonal and institutional interactions may limit a child's abilities reflects a 'social model' of disability. In this model, emphasis is shifted from the level of the individual to the disabling effects of society and stigma. The social model helps to explain, for instance, how the challenges of autism are in part defined by the hardships faced by children and adults in accessing the human, material, and temporal resources necessary to receive a diagnosis (particularly among girls and women, non-white individuals, and those in developing countries), and the significant economic, cultural, and geographic barriers to getting adequate support services.

Obtaining an autism diagnosis however is distinct from identifying with autistic culture (Straus, 2013). Many autistic adults today did not receive formal diagnoses as children or were misdiagnosed in the past. A more 'political/relational' model of disability (Kafer, 2013) recognises faults in both the medical and social models for denying either the lived pleasures or pains of disability. Drawing on work from feminism and crip theory, disability is defined in the political/relational model in part by the collective actions undertaken by people with disabilities as they develop new alliances and forms of kinship in efforts to thrive and survive in a largely ableist world. The self-advocacy movement around 'neurodiversity', the idea that neurological differences are authentic forms of diversity, challenges the conception that autistic people should socially conform to a clinical ideal (Kapp et al., 2013).

Just as there are various perspectives on what disability means for medicine, society, and disabled people themselves, there are many answers to the question of what it means to be social – more than can be discussed here. The most relevant for this chapter's purposes comes from the field of cultural anthropology, specifically the work of Elinor Ochs and Olga Solomon (2010). They offer the notion of 'autistic sociality', meaning a sociality shared by autistic individuals that is not quantitatively less social than non-autistic people, but rather, qualitatively different. Human sociality, according to Ochs and Solomon, encompasses a range of possibilities for social coordination shaped by situational contexts, material objects, and the dynamics of groups and individuals. From this perspective, teaching autistic children 'pro-social skills' and promoting their 'social-emotional development' is not value neutral (e.g., promoting agreeability and compliance over resistance and non-compliance), especially not in the context of digital media and communication technologies designed for the socialisation of autistic children.

Socialisation through Digital Media

Digital socialisation refers to technologies and tools that, at the less extreme end, are used to help autistic children better adapt into neurotypical society through social learning and imitation, helping them to reduce anxiety or uncertainty when encountering novel social situations. From the more extreme angle, these technologies are implicitly or explicitly designed to make children appear 'less autistic' and more neurotypical in their communication and behaviour. Used in tandem with human educators and clinical professionals, these digital media focus on educational and therapeutic goals such as teaching children turn-taking in play, rules in games, and reciprocity in face-to-face conversation.

One of the major socialisation technologies for autistic children in educational settings are social narrative apps. Social narratives (or Social Stories™) prepare individuals for unfamiliar social situations by depicting future interactions or events so that a person can predict what might happen or be more aware of social expectations in a given circumstance, thereby reducing anxiety. They may emphasise a social behaviour, like making eye contact or addressing people when speaking. Like picture books, social narratives present visual information through photographs, illustrated symbols, and written words (Howley & Arnold, 2005). Digital tools and apps for creating social narratives allow for audio and video to supplement pictures, support a child's independent navigation of the text, and offer a cost-effective method of customising narratives for different circumstances (Doody, 2015).

Virtual reality (VR) has also been used for socialisation in education, as it provides dynamic social settings and controlled environments for children to work on specific social communication skills and for educators to quantitatively track gains in skills over time. Through the use of VR, children can learn to recognise body language or facial expressions and gauge emotional environments, all in a digital space that can be customised to their needs and without real-world social ramifications. Studies have shown that VR, for example, can aid autistic children in adapting to pretend play situations with a peer (Herrera et al., 2008).

In terms of therapeutic and medical contexts, digital media for socialisation includes robots that mimic humans and wearable technologies to enhance social-emotional learning. Robots can be programmed to predictably perform simple social interactions based on the principles of cognitive behavioural therapy (CBT) or applied behavioural analysis (ABA).[2] They can be used to practise joint attention, reading facial expressions, and imitation in specific contexts (e.g., listening to and telling a story). While robots with faces are effective for building these skills, those that can also talk are used for such purposes as increasing comfort discussing an expanded range of conversational topics among children with narrow interests (Aresti-Bartolome & Garcia-Zapirain, 2014).

Wearable devices like Google Glass provide opportunities for adolescents and teenagers to work on skills in active social situations. Through speech recognition and various algorithms, spoken words can be translated into text and paired with an appropriate social response, which is then projected onto the lens of the glasses in the user's line of sight. Such 'heads-up technologies' allow users to observe and participate in the social world around them, potentially more so than 'heads-down technologies' like iPads (Keshav et al., 2017). At the moment though, iPads blend in more easily than Google Glass and are more socially acceptable in public spaces.

These technologies for promoting socialisation come with a host of limitations, including a lack of empirical support even if one accepts their rationale (Bottema-Beutel, Park, & Kim, 2018). Critics contend that these technologies treat autistic children like machines themselves and perpetuate the idea that they are robotic in their movement, language, and emotions (Kobie, 2018). They can ultimately be socially isolating if not integrated into inclusive learning settings (Sobel et al., 2016). And though there is strong evidence indicating that art, nature, and animal-based therapies are enjoyed by autistic children and can support social interactions by reducing anxiety, funding for 'innovative' research tends to go towards technological interventions (Richardson et al., 2018).

Anti-Sociality through Digital Media

The view of autistic children's social expression as something biomedical also extends to a focus on negative health outcomes in their use of digital media, and on recreational technology use as something that requires intervention from medical and clinical professionals (Mello, Alper, & Allen, 2020). Anti-sociality is characterised in this context by improper and problematic screen use, addiction, and the development of maladaptive and harmful behaviours (e.g., Mazurek et al., 2012). Outcomes include diminished ability to read facial expressions, lower friendship trust, and feelings of alienation (Blais et al., 2007). Such pathologised framing reflects broader concerns about smartphones 'rewiring' the brains of neurotypical children; specifically, neurologically diverging from typical development by reducing empathy, causing the avoidance of eye contact, and being unable to handle spontaneous social interactions such as talking on the phone (Browning, 2011). At its most alarmist, this rhetoric warns of "'Virtual Autism', or autism induced by screens" among neurotypical children (Cytowic, 2017).

The majority of published research on how autistic children use screen and interactive media has focussed on the negative effects of television and video games. Children on the spectrum spend more time with screen-based media than any other leisure activity, averaging about 4.5 hours per day (Mazurek & Wenstrup, 2013). Due to the nature of autism, children may also have difficulty disengaging from digital devices (Harrison et al., 2019). Interviews with parents have indicated that an autistic child's TV viewing preferences and routines are prioritised in households, potentially side-lining siblings and putting a strain on relationships (Nally, Houlton, & Ralph, 2000). However, since today's households tend to contain multiple screens, sometimes more than one per family member, a child on the autism spectrum may be able to be co-located with family members while wearing headphones and watching programming of their choice on a mobile device.

Autistic adolescents also report a preference for video games in comparison with other leisure activities (Kuo et al., 2013) and spend on average one hour more per day playing than their typically developing peers (Mazurek et al., 2012). Little of that time is reportedly spent on games with an element of social interaction (Mazurek & Wenstrup, 2013). Even within games that contain some opportunity to interact with others, those online exchanges are not always positively associated with quality relationships. They can lead to negative social consequences like cyberbullying and online harassment, which is further exacerbated by challenges that autistic children encounter in registering emotional cues.

Socialising through Digital Media

There is a pressing need to move beyond the rhetoric above that characterises technology as either social cure or social harm for children on the autism spectrum. It is just as, if not more, important to study the mundane and ordinary uses of media and technology in autistic children's everyday lives, pre-existing environments into which novel tools like robots would conceivably enter. There is a pervasive belief that there must be therapeutic benefits from screens in order for them to be seen as worthwhile for autistic children. It is worth arguing however that children with disabilities should be able to experience things that they enjoy, regardless of any perceived benefit (Goodley & Runswick-Cole, 2010). Digital socialising encompasses all social spaces where the digital is present, ubiquitous mobile technologies in the public and private sphere, and digital environments that can both limit and support social well-being. These social practices also draw upon digital tools designed for and by autistic people, and the ways in which autistic people adapt tools for autistic sociality (van Schalkwyk et al., 2017).

New media technologies can reduce barriers to social and cultural participation. For instance, Ringland and colleagues (2016) have studied Autcraft, a private server of the popular video game Minecraft created by an autistic father of an autistic son who enjoyed the game but faced targeted bullying on public Minecraft servers. Autcraft generally provides a safe and supportive space for autistic children to play the game (Ringland et al., 2015). The server models a strengths-based approach to autism while also being responsive to realistic challenges (e.g., scaffolded content moderation within Minecraft's chat feature). Through their digital ethnographic work, Ringland et al. argue for more grounded and expansive approaches to digital sociality among autistic youth; for example, recognising the value of YouTube video creation on topics of deep personal interest that additionally support an autistic child's confidence and communication skills.

Digital socialising among autistic children is also influenced by their sensory processing and perception, and the extent to which digital media is able to meet autistic children's sensory needs (Alper, 2018; Harrison et al., 2019). Many autistic people report over or under reactivity to sensory stimuli (Donnellan, Hill, & Leary, 2010). Autistic children will often self-stimulate (or 'stim') while engaging with digital media as well as use media to experience pleasurable sensory stimuli; for example, "trampoline jumping while listening to music on headphones and watching television, [and] bringing [their] face close to [the] video screen and tensing [their] whole body" (Kirby et al., 2017, p. 148). They may use media and technology to adapt a physical experience in order to remove an unpleasant sensory aspect (Ringland et al., 2017), such as watching a boisterous sporting event on TV instead of in person (Kirby, Dickie, & Baranek, 2015).

Environmental modifications with and around media can allow children on the autism spectrum to avoid sensory discomfort and in turn support their everyday functioning in the social world.

Lastly, socialisation and socialising are not wholly distinct from one another and are highly contextual. One prime example of this entwinement is the dual use of tablet computers and apps by non-, minimally, and selectively speaking autistic youth as both assistive speech devices (also known as augmentative and alternative communication or AAC) and as tools for learning and leisure through additional educational and entertainment apps (Alper, 2017). AAC apps exist in tension with other ways in which media content, like playing aloud a song on the Spotify app, can be used to communicate cultural meaning. Children without access to adequate means of sharing their needs, desires, and thoughts with others often enact behaviour that might be considered anti-social. AAC as a communication system and means of social participation is bound up in complex ways with educational and medical discourses.

Future Directions

While not everything that autistic children do with digital media can be explained by their autism, in the future society needs to better understand how neurotypical and neurodivergent children may be both similar and different in their usage.[3] There has been considerably less research on autistic youth's digital socialising than on their digital socialisation and anti-sociality through digital media. This neglect in part reflects a greater focus on harms than benefits in research on children, media, and technology. While these different types of technologies are usually studied separately, they are all part of autistic children's digital ecologies (Takeuchi & Levine, 2014), which includes wearable GPS tracking devices for autistic children with a tendency to run suddenly into dangerous situations, as well as resulting discussions about digital rights, negotiating privacy and safety in society, and the free movement of people with disabilities through public space (Alper & Goggin, 2017).

Future research needs to be more representative, longitudinal, qualitative, and global in nature (Stiller & Mößle, 2018). Efforts should be made to generate knowledge drawn from the media experiences of autistic girls and non-white children on the spectrum. Beyond a given medium or platform, content is understudied as a central aspect of media usage (Martins, King, & Beights, 2019). Considering that a great deal of research is drawn from parent report and surveys, more inroads should be made to conduct ethnographic work embedded in the everyday lives of autistic children and adolescents. This includes directly engaging with them in a manner that best accommodates their diverse cognitive, behavioural, and communication profiles. Lastly, more work should also grapple with the morality and ethics of technologies for digital socialisation, especially with marginalised and vulnerable groups (Richardson et al., 2018).

One concluding example from fieldwork highlights the complexities of autistic children's engagement with digital technologies, and how future research directions might explore these layered interactions, specifically as they pertain to how social norms and social inequalities are maintained through media technologies. Ryan is a three-year-old middle-class white boy on the autism spectrum.[4] During Alper's visit to his home, he had a meltdown after his mom, Tara, refused to let him watch continuous YouTube videos on the large flatscreen TV in their living room. She wanted him instead to play with an ABA app on the iPad designed to teach autistic children about professions and their societal roles. "Who helps keep neighbourhoods safe?" asked the app's voiceover while the screen displayed illustrations of different professionals. Ryan initially selected the firefighter on-screen but the correct response, according to the app, was police officer. "A firefighter technically does too", Alper quietly interjected. Tara replied, "Yeah but, in the wording that ABA uses, it's 'Who puts out fires, is the firefighter' and 'Who keeps us safe, the police officer'". According to whoever wrote, programmed, and produced the app, police officers keep us safe, while firefighters do not.

Immediately notable was the implied 'us' in the app, particularly with respect to race, disability, and intersectionality (Brown, Ashkenazy, & Onaiwu, 2017). The visit to Ryan's house in March 2017 came a few years into the Black Lives Matter movement protests in the United States against police killings of Black people and broader issues of police brutality. Who did the universal 'us' represent? Did it include autistic people, and specifically autistic people of colour? Nearly 20% of young people on the spectrum have had an encounter with police by age 21, and about half of those by age 15 (Crane et al., 2016). The belief that police officers keep us safe is not morally or ethically neutral; it is an inherently political one, and Ryan's social skills app was not outside of those politics. While the same can be said for any curricular material that children encounter throughout their informal and formal learning, what distinguished this interaction was that it occurred within the context of a therapy app and was bound up with medical authority that is largely off-limits to wide swathes of society. Learning about social institutions was tied to therapeutic treatment – treatment which constituted being able to select a single 'correct' answer, which was not in fact correct – and all of this took place against the backdrop of a child's desire to stream YouTube videos.

The above discussion and the literature reviewed in this chapter are all intended to generate more questions than answers about digital media, children, and autism. For example, what does it mean for technologies to be 'social', and for society – including autistic children – to make use of them through all that is associated with the 'sociotechnical', including digital interactions, norms, and networks? What unquestioned beliefs about sociality underpin the design and deployment of social media technologies generally? And in what ways are these assumptions similar or different from those programmed into technologies explicitly designed to teach autistic children how to be social? Much more work is needed to fully understand how young people on the autism spectrum engage in digital socialising, and how it in turn shapes and is shaped by socialisation and anti-sociality.

Acknowledgements

The authors would like to thank Kristen Bottema-Beutel, the Northeastern Humanities Center 2018–2019 Faculty Fellows, the editors, and two anonymous reviewers for their invaluable feedback on earlier drafts of this chapter.

Notes

1 This chapter uses the language of 'autistic child', 'child on the (autism) spectrum', and 'autism'. These terms are largely preferred by autism self-advocates over 'person with autism' and 'autism spectrum disorder', which tend to be preferred by parents and clinicians (Kenny et al., 2016). It should also be noted that the notion of autism as a 'spectrum' is itself imperfect and may reinforce a hierarchy of abilities (e.g., 'high' and 'low' functioning); see Thomas and Boellstorff (2017).
2 The ethics of CBT and ABA techniques are greatly debated within and outside the autism community (Kirkham, 2017).
3 Neurodivergence encompasses other variations in the human brain besides autism resulting in differences in sociability, mood, learning, attention, and other mental functions (i.e., ADHD, dyslexia) (Silberman, 2015).
4 All participant names are pseudonyms.

References

Alper, M. (2017). *Giving voice: Mobile communication, disability, and inequality*. Cambridge, MA: MIT Press.
Alper, M. (2018). Inclusive sensory ethnography: Studying new media and neurodiversity in everyday life. *New Media & Society, 20*(10), 3560–3579.

Alper, M., & Goggin, G. (2017). Digital technology and rights in the lives of children with disabilities. *New Media & Society*, *19*(5), 726–740.

American Psychiatric Association. (2013). *Diagnostic and statistical manual of mental disorders, fifth edition (DSM-5)*. Arlington, VA: American Psychiatric Association.

Aresti-Bartolome, N., & Garcia-Zapirain, B. (2014). Technologies as support tools for persons with autistic spectrum disorder: A systematic review. *International Journal of Environmental Research and Public Health*, *11*(8), 7767–7802.

Bettelheim, B. (1967). *The empty fortress: Infantile autism and the birth of the self*. New York: Free Press.

Biklen, D. (2005). *Autism and the myth of the person alone*. New York: NYU Press.

Blais, J. J., Craig, W. M., Pepler, D., & Connolly, J. (2007). Adolescents online: The importance of internet activity choices to salient relationships. *Journal of Youth and Adolescence*, *37*(5), 522–536.

Bottema-Beutel, K., Park, H., & Kim, S. Y. (2018). Commentary on social skills training curricula for individuals with ASD: Social interaction, authenticity, and stigma. *Journal of Autism and Developmental Disorders*, *48*(3), 953–964.

Brown, L. X. Z., Ashkenazy, E., & Onaiwu, M. G. (Eds.). (2017). *All the weight of our dreams: On living racialized autism*. Lincoln, NE: DragonBee Press.

Browning, D. (2011, December 4). Talking face to face is so . . . yesterday. *New York Times*, p. SR5. Retrieved from: www.nytimes.com/2011/12/04/opinion/sunday/actual-conversation-so-yesterday.html.

Crane, L., Maras, K. L., Hawken, T., Mulcahy, S., & Memon, A. (2016). Experiences of autism spectrum disorder and policing in England and Wales: Surveying police and the autism community. *Journal of Autism and Developmental Disorders*, *46*(6), 2028–2041.

Cresswell, L., Hinch, R., & Cage, E. (2019). The experiences of peer relationships amongst autistic adolescents: A systematic review of the qualitative evidence. *Research in Autism Spectrum Disorders*, *61*, 45–60.

Cytowic, R. E. (2017). There is a new link between screen-time and autism. *Psychology Today*. Retrieved from: www.psychologytoday.com/us/blog/the-fallible-mind/201706/there-is-new-link-between-screen-time-and-autism.

Donnellan, A. M., Hill, D. A., & Leary, M. R. (2010). Rethinking autism: Implications of sensory and movement differences. *Disability Studies Quarterly*, *30*(1). Retrieved from: http://dsq-sds.org/article/view/1060/1225.

Doody, K. R. (2015). GrAPPling with how to teach social skills? Try tapping into digital technology. *Journal of Special Education Technology*, *30*(2), 122–127.

Eyal, G., Hart, B., Onculer, E., Oren, N., & Rossi, N. (2010). *The autism matrix: The social origins of the autism epidemic*. Cambridge, UK: Polity.

Fletcher-Watson, S., & Happé, F. (2019). *Autism: A new introduction to psychological theory and current debate* (2nd ed.). London: Routledge.

Goodley, D., & Runswick-Cole, K. (2010). Emancipating play: Dis/abled children, development, and deconstruction. *Disability and Society*, *25*(4), 499–512.

Harrison, K., Couture, A., Wenhold, H., Vallina, L., & Moorman, J. (2019). Sensory curation: Theorizing media use for sensory regulation and implications for family media conflict. *Media Psychology*, *22*(4), 653–688.

Herrera, G., Alcantud, F., Jordan, R., Blanquer, A., Labajo, G., & De Pablo, C. (2008). Development of symbolic play through the use of virtual reality tools in children with autistic spectrum disorders. *Autism*, *12*(2), 143–157.

Howley, M., & Arnold, E. (2005). *Revealing the hidden social code: Social Stories™ for people with autistic spectrum disorders*. London: Jessica Kingsley.

Jaswal, V. K., & Akhtar, N. (2019). Being vs. appearing socially uninterested: Challenging assumptions about social motivation in autism. *Behavioral and Brain Sciences*, *42*(e82), 1–73.

Kafer, A. (2013). *Feminist, queer, crip*. Bloomington, IN: Indiana University Press.

Kanner, L. (1943). Autistic disturbances of affective contact. *Nervous Child*, *2*, 217–250.

Kapp, S. K. (2018). Social support, well-being, and quality of life among individuals on the autism spectrum. *Pediatrics*, *141*(Supplement 4), S362–S368.

Kapp, S. K., Gillespie-Lynch, K., Sherman, L. E., & Hutman, T. (2013). Deficit, difference, or both? Autism and neurodiversity. *Developmental Psychology*, *49*(1), 59–71.

Kenny, L., Hattersley, C., Molins, B., Buckley, C., Povey, C., & Pellicano, E. (2016). Which terms should be used to describe autism? Perspectives from the UK autism community. *Autism*, *20*(4), 442–462.

Keshav, N. U., Salisbury, J. P., Vahbzadeh, A., & Sahin, N. T. (2017). Social communication coaching smartglasses: Well tolerated in a diverse sample of children and adults with autism. *JMIR Mhealth and Uhealth*, *5*, 9.

Kirby, A. V., Boyd, B. A., Williams, K. L., Faldowski, R. A., & Baranek, G. T. (2017). Sensory and repetitive behaviors among children with autism spectrum disorder at home. *Autism, 21*(2), 142–154.

Kirby A.V., Dickie, V. A., & Baranek, G.T. (2015). Sensory experiences of children with autism spectrum disorder: In their own words. *Autism, 19*(3), 316–326.

Kirkham, P. (2017). 'The line between intervention and abuse' – Autism and applied behaviour analysis. *History of the Human Sciences, 30*(2), 107–126.

Kobie, N. (2018). The questionable ethics of treating autistic children with robots. *Wired (UK)*. Retrieved from: www.wired.co.uk/article/autisim-children-treatment-robots.

Kuo, M. H., Orsmond, G. I., Coster, W. J., & Cohn, E. S. (2013). Media use among adolescents with autism spectrum disorder. *Autism, 18*(8), 914–923.

Martins, N., King, A., & Beights, R. (2019, March). Audiovisual media content preferences of children with autism spectrum disorders: Insights from parental interviews. *Journal of Autism and Developmental Disorders*. doi.org/10.1007/s10803-019-03987-1.

Mazurek, M. O., Shattuck, P. T., Wagner, M., & Cooper, B. P. (2012). Prevalence and correlates of screen-based media use among youths with autism spectrum disorders. *Journal of Autism and Developmental Disorders, 42*(8), 1757–1767.

Mazurek, M. O., & Wenstrup, C. (2013). Television, video game and social media use among children with ASD and typically developing siblings. *Journal of Autism and Developmental Disorders, 43*(6), 1258–1271.

Mello, S., Alper, M., & Allen, A. (2020, July). Physician mediation theory and pediatric media guidance in the digital age: A survey of autism medical and clinical professionals. *Health Communication, 35*(8), 955–965. doi.org/10.1080/10410236.2019.15987441.

Nally, B., Houlton, B., & Ralph, S. (2000). Researches in brief: The management of television and video by parents of children with autism. *Autism, 4*(3), 331–337.

Ochs, E., & Solomon, O. (2010). Autistic sociality. *Ethos, 38*(1), 69–92.

Richardson, K., Coeckelbergh, M., Wakunuma, K., Billing, E., Ziemke, T., Gomez, P., Vanderborght, B., & Belpaeme, T. (2018). Robot enhanced therapy for children with autism (DREAM): A social model of autism. *IEEE Technology and Society Magazine, 37*(1), 30–39.

Ringland, K. E., Boyd, L., Faucett, H., Cullen, A., & Hayes, G. R. (2017). Making in Minecraft: A means of self-expression for youth with autism. In *Proceedings of the 2017 Conference on Interaction Design and Children* (pp. 340–345). New York: ACM.

Ringland, K. E., Wolf, C. T., Dombrowski, L., & Hayes, G. R. (2015) Making "safe": Community-centered practices in a virtual world dedicated to children with autism. In *Proceedings of the 2015 ACM International Conference on Computer Supported Collaborative Work (CSCW)* (pp. 1788–1800). New York: ACM.

Ringland, K. E., Wolf, C. T., Faucett, H., Dombrowski, L., & Hayes, G. R. (2016). "Will I always be not social?": Re-conceptualizing sociality in the context of a Minecraft community for autism. In *Proceedings of the 2016 ACM CHI Conference on Human Factors in Computing Systems* (pp. 1256–1269). New York: ACM.

Robison, J. E. (2008). *Look me in the eye: My life with Asperger's*. New York: Random House.

Silberman, S. (2015). *NeuroTribes: The legacy of autism and the future of neurodiversity*. New York: Avery.

Silverman, C. (2012). *Understanding autism: Parents, doctors, and the history of a disorder*. Princeton, NJ: Princeton University Press.

Sinclair, J. (1993). Don't mourn for us. *Our Voice, 1*(3), 3–6.

Sobel, K., Rector, K., Evans, S., & Kientz, J. (2016). Incloodle: Evaluating an interactive application for young children with mixed abilities. In *Proceedings of the 2016 ACM CHI Conference on Human Factors in Computing Systems* (pp. 165–176). New York: ACM.

Stiller, A., & Mößle, T. (2018). Media use among children and adolescents with autism spectrum disorder: A systematic review. *Review Journal of Autism and Developmental Disorders, 5*(3), 227–246.

Straus, J. N. (2013). Autism as culture. In L. Davis (Ed.), *The disability studies reader* (4th ed., pp. 460–484). New York: Routledge.

Takeuchi, L. M., & Levine, M. H. (2014). Learning in a digital age: Toward a new ecology of human development. In A. B. Jordan & D. Romer (Eds.), *Media and the well-being of children and adolescents* (pp. 20–43). New York: Oxford University Press.

Thomas, H., & Boellstorff, T. (2017). Beyond the spectrum: Rethinking autism. *Disability Studies Quarterly*. Retrieved from: http://dsq-sds.org/article/view/5375/4551.

van Schalkwyk, G. I., Marin, C. E., Ortiz, M., Rolison, M., Qayyum, Z., McPartland, J. C., Lebowitz, E.R., Volkmar, F.R., & Silverman, W. K. (2017). Social media use, friendship quality, and the moderating role of anxiety in adolescents with autism spectrum disorder. *Journal of Autism and Developmental Disorders, 47*(9), 2805–2813.

Wagner, M., Cadwallader, T. W., Garza, N., & Cameto, R. (2004). Social activities of youth with disabilities. *NLTS2 Data Brief: A Report from the National Longitudinal Transition Study-2, 3*(1), 1–4.

Whitehouse, A. J., Durkin, K., Jaquet, E., & Ziatas, K. (2009). Friendship, loneliness and depression in adolescents with Asperger's syndrome. *Journal of Adolescence, 32*, 309–322.

Yergeau, M. (2017). *Authoring autism: On rhetoric and neurological queerness*. Durham, NC: Duke University Press.

34
DISABILITY, CHILDREN, AND THE INVENTION OF DIGITAL MEDIA

Katie Ellis, Gerard Goggin, and Mike Kent

Introduction

Much research, policy, and practice on digital media has struggled to move beyond the powerful dominant framing of children as humans in development, in need of protection, regulation, and guidance, especially in the face of the dystopian and threatening perceptions and realities of how social life is being recomposed via varieties of internet, mobile, and social media (Lahikainen et al., 2017). As Sonia Livingstone and Kirsten Drotner noted over a decade ago:

> In many parts of the world, and for many decades, children have been early and avid adopters of new media. Indeed, they often challenge normative socio-cultural practices through the ways in which they use media. Yet, at the same time, many parents, educationalists and marketers consider that media permeate, even control, children's lives to a degree that was unknown just a generation ago.
>
> *(Drotner & Livingstone, 2008, p. 1)*

They make the telling and still relevant point that "debates over children and media throw into relief our basic understandings of childhood and, additionally, of media" (Drotner & Livingstone, 2008, p. 4). While much has changed in media, these propositions ring true – even more so – when it comes to children with disabilities and digital media.

Children with disabilities have tended to be overlooked in discussions of media. With the advent of digital media, and the various ways in which children have figured as key users, innovators, and sites of social anxiety and discussions of risk, attention has also been drawn to disability as an important dimension. There is now a notable sea change in children and media research (see, for instance, work by Meryl Alper, notably her key 2017 book *Giving Voice*; Golos, 2010; Hynan et al., 2015; Manhique & Giannoumis, 2019; Meredith et al., 2018; Smith & Abrams, 2019; Third et al., 2013, 2017; Tsaliki & Kontogianni, 2014). Various influential figures have acknowledged disability as a notable gap in research – and an important area to address for its potential contribution to the emerging agenda of intersectionality, diversity, equality for children, and digital media. As Meryl Alper, Vikki Katz, and Lynn Schofield Clark put it, "[g]iving full consideration to the identity, inequality, and marginality that affect children's and adolescents' experiences with media better enables researchers and other stakeholders to advance the rights of young people across various forms of social distinctiveness" (Alper et al., 2016, p. 109). In their call for work on the "invisible children in media research" (Jordan & Prendella, 2019), Amy Jordan and Kate Prendella note that: "[a]nother significant part of the child population under-represented in CAM [Children and Media] research is children with disabilities" (Jordan & Prendella, 2019, p. 236). They emphasise that "a lack of diversity within research can lead to a tilting of the questions we ask" (Jordan & Prendella, 2019, p. 237). Researchers on children's rights have been pioneers in this regard, with Sonia Livingstone and Amanda Third, for instance, underscoring how:

> the persistent exclusion of children living with disability illustrates a host of challenges associated with intersectionality online as offline. Such challenges are particularly acute online because of the hitherto lack of flexibility or contingency in the regulation of digital resources and infrastructure by comparison with the nuanced possibilities for shaping social norms and opportunity structures offline.
> *(Livingstone & Third, 2017, p. 665; see also Livingstone & Bulger, 2014)*

If the scene is set for the late flourishing of research and children with disabilities and digital media, three questions need answering:

1 Do the frameworks, concepts, approaches, resources, and partnerships exist that are needed?
2 What might hold back work (or constrain the terms upon which it unfolds)?
3 What research, approaches, relationships, and engagement might/should emerge and be encouraged?

With this backdrop in mind, this chapter aims to put the topic of children with disabilities on the agenda for digital media research. The discussion is underpinned by two linked ideas, namely that: 1) children with disabilities are an important group to include when aiming to gain a comprehensive understanding of digital media and children; 2) beyond that, critical understandings of disability offer us important theoretical, policy, and practice insights into how to approach digital media, especially in relation to children.

The discussion below structured as follows. First, this chapter brings into dialogue the state-of-the-art research and conceptualisations of children and digital media with accounts of children with disabilities, and considers how disability and digital media might be understood. Sketching this kind of theoretical synthesis leads us to draw attention to: the diversity of disabilities and impairments; the sense in which, if children figure as still-to-become full subjects and human, then children with disabilities are even further behind such a liminal position; the ways in which emergent, dynamic conceptions of children with disabilities are entangled with socio-technical arrangements of digital media. Second, the authors discuss the ways in which children with disabilities are imagined in relation to digital media. A central issue is that underpinning much discourse, ideas, and arrangements of digital media are problematic 'disabling' concepts about what 'normal' communication entails. As disability and technology scholars have suggested, this is a serious problem for understanding media and communication when people – such as children with disabilities – do not fit into the default concept of human (as able-bodied). The chapter then contrasts these often limited, particular, and misleading imaginaries with the materialities of affordances, use, innovation, and contexts of children with disabilities' appropriation and enlistment in digital media. Here the authors offer an overview and discussion of key aspects of children with disabilities' use of digital media. The chapter concludes with suggestions for the research agenda in relation to children with disabilities and digital media.

Children, Disabilities, and Digital Media: "Something Strange Happens"

The study of children with disabilities has been highly influenced by particular concerns, including the imperative of understanding the developmental, social, educational, and other challenges of children – by dint of their impairment, the power relations of disability, and the disparities in resources – that they themselves, their families, and communities experience in supporting them in the face of adverse, oppressive, or unequal situations. Across social life and research, the discourse and conceptualisation of children with disabilities has been profoundly shaped by ideologies and institutions of disabilities, in which narrow and partial ideas of disabled childhoods have predominated.

As disability studies has developed in recent years to challenge inadequate and problematic models of disability, there has also been an important movement to rethink research on children with disabilities. In 2014, Tillie Curran and Katherine Runswick-Cole proposed the need for a distinct domain of "disabled children's childhood studies" founded on three key principles:

> 1. [Such research would] take a very different starting point from other studies of disabled children by moving beyond the discussion of impairment, inequality and abuse to enable disabled children to step out from under the shadows of normative expectations that have clouded their lives. 2. Disabled children's childhood studies demands an ethical research design that seeks to position the voice and experiences of disabled children at the centre of the inquiry. 3. Disabled children's childhood studies seeks to trouble these practices in their local, historical and global locations.
>
> *(Curran & Runswick-Cole, 2014)*

The research gathered together under this banner (showcased in Curran & Runswick-Cole, 2013; Runswick-Cole et al., 2018) represents a major step forward, indicating from a contemporary disability-studies-inflected location the major dimensions of the lives of children with disabilities, the way their worlds are made, inhabited, and imagined, and exploring the ways that researchers might respond.

Armed with this new understanding, if the research landscapes and literatures that study children with disabilities and digital media are re-entered, readers are apt to be disoriented and disappointed. While a full discussion lies outside the scope of this chapter, it is fair to say that still, most surprisingly, the bulk of work focusses on particular issues, and from a limited range of frames. In addition, disciplines such as education, social work, medical and health sciences, rehabilitation engineering, and Human–Computer Interaction (HCI), have produced much of the research on children with disabilities and digital media. For their part, disciplines such as media, communication, and cultural studies, internet, mobile media and communication, games, social media studies, sociology, anthropology, science and technology studies, and other associated disciplines have rarely produced research. Overall, common foci of research relating to children with disabilities and digital media include: where digital technology fits into rehabilitation; accessible and inclusive design; use of digital media to extend children with disabilities' participation in educational settings; the role of emerging digital media in enhancing augmentative and alternative communication for children; digital media's potential to support social support and inclusion in families, friendships, and communities for children with disabilities.

Since the late 1990s, the body of work produced has increased dramatically and includes many important insights and advances in knowledge. To be sure, these are vital issues. However, the way that children with disabilities and their engagement with media are conceptualised, studied, and engaged leaves great swathes of their experiences relatively untouched, and lacking acknowledgement, exploration, and reflection as to what significance their 'invention' of digital media holds. The frustration with these orthodox approaches is nicely expressed in a recent study of young people with disabilities and gaming:

> But when researchers address a certain subcategory of young people – those living with disabilities – something strange happens. Now, digital arenas are defined in terms of potentialities to directly alleviate troubles linked to their disabilities, and users are defined in terms of treatment-receiving objects. Electronic games plus disability build up a striking case; research in this field tend to overlook how digital activities – also for gamers with disabilities – belong to young people's construction of meaning and connectedness ... Researchers now tend to define gaming as a sort of instrumental 'disability-help' and show little interest in young people's gaming engagement as persons rather than clients.
>
> *(Wästerfors & Hansson, 2017, pp. 1143–4)*

Wästerfors and Hansson are among a growing group of researchers who make a persuasive case that the current research is simply not good enough, first and foremost because it leaves us lacking fundamental and vitally important insights and knowledge into the lives of children with disabilities. All in all, there is as yet little work that explicitly responds to or brings together the dual imperatives represented by disabled children's childhood studies, as set out by Runswick-Cole and collaborators, and various other scholars, and the new trajectories and approaches for work sketched by key researchers in children and media that would take international, intersectional disabilities as a cutting-edge future topic. There is every reason to think digital media is more than ever central to the lives of very many children with disabilities – as often remarked in relation to digital media and social life generally; but researchers do not know as yet in what ways, and with what significance. So, it is a priority to consider how to transform research in this area, and secure its integral and generative contribution to research and conversations on children and media generally.

Imagining Digital Media and Children with Disabilities

To understand the layers of deep conceptual and attitudinal bedrock that needs dismantling, some basic understanding about how disabilities are still imagined in relation to digital media is required. A good place to start is at the heart of things, by identifying and interrogating problematic 'disabling' concepts about so-called 'normal' communication (Alper et al., 2015). These concepts underpin much discourse, ideas, and arrangements of digital media and, as disability and technology scholars have suggested, are a serious problem for understanding media and communication when people – such as children with disabilities – do not fit into the default concept of human (as able-bodied) (Alper, 2017b; Ellcessor, 2016; Ellis & Kent, 2011; Roulstone, 2016). Following this, the chapter explores three key approaches to the study of children and digital media and their relationship to deficit approaches to both disability and childhood.

From the time they are born, children are subject to a series of tests and assessments to ensure they are developing along a 'normal' continuum. There are many online checklists parents can consult about their child's development, particularly with reference to communication. Communication is both a key site of assessment and a mechanism through which to assess. For example, the Victorian State government in Australia offers this list of problems that should prompt parents to seek help:

- You think your baby or child has difficulty hearing;
- Your toddler isn't speaking at all by two years of age;

- Your child doesn't understand what you say by two years of age;
- Your child stutters or has some other form of speech difficulty;
- You have problems communicating with your child.

(Better Heath Channel, 2018).

The role of digital communications in assessing these milestones is suggested by work on pivotal elements of emerging digital media, such as algorithms. Consider, for instance, Michele Willson's interrogation of the intersection between algorithms that "surveil, interrogate, manipulate and anticipate activities and outcomes", on the one hand, and the "social, cultural and political discourses that imagine the 'ideal' child" (Willson, 2018, p. 1), on the other hand. While Willson does not focus on the disabled child in this paper, her account is helpful because it underscores the way in which families, businesses, and governments all make use of algorithms within a health framework (amongst others) to recognise normal development and facilitative diagnosis and intervention. This is a potential new front opening up in the profoundly normative ways that communication is conceived and operationalised for children with disabilities – where disability meets health in the new landscapes of digital media and consumption, raising many questions about their digital citizenship (Goggin, 2016; Third & Collin, 2016).

The underlying structural dynamic in communication flows from the way in which both the ideal and the norm are defined in opposition to disability (Davis, 1995; Garland-Thomson, 1997; Goggin et al., 2017; Kumari Campbell, 2009; McRuer, 2006). Davis argues that because no one human can meet the ideal, people strive for the norm or rely on other bodies deemed less like the norm than their own to feel better about not achieving the ideal (Davis, 1995, p. 25). Similarly Rosemarie Garland-Thomson delineates between the normate and extraordinary bodies. While the normate is defined as "the corporeal incarnation of culture's collective, unmarked, normative characteristics" (Garland-Thomson, 1997, p. 8), extraordinary bodies, such as the disabled body in its various forms, act as a metaphor for society's concerns, preoccupations, and anxiety. The fundamental issue, explored by many disability studies scholars, is the unsettling ways in which incidence and experience of impairment upturns accepted concepts of humanness (Garland-Thomson, 2019; Goggin & Newell, 2005; Kumari Campbell, 2009; Taylor, 2017). Consideration of children's use of digital media reveals the ways childhood functions as a repository for ideologies of disability (Alper & Goggin, 2017). For example, children with disabilities are framed in popular discourse as beneficiaries of digital media (Alper, 2014). Affordable and portable tablet computers present new opportunities for children with disabilities to communicate. While this is a real phenomenon, it is often only heard about through uncritical celebratory popular news media narratives in which these children are presented as a homogeneous group with little recognition of differences related to class, cultural capital, and other forms of privilege (for a critique of this phenomenon see Alper, 2017a).

Within current discussions of digital media it is common for a normative approach to be taken, excluding people along age, race, ability, nationality, and generational lines (Livingstone & Third, 2017). Indeed, the preferred user of digital media typically upholds an able-bodied norm (Ellcessor, 2016; Johnson, 2019; White, 2006). Thus, the debate surrounding children and digital media has been imagined and framed in particular ways – typically proceeding from a medical model framework and focussing on particular, narrow notions of risk. Again, the discussion excludes children with disability and assumes the child potentially accessing digital media possesses a normative body and mind – with the result that important specific issues for children with disabilities can be overlooked (for example, see the discussion of information ethics and privacy issues for children with communication disability in Meredith et al., 2018).

A common example lies in often-expressed concerns for the impacts of 'screen time' on children's brains, a frequent source of moral panic. Children's use of digital media is an interdisciplinary concern; scholars within cultural and media studies, education, health, psychology, and medicine all focus attention on this topic. Deficit approaches cataloguing the negative or antisocial consequences of media usage popularised during the early twentieth century continue to dominate many of these disciplines. As Meryl Alper reflects:

> [I]nstead of the lopsided concern with the internet 'changing' children's brains, we need to take a step back and identify societal biases in how we think about minds and bodies, reflect on how these assumptions inform research questions (and research funding), and ultimately shift understandings of the 'normal' brain in order to more fully account for the neurodiversity of all children and their uses of new media.
>
> *(Alper, 2016)*

The broader issue is highlighted in the criticism levelled by scholars that childhood media studies remains characterised by a skewed focus on so-called 'WEIRD' families (Western, Educated, Industrialised, Rich, and Democratic) at the expense of other groups, including children with disability (Alper et al., 2016).

What we find is that the disabled child is both absent and hyper-visible in the discussion of society, individuals, and digital media – a peculiar resonance of a long-observed overarching dynamic in the economies of visibility in disability (Ellis & Goggin, 2015; Hirschmann, 2015). For example, in a study of digital media usage by children and adolescents published in *Paediatrics*, digital media, following in the wake of traditional media before it, is seen to have negative consequences on children and adolescents who are framed in normative ways (Reid Chassiakos et al., 2016). Disability enters the discussion only when the researchers turn to a consideration of health and recognise the benefits of community belonging in social media spaces dedicated to particular illnesses, disability, and other marginalised identifications (Reid Chassiakos et al., 2016, p. 6).

Use of digital media by children with Autism Spectrum Disorder (ASD) is of concern within both medical and educational fields (Desch & Gaebler-Spira, 2008; Odom et al., 2015). In a review of literature published between 1990 and 2013 (Odom et al., 2015) regarding use of technology at school, home, and in the community by adolescents with ASD, Odom et al. acknowledge the efficacy of technological support including digital technologies but call for continual reassessment and systematic revaluation. However, some researchers still foreground the primacy of risk in arguments for limiting screen time for youth with disability, even when digital media is used to augment communication (Reid Chassiakos et al., 2016, p. 6). Such work neglects the rich research and alternative theorisations of autism that have emerged in research and disability activism (see, for instance, Alper, 2017b; Jack, 2014). In addition to this medicalised deficit discourse, digital media use by children with disability is explored within a narrowly conceptualised educational context. On the one hand the benefits of the use of digital technology is considered 'self-evident', yet, on the other hand, questions remain regarding quality for children with disabilities in educational contexts, especially if we have in mind the full range of international settings (Larsen, 1995; Musengi & Nyangairi, 2019).

A major challenge to the continuing primacy of legacy 'deficit' approaches – such as the medicalised approaches to disability we have discussed, or the evolution of concepts and canonical topics associated with disability developed in only partially decolonised fields such as 'special education' (now often renamed as 'inclusive education') – has come from the rise of disability human rights – and the central place it accords digital technology in the present conjuncture. The United Nations Convention on the Rights of Persons with Disabilities

(CRPD) defines people with disability as "those who have long-term physical, mental, intellectual or sensory impairments which in interaction with various barriers may hinder their full and effective participation in society on an equal basis with others" (United Nations, 2006). This recognition of the disabling impacts of both the body (impairment) and society therefore proceeds from the so-called social model of disability. The social model is one of a number of approaches that have developed since the 1970s that offer a direct contrast, and challenges, to the more pervasive biomedical and charity models of disability. Digital media features prominently throughout the CRPD (Alper & Goggin, 2017; Ellis, 2019) – with the result that governments, civil society, and technology providers alike have been paying greater attention to questions of disability and digital technology. What is especially promising are the ways that the CRPD builds on, combines with, and indeed goes beyond the Convention on the Rights of the Child (CRC) (Alper & Goggin, 2017; Livingstone & Third, 2017). As Ralph Sandland suggests

> the way the CRPD restructures orthodox understandings of rights and their limits, rejects tests of capacity as disempowering and discriminatory, and does so on the philosophical basis of a 'social model' of disability, raises far-reaching and awkward questions regarding the continued viability of an essentialist, status-based and non-socialised construction of children and their rights.
>
> *(Sandland, 2017, p. 126)*

The prominence of rights as a frame in contemporary disability research, practice, policy, and politics makes it the most readily available approach for breaking the lock held on research on children with disabilities and digital media by the disabling paradigms of previous traditions (see, for example, Bosman et al., 2015). However, rights too have their shortcomings and exclusions – as an often critically unexamined lens that overlooks many aspects of the topic. Rights approaches to children with disabilities, then, can be complemented and extended by many other productive approaches, including work that seeks to rethink citizenship (Goggin, 2016; Third & Collin, 2016), social inclusion, ethnographic work (including the new area of digital ethnography), and research on the complex intersectional cultural and social dimensions at play (e.g., Atkin & Hussain, 2003; Bachen, 2015; Banaji, 2017).

Conclusion and Future Agenda

An archaic adage holds that children should be seen but not heard. For children with disability it is often the case that they are also not expected to be seen, particularly in the case of digital media (cf. Renwick, 2016). Children and their impairments can disappear on the other side of the screen, rendering their disability invisible along with the unspoken demands for universal design and digital inclusion that disability visibility and advocacy champion.

Future directions in research for this group need to start by acknowledging and exploring from the perspectives of children with disabilities regarding what their digital media concerns are, and not assuming that they directly map onto other children's or adults' issues. There needs to be a greater understanding of how children with disabilities fit and reconfigure the full range of existing and emerging digital media and platforms. What are their preferred and specific formats, media, social and digital practices, meanings, and platforms? A fuller understanding of the 'invention' of digital media by children with disabilities across all settings is essential. In keeping with a general imperative in media studies, this includes more international work (Sakr & Steemers, 2017; Watermeyer & Goggin, 2018) and theorisation and research on non-traditional issues of pleasure, fun, play in/with digital media for children with disabilities.

To make this transformative project possible, there needs to be greater engagement with policymakers, children with disabilities and their families, partners, allies, and supporters around rights for children with disabilities in the digital age and a greater level of engagement and ownership of co-research with this diverse group to extend the disability activists' dictum of "nothing about us without us" (Liddiard et al., 2019). Scholars must develop intersectional children's media research that is transformed by embracing the perspectives of children with disabilities and champion the ensuing innovative approaches, concepts, methods, and, above all, relationships.

Happily, such an overdue shift will help researchers and society more broadly rethink children and digital media via the insights provided through this sharpened, deepened, and enriching focus on disability.

References

Alper, M. (2014). *Digital youth with disabilities*. Cambridge, MA: MIT Press.
Alper, M. (2016, April 21). What constant screen time does to kids' brains. *Zócalo Public Square*. Retrieved from: http://zocalo-on.kcrw.com/2016/04/what-constant-screen-time-does-to-kids-brains.
Alper, M. (2017a). *Giving voice: Mobile communication, disability, and inequality*. Cambridge, MA: MIT Press.
Alper, M. (2017b). Inclusive sensory ethnography: Studying new media and neurodiversity in everyday life. *New Media & Society*, *20*(10), 3560–3579.
Alper, M., Ellcessor, E., Ellis, K., & Goggin, G. (2015). Reimagining the good life with disability: Communication, new technology, and humane connections. In H. Wang (Ed.), *Communication and the "good life"* (pp. 197–212). New York: Peter Lang.
Alper, M., & Goggin, G. (2017). Digital technology and rights in the lives of children with disabilities. *New Media & Society*, *19*(5), 726–740.
Alper, M., Katz, V. S., & Schofield Clark, L. (2016). Researching children, intersectionality, and diversity in the digital age. *Journal of Children and Media*, *10*(1), 107–114.
Atkin, K., & Hussain, Y. (2003). Disability and ethnicity: How young Asian disabled people make sense of their lives. In S. Riddell & N. Watson (Eds.), *Disability, culture, identity* (pp. 161–179). London: Routledge.
Bachen, C. (2015). Out of the mainstream: Viewing media and communication through the lens of children of immigrants and youth with disabilities. *Journal of Children and Media*, *9*(3), 394–397.
Banaji, S. (2017). *Children and media in India: Narratives of class, agency, and social change*. New York: Routledge.
Better Heath Channel. (2018). Young children and communication. Retrieved from: www.betterhealth.vic.gov.au/health/HealthyLiving/young-children-and-communication.
Bosman, J., Bayraktar, F., & d'Haenens, L. (2015). Children's digital media practices within the European family home: Does perceived discrimination matter? *Journal of Children and Media*, *9*(1), 77–94.
Curran, T., & Runswick-Cole, K. (Eds.). (2013). *Disabled children's childhood studies: Critical approaches in a global context*. Basingstoke, UK: Palgrave Macmillan.
Curran, T., & Runswick-Cole, K. (2014). Disabled children's childhood studies: A distinct approach? *Disability & Society*, *29*(10), 1617–1630.
Davis, L. (1995). *Enforcing normalcy: Disability, deafness, and the body*. London: Verso.
Desch, L. W., & Gaebler-Spira, D. (2008). Prescribing assistive-technology systems: Focus on children with impaired communication. *Pediatrics*, *121*(6), 1271–1280.
Drotner, K., & Livingstone, S. (2008). Editor's introduction: Questioning childhood, media, and culture. In K. Drotner & S. Livingstone (Eds.), *International handbook of children, media, & culture* (pp. 1–16). London: Sage.
Ellcessor, E. (2016). *Restricted access: Media, disability, and the politics of participation*. New York: New York University Press.
Ellis, K. (2019). *Disability and digital television cultures: Representation, access, and reception*. New York: Routledge.
Ellis, K., & Goggin, G. (2015). *Disability and the media*. Houndmills, UK: Palgrave Macmillan.
Ellis, K., & Kent, M. (2011). *Disability and new media*. London and New York: Routledge.
Garland-Thomson, R. (1997). *Extraordinary bodies: Figuring physical disability in American culture and literature*. New York: Columbia University Press.
Garland-Thomson, R. (2019). World building, citizenship, and disability: The strange world of Kazuo Ishiguro's never let me go. In B. Watermeyer, J. McKenzie, & L. Swartz (Eds.), *Palgrave handbook of disability and citizenship in the global south* (pp. 27–44). Houndmills, Basingstoke, UK: Palgrave Macmillan.

Goggin, G. (2016). Reimagining digital citizenship via disability. In A. McCosker, S. Vivienne, & A. Johns (Eds.), *Negotiating digital citizenship: Control, contest, culture* (pp. 61–80). London: Rowman & Littlefield.

Goggin, G., & Newell, C. (2005). *Disability in Australia: Exposing a social apartheid*. Sydney: UNSW Press.

Goggin, G., Steele, L., & Cadwallader, J. R. (2017). Normality and disability: Intersections among norms, law, and culture. *Continuum*, 31(3), 337–340.

Golos, D. B. (2010). The representation of deaf characters in children's educational television in the US: A content analysis. *Journal of Children and Media*, 4(3), 248–264.

Hirschmann, N. J. (2015). Invisible disability: Seeing, being, power. In N. J. Hirschmann & B. Linker (Eds.), *Civil disabilities: Citizenship, membership, and belonging* (pp. 204–222). Philadelphia, PA: University of Pennsylvania Press.

Hynan, A., Goldbart, J., & Murray, J. (2015). A grounded theory of Internet and social media use by young people who use augmentative and alternative communication (AAC). *Disability & Rehabilitation*, 37(17), 1559–1575.

Jack, J. (2014). *Autism and gender: From refrigerator mothers to computer geeks*. Chicago, IL: University of Illinois Press.

Johnson, M. R. (2019). Inclusion and exclusion in the digital economy: Disability and mental health as a live stream on Twitch.tv. *Information, Communication & Society*, 22(4), 506–520.

Jordan, A., & Prendella, K. (2019). The invisible children of media research. *Journal of Children and Media*, 13(2), 235–240.

Kumari Campbell, F. (2009). *Contours of ableism: The production of disability and abledness*. New York: Palgrave Macmillan.

Lahikainen, A. R., Mälkiä, T., & Repo, K. (Eds.). (2017). *Media, family interaction, and the digitalization of childhood*. Cheltenham, UK: Edward Elgar.

Larsen, S. (1995). What is "quality" in the use of technology for children with learning disabilities? *Learning Disability Quarterly*, 18(2), 118–130.

Liddiard, K., Runswick-Cole, K., Goodley, D., Whitney, S., Vogelmann, E., & Watts, L. (2019). "I was excited by the idea of a project that focuses on those unasked questions": Co-producing disability research with disabled young people. *Children & Society*, 33(2), 154–167.

Livingstone, S., & Bulger, M. (2014). A global research agenda for children's rights in the digital age. *Journal of Children and Media*, 8(4), 317–335.

Livingstone, S., & Third, A. (2017). Children and young people's rights in the digital age: An emerging agenda. *New Media & Society*, 19(5), 657–670.

Manhique, J., & Giannoumis, A. G. (2019). Experiences of disabled people in using information and communication technology in Mozambique. In T. Chataika (Ed.), *Routledge handbook of disability in Southern Africa* (pp. 69–81). London and New York: Routledge.

McRuer, R. (2006). *Crip theory: Cultural signs of queerness and disability*. New York and London: New York University Press.

Meredith, J., McCarthy, S., & Hemsley, B. (2018). Legal and ethical issues surrounding the use of older children's electronic personal health records. *Journal of Law and Medicine*, 25(4), 1042–1055.

Musengi, M., & Nyangairi, B. (2019). Educating deaf children in mainstream and special secondary school settings: Inclusive mirage or reality? In T. Chataika (Ed.), *Routledge handbook of disability in Southern Africa* (pp. 97–108). London and New York: Routledge.

Odom, S. L., Thompson, J. L., Hedges, S., Boyd, B. A., Dykstra, J. R., Duda, M. A., & Bord, A. (2015). Technology-aided interventions and instruction for adolescents with Autism Spectrum Disorder. *Journal of Autism and Developmental Disorders*, 45(12), 3805–3819.

Reid Chassiakos, Y., Radesky, J., Christakis, D., Moreno, M. A., & Cross, C. (2016). Children and adolescents and digital media. *Pediatrics*, 138(5), e20162593. doi:10.1542/peds.2016-2593.

Renwick, R. (2016). Rarely seen, seldom heard: People with intellectual disabilities in the mass media. In K. Scior & S. Werner (Eds.), *Intellectual disability and stigma: Stepping out from the margins* (pp. 61–75). London: Palgrave Macmillan.

Roulstone, A. (2016). *Disability and technology: International and interdisciplinary perspectives*. Basingstoke, UK: Palgrave Macmillan.

Runswick-Cole, K., Curran, T., & Liddiard, K. (Eds.). (2018). *Palgrave handbook of disabled childhood studies*. London: Palgrave Macmillan.

Sakr, N., & Steemers, J. (Eds.). (2017). *Children's TV and digital media in the Arab world: Screen culture and education*. London and New York: I. B. Tauris.

Sandland, R. (2017). Lessons for children's rights from disability rights? In E. Brems, E. Desmet, & W. Vandenhole (Eds.), *Children's rights law in the global human rights landscape* (pp. 109–128). London: Routledge.

Smith, K., & Abrams, S. S. (2019). Gamification and accessibility. *International Journal of Information and Learning Technology, 36*(2), 104–123.

Taylor, S. (2017). *Beasts of burden: Animal and disability liberation.* New York: New Press.

Third, A., Bellerose, D., Diniz De Oliveira, J., Lala, G., & Theakstone, G. (2017). *Young and online: Children's perspectives on life in the digital age. The state of the world's children 2017 companion report.* Sydney: Western Sydney University. doi:10.4225/35/5a1b885f6d4db.

Third, A., & Collin, P. (2016). Rethinking (children's and young people's) citizenship through dialogues on digital practice. In A. McCosker, S. Vivienne, & A. Johns (Eds.), *Negotiating digital citizenship: Control, contest, and culture* (pp. 41–59). London: Rowman & Littlefield International.

Third, A., Kelly-Dalgety, E., & Spry, D. (2013). *Real livewires: A research report on the role of chat hosts in the Livewire online community for young people living with a chronic illness or disability.* Melbourne: Young and Well Cooperative Research Centre. Retrieved from: www.westernsydney.edu.au/__data/assets/pdf_file/0015/542211/Real_Livewires_December_2013.pdf.

Tsaliki, L., & Kontogianni, S. (2014). Bridging the disability divide? Young children's and teenager's with disability Internet experiences in Greece. *Journal of Children and Media, 8*(2), 146–162.

United Nations. (2006). *Convention on the rights of persons with disabilities.* Retrieved from: www.un.org/development/desa/disabilities/convention-on-the-rights-of-persons-with-disabilities.html.

Wästerfors, D., & Hansson, K. (2017). Taking ownership of gaming and disability. *Journal of Youth Studies, 20*(9), 1143–1160.

Watermeyer, B., & Goggin, G. (2018). Digital citizenship in the global south: 'Cool stuff for other people'? In B. Watermeyer, J. McKenzie, & L. Swartz (Eds.), *Palgrave handbook of disability and citizenship in the global south* (pp. 167–181). Houndmills, Basingstoke, UK: Palgrave Macmillan.

White, M. (2006). Where do you want to sit today? Computer programmers' static bodies and disability. *Information, Communication & Society, 9*(3), 396–416.

Willson, M. (2018). Raising the ideal child? Algorithms, quantification and prediction. *Media, Culture & Society*. Advance online publication. doi:10.1177/0163443718798901.

35
CHILDREN'S MORAL AGENCY IN THE DIGITAL ENVIRONMENT

Joke Bauwens and Lien Mostmans

Introduction

For many children, intersubjectivity has firmly settled in 'the digital', understood as something that is not separate, but "increasingly embedded in the infrastructure of society" (Livingstone, Lansdown, & Third, 2017, p. 11). If communicating with other people, telling and listening to stories about other human beings and sharing one's feelings and thoughts with other persons is pivotal to the construction of the moral self (Luckmann, 1995), it can be argued that the digital has become a crucial practise ground where children make sense of, reflect, and act upon ethical questions on reformulating (Wall, 2011, pp. 7–9) what it means to be human (ontology); what human relations and societies they should try to aim toward (teleology); and how they should treat one another (deontology).

However, the technological affordances of digital media also seem to produce distinct instances of moral uncertainty, disengagement, and harm. For example, extreme cases of cyberbullying have shown that a one-off intimate selfie, revealing video, or outspoken statement can become a massively exposed 'faux pas', condemned by the 'networked public' (boyd, 2008) with tremendously serious or even tragic consequences. Many suggest that the affordances of digital media in terms of anonymity, searchability, connectivity, instantaneity, ephemerality, replicability, persistence, manipulation, visibility, etc., rearrange the distance between the self and other, reconfigure a sense of moral responsibility and recalibrate the meaning of obligations to other people and oneself (boyd, 2014; James et al., 2009; Jenkins, Clinton, Purushotma, Robison, & Weigel, 2006; Lenhart et al., 2011; Livingstone & Sefton-Green, 2016; Ringrose, Harvey, Gill, & Livingstone, 2013; Silverstone, 2007; Turkle, 2011).

This chapter brings these two observations into dialogue and addresses the question of how children and young people themselves are addressing the ethical complicatedness of the digital. The terms children and young people will be used from now on interchangeably to refer to youth aged 10–19. In line with recent approaches to moral agency, this chapter highlights the importance of children's lived-experience accounts for learning how they construe their *moral agency* in interaction with their own goals and beliefs and their social surroundings (Wall, 2011). Such an approach has not previously been the central focus in the vast field of literature that deals with children, digital media, and morality. In fact, despite more than two decades of a growing recognition that children are agentive participants to their lives, very little attention has been paid to children's *moral* agency in connection with digital media. Instead, the developmental model remains quite influential, typically resulting in experimental and behaviourist research that ignores the lived experiences of children (as noticed by Frankel, 2012; Krcmar, 2015; Niemi, 2016).

This chapter approaches this debate from a different angle and argues that a focus on the lived moral experiences of young people provides a more constructive approach for understanding how young people themselves are addressing the moral difficulties they face in their everyday life, that is ipso facto digital. Leaving aside the research literature that considers children as "merely undeveloped adults, passive recipients of care, occupying a separate innocence, or, perhaps, in need of being civilised" (Wall, 2011, p. 1), the analysis here is interested in how children navigate trade-offs between what's morally wrong and socially accepted among peers. Given the key role digital media play in young people's need for connection, communication, and sharing, the chapter pays particular attention to the 'moral horizons' (Taylor, 1989) they rely on in their peer interactions. Across the large range of social media platforms, messenger apps, game chats, and mobile phone texting, issues of identity, participation, and privacy – the latter also identified as one of children's most important concerns in terms of rights in the digital age (Livingstone et al., 2017, p. 20) – have emerged as ethically significant themes in peer-to-peer interactions (James et al., 2009).

There is little research that specifically investigates the children–digital–moral agency triptych from the perspective of their own worlds, but the growing field of qualitative research that provides a glimpse into children's feelings and thoughts about their *everyday* digital media experiences regularly touches upon moral agency. Given the authors' own 'social situatedness' (Vygotsky, 1978), the analysis will focus on the perspectives of young people growing up in the Global North with regular, seemingly uninterrupted access to digital media, living relatively flourishing lives. Based on this literature and the authors' own research, the analysis argues that children are not only active moral agents, who are *already* capable of moral experience (i.e., 'full' moral beings), but also moral 'becomings' who are exploring the "horizons of issues of importance, which help define the respects in which self-making is significant" (Taylor, 1991, pp. 39–40). In doing so, this chapter links to scholarship that has pointed to the ethical complicatedness of the internet, and the ways in which children already actively explore and negotiate norms and values (Flores & James, 2012; Gardner & Davis, 2013; James et al., 2009).

The chapter is divided into three sections. The first section sets out a definition of moral agency that contributes to the study of children's moral experiences in their own right, independent of adult-centric perspectives and concerns (Jenks, 2005). The second section considers young people's moral agency as the result of the intricate relationship between the moral and the social in digitised peer cultures. The third section discusses young people's remarkable amount of self-regulation in their narratives, illustrating how they fall back on the given moral horizons of the age of neoliberalism and insecurity. Throughout the chapter, we look at the level of diversity found in moral agency. While gender differences are often discussed in the research literature, there is no systematic examination of questions about how other structural differentials interact with moral agency.

Reconsidering Children's Moral Agency

In various disciplines there is growing recognition that other approaches, methodologies, and vocabularies are needed to comprehend how children are handling the moral tasks and ethical challenges in the textures of their everyday life (Frankel, 2012; Montreuil, Noronha, Floriani, & Carnevale, 2018; Niemi, 2016; Wall, 2011). In contrast to the developmental approach, childhood studies scholars (working at the interface) have argued that an understanding of children's morality, which takes its departure from their lived experiences, contributes to a more constructive theoretical framework which does justice to children's agency (Frankel, 2012; Niemi, 2016; Wall, 2011). Although they agree upon the importance of mundane meaning-formation, these scholars have also displayed a strong sensitivity for the wider social arrangements and power relations with which children are interacting (Buckingham & Jensen, 2012; Frankel, 2012; Livingstone & Sefton-Green, 2016; Silcock, Payne, & Hocking, 2016; Tisdall & Punch, 2012).

Complementary to this perspective, recent psychological and ethical theory on moral agency has explained that children's own stories are pivotal for learning about how they develop their moral agency. Concurring with childhood studies, they have argued that children are already full moral beings "who actively participate and contribute to moral life instead of passively conforming to pre-established moral norms" (Montreuil et al., 2018, p. 25). Narrative approaches define moral agency as a process that is always under construction by way of sense-making processes (Pasupathi & Wainryb, 2010, pp. 56–9). The crucial point here is that conversations with others are considered as pivotal to the formation of the moral self, for both adults *and* children (Pasupathi & Wainryb, 2010, p. 64). As a consequence, rather than considering children as exceptional, a strategy so often applied in research on children (Livingstone & Third, 2017), this definition of moral agency leaves room for the much-advocated view of children as both moral beings *and* moral becomings, actively constructing moral meanings in larger circumstances not shaped by themselves; already demonstrating ethical responsibility but, at the same time, vulnerable due to lack of power resources (Lee, 2001; Wall, 2011).

Besides, narrative psychological research has indicated that moral agency is a complicated phenomenological experience, also for adults for that matter, and that people's understanding of moral harm is very often the imperfect result of difficult trade-offs between obligations to other people and oneself and problematical choices between one's own desires and those of others (Pasupathi & Wainryb, 2010). An approach that starts from the social situatedness of children's online experiences therefore offers a more adequate entry point to the distinct moral uncertainties that come with digital technologies (Puech, 2016; Silverstone, 2007).

The Trade-Off Between the Moral and the Social

Young people's narratives display an unremitting negotiation between, on the one hand, the routine social practices that give meaning to their lives, and, on the other hand, the broader horizons about 'good' behaviour which constitute their activities and are shaped by societal expectations, requirements, norms, and power imbalances. Although it is often suggested that there are differences between young people's offline and online moral decision-making, most of the studies that we reviewed for this chapter point out that the online and offline worlds of young people are so interconnected that it is in fact more truthful to acknowledge both the complex and 'naturalised' ways in which "the digital bleeds into the material space of peer culture" (Ringrose & Harvey, 2015, p. 210), and vice versa (Lenhart et al., 2011; Marwick & boyd, 2014; Miegel & Olsson, 2012; Pabian et al., 2018; Salter, 2016).

Peer culture has always been very important for children's *becoming* (identity development, learning) and *belonging* (companionship, peer culture); digital media, however, afford constant sharing, connectivity, and performativity which break through boundaries between home and school, known and unknown others, privacy and publicity (Albury, 2015; Bond, 2010; Livingstone, 2006; Riva, 2018). Not only have digital media amplified the communicative scope of peer culture, they are pivotal to young people's social well-being (e.g., integration, acceptance, actualisation) (Adorjan & Ricciardelli, 2019; boyd, 2014). Consequently, research shows that navigating trade-offs between the social importance of digitised peer culture and the ethical questions it produces is inherent to young people's everyday life (Adorjan & Ricciardelli, 2019;

Berriman & Thomson, 2014; Betts & Spenser, 2017; Davis & James, 2013). "This navigational complexity", as Lenhart et al. (2011, p. 12) put it, is at the heart of teenagers' work "to incorporate norms into their lives at the same time the teen is trying to craft a personal identity".

In particular, regarding digital exploration of sexual identity, teenage girls' talk indicates that their own and others' decisions to share or not to share sexually suggestive images or 'nudes' with boys are the result of an intricate negotiating process between social and moral acceptance. In teen cultures and schools especially, where there is an articulate ethos of heteronormativity, girls must become proficient in navigating the social and moral complexities of whether or not to send these type of images (Ringrose & Harvey, 2015; Ringrose et al., 2013). While it is clear that in some peer cultures and school settings, social pressure to digitally perform can be substantial, research also reveals that from the age of 12, girls and boys scan the moral discourses that society and culture provide (Ringrose et al., 2013). Feminist research points in this respect to the pivotal role of gender differences and discourses. Girls reflect profoundly upon the consequences that digital sexual performances can have on what it means to be a girl – mostly expressed in terms of 'reputation' – and exploit the affordances of digital media (e.g., by cutting off their heads or greying out their faces in the photos or videos) to resolve the conflict between teen sociality and its social rewards, on the one hand, and conventional gendered norms, on the other. But boys' narratives also show this kind of 'negotiating work', by not sharing with other boys the images they receive from girls – even though some images could promote their status in peer hierarchy – and investing in trustful engagements with girls (Ringrose & Harvey, 2015; Ringrose et al., 2013).

Although 'sexting' practices are often regarded as worrisome examples of amoral and immoral behaviour (Gill-Peterson, 2015), they provide a tremendously challenging training ground for moral agency, as they seem to generate a lot of talk among young people (Adorjan & Ricciardelli, 2019); talk that contributes to the formation of moral agency (Pasupathi & Wainryb, 2010, p. 64). Besides, very often teenagers are exchanging self-produced sexual images through smartphones or the internet in consensual contexts of romance and friendship (Albury & Crawford, 2012; Döring, 2014; Hasinoff, 2012; Lenhart, 2009). The fact that these "risky opportunities" (Livingstone, 2008) are labelled in deviant and criminal terms (cf. the application of child pornography legislation and conviction of minor offenders in countries such as the US and Australia) contrasts with the actual moral negotiation and learning that takes place through this type of social intercourse, in terms of how to treat others with goodness and care, or how to sound out 'permissible' gendered moralities (Salter, 2016).

Another related realm of practices which is instructive here, is how young people understand privacy. Much inconsistency has been found in the way children feel about their own and other people's privacy as part of their larger development as a moral self. Young people are concerned about their online privacy, but this does not always show in their disclosing behaviour (boyd & Hargittai, 2010; Davis & James, 2013; Taddicken, 2014). In trying to explain how children are both concerned about their privacy and, at the same time, willing to share personal information online, researchers have suggested that children's conception of privacy online has less to do with the types of information they disclose than with their desire to exert control over this information and who has access to it (Adorjan & Ricciardelli, 2019; Livingstone, 2008). Moral conceptions and sensitivities regarding self-disclosure are embedded in a general concern about their vulnerability to other, more powerful children and adults in their social networks (Mostmans, Bauwens, & Pierson, 2014).

From children's stories we learn that their moral understanding of privacy and self-disclosure is inherently "context-sensitive" (Nissenbaum, 2009). During childhood, children's social and relational contexts change significantly, and increasingly become peer-oriented (boyd, 2014). Knowing the inner ways of a group, with its specific codes, jokes, languages, and routines, can offer a sense of belonging that many children find appealing (Livingstone, 2006). Humour, playfulness, banter, and drama can sometimes afford social interactions that might be negatively interpreted by adults, but not necessarily by young people themselves (Albury, 2015; Betts & Spenser, 2017; Marwick & boyd, 2014). However, disclosures that are not accepted within peer groups can lead to strong moral judgements, negative evaluation, and even social exclusion. In the authors' own research (Mostmans, 2017; Mostmans et al., 2014), children repeatedly described how implicit, unwritten rules of self-disclosure within peer groups guide their behaviour. They also explained how not subscribing to these rules, for instance how to deal with each other's photos, could have significant social consequences offline, as one ten-year-old girl illustrated:

> If someone would ever write negative comments to my pictures, even if it would be your best friend in class, one day he'll notice that he doesn't have a friend left. He wouldn't be our best friend anymore. And it would be his own fault.

Risk, Responsibility, and Reputation

Despite children's capacity to interact with and respond in agentic, meaningful ways to the worlds they are living in, these worlds are nevertheless designed and coordinated by adults (Livingstone & Sefton-Green, 2016; Niemi, 2016; Wall, 2011). This not only shows in the power adults have to impose explicit moral rules, but also in dominant discourses of childhood and 'appropriate and inappropriate conduct' that circulate in spheres of parenting, teaching, counselling, youth work, industry, policy, media, and research (Buckingham, 2000; Haddon, 2012; Turow & Nir, 2000). From a Foucauldian perspective, these societal discourses can be understood as governmental means to producing moral subjects; trained to a life that meets societal demands and expectations (Guigni, 2011; Silcock et al., 2016). In that way, children are indeed becomings, not in the developmental but in the social sense of the word, as they discover through their encounters and negotiations with these social spheres (and their discourses) what it means to comply, or not, with moral rules (Frankel, 2012; Guigni, 2011; Livingstone & Sefton-Green, 2016).

In the Global North, children's narratives about their digitised social lives unfold a set of critical concepts they draw upon to explain – to adults though – why they engage in behaviour that gives rise to adult concerns and societal dread. Findings suggest that even though children's moral agency can seem unruly and inconsistent, young people fall back on given frameworks or, as Taylor (1989, p. 19) puts it, horizons that incorporate "a crucial set of qualitative distinctions" helping them "to function with the sense that some actions, or mode of life, or mode of feeling are incomparably higher than the others which are more readily available" to them. From studies on young people's experiences with sexting and illegal downloading, we learn that these frameworks are not necessarily complicit with the law; teenagers see no harm, for example, in sending and receiving nude, or semi-nude images in romantic contexts (Albury & Crawford, 2012) or in illegal downloading and sharing of copyrighted material (Flores & James, 2012; Miegel & Olsson, 2012). But, the moral categories that young people fall back on are highly contingent; reflecting the neoliberal and risk-obsessed temporalities (Hasinoff, 2012). Three interrelated concepts, in particular, are at the heart of children's and young people's narratives about moral agency. These critical concepts are: risk, responsibility, and reputation.

The practises children display when confronted with liminal digital interactions are profoundly articulated in terms of keeping oneself safe and minimising potential risks. Risk awareness is an important moral compass to fend off dubious digital activities (Berriman & Thomson, 2014). Especially for girls (Adorjan & Ricciardelli, 2019; Albury & Crawford, 2012) and for children growing up in families where moral rules are not always clearly defined and sanctions are rather limited (Frankel, 2012, p. 186; Livingstone & Sefton-Green, 2016), young people are increasingly encouraged to rely on their own sense of responsibility, from which boundaries can indeed be explored and tested and standards readily internalised (Thomson & Holland, 2004). This results in a high degree of self-governance through the enactment of responsible, prudent, and conservative subjectivities (Adorjan & Ricciardelli, 2019; Livingstone & Sefton-Green, 2016; Salter, 2016). For example, European evidence covering the past decade suggests that most children have become more cautious and have learned that it is 'unwise' to post identifying information on their social networking profiles, such as a photo that shows one's face or their surname, address, and phone number (Livingstone, Haddon, Görzig, & Ólafsson, 2011).

It is argued that the ethical self-responsibility which children articulate in their everyday engagement with digital technologies is congruent with the neoliberal discourses of childhood generally found in Western societies (Silcock et al., 2016), built on entrepreneurship, consumerism, and sovereignty (Cradock, 2007). Researchers point out that children too are appropriating the "individualised neoliberal morals of self-creation and self-responsibility" (Bond, 2010, p. 590; Hope, 2015). Looking back on their digital media practises as a child, adolescents' talk often echoes the postmodern 'well-tempered self' (Miller, 1993); here moral agency amounts to questioning what it means to act responsibly or irresponsibly, and how they have learned to become more in charge of their digital performances. This shows clearly in girls' talk on sexting (Ringrose & Harvey, 2015; Ringrose et al., 2013; Salter, 2016). But also, regarding larger privacy issues, both boys and girls in a range of age groups regularly use vocabulary that resonates with choice, self-monitoring, and self-surveillance (Adorjan & Ricciardelli, 2019; Berriman & Thomson, 2014; Davis & James, 2013).

Taking ethical responsibility for oneself is closely connected to what Flores and James (2012, p. 837) call 'individualistic thinking', i.e., 'focusing on consequences for oneself'. In young people's narratives, this form of moral agency crystallises mainly into a sincere concern about one's reputation and the potential consequences of their digital practices for that reputation. Again, when it comes to digital sexual performances, girls articulate more often than boys a strong concern about self-respect and distinction from girls with 'loose' morality (Flores & James, 2012); in certain peer cultures and school settings sometimes labelled in harsh judgemental terms such as 'skets' and 'sluts' (Ringrose & Harvey, 2015; Ringrose et al., 2013). But also concern about future reputation in the professional and personal life they aspire to carefully guides young people's moral decisions (Berriman & Thomson, 2014; Salter, 2016). Because a large part of digitised teen sociality has the property of constant visibility and persistence, these findings echo Taylor's (1989, p. 15) analysis of 'dignity' as inherent to the making of modern identity, to

> our very comportment. The very way we walk, move, gesture, speak is shaped from the earliest moments by our awareness that we appear before others, that we stand in public space, and that this space is potentially one of respect or contempt, of pride or shame.

Conclusion

This chapter reviewed the growing body of qualitative work that provides a glimpse into young people's lived accounts of moral experiences in the digital. This field of research is not only relevant in terms of building more knowledge about the ways in which children actually make sense of their ethical responsibilities to themselves, to others, and to society, but also to children's moral agency itself. If the "creation of narratives in conversations with others is a paramount developmental process for the formation of a sense of self", then giving children the opportunity to construct narratives about their moral experiences as "a critical process by which moral agency can develop" (Pasupathi & Wainryb, 2010, p. 59) is indeed a crucial task.

Whereas the starting point for this chapter was *everyday* rather than problematic digital media use, research on young people's moral agency remains particularly occupied with practises that can typically be categorised as 'moral crisis' (Hasinoff, 2012, p. 450), such as 'sexting' and 'cyber-bullying'. Remarkably little attention has been paid to the less controversial and more positive aspects of digitised teen sociality that are also a part of their moral lives and which enable them to explore questions, as Taylor (1989, p. 4) puts it, "about what makes our lives meaningful or fulfilling". Research needs to be more open to seeing the moral possibilities digital cultures offer for children's moral self, even though building this takes place in worlds and structures not of their own making.

This chapter opted to take a helicopter view to discuss key trends in research on children's moral agency in their digitised social worlds. It reflected the perspectives of young people living in technologically affluent societies in the Global North. A considerable part of the research published in English stems from the Anglo-Saxon regions (USA, Canada, UK, Ireland, Australia, New Zealand). This can be seen as a serious limitation of the knowledge on young people's moral agency in the digital; many questions on young people's values and horizons in other parts of the world remain unanswered (notable exceptions are, e.g., Arora & Scheiber, 2017; Livingstone, Nandi, Banaji, & Stoilva, 2017).

Focussing on a large age group was a way to avoid the developmental perspective so dominant in discussions on children and moral agency. Although it can be argued that the more older children grow, the more experiences they acquire in "traversing life's moral terrain" (Wall, 2011, p. 10) and understanding the social complexities of digital media (Davis & James, 2013, p. 21), blindness to age differences contributes to a contextualised understanding of children and young people's moral agency. Context-sensitivity is certainly inherent to many qualitative investigations on young people's moral agency; and social stratification and multicultural diversity among children in Western societies and schools are increasingly acknowledged by scholars as a social fact. However, based on the research discussed in this chapter, it is difficult to draw conclusions on how social and cultural differences materialise in children's moral engagement with digital media. One notable exception is the field of feminist research, which sharply reveals how the frameworks children use to make discriminations between "what is honourable and dishonouring, what is admirable, what is done and not done" (Taylor, 1989, p. 20) are profoundly shaped by gender norms and the common-sense discourses that trickle down through girls' and boys' narratives.

Some scholars have argued that children's moral experiences bear the promise of expanding moral horizons in new ways and destabilising the foundations of established beliefs and values in society (Miegel & Olsson, 2012; Wall, 2011). It is unclear whether the empirical evidence available today can support this claim. Research on sexting and privacy suggests that young people sometimes articulate conservative, harsh normative judgements on feminine and masculine digital performances. However, other realms of digitised peer sociality, such as the recent upsurge of Global North climate activists, reveal that young people traverse life's moral terrain with creativity and dynamism, and that they negotiate the specific affordances of the various digital media not only in terms of convenience and sociality (Livingstone, 2008; Marwick, Murgia-Diaz, & Palfrey, 2010), but also in terms of morality.

References

Adorjan, M., & Ricciardelli, R. (2019). A new privacy paradox? Youth agentic practices of privacy management despite "nothing to hide" online. *Canadian Review of Sociology*, *56*(1). doi:10.1111/cars.12227.

Albury, K. (2015). Selfies, sexts, and sneaky hats: Young people's understandings of gendered practices of self-representation. *International Journal of Communication*, *9*, 1734–1745.

Albury, K., & Crawford, K. (2012). Sexting, consent and young people's ethics: Beyond Megan's story. *Continuum*, *26*(3), 463–473. doi:10.1080/10304312.2012.665840.

Arora, P., & Scheiber, L. (2017). Slumdog romance: Facebook love and digital privacy at the margins. *Media, Culture & Society*, *39*(3), 408–422. doi:10.1177/0163443717691225.

Berriman, L., & Thomson, R. (2014). Spectacles of intimacy? Mapping the moral landscape of teenage social media. *Journal of Youth Studies*, *18*(5), 583–587.

Betts, L. R., & Spenser, K. A. (2017). "People think it's a harmless joke": Young people's understanding of the impact of technology, digital vulnerability and cyberbullying in the United Kingdom. *Journal of Children and Media*, *11*(1), 20–35. doi:10.1080/17482798.2016.1233893.

Bond, E. (2010). The mobile phone = *bike shed*? Children, sex and mobile phones. *New Media & Society*, *13*(4), 587–604. doi:10.1177/1461444810377919.

boyd, d. (2008). *Taken out of context: American teen sociality in networked publics* (Doctoral thesis, University of California, US). Retrieved from: www.danah.org/papers/TakenOutOfContext.pdf.

boyd, d. (2014). *It's complicated: The social lives of networked teens*. New Haven, CT: Yale University Press.

boyd, d., & Hargittai, E. (2010). Facebook privacy settings: Who cares? *First Monday*, *15*(8), 2.

Buckingham, D. (2000). *After the death of childhood: Growing up in the age of electronic media*. Cambridge, UK: Polity Press.

Buckingham, D., & Jensen, H. (2012). Beyond "media panics". *Journal of Children and Media*, *6*(4), 413–429. doi:10.1080/17482798.2012.740415.

Cradock, G. (2007). The responsibility dance: Creating neoliberal children. *Childhood*, *14*(2), 153–172. doi:10.1177/0907568207078325.

Davis, K., & James, C. (2013). Tweens' conceptions of privacy online: Implications for educators. *Learning, Media and Technology*, *38*(1), 4–25. doi:10.1080/17439884.2012.658404.

Döring, N. (2014). Consensual sexting among adolescents: Risk prevention through abstinence education or safer sexting? *Cyberpsychology: Journal of Psychosocial Research on Cyberspace*, *8*(1), article 9. doi:10.5817/CP2014-1-9.

Flores, A., & James, C. (2012). Morality and ethics behind the screen: Young people's perspectives on digital life. *New Media & Society*, *15*(6), 834–852. doi:10.1177/1461444812462842.

Frankel, S. (2012). *Children, morality and society*. Basingstoke, UK: Palgrave Macmillan.

Gardner, H., & Davis, K. (2013). *The app generation: How today's youth navigate identity, intimacy, and imagination in a digital world*. New Haven, CT: Yale University Press.

Gill-Peterson, J. (2015). Sexting girls: Technological sovereignty and the feminine-digital. *Women & Performance: A Journal of Feminist Theory*, *25*(2), 143–156. doi:10.1080/0740770X.2015.1057010.

Guigni, M. (2011). "Becoming worldy with": An encounter with the Early Years Learning Framework. *Contemporary Issues in Early Childhood*, *12*(1), 11–27. doi:10.2304/ciec.2011.12.1.11.

Haddon, L. (2012). Parental mediation of internet use: Evaluating family relationships. In E. Loos, L. Haddon, & E. Mante-Meijer (Eds.), *Generational use of new media* (pp. 119–136). Farnham, UK: Ashgate.

Hasinoff, A. A. (2012). Sexting as media production: Rethinking social media and sexuality. *New Media & Society*, *15*(4), 449–465. doi:10.1177/1461444812459171.

Hope, A. (2015). Schoolchildren, governmentality and national e-safety policy discourse. *Discourse: Studies in the Cultural Politics of Education*, *36*(3), 343–353. doi:10.1080/01596306.2013.871237.

James, C., Davis, K., Flores, A., Francis, J. M., Pettingill, L., Rundle, M., & Gardner, H. (2009). *Young people, ethics, and the new digital media: A synthesis from the GoodPlay Project*. Cambridge, MA: MIT Press.

Jenkins, H., Clinton, R., Purushotma, A. J., Robison, A. J., & Weigel, M. (2006). *Confronting the challenges of participatory culture: Media education for the 21st Century. (The John D. and Catherine T. MacArthur Foundation reports on digital media and learning)*. Cambridge, MA: The MIT Press.

Jenks, C. (2005). *Childhood*. Abingdon, UK: Routledge.

Krcmar, M. (2015). Examining the assumptions in research on children and media. In D. Lemish (Ed.), *The Routledge international handbook of children, adolescents and media* (pp. 39–45). New York, NY: Routledge.

Lee, N. (2001). *Childhood and society: Growing up in an age of uncertainty*. Buckingham, UK: Open University Press.

Lenhart, A. (2009). *Teens and sexting: How and why minor teens are sending sexually suggestive nude or nearly nude images via text messaging*. Retrieved from: http://pewinternet.org/Reports/2009/Teens-and-Sexting.aspx.

Lenhart, A., Madden, M., Smith, A., Purcell, K., Zickuhr, K., & Rainie, L. (2011). *Teens, kindness and cruelty on social network sites: How American teens navigate the world of "digital citizenship"*. Retrieved from: www.pewinternet.org/2011/11/09/teens-kindness-and-cruelty-on-social-network-sites.

Livingstone, S. (2006). Children's privacy online: Experimenting with boundaries within and beyond the family. In R. Kraut, M. Brynin, & S. Kiesler (Eds.), *Computers, phones, and the Internet: Domesticating information technology* (pp. 128–144). Oxford, UK: Oxford University Press.

Livingstone, S. (2008). Taking risky opportunities in youthful content creation: Teenagers' use of social networking sites for intimacy, privacy and self-expression. *New Media & Society, 10*(3), 393–411. doi:10.1177/1461444808089415.

Livingstone, S., Haddon, L., Görzig, A., & Ólafsson, K. (2011). *Risks and safety on the internet: The perspective of European children: Full findings and policy implications from the EU Kids Online survey of 9–16 year olds and their parents in 25 countries. EU Kids Online, Deliverable D4.* London, UK: EU Kids Online Network.

Livingstone, S., Lansdown, G., & Third, A. (2017). *The case for a UNCRC general comment on children's rights and digital media (a report prepared for Children's Commissioner).* London, UK: LSE Consulting. Retrieved from: www.childrenscommissioner.gov.uk/wp-content/uploads/2017/06/Case-for-general-comment-on-digital-media.pdf.

Livingstone, S., Nandi, A., Banaji, S., & Stoilova, M. (2017). *Young adolescents and digital media: Uses, risk and opportunities in low- and middle-income countries. A rapid evidence review.* London, UK: Gage.

Livingstone, S., & Sefton-Green, J. (2016). *The class: Living and learning in the digital age.* New York, NY: New York University Press.

Livingstone, S., & Third, A. (2017). Children and young people's rights in the digital age: An emerging agenda. *New Media & Society, 19*(5), 657–670. doi:10.1177/1461444816686318.

Luckmann, T. (1995). On the Intersubjective Constitution of Morals. In S. G. Crowell (Ed.), *The prism of the self: Contributions to phenomenology* (pp. 73–91). Dordrecht, Netherlands: Springer.

Marwick, A., & boyd, d. (2014). "It's just drama": Teen perspectives on conflict and aggression in a networked era. *Journal of Youth Studies, 17*(9), 1187–1204. doi:10.1080/13676261.2014.901493.

Marwick, A., Murgia-Diaz, D., & Palfrey, J. G. (2010). *Youth, privacy and reputation: Literature review.* Retrieved from: http://papers.ssrn.com/sol3/papers.cfm?abstract_id=1588163.

Miegel, F., & Olsson, T. (2012). A generational thing? The internet and new forms of social intercourse. *Continuum: Journal of Media & Cultural Studies, 26*(3), 487–499. doi:10.1080/10304312.2012.665842.

Miller, T. (1993). *The well-tempered self: Citizenship, culture and the postmodern subject.* Baltimore, MD: John Hopkins University Press.

Montreuil, M., Noronha, C., Floriani, N., & Carnevale, F. (2018). Children's moral agency: An interdisciplinary scoping review. *Journal of Childhood Studies, 43*(2), 17–30.

Mostmans, L. (2017). *Under the radar: Preadolescents' moral conceptions about online self-disclosure* (Doctoral thesis). Vrije Universiteit Brussel, Belgium.

Mostmans, L., Bauwens, J., & Pierson, J. (2014). "I would never post that": Children, moral sensitivity and online disclosure. *Communications, 39*(3), 347–367. doi:10.1515/commun-2014-0112.

Niemi, K. (2016). *Moral beings and becomings: Children's moral practices in classroom peer interaction* (Doctoral thesis, University of University of Jyväskylä, Finland). Retrieved from: https://jyx.jyu.fi/handle/123456789/48975.

Nissenbaum, H. (2009). *Privacy in context: Technology, policy, and the integrity of social life.* Stanford, CA: Stanford University Press.

Pabian, S., Erreygers, S., Vandebosch, H., Van Royen, K., Dare, J., Costello, L., ... Cross, D. (2018). "Arguments online, but in school we always act normal": The embeddedness of early adolescent negative peer interactions within the whole of their offline and online peer interactions. *Children and Youth Services Review, 86*, 1–13. doi:10.1016/j.childyouth.2018.01.007.

Pasupathi, M., & Wainryb, C. (2010). Developing moral agency through narrative. *Human Development, 53*, 55–80. doi:10.1159/000288208.

Puech, M. (2016). *The ethics of ordinary technology.* New York, NY: Routledge.

Ringrose, J., & Harvey, L. (2015). Boobs, pack-off, six packs and bits: Mediated body parts, gendered reward, and sexual shame in teens' sexting images. *Continuum: Journal of Media & Cultural Studies, 29*(2), 205–217. doi:10.1080/10304312.2015.1022952.

Ringrose, J., Harvey, L., Gill, R., & Livingstone, S. (2013). Teen girls, sexual double standards and "sexting": Gendered value in digital image exchange. *Feminist Theory, 14*(3), 305–323. doi:10.1080/10304312.2015.1022952.

Riva, C. (2018). Outlooks, gaps or boundaries: Adults' and young people's relationship with the media. *Interdisciplinary Journal of Family Studies, 23*(2), 39–53.

Salter, M. (2016). Privates in the online public: Sex(ting) and reputation on social media. *New Media & Society, 18*(11), 2723–2739. doi:10.1177/1461444815604133.

Silcock, M., Payne, D., & Hocking, C. (2016). Governmentality within children's technological play: Findings from a critical discourse analysis. *Children & Society, 30*, 85–95. doi:10.1111/chso.12123.

Silverstone, R. (2007). *Media and morality: On the rise of the mediapolis.* Cambridge, UK: Polity Press.

Taddicken, M. (2014). The "privacy paradox" in the social web: The impact of privacy concerns, individual characteristics, and the perceived social relevance on different forms of self-disclosure. *Journal of Computer-Mediated Communication, 19*(2), 248–273. doi:10.1111/jcc4.12052.

Taylor, C. (1989). *Sources of the self: The making of the modern identity*. Cambridge, MA: Harvard University Press.

Taylor, C. (1991). *The ethics of authenticity*. Cambridge, MA: Harvard University Press.

Thomson, R., & Holland, J. (2004). *Youth values and transitions to adulthood: An empirical investigation*. London, UK: Families & Social Capital ESRC Research Group.

Tisdall, K., & Punch, S. (2012). Not so "new"? Looking critically at childhood studies. *Children's Geographies, 10*(3), 249–264. doi:10.1080/14733285.2012.693376.

Turkle, S. (2011). *Alone together: Why we expect more from technology and less from each other*. New York, NY: Basic Books.

Turow, J., & Nir, L. (2000). *The Internet and the family: The view from parents, the view from kids (Report No. 13)*. Retrieved from: http://repository.upenn.edu/cgi/viewcontent.cgi?article=1409&context=asc_papers.

Vygotsky, L. S. (1978). *Mind in society: The development of higher psychological processes*. Cambridge, MA: Harvard University Press.

Wall, J. (2011). *Ethics in light of childhood*. Washington, DC: Georgetown University Press.

36
CHILDREN'S RIGHTS IN THE DIGITAL ENVIRONMENT

A Challenging Terrain for Evidence-Based Policy

Sonia Livingstone, Amanda Third, and Gerison Lansdown[1]

Applying the UNCRC in the Digital Age: A Short History

When children's social environment is no longer only physical but also digital … a CRC for the Digital Age … [could tell States the] most important things that you need to do to ensure that your young people's engagement is constructive, rather than destructive or worrying.

(Christopher de Bono, UNICEF East Asia and Pacific Regional Office)

The United Nations Convention on the Rights of the Child (UNCRC) (UN, 1989) affirms children as independent rights-holders and delineates the particular rights of children to ensure they develop to their full potential, together with the special mechanisms needed to deliver them. But why is interpreting and implementing the UNCRC for the digital age needed, what does it require, and what are the challenges?

De Bono's comment dates from 2013, when UNICEF's Office of Research-Innocenti asked Sonia Livingstone and Monica Bulger (2013) to interview experts on how its research agenda should embrace the risks and opportunities of the digital age. Noting the paucity of evidence in the Global South, where already one in three children were online (Livingstone, Carr, & Byrne, 2015), their report called urgently for new research that is comparable across countries and yet flexibly implemented to recognise local contexts and concerns. This led to the Global Kids Online project which, by 2018, had surveyed over 25,000 children and many of their parents in countries on all continents, with follow-up work to ensure that policies and practices are evidence-based and impactful in advancing a child rights agenda on the digital environment.[2]

Building on the work of EU Kids Online (O'Neill, Staksrud, & McLaughlin, 2013), Global Kids Online evidence shows that children start using the internet younger and spend more time online the more available the internet becomes, and they are likely to face ever more opportunities and risks. The trend towards personalised devices intensifies digital experiences, enabling children to be more independent users, but making parental supervision more difficult. However, while the internet can have a positive impact on children's learning, social relationships, and participation, its use can also bring pornography, cyberbullying, sexual exploitation and abuse, online hate, and other potential harms. Importantly, too, not all children have equal access to the opportunities: social, cultural, and economic divides, especially in the Global South, continue to prevent many children from benefiting from the digital environment.

UNICEF devoted its annual 2017 *State of the World's Children* report to "children in a digital world", revealing the benefits for the realisation of children's rights but also the new threats emerging as digitalisation, datafication, and global networks become embedded in the infrastructure of children's lives. Among all those with views on the societal transformations brought about by digital technologies, children are the most vocal, as revealed by a consultation with children around the world conducted by Amanda Third and her colleagues for UNICEF (2017): children are calling for new rights of access and digital literacy because, they are clear, these increasingly mediate their participation, provision, and protection rights in the digital age (see Third, Bellerose, Diniz de Oliveira, Lala, & Theakstone, 2017).[3]

While the sometimes hyperbolic excitement regarding the benefits for children of digital engagement continues to drive the market and take-up by families, it is the threats that drive policy and regulation. Recent threats include the growth of web streaming of child sexual abuse and exploitation, whereby children typically in a Global South country are abused 'to order' via live web streaming services, typically by men located in the Global North, and sometimes with the knowing cooperation of the child's parents. Also gathering controversy, consider the sale of 'smart' toys (dolls, teddies) and other domestic products (e.g., baby monitors, rucksacks, socks, among other instances of the 'internet of things') that collect children's personal data (including their conversations) in ways that parents do not understand, leaving them vulnerable to privacy abuses when data are profiled for commercial gain or hacked by criminals (Mascheroni & Holloway, 2019). As a third example, policy makers are increasingly worried about the explosion in 'fake news', and other forms of bias and misinformation, deliberate or otherwise, that favour manipulative persuasion over knowledge and decision-making for the public – and children's – good.

The UN Committee on the Rights of the Child is the body responsible for promoting, interpreting, and monitoring the implementation of the UNCRC. In 2014, in the year of the 25th anniversary of the UNCRC and, coincidentally, of the World Wide Web, it held a Day of General Discussion on the rights of the child and digital media (OHCHR, 2014). Following a lively discussion among experts, underpinned by a consultation with children (Third, Bellerose, Dawkins, Keltie, & Pihl, 2014), a strong set of recommendations emerged for all States that have ratified the UNCRC (every state, bar the US). In a fast-moving, complex, global policy terrain, who is responsible for the needed actions?

The Committee produces General Comments to

> provide interpretation and analysis of specific articles of the CRC or deal with thematic issues related to the rights of the child. General Comments constitute an authoritative interpretation as to what is expected of States parties as they implement the obligations contained in the CRC.[4]

In 2017, the present authors were asked by the Children's Commissioner for England to prepare a case for a General Comment on the digital environment (Livingstone, Lansdown, & Third, 2017). Recognising that society's growing reliance on the digital environment has profound consequences for children's rights, and that States around the world are struggling to address children's provision, protection, and participation in the face of rapid technological transformation, in 2018 the Committee accepted the case made by the authors, working with the 5Rights Foundation with a view to publishing the new General Comment in 2021. In March 2019, the UN Committee on the Rights of the Child issued a global call for submissions to inform the Committee's development of the General Comment. There was a global call for submissions. Contributions are currently under consideration as part of the Committee's development of the General Comment.

Interpreting the UNCRC in Relation to the Digital Environment

What is it about the digital environment that poses new challenges for evidence-based policy and practice in realising children's rights? Digital technologies – including not only the internet and mobile technologies but also digital networks and databases, digital contents and services, as well as developments in artificial intelligence, robotics, algorithms, and 'big data' and the 'internet of things' – are globally networked, enabling extensive and rapidly scalable connectivity that can operate beyond top-down control. Taken together, digital technologies are increasingly connected through a complicated, transnational value chain;[5] hence the reference to the 'digital environment'.

Consequently, children's rights in research, policy, and practice can be conceived in three ways (Third & Collin, 2016). First, children's uses of digital technologies raise questions of children's *right to* digital devices, content, and services. Second, promoting children's *rights in* digital environments invites consideration of how children can realise their rights in online spaces and how society can counter ways in which their rights are infringed or violated. The third category is the most ambitious, namely, addressing children's *rights in the digital age* by recognising that digital technologies are reshaping society so that multiple dimensions of children's lives – from education to health, from family to future life chances – are being reconfigured (Livingstone & Third, 2017). All three categories intersect, building on each other to intensify connections and disconnections of many kinds.

Children's rights can be affected by a range of policies – for example, the outsourcing, at a national level, of educational technology or school information management systems or the privatisation of medical records and health information systems. In such domains, child rights considerations (e.g., in relation to privacy) easily and often go unrecognised unless specific measures are taken to 'mainstream' child rights within policy and practice.[6] Indeed, technological developments can reshape children's rights in a host of ways as yet little understood. For example, what are the implications for children's freedom of expression or safety of encrypted or anonymous digital services? Where such technological developments are examined in terms of their human rights implications or in relation to internet governance processes, there is often little or no recognition of child-specific issues. For example, practical approaches to protecting child rights in digital environments are often based on setting a minimum age for use of a service, but this tends to treat all children as reaching levels of maturity at the same ('average') age, which doesn't address their individual interests well, and can even be detrimental for some. Insofar as such age limits are operated by global companies (for example, the age of 13 for social media services), they also have the effect of applying internationally a standard set in the Global North. Moreover, some child rights are particularly impacted by the digital age and should be newly interpreted: for example, Article 17, the right to information, takes on significant additional implications for children's education, given how frequently they now use the internet for informal learning (Third et al., 2017) – consider, further, how access to the internet can facilitate children's right to sexuality and health information and their positive right to communicate online (see Albury, 2017).

The UNCRC includes four rights that are also recognised as general principles with cross-cutting applicability:

1. Right to non-discrimination (Article 2);
2. Best interests of the child (Article 3(1));

3 Right to life, survival, and fullest development of the child (Article 6);
4 Right to be heard (Article 12).

What might these mean in relation to the digital environment? Non-discrimination has mainly been applied to children's access to digital technologies, but the implications for equality in digital environments and, more widely, in the digital age are far-reaching. This is especially the case because digital exclusion tends to mirror social, economic, and cultural exclusion, with special efforts needed, for example, regarding girls' empowerment, children with disabilities, refugees and asylum-seekers, children in extreme poverty, and children in institutions. Interestingly, public and third sector institutions are hopeful that digital inclusion can offer a workaround to traditional forms of exclusion. But the digital environment's commercial infrastructure and algorithmic logics may undermine such hopes, with existing and emerging business models increasingly relying on privatised processes that risk exclusionary, discriminatory, or commodifying effects rather than outcomes in the public interest (Mansell, 2017).

The obligation to ensure that the best interests of the child are a primary consideration in all actions concerning the child poses a regulatory challenge in the digital age, calling for a nuanced and context-dependent balance between rights to protection and civil rights and freedoms. This might best be achieved through a mix of regulation of the media industry, provision of appropriate protection, interpretation of confidentiality and privacy rules, and emergence of new social norms and institutional practices. Only thus can Article 6 become feasible, namely, that children should be able to benefit positively from their experiences of the digital environment without detriment to their wellbeing. How this can occur will vary for different individuals or groups of children in different national or cultural settings. For example, for children with disabilities, opportunities for online learning can be particularly important, as their offline opportunities may be restricted (Council of Europe, 2019).

As a guide in interpreting the UNCRC in all contexts including the digital, it is important to recognise the right of every child capable of forming a view to express their views and have them taken seriously, whilst also recognising the diversity of obstacles children in different settings experience to this right. In the digital context, this right implies not only harnessing the particular affordances of digital technologies as a means of consulting and collaborating with children in the development of legislation and policy with regard to digital participation and protection, but also across diverse policy domains. It also means promoting children's digital citizenship and opportunities for social and educational participation, enabling and empowering children to enact their political citizenship online and through social media, and educating children regarding their rights in digital and other environments.

Of the remaining articles in the UNCRC, several are highly relevant to the digital environment:

5 Right to freedom of expression and information (Article 13);
6 Right to freedom of association (Article 15);
7 Right to privacy (Article 16);
8 Right to information and protection from harmful content (Article 17);
9 Right to protection from exploitation and violence (Articles 19, 32, 33, 34, 35, 36, 37(a) and 39);
10 Right to physical and mental health and access to healthcare services (Article 24);
11 Right to education and literacy (Articles 28 and 29);
12 Right to engage in play and recreational activities (Article 31).

Space restrictions prevent elaborations upon the interpretation of these and related articles (see Lievens, Livingstone, McLaughlin, O'Neill, & Verdoodt, 2018; Third, Livingstone, & Lansdown,

2019), but it is possible to draw attention to some emerging concerns. As regards children's right to freedom of expression and information, this is too often neglected by policy-makers more concerned with negotiating the thorny relation between child protection and adult speech rights (O'Neill et al., 2013). Yet children share in these fundamental human rights, even though many online spaces of discussion are barred to them or hazardous for them. Access to digital information, for instance, is highly valued by children for many reasons including, as Global Kids Online has shown (Livingstone, Kardefelt Winther & Hussein, 2019), for health information that is otherwise hard to obtain.

As quoted in Third et al. (2017), children say:

> If someone is sick in the family, we can use the internet to match symptoms to the sickness and determine its severity.
>
> *(Bhutan, girl, 18)*

> If we do not use the computer, if we do not know the computer, then we do not know anything, including . . . the good things for our lives.
>
> *(Timor-Leste, girl, 14)*

Digital opportunities for expression and information also have consequences for children's civil rights and freedoms, including their right to freedom of association. Additionally, there are benefits for their rights to education and literacy. As children told Third et al. (2017):

> Technology helps me to do research for my homework and also, if I miss a class, I can contact a friend on WhatsApp to get information or work together.
>
> *(Burundi, girl, 18)*

> I learnt coding through YouTube. I watched so many videos about coding and thus I have learned coding.
>
> *(Bangladesh, girl, 17)*

In relation to education, however, children demand more of their school, in both wealthier and poorer countries:

> School should help me know the bad and good effects of technology, the impacts.
>
> *(Fiji, girl, 12)*

> Teachers should teach classes that help us use digital technology appropriately.
>
> *(Japan, girl, 17)*

Policy-makers have been far more active in relation to the risk of harm, seeking solutions to provide appropriate protection, including policies and training for schools, as well as positive measures to engage children in strategies to raise awareness and engage as partners in addressing cyberbullying, for example. Some initiatives have been targeted at specifically vulnerable groups such as LGBTQI children, children with disabilities or children from minority religious or ethnic groups, though more often interventions are generic. In relation to sexual abuse and exploitation, policy solutions have been more legislative, focussed on the capacity and actions of law enforcement to enable identification of victims, remove images, and prosecute perpetrators. Yet children remain concerned about online risks:

> I'm worried about my safety on the internet because my information can be viral anywhere.
>
> *(Bangladesh, girl, 17)*

> I don't upload certain pics with which bad people can make dirty videos of us.
>
> *(Bhutan, girl, 16)*

> It is very distressing when you publish something [online] and suddenly others attack you with no reason, without knowing you.
>
> *(Uruguay, girl, 14)*

> Sometimes, when we use Google or social media on the laptop then there was like a popup of a porn website.
>
> *(Malaysia, girl, 16)*

> I think that adults worry for our own good because it is also through the internet that many young people join terrorist groups, because the internet helps but on the other hand it destroys.
>
> *(Central African Republic, boy, 15)*

Underpinning both opportunities and risks is the management of privacy in digital environments. This encompasses not only interpersonal privacy, of considerable importance to young people, but also privacy from the State and from business (Livingstone, Stoilova, & Nandagiri, 2018).

> I am concerned about leakage of my personal information – because this means leakage of my money and personal information.
>
> *(Republic of Korea, boy, 14)*

In the digital environment, data protection regulation is making some inroads into preventing infringements of children's privacy rights, although it seems likely that further policy steps will be required.

Implementing the UNCRC in Relation to the Digital Environment

The UNCRC includes a series of articles specifying general measures of implementation by States. For instance, the 2014 Day of General Discussion on "Digital media and children's rights" held by the UN Committee on the Rights of the Child (OHCHR, 2014, p. 19) concluded that:

> States should adopt a national coordinating framework with a clear mandate and sufficient authority to coordinate all activities related to children's rights and digital media and ICTs at cross-sectoral, national, regional and local levels and facilitate international cooperation.

Also needed is training for all professionals working with and for children to raise awareness and improve technical skills, along with appropriate budgetary allocation to ensure digital protection and access. Trusted and effective systems are needed to provide child-friendly forms of remedy and redress, and such measures should be independently monitored and evaluated, as well as evidence-based and informed by consultation with children. This raises a series of challenges discussed below.

Most generally, the use of digital technologies – by public and private bodies as well as by individuals – amplifies and intensifies both risks and opportunities for children. Consider, for example, the current imperative for refugee children to have access to mobile technology to sustain vital family connections and sources of information, even though this same technology can put them at risk of abuse from people traffickers. Those building digital opportunities need a framework to alert them to unintended risks; those addressing risks need a framework to ensure they do not inadvertently curtail children's opportunities.

The UN more broadly recognises that the digital environment offers huge opportunities for the implementation and monitoring of the Sustainable Development Goals in realising children's rights (Wernham, 2016). For example, appropriate deployment of digital technology can enable children to gain much-needed information at low cost, to engage with affordable educational resources and knowledge, to overcome forms of discrimination or exclusion, to participate and be heard in meaningful decision-making processes, and much more. There is, in short, considerable enthusiasm among States and child rights organisations for initiatives that seek to capitalise on the attractive and scalable possibilities of using digital media to deliver health information, community resources, emergency response, or other programme initiatives to children in hard-to-reach settings (Kleine, Hollow, & Poveda, 2014). Hence it is important not to be swayed by the new risks into taking an overly protectionist approach. Indeed, without clear guidance on managing conflicting rights and attending to children's civil rights and freedoms, policies can quickly revert to a predominant focus on protection which, important as it is, can tend to override efforts to support positive rights.

Challenges of both principle and practice regarding the implementation of the UNCRC in relation to the digital environment were explained in the expert interviews conducted when preparing the case for the General Comment. Key experts from civil society, business, and international and national non-governmental organisations around the world were interviewed individually for between 30 and 60 minutes in person or by Skype during December 2016–February 2017 for the original report (Livingstone et al., 2017). The interview guide examined the practical challenges and concerns, regional or contextual considerations, and priorities for the scope of what a General Comment would cover, as well as practicalities concerning steps to implementation. Quotations from experts in this chapter come from this report.

One practical challenge much discussed by the experts is that often a platform or online service is unable to determine whether a user is a child, so, in effect, children are often treated online as adults rather than in an age-appropriate way. This is especially problematic insofar as children are often the first to engage with fast-developing digital environments, ahead of the adults around them. Consequently, their wellbeing can be inadvertently overlooked as States rush to embrace new economic opportunities.

This, in turn, raises a further difficulty discussed by experts – the relation between the State and parents in adjudicating

> with respect to the boundaries between parental responsibilities to protect children vis-à-vis the child's evolving capacity to make decisions about in what way they interact with the internet.
>
> *(Amihan Abueva, Child Rights Coalition Asia)*

In addition,

> while parents have valid concerns (about their children's safety online), they could also unwittingly be the people who put their own children or even their children's friends at risk.
>
> *(Indra Kumari Nadchatram, UNICEF Malaysia)*

Alongside guiding parents in their responsibilities, and respecting the rights of children when these conflict with their parents, States must also consider potential conflicts between adult freedoms and child rights more generally. On occasion, and somewhat perversely, the call to attend to child rights becomes problematic if used as a justification for introducing unwarranted censorship or surveillance; here the experts suggested that a General Comment should guide States in order that child protection does not violate other rights (La Rue, 2014).

In addition to the challenge of addressing the attendant and ever-emerging risks of harm, States must promote digital literacy education and child-centred design alongside top-down policy initiatives. They must also attend to children's voices and concerns in planning new digital resources. Last, they must ensure that business-led innovation is subject to effective national and international regulation that recognises children's rights and is informed by risk impact assessments. This last point is currently proving almost-overwhelming for States: digital transformation is being driven by both major corporations and a multitude of small and medium-sized businesses, often fast-moving start-ups, often led by young developers, and often with little awareness of child rights and with commercial priorities that mitigate against efforts towards safety- or privacy-by-design. Indeed, there is a widespread relocation of communication, learning, health, civic participation, social relationships, and other societal processes onto proprietary platforms primarily motivated by profit. While many constructive initiatives for children are instigated by business, others collect and monetise children's data in ways that seemingly evade State oversight and regulation. The UN Committee on the Rights of the Child's General Comment No. 16 on State obligations regarding the impact of the business sector on children's rights:

> recognises that duties and responsibilities to respect the rights of children extend in practice beyond the State and State-controlled services and institutions and apply to private actors and business enterprises. Therefore, all businesses must meet their responsibilities regarding children's rights and States must ensure they do so. In addition, business enterprises should not undermine the States' ability to meet their obligations towards children under the Convention and the Optional Protocols thereto.
>
> *(paragraph 8)*

But calling for something is not the same as achieving it:

> The feeling is that, you know, these big companies are much bigger than the States, and I think the other dilemma as well is that the technologies are developing so fast that the legislation is oftentimes not able to keep pace with the development of technology.
>
> *(Amihan Abueva, Child Rights Coalition Asia)*

States must find new ways to incentivise and coordinate the actions of multiple relevant stakeholders across the public, private, and third sectors. Yet problematically, digital technologies have cross-cutting and intersecting consequences across the full range of children's rights. Not only do these not fall neatly into the domain or expertise of one particular ministry or regulator, they are too easily neglected altogether by being passed from one ministry to another (e.g., the Ministry of Justice, Education, Family Welfare, Telecommunications, or Business) or by ministries advancing mutually contradictory approaches. This adds weight to the call for an integrated approach:

> Digital influences almost all spheres of children's everyday lives. It is broad and pretty much all-encompassing that it is impossible to focus only on a few specific issues.
>
> *(Indra Kumari Nadchatram, UNICEF Malaysia)*

Yet while it might be feared that the technology is developing too fast to be managed, the experts who were interviewed urged the contrary. In short, they believed it is possible and now urgent to encourage and enable States to recognise and identify key trends, to take the steps they can, to marshal their resources to address early the problems that can be foreseen, and to build the competent and trusted institutions required to anticipate future innovations and challenges as they unfold. Digital technologies

> will continue to be a kind of moving target. I don't think things are going to settle necessarily in the next 20 years. I think we're in an epoch of continued evolution and so one needs ongoing guidance.
>
> *(Guy Berger, UNESCO)*

Several experts therefore recommended a 'technologically neutral', principled approach, insofar as possible, rather than tying recommendations or policies to particular technologies or social practices that will soon change. But, as the experts argued, it would be wrong to do nothing now:

> The world evolves. Problems evolve. They take a different shape. I mean, maybe the name is the same but the shape is different. And the societies evolve, and so do the solutions, especially when you link that to the digital world. So there is need for a constant thinking, rethinking and questioning of what's going on, to look at this in a different way. I mean that's an obligation we have.
>
> *(Marie-Laure Lemineur, ECPAT International)*

Because the drafting of the UNCRC preceded the emergence of widespread uses of digital technology, it is throwing up new challenges that need to be interpreted in light of the significant impact these phenomena are having on the lives of children globally. As one expert observed:

> The Convention was created in a time when digital technology was not yet that well known or not yet that advanced, so it would be the General Comment that can provide guidance on how to apply these rights in the age that we have right now.
>
> *(Hazel Bitaña, Child Rights Coalition Asia)*

The nascent General Comment will, in short, provide a defence against those who say the UNCRC is out of date, reasserting it instead as a timely, legitimate, and useful instrument for realising children's rights in the digital age.

Effective implementation of child rights depends substantially on national legislation, and States could lead the way in terms of ethical, rights-respecting treatment of children's data (e.g., birth registration, case management, government records), setting standards by which to raise expectations for other stakeholders. Experts were of the view that international coordination and cooperation is particularly challenging for States given the global businesses and networked processes which characterise the digital environment. For instance, increasingly child protection depends on the availability of and jurisdiction over forms of digital evidence, making international cooperation in law enforcement processes vital. Potentially, the General Comment will serve to prioritise the effort to manage and share evidence in and across digital platforms and national boundaries.

Conclusion

New policy and practice is urgently needed so that the UNCRC can be effectively interpreted and implemented in relation to digital technologies, since "we can't separate any longer our on- and offline lives, and children even less than we can" (Sheila Donovan, Child Helpline International). Further, since the internet transcends national boundaries, the forthcoming global protocol responds to an urgent need:

> The internet is a transnational technology. Individual nation states can make advances but children's rights in the digital environment must be set out clearly and established on an international basis. A General Comment on the CRC is the necessary first step to protecting children's rights in the 21st century.
>
> *(Beeban Kidron, 5Rights)*

Digital technologies are increasingly embedded in the infrastructure of society rather than something discrete and set apart. Thus it is not so much new digital rights but, rather, children's fundamental human rights that are at stake in new ways in the digital age. Echoing the argument of former UN Special Rapporteur on the promotion and protection of the right to freedom of opinion and expression, Frank La Rue (2014), Jenny Thomas (Child Rights International Network) suggests of internet access, "I would not frame it as a right in itself but a way of implementing other rights". One can make the same argument about digital literacy – as not a right in itself, but as an enabler for achieving rights in the digital age.

At present, policy and practice designed to optimise children's engagement with the digital environment is not always rights-focussed and so may not recognise the full range of children's rights in ways that are both holistic and authoritative. Experts interviewed also suggested that a General Comment would carry significant political weight, adding strength to child rights organisations' demands, and fostering States' accountability to children by requiring States to report on their compliance to the Committee:

> A General Comment is a useful guide for those of us who are working at the regional and country levels because it helps us to push governments. When the reporting time comes, if we have General Comments, we can take them to task, or we can challenge them to make sure that policies are in place or make sure that programmes are implemented.
>
> *(Amihan Abueva, Child Rights Coalition Asia)*

> It would mean that countries that don't have legislation in place or if they do it's not enforced, would be then somehow put on the spot to either implement existing legislation or enact legislation, and to enforce the legislation ... [the Committee] has moral persuasion influence and it probably is the only one that does.
>
> *(Sheila Donovan, Child Helpline International)*

> From an NGO perspective, they are very useful for our advocacy work. We draw on General Comments all the time in submissions to the UN and to governments.
>
> *(Jenny Thomas, Child Rights International Network)*

> It's not just any old wish list, it is authoritative. (Guy Berger, UNESCO)

Without the principled, coherent, and authoritative guidance of the General Comment currently under development, States would continue to struggle to meet their obligations to children, including instituting the vital regulatory checks and balances to ensure that businesses meet their responsibilities to protect and enhance children's rights. Taking action now enables States to face the challenges of the digital age in its early stages. The sooner child rights issues are recognised and addressed as part of the wider rush to embrace digital and business innovations – rather than being tacked on belatedly or even too late – the more secure a foundation can be laid for a present and a future in which the digital environment is inseparable from any other environment. The forthcoming General Comment is required to fulfil ethical obligations to children. It is also a matter of practical necessity.

Notes

1. This chapter draws on a report produced by the authors that was commissioned and funded by the Office of the Children's Commissioner of England (Livingstone et al., 2017). The authors thank the children and experts who contributed their insights to this publication. See www.childrenscommissioner.gov.uk/wp-content/uploads/2017/06/Case-for-general-comment-on-digital-media.pdf.
2. See www.globalkidsonline.net.
3. Quotations from children in this chapter are taken from Third et al. (2017); see also UNICEF (2017). Children and adolescents aged 10–19 were consulted on their rights in the digital environment in in-depth, child-centred, multi-method workshops held in 26 countries concentrated in the Global South.
4. See UNCRC General Comments, Child Rights International Network (CRIN) (www.crin.org/en/library/publications/crc-general-comments).
5. See, for example, the resources available at the Global Commission on Internet Governance at www.ourinternet.org/research and the Internet Society at www.internetsociety.org/publications.
6. See www.consilium.europa.eu/en/meetings/fac/2017/03/st06846_en17_pdf.

References

Albury, K. (2017). Just because it's public doesn't mean it's any of your business: Adults' and children's sexual rights in digitally mediated spaces. *New Media & Society*, *19*(5), 713–725.

Council of Europe. (2019). *Rights of children with disabilities and the digital environment*. Strasbourg: Council of Europe. Retrieved from: www.coe.int/en/web/portal/-/-two-clicks-forward-and-one-click-back-children-with-disabilities-reveal-their-experiences-in-the-digital-environment.

Kleine, D., Hollow, D., & Poveda, S. (2014). Children, ICT and development: Capturing the potential, meeting the challenges. Florence: UNICEF Office of Research-Innocenti. Retrieved from: www.unicef-irc.org/publications/pdf/unicef_royalholloway_ict4dreport_final.Pdf.

La Rue, F. (2014). *Report of the Special Rapporteur on the promotion and protection of the right to freedom of opinion and expression*. A/69/335. United Nations General Assembly. Retrieved from: www.ohchr.org/en/issues/freedomopinion/pages/annual/aspx.

Lievens, E., Livingstone, S., McLaughlin, S., O'Neill, B., & Verdoodt, V. (2018). Children's rights and digital technologies. In T. Liefaard & U. Kilkelly (Eds.), *International children's rights law*. Berlin: Springer. doi:10.1007/978-981-10-3182-3_16-1. Retrieved from: http://eprints.lse.ac.uk/84871.

Livingstone, S., & Bulger, M. (2013). *A global agenda for children's rights in the digital age: Recommendations for developing UNICEF's research strategy*. Florence: UNICEF Office of Research. Retrieved from: www.unicef-irc.org/publications/702-a-global-agenda-for-childrens-rights-in-the-digital-age-recommendations-for-developing.html.

Livingstone, S., Carr, J., & Byrne, J. (2015). *One in three: The task for global internet governance in addressing children's rights*. Global Commission on Internet Governance, Paper Series. London: Centre for International Governance Innovation (CIGI) and Chatham House. Retrieved from: www.cigionline.org/publications/one-three-internet-governance-and-childrens-rights.

Livingstone, S., Kardefelt Winther, D., & Hussein, M. (2019). *Global kids online comparative report, Innocenti research report*. UNICEF Office of Research – Innocenti, Florence. Retrieved from: www.unicef-irc.org/publications/1059-global-kids-online-comparative-report.html.

Livingstone, S., Lansdown, G., & Third, A. (2017). *The case for a UNCRC General Comment on children's rights and digital media. A report prepared for the Children's Commissioner for England*. London: Office of the Children's Commissioner. Retrieved from: www.childrenscommissioner.gov.uk/publication/the-case-for-a-uncrc-general-comment-on-childrens-rights-and-digital-media.

Livingstone, S., Stoilova, M., & Nandagiri, R. (2018). *Children's data and privacy online: Growing up in a digital age. Evidence review*. London: London School of Economics and Political Science. Retrieved from: www.lse.ac.uk/media-and-communications/assets/documents/research/projects/childrens-privacy-online/Evidence-review-final.pdf.

Livingstone, S., & Third, A. (2017). Children and young people's rights in the digital age: An emerging agenda. *New Media & Society*, *19*(5), 657–670. Retrieved from: http://eprints.lse.ac.uk/68759.

Mansell, R. (2017). Inequality and digitally mediated communication: Divides, contradictions and consequences. *Javnost – The Public*, *24*, 146–161.

Mascheroni, G., & Holloway, D. (2019). *The internet of toys: Practices, affordances and the political economy of children's smart play*. Cham: Palgrave Macmillan.

O'Neill, B., Staksrud, E., & McLaughlin, S. (Eds.). (2013). *Children and internet safety in Europe: Policy debates and challenges*. Gothenburg, Sweden: Nordicom.

OHCHR (Office of the United Nations High Commissioner for Human Rights). (2014). *Committee on the rights of the child: Report of the 2014 Day of General Discussion "Digital media and children's rights"*. Retrieved from: www.ohchr.org/Documents/HRBodies/CRC/Discussions/2014/DGD_report.pdf.

Third, A., Bellerose, D., Dawkins, U., Keltie, E., & Pihl, K. (2014). *Children's rights in the digital age – A download from children around the world*. Melbourne, VIC: Young and Well Cooperative Research Centre. Retrieved from: www.westernsydney.edu.au/__data/assets/pdf_file/0003/753447/Childrens-rights-in-the-digital-age.pdf.

Third, A., Bellerose, D., Diniz de Oliveira, J., Lala, G., & Theakstone, G. (2017). *Young and online: Children's perspectives on life in the digital age (The state of the world's children 2017 companion report)*. Sydney, NSW: Western Sydney University. doi:10.4225/35/5a1b885f6d4db.

Third, A., & Collin, P. (2016). Rethinking (children's and young people's) citizenship through dialogues on digital practice. In A. McCosker, S. Vivienne, & A. Johns (Eds.), *Negotiating digital citizenship: Control, contest and culture* (pp. 41–60). London and New York, NY: Rowman & Littlefield.

Third, A., Livingstone, S., & Lansdown, G. (2019). Recognising children's rights in relation to digital technologies: Challenges of voice and evidence, principle and practice. In M. Kettermann, K. Vieth, & B. Wagner (Eds.), *Research handbook on human rights and digital technology* (pp. 376–410). London: Edward Elgar.

UN (United Nations). (1989). *Convention on the Rights of the Child*. Retrieved from: www.ohchr.org/Documents/ProfessionalInterest/crc.pdf.

UNICEF. (2017). *The State of the world's children 2017: Children in a digital world*. New York, NY: UNICEF. Retrieved from: www.unicef.org/publications/index_101992.html.

Wernham, M. (2016). *Mapping the global goals for sustainable development and the Convention on the Rights of the Child*. UNICEF. Retrieved from: www.unicef.org/agenda2030/files/SDG-CRC_mapping_FINAL.pdf.

PART V

Changing and Challenging Circumstances

37

CARING DATAVEILLANCE

Women's Use of Apps to Monitor Pregnancy and Children

Deborah Lupton

Introduction

Apps for pregnancy and motherhood are part of a wider group of digital technologies that have been grouped under the term 'femtech' (Rosas, 2019). Femtech incorporates a panoply of technologies directed at supporting women's health, including smartphone apps, wearable devices for self-tracking that have been designed specifically for women (often made to look like women's jewellery), digitised breast pumps, and insertible devices to help women master pelvic floor exercises (Lupton, 2016b; Rosas, 2019). While some femtech is targeted at women's general health, many devices focus on their reproductive health and fertility. Parents, and particularly mothers, are increasingly using digital media and devices to monitor the progress of pregnancy and the health and development of their children.

A plethora of apps is available for these purposes, including those designed for monitoring pregnancy and the health, development, and well-being of infants and young children (Barassi, 2017; Johnson, 2014; Lupton & Thomas, 2015; Thomas & Lupton, 2016). The vast majority of these apps are explicitly designed for the use of mothers, because it is assumed they are more interested and active in caring for infants and young children than are fathers. Monitoring opportunities related to foetal development begin from pre-conception, where devices and apps help women track their ovulation and menstrual cycles and prepare for conception by optimising the health of their bodies (Lupton, 2015, 2016b; Rosas, 2019; Wilkinson, Roberts, & Mort, 2015). Once pregnancy is achieved, another range of apps encourages women who are expecting a baby to monitor the development of their foetus, often involving customisation such as providing a name for the foetus and the expected date of delivery, and the opportunity to enter into the app details of doctors' visits and tests. Some apps allow women to monitor and record foetal movements and heartbeats (Lupton & Thomas, 2015; Thomas & Lupton, 2016). Many other apps are available for caregivers to track their infants' sleeping, feeding, growth, and development (Johnson, 2014; Leaver, 2017; Lupton & Williamson, 2017).

Only a small number of studies thus far have addressed how women during pregnancy and the early years of motherhood are using apps. Existing studies have shown that they are beginning to be used by women in countries as diverse as Germany (Goetz et al., 2017; Wallwiener et al., 2016), Ireland (O'Higgins et al., 2015), Turkey (Şat & Sozbİr, 2018), South Korea (Lee & Moon, 2016), China (Wang, Deng, Wen, Ding, & He, 2019), and the USA (Tomfohrde & Reinke, 2016) as well as Australia (Johnson, 2014; Rodger et al., 2013). The findings from these studies show that apps for pregnancy and parenting are appreciated by women in these countries to help them learn more about their bodies and those of their foetuses or children. However, few focus in great detail on how women use these apps for monitoring their pregnancies or their infants' health and development and how women feel about the apps.

This chapter examines and analyses the implications of these types of monitoring apps for women's experiences of pregnancy and the care of children, drawing on the findings of the researcher's two empirical studies involving Australian women. In doing so, two literatures – those on dataveillance and feminist new materialism – are brought together to offer new insights into digitised caring practices in relation to foetuses and children. The chapter begins with an overview of this scholarship before discussion of some of the key findings of the projects.

Dataveillance and Feminist New Materialism Theory

The term 'dataveillance' refers to conducting watching of people by gathering information about them, often these days using digital technologies to generate, store, and process these personal data (Clarke & Greenleaf, 2018; Raley, 2013; van Dijck, 2014). Digitised and other forms of surveillance are often understood in negative terms as an authoritarian restriction of autonomy and privacy of those who are being watched (Lupton, 2016a). In the wake of numerous scandals about the leaking or breaching of people's digital data, originating with Edward Snowden's 2013 revelations about the dataveillance of unwitting citizens by national security authorities in the USA, UK, Canada, and Australia (Lyon, 2014), many scholarly critiques of dataveillance have focussed on the negative features of dataveillance. They tend to adopt a view that positions it as repressive, invasive, or exploitative, conducted by those with power on less-powerful citizens (Andrejevic, 2013, 2014; Clarke & Greenleaf, 2018) as part of the digitised 'control society' (Best, 2010). This is a macro-political position on dataveillance which pays little attention to the micro-politics of how people live with and through devices and practices related to the datafication of their selves and bodies, and how they might seek to generate digital data about people with whom they have intimate and caring relationships (Lupton, 2018).

Dataveillance need not be conducted from an authoritarian, repressive, or coercive position, however. While these uses of people's personal data certainly exist and are worthy of critique, the more benign modes of dataveillance tend to be ignored. Many contemporary forms of dataveillance target children, from pre-birth into adolescence, including the use of apps by mothers for monitoring foetuses and young children as well as various forms of educational monitoring once children start attending school (Gard & Lupton, 2017; Lupton & Williamson, 2017). When dataveillance is employed as part of familial relationships and caring practices, the power dynamics can be very different. At the micro-political level, dataveillance conducted as part of intimate family relationships or other types of nurturing relationships can be an expression of love and attentiveness to others who need this kind of care because of illness (Essén, 2008) or physical dependency, including infants and children (Leaver, 2017; Levy, 2015) and companion animals (Richardson, Hjorth, Strengers, & Balmford, 2017).

Richardson and colleagues (2017) have drawn attention to what they entitle the 'careful surveillance' undertaken of companion animals by the humans who live with them, some of whom use at-home monitoring cameras to check on the activities of both their children and their pets. This chapter adopts instead the term 'caring dataveillance' as a means of working across the concepts of dataveillance and caring practices as they are experienced in and with the use of apps for pregnancy and parenting. Caring is used as a term instead of careful, as the author wanted to clarify that the practices are about engaging in care, whereas the word careful has multiple meanings (including being cautious). The term 'dataveillance' was used instead of 'surveillance' to signal that the watching involved uses digital data.

Adopting a feminist materialist perspective draws attention to these material dimensions of these forms of dataveillance by acknowledging the more-than-human worlds in which intimate relationships such as those between mothers and their children are conducted. Human bodies/selves are viewed as entangled with other humans and with nonhumans such as digital technologies, and as unbounded and emergent (Barad, 2007; Bennett, 2004, 2010; Braidotti, 2016; Haraway, 2016). These human-nonhuman assemblages configure a 'thing-power' (Bennett, 2004) that is dynamic and contingent on the time and space through and in which humans move and the other humans, other living creatures, and objects with which they come into contact. Working together, humans and nonhumans generate thing-power. Relational connections, affective forces, digital and bodily affordances, and agential capacities are part of this thing-power, inspiring and enacting action, knowledge, and responses. This perspective invites considerations of caring practices that acknowledge that they are more-than-human and more-than-digital. Viewed through the lens of feminist new materialism approaches, dataveillance involves continually changing assemblages of humans–technologies–data as humans learn to become and live with data (Lupton, 2018).

Details of Projects

Findings from two research projects involving Australian women are discussed in this chapter.

Project 1, 'Australian Women's Use of Digital Media for Pregnancy and Parenting', involved a survey and focus groups with women who were either pregnant at the time they participated or caring for a young child aged three or younger. The online survey was completed in late 2014 by 410 women around Australia. The participants were diverse in terms of their ethnicity and geographical location (from all states and territories of Australia, including rural regions), but had higher levels of education compared with the Australian population as a whole. The survey found that almost three-quarters of respondents said that they were using pregnancy apps, while half reported using a parenting app (Lupton & Pedersen, 2016). Following the survey, a focus group study was conducted in mid-2015 in Sydney, involving four groups with a total of 36 Sydney women. The focus groups were designed to follow up in more detail why women used pregnancy and parenting apps and other digital media and devices. These women were also mostly university educated (findings are outlined in Lupton, 2016c, 2017).

Project 2, 'Australian Women and Digital Health' took place between late 2016 and mid-2017. It included women living across Australia and at a range of life-stages in interviews and focus groups, and had a broader focus, asking them about their use of digital technologies for health-related purposes. A total of 66 women participants across Project 2 were involved in either interviews or focus groups about their use of digital health technologies. Among the participants were women who were pregnant or caring for young children, including two focus groups of mothers with infants. It is these participants' experiences with digital health related to pregnancy and parenting that are discussed in this chapter (overviews of findings from all participants can be found in Lupton, 2019; Lupton & Maslen, 2019), together with the focus group discussions from Project 1. Combining qualitative investigations from both projects allows for an analysis that incorporates women's experiences elicited between mid-2015 and mid-2017 in different geographical locations.

Findings

Across the focus groups and interviews conducted for the two different projects, it emerged that using digital media for pregnancy and parenting, as well as for general health-related purposes, was very common. The findings of Project 1 revealed that digital media were very important to the participants. They used mobile apps, social media, content-sharing platforms and online discussion forums to connect with each other and with family members, post images and other information about their pregnancy and children, track their pregnancy or their children's behaviours and development, and learn about pregnancy, infants, and childcare. They commented that they were constantly googling to find information about their children. Project 2, which included women across the life-stages, revealed that all of them, regardless of their age, went online to look for health-related information not just for themselves but for their partners and family members, including young and adult children, grandchildren, and elderly parents. The women were highly digitally engaged in their health- and caring-related practices, willing and able to conform to the ideal of the self-responsible citizen who not only managed her own health but also that of her family members.

Both projects found that many participants who were pregnant or caring for infants and young children had used pregnancy or parenting apps. Participants also talked about using period and ovulation tracking apps when they were trying to conceive. This practice had encouraged them to carefully monitor their own bodies in the effort to achieve conception, almost to the point of obsession, as some of the women in a focus group (Project 2) noted.

Participant: I was very diligent with recording my health when I was trying to get pregnant. So, you can use an app to record like literally daily symptoms of like, put in your period and then all kinds of – if there's any signs of discharge, if you've got a temperature, you put in all of your details and it tells you when you are at your most fertile.

Participant: I got a bit obsessive about it. I was told that I wouldn't be able to fall pregnant, so I was like obsessively putting information in and checking it. And I don't think I would want to use it again, because it was a bit – I was a bit addicted to it.

Participant: I was using it daily and ticking if I took my vitamins and ticking off this and that, and it kind of make trying to fall pregnant very scientific and mechanical and it wasn't fun. For me it was all about having a baby.

Women in both projects who were pregnant or had young children had used apps for tracking the progress of their pregnancy and finding information (apps such as Ovia and What to Expect When You're Expecting), child vaccination records, infant development monitoring (in particular, the Wonder Weeks app), and parenting advice (for example, Baby Center). These apps served a combination of information provision and generating new data about their infants' health and development. Some participants mentioned pregnancy apps, including those that showed the size of the foetus as it grew, comparing it with fruit as a way of helping users conceptualise the foetus in visual terms. Women who used these kinds of apps described how the apps helped them to develop a relationship and bond with their foetuses and generate a sense of excitement about their pregnancy.

Participant: I think it was Pregnancy [app], the one that tracks your – you know, how far along you are, what's happening, what's happening with baby. Yeah, because it kind of made me feel excited as well, month by month seeing baby grow and all that kind of stuff.

Participant: I like the app where it says, 'the baby's the size of an avocado'. Like that sort of inspires me, it just makes it a little bit – because you can't see [the foetus] and when it's early you can't necessarily feel it – so it just kind of – I'm a visual person, so it just helps. (Project 1)

Some of the new mothers in one of the focus groups in Project 2 had a conversation in which they talked about apps for tracking feeding, nappy changes, and sleep. They said that they found these apps helpful because "we're still new mums", as one woman put it, and "you're just so tired all the time" as another added. A participant in this group went on to note that apps for tracking their babies can be helpful when they are dealing with trying to note the routines and behaviour of their babies:

> You're thinking about so many different things, it's so easy to forget to look at the clock when they get up from their sleep. Or yeah, to pay attention to the clock. So it can really help if you're like, 'Why are you [the baby] cranky? Maybe you're tired?'... So it gives you that information that you might not have kind of been able to keep track of yourself.

These participants went on to describe how they were 'offloading information' from their brains to the app, "so you don't have to rely on your brain so much". One woman said that if she went to a child health centre for her baby's check-up and was asked how many nappies she went through a day, she could pull out her phone and check it on the app. These participants described inputting these data in the middle of the night, when changing or feeding their babies, or first thing in the morning.

In a different focus group in Project 2, another participant described the distress and tiredness she had experienced in dealing with her new baby's needs. For this woman, using infant monitoring apps was a significant means of coping with these feelings and managing the chaos of her life. Using digitised monitoring of what appeared to be highly unpredictable and mysterious behaviour of the infant helped her to gain an understanding of her baby's needs and patterns, as well as working towards finding some respite from lack of sleep.

> Like when your baby's screaming when you try to put him to sleep and you don't realise you'd only fed him two hours ago, so it's gone from screaming because he doesn't want to sleep to screaming, 'I'm hungry!' By inputting all that into the apps, like I know when it was changed last week, when it fed last, how long it slept during the day, if it's teething, then it sleeps less or if it's having a good day, it sleeps more. It's really good for understanding what's going on with the baby. Yeah, so I – at the moment I just do it for sleep because I'm obsessed with sleep as most mothers are and you can just like – so for me, it makes it easy to see like if he's a bit cranky, I'll look at the phone and 'Oh yeah, he's due for a nap'. So, he has a pattern that's emerged so he can only really stay awake for two hours before he gets tired. But otherwise I would lose track of that.

Several women in both projects made specific mention of using the Wonder Weeks app, which provides information on the cognitive development of infants in terms of 'leaps' and how this affects their behaviour. The women found this app reassuring, as it helped to explain why their infants may be particularly unsettled:

Participant: So I don't have the notifications on it or anything, but if [my baby's] been real crazy, shitty for no apparent reason, sometimes I'll check that and be like, 'Oh she's going through a developmental leap this week and I don't have to worry about it – she's okay, so she's not sick or anything, she's just having a mental growth spurt'. Which is great.
Participant: Yeah, it's reassurance isn't it?
Participant: Yeah, it's reassuring to be like, 'Oh!' And it makes sense because they change so much!
Participant: It's happened to me a couple of times, where I just genuinely do not know what's wrong with this child. And then you're thinking, 'Is she teething, is she sick, is there is she constipated?' Then you'll [think], OK, well she's going through a leap so that is probably the reason. (Project 2)

It was evident from the focus group discussions that new mothers spend far less time thinking about their own health or searching for information about it online, as they are currently preoccupied with their infants' health and well-being. As one woman in Project 2 explained:

> I know if I'm not feeling well, whereas with [my baby] I don't know. Is he just being a baby or is he unwell? Is there something wrong? Whereas with myself, I know if I've got a cold or whatever. So it's much more about him than about me.

Those women who had been using self-tracking apps to monitor their health and fitness before the birth of their babies said that since the birth they have not been interested in using these devices because their attention has been diverted to their infants' health and well-being. Their lives had changed so significantly that there was no longer any time or interest in continuing these practices. Their self-monitoring had become devolved to monitoring of their infants' bodies.

Affective responses were key to women's explanations of their relinquishment of self-tracking. One woman in a Project 2 focus group noted that she had de-activated a fitness tracking app on her phone because she kept receiving notifications from it that she had not reached her goals, and she simply wasn't able to engage any more. Other participants in the same focus group agreed that such apps 'make you feel bad about yourself' or 'guilty'. One woman suggested that there should be a 'baby option' programmed in the app ('like holiday mode') that changed expectations about step counts or calories expended for new mothers:

> Like [my baby's] having a clingy day today. I could barely put him down this morning. As if I'm going to get 10,000 steps!

The participants in this group also commented that they didn't want to track their sleep, because it would simply be too confronting to document exactly how badly they slept when they were disturbed by the needs of their infants. As they found it difficult to eat meals at regular times and to ensure they were eating nutritious food, these women also didn't see a reason to track their own food intake. They felt as if they had not yet 'had their body back' and it was difficult to return to the same kinds of fitness routines or eating habits they kept up before becoming pregnant, because they now had to respond to the demands and needs of their babies.

> I'd like to be able to go out for runs in the morning like I used to, but I can't, because most of the time we're still asleep because that's his best sleep, around 7 a.m. Then I can't leave him at home and I can't go running with him. So I don't go running.

One focus group in Project 2 included women who were struggling with mental health conditions, such as post-natal anxiety. They suggested that an app that sent them friendly, supportive reminders to care or take time for themselves and their own health and well-being would be an ideal replacement for the self-tracking apps they had given up using.

Participant: It'd be nice if you had someone to just – if you could put an app on your phone that sends you really lovely friendly messages that were just sporadic reminders to drink water.
Participant: Just like …
Participant: Eat something healthy today.
Participant: That didn't make you feel bad about yourself.

Discussion

Any discussion of the ethics of caring needs to acknowledge that the agential capacities generated in and through these practices can both open and restrict freedoms for the watched subjects and those who engage in watching (Puig de la Bellacasa, 2017). As Richardson et al. (2017) point out, this form of monitoring may be asymmetrical and non-reciprocal, involving the watching of one subject by another, but it is also 'careful', incorporating both caring affects and practices and notions of maintaining responsibility for the close monitoring of the health, safety, and well-being of those humans or nonhumans under one's care. Richardson and colleagues call for attention to be paid to the ethics of how this digitised form of care is achieved, and the tension between care and the restriction of freedom of those who are subjected to dataveillance.

The findings of the two projects provide insights into women's experiences of engaging in dataveillance related to pregnancy and motherhood using apps. Using pregnancy and child monitoring apps, as well as other forms of digital media such as social media and online discussion forums, women can actively generate information about their foetuses and children. They are not simply passively accessing information, therefore, but creating very personal datasets about their children, some of which may be shared with others online. Expectations that women should aspire to the ideal of the 'good' mother who seeks out knowledge and intensely monitors the health and well-being of her foetus or children existed for decades prior to the emergence of digital technologies. However, the close and continual tracking that digital media such as apps can offer provides new opportunities for women to practise this kind of caring labour, as well as manage the often chaotic and physically demanding experiences of living with infants.

The broader sociocultural context in which these apps are developed and marketed is that in which foetuses and young children are represented as vulnerable and precious, requiring high levels of care and attention to protect them from harm, and where the 'good mother' takes steps to do so (Doshi, 2018; Johnson, 2014; Lupton, 2012, 2014, 2016b). Women in their reproductive and child-caring life stages are under intense pressure to conform to the ideal of the 'digitised reproductive citizen' who takes responsibility for finding, generating, and using digitised information about pregnancy and childcare in the interests of protecting and promoting their health, development, and well-being (Lupton, 2016b). Critical analysis of the content of pregnancy and parenting apps has demonstrated that they tend to reproduce and reinforce these norms and expectations about 'good' mothers (Barassi, 2017; Doshi, 2018; Lupton, 2016b; Lupton & Thomas, 2015; Thomas & Lupton, 2016). In her analysis of apps designed specifically for women, for example, Doshi (2018) noted that the subject position of the 'earth goddess' was frequently portrayed in apps for pregnancy and motherhood. This archetype promoted the normative feminine body as naturally fertile, maternal, and devoted to caring for others. Lupton and Thomas' analysis of pregnancy apps (Lupton & Thomas, 2015; Thomas & Lupton, 2016) found that the app visuals tended to aestheticise pregnancy and the foetal subject, and represented foetuses as already infants that required the greatest of care and attention from women to protect them from harm. Pregnancy was simultaneously presented as a joyous and exciting experience and replete with risks that must be assiduously avoided.

Digital devices, in these contexts, become part of the materialities of care, or the spaces and things that are imbricated in and with caring labour and caring affects (Brownlie & Spandler, 2018; Buse, Martin, & Nettleton, 2018). The projects' findings demonstrate the centrality of relational connections such as those between a woman and her unborn or her children to the thing-power of these digitised assemblages. Affective forces such as the desire for better knowledge and understanding of their foetuses and babies as well as for intimacy and to successfully perform caring impelled and were generated in and through women's app use. Women often took up pregnancy or parenting monitoring apps to counter their feelings of anxiety, inadequacy, uncertainty, fatigue, and loss of control, and they reported that apps helped them manage and cope with these affects.

The women's use of these types of apps enabled them to perform acts of maternal caring by actively preparing their bodies for pregnancy and monitoring the progress of pregnancy and the behaviours and well-being of their infants. The apps helped women develop a sense of connection with their foetuses and build on their relationships with their infants, supporting them to better know and understand their foetuses and children. When women were dealing with the unpredictable and changeable behaviour of their infants, apps that could discern patterns in the babies' behaviours and emotional responses enabled them to feel reassured and more confident in a context in which their own bodies were struggling with tiredness and coping with the unfamiliar physical demands of providing care to a new infant. Some of this intense work, including monitoring infants and remembering when they should be next fed, or put down for a nap, could be devolved to the app.

These findings, therefore, also demonstrate the shared capacities of dataveillance that involve entanglements of sensory and technological capacities between women, foetus or infant, device and the data that were generated in and with these assemblages. Maternal caring involves a set of interembodied practices and affects that is distributed between the foetal/infant body and that of the mother (Lupton, 2013a, 2013b). By using monitoring apps to track their reproductive cycles, pregnancies, and infants' bodies, women were simultaneously monitoring themselves and their children. Caring dataveillance, in this context, was much more than vigilant watching on the part of women to protect the health of their children. It was a practice directed at attempting to regain a sense of control over their lives and lessen some of the burden of caring labour. In this way, caring dataveillance could engender some forms of self-care, while closing off others. For some women, previous habits of self-tracking their bodies were re-directed to their babies' bodies. They had become aware that their lives and bodies had changed so much that these apps were no longer useful and were generating distressing affects of guilt and shame, emphasising the negative ways in which their lives had changed following the birth of their infants.

As the findings demonstrate, when the participants became mothers, the focus on conducting dataveillance on their own bodies shifted to the bodies of their infants. Indeed, their capacity to engage in self-surveillance of their own bodies became limited, as their interests and energies became absorbed into attempting to understand their babies' behaviours and meeting their needs. The dataveillance apps generated good but also bad feelings. In this context, the thing-power of the apps worked positively towards enhancing the caring surveillance of pregnancies and infants but against dataveillance of the post-birth body. One solution to this, as suggested by the focus group of women coping with mental health conditions, was an imagined app that would encourage new mothers to turn their attention for a while away from their infants and focus again on themselves, encouraging a benevolent and supportive mode of self-caring dataveillance.

Acknowledgement

The funding for both projects was provided to the author by the University of Canberra as part of her Centenary Professor appointment.

References

Andrejevic, M. (2013). *Infoglut: How too much information is changing the way we think and know*. New York, NY: Routledge.

Andrejevic, M. (2014). The big data divide. *International Journal of Communication, 8*, 1673–1689.

Barad, K. (2007). *Meeting the universe halfway: Quantum physics and the entanglement of matter and meaning*. Durham, NC: Duke University Press.

Barassi, V. (2017). BabyVeillance? Expecting parents, online surveillance and the cultural specificity of pregnancy apps. *Social Media + Society*, *3*(2). Retrieved from: https://journals.sagepub.com/doi/full/10.1177/2056305117707188.

Bennett, J. (2004). The force of things: Steps toward an ecology of matter. *Political Theory*, *32*(3), 347–372.

Bennett, J. (2010). A vitalist stopover on the way to a new materialism. In D. Coole & S. Frost (Eds.), *New materialisms. Ontology, agency and politics* (pp. 47–69). Durham, NC and London: Duke University Press.

Best, K. (2010). Living in the control society: Surveillance, users and digital screen technologies. *International Journal of Cultural Studies*, *13*(1), 5–24.

Braidotti, R. (2016). Posthuman critical theory. In D. Banerji & M. Paranjape (Eds.), *Critical posthumanism and planetary futures* (pp. 13–32). Berlin: Springer.

Brownlie, J., & Spandler, H. (2018). Materialities of mundane care and the art of holding one's own. *Sociology of Health & Illness*, *40*(2), 256–269.

Buse, C., Martin, D., & Nettleton, S. (2018). Conceptualising 'materialities of care': Making visible mundane material culture in health and social care contexts. *Sociology of Health & Illness*, *40*(2), 243–255.

Clarke, R., & Greenleaf, G. (2018). Dataveillance regulation: A research framework. *Journal of Law and Information Science*, *25*(1). Retrieved from: www.scribd.com/document/371829503/Dataveillance-Regulation-A-Research-Framework-Roger-Clarke-and-Graham-Greenleaf#fullscreen=1.

Doshi, M. J. (2018). Barbies, goddesses, and entrepreneurs: Discourses of gendered digital embodiment in women's health apps. *Women's Studies in Communication*, *41*(2), 183–203.

Essén, A. (2008). The two facets of electronic care surveillance: An exploration of the views of older people who live with monitoring devices. *Social Science & Medicine*, *67*(1), 128–136.

Gard, M., & Lupton, D. (2017). Digital health goes to school: Implications of digitising children's bodies. In E. Taylor & T. Rooney (Eds.), *Surveillance futures: Social and ethical implications of new technologies for children and young people* (pp. 36–49). London: Routledge.

Goetz, M., Muller, M., Matthies, L. M., Hansen, J., Doster, A., Szabo, A., & Wallwiener, S. (2017). Perceptions of patient engagement applications during pregnancy: A qualitative assessment of the patient's perspective. *JMIR mHealth and uHealth*, *5*(5). Retrieved from: http://mhealth.jmir.org/2017/5/e73.

Haraway, D. (2016). *Staying with the trouble: Making kin in the Chthulucene*. Durham, NC: Duke University Press.

Johnson, S. (2014). "Maternal devices", social media and the self-management of pregnancy, mothering and child health. *Societies*, *4*(2), 330–350.

Leaver, T. (2017). Intimate surveillance: Normalizing parental monitoring and mediation of infants online. *Social Media + Society*, *3*(2). Retrieved from: https://journals.sagepub.com/doi/full/10.1177/2056305117707192.

Lee, Y., & Moon, M. (2016). Utilization and content evaluation of mobile applications for pregnancy, birth, and child care. *Healthcare Informatics Research*, *22*(2), 73–80.

Levy, K. (2015). Intimate surveillance. *Idaho Law Review*, 679. Retrieved from: www.uidaho.edu/law/law-review/articles.

Lupton, D. (2012). 'Precious cargo': Risk and reproductive citizenship. *Critical Public Health*, *22*(3), 329–340.

Lupton, D. (2013a). Infant embodiment and interembodiment: A review of sociocultural perspectives. *Childhood*, *20*(1), 37–50.

Lupton, D. (2013b). *The social worlds of the unborn*. Houndmills: Palgrave Macmillan.

Lupton, D. (2014). Precious, pure, uncivilised, vulnerable: Infant embodiment in Australian popular media. *Children and Society*, *28*(5), 341–351.

Lupton, D. (2015). Quantified sex: A critical analysis of sexual and reproductive self-tracking using apps. *Culture, Health & Sexuality*, *17*(4), 440–453.

Lupton, D. (2016a). The diverse domains of quantified selves: Self-tracking modes and dataveillance. *Economy and Society*, *45*(1), 101–122.

Lupton, D. (2016b). 'Mastering your fertility': The digitised reproductive citizen. In A. McCosker, S. Vivienne, & A. Johns (Eds.), *Negotiating digital citizenship: Control, contest and culture* (pp. 81–93). London: Rowman & Littlefield.

Lupton, D. (2016c). The use and value of digital media for information about pregnancy and early motherhood: A focus group study. *BMC Pregnancy and Childbirth*, *16*(1), 171. Retrieved from: https://bmcpregnancychildbirth.biomedcentral.com/articles/10.1186/s12884-016-0971-3.

Lupton, D. (2017). 'It just gives me a bit of peace of mind': Australian women's use of digital media for pregnancy and early motherhood. *Societies*, *7*(3). Retrieved from: www.mdpi.com/2075-4698/7/3/25.

Lupton, D. (2018). How do data come to matter? Living and becoming with personal data. *Big Data & Society*, *5*(2). Retrieved from: https://journals.sagepub.com/doi/full/10.1177/2053951718786314.

Lupton, D. (2019). *The Australian women and digital health project: Comprehensive report of findings*. Retrieved from: https://apo.org.au/node/220326.

Lupton, D., & Maslen, S. (2019). How women use digital technologies for health: Qualitative interview and focus group study. *Journal of Medical Internet Research*, *21*(1). Retrieved from: www.jmir.org/2019/1/e11481.

Lupton, D., & Pedersen, S. (2016). An Australian survey of women's use of pregnancy and parenting apps. *Women and Birth*, *29*(4), 368–374.

Lupton, D., & Thomas, G. M. (2015). Playing pregnancy: The ludification and gamification of expectant motherhood in smartphone apps. *M/C Journal*, *18*(5). Retrieved from: http://journal.media-culture.org.au/index.php/mcjournal/article/viewArticle/1012.

Lupton, D., & Williamson, B. (2017). The datafied child: The dataveillance of children and implications for their rights. *New Media & Society*, *19*(5), 780–794.

Lyon, D. (2014). Surveillance, snowden, and big data: Capacities, consequences, critique. *Big Data & Society*, *1*(2). Retrieved from: http://bds.sagepub.com/content/1/2/2053951714541861.

O'Higgins, A., Murphy, O., Egan, A., Mullaney, L., Sheehan, S., & Turner, M. (2015). The use of digital media by women using the maternity services in a developed country. *Irish Medical Journal*, *108*(10), 313–315.

Puig de la Bellacasa, M. (2017). *Matters of care: Speculative ethics in more than human worlds*. Minneapolis, MN: University of Minnesota Press.

Raley, R. (2013). Dataveillance and countervailance. In L. Gitelman (Ed.), *"Raw data" is an oxymoron* (pp. 121–145). Cambridge, MA: MIT Press.

Richardson, I., Hjorth, L., Strengers, Y., & Balmford, W. (2017). Careful surveillance at play: Human-animal relations and mobile media in the home. In E. G. Cruz, S. Sumartojo, & S. Pink (Eds.), *Refiguring techniques in digital visual research* (pp. 105–116). Houndmills: Palgrave Macmillian.

Rodger, D., Skuse, A., Wilmore, M., Humphreys, S., Dalton, J., Flabouris, M., & Clifton, V. L. (2013). Pregnant women's use of information and communications technologies to access pregnancy-related health information in South Australia. *Australian Journal of Primary Health*, *19*(4), 308–312.

Rosas, C. (2019). The future is femtech: Privacy and data security issues surrounding femtech applications. *Hastings Business Law Journal*, *15*(2), 319.

Şat, S. Ö., & Sozbİr, Ş. Y. (2018). Use of mobile applications and blogs by pregnant women in Turkey and the impact on adaptation to pregnancy. *Midwifery*, *62*(July 2018), 273–277.

Thomas, G. M., & Lupton, D. (2016). Threats and thrills: Pregnancy apps, risk and consumption. *Health, Risk & Society*, *17*(7–8), 495–509.

Tomfohrde, O. J., & Reinke, J. S. (2016). Breastfeeding mothers' use of technology while breastfeeding. *Computers in Human Behavior*, *64*, 556–561.

van Dijck, J. (2014). Datafication, dataism and dataveillance: Big data between scientific paradigm and ideology. *Surveillance & Society*, *12*(2), 197–208.

Wallwiener, S., Müller, M., Doster, A., Laserer, W., Reck, C., Pauluschke-Fröhlich, J., & Wallwiener, M. (2016). Pregnancy eHealth and mHealth: User proportions and characteristics of pregnant women using web-based information sources – a cross-sectional study. *Archives of Gynecology and Obstetrics*, *294*(5), 937–944.

Wang, N., Deng, Z., Wen, L. M., Ding, Y., & He, G. (2019). Understanding the use of smartphone apps for health information among pregnant Chinese women: Mixed methods study. *JMIR Mhealth Uhealth*, *7*(6). Retrieved from: http://mhealth.jmir.org/2019/6/e12631.

Wilkinson, J., Roberts, C., & Mort, M. (2015). Ovulation monitoring and reproductive heterosex: Living the conceptive imperative? *Culture, Health & Sexuality*, *17*(4), 454–469.

38
DIGITAL MEDIA AND SLEEP IN CHILDREN

Alicia Allan and Simon Smith

Introduction

Digital media are a ubiquitous part of modern childhood. The integration of digital devices into all aspects of daily life means that the potential benefits and opportunities of digital media are accompanied by, and tempered against, concerns regarding the impact on children's social, emotional, and cognitive development. Healthy sleep is a fundamental component of well-being in childhood, and children have a high need for sleep. Current recommendations suggest that healthy sleep durations gradually reduce from 12–16 hours (per 24 hours) in children aged 4–12 months, to 10–13 hours for children aged 3–5, and 8–10 hours for teenagers (Paruthi et al., 2016). Sleep gradually consolidates across the early childhood years as children reduce their daytime napping and achieve the majority of their sleep at night (Galland, Taylor, Elder, & Herbison, 2012).

Sleep is integral to many social, emotional, and cognitive dimensions of growth and development, and poor or disrupted sleep has been associated with poorer health, well-being, and educational outcomes (Chaput et al., 2016). Sleep quality, duration, timing, and regularity can each affect a child's developmental trajectory, with immediate and long-term consequences for everyday behaviour, learning, and health (Miller, Kruisbrink, Wallace, Ji, & Cappuccio, 2018; Quach, Hiscock, Canterford, & Wake, 2009; Sadeh, Gruber, & Raviv, 2002; Vriend et al., 2013). New learning, in particular, strongly depends on processes of memory consolidation and generalisation that occur during sleep (Gómez & Edgin, 2015). For these reasons, good sleep in childhood needs to be protected and promoted.

Available evidence suggests a relationship between increased digital media use and poor sleep in children. Two systematic reviews (Cain & Gradisar, 2010; Hale & Guan, 2015) and subsequent meta-analyses (Bartel, Gradisar, & Williamson, 2015; Carter, Rees, Hale, Bhattacharjee, & Paradkar, 2016) have found that children with greater exposure to screen media in the evening hours show significantly shorter night-time sleep duration, poorer sleep quality, and increased daytime sleepiness when compared with those with no, or little, evening screen exposure. Further, preliminary intervention evidence suggests that reducing evening screen use can improve sleep in adolescents (Perrault et al., 2019). A number of potential mechanisms have been proposed to explain this relationship, however the causal evidence base for these mechanisms is still developing (LeBourgeois et al., 2017). This chapter describes pathways via which digital media may impact sleep in children, summarises available evidence regarding each of these mechanisms, and outlines limitations in order to inform future research. Although this chapter focusses on children up to early adolescence, findings in adolescent and adult populations are discussed when they illustrate plausible pathways and where data is scarce for younger groups.

Possible Mechanisms

Experiences across the entire waking day can influence children's night-time sleep, but the period just before sleep is particularly important (Mindell & Williamson, 2018). Digital media exposure in the evening could negatively impact children's sleep via three potential mechanisms (Hale et al., 2018; LeBourgeois et al., 2017). These are a) increased evening light exposure; b) pre-sleep arousal; and c) sleep displacement. Currently, none have a strong causal evidence base in children, however many of the underlying processes are supported by considerable experimental and observational evidence. Figure 38.1 shows these predicted processes, each of which could work independently or together to affect sleep quantity, quality, timing, and regularity.

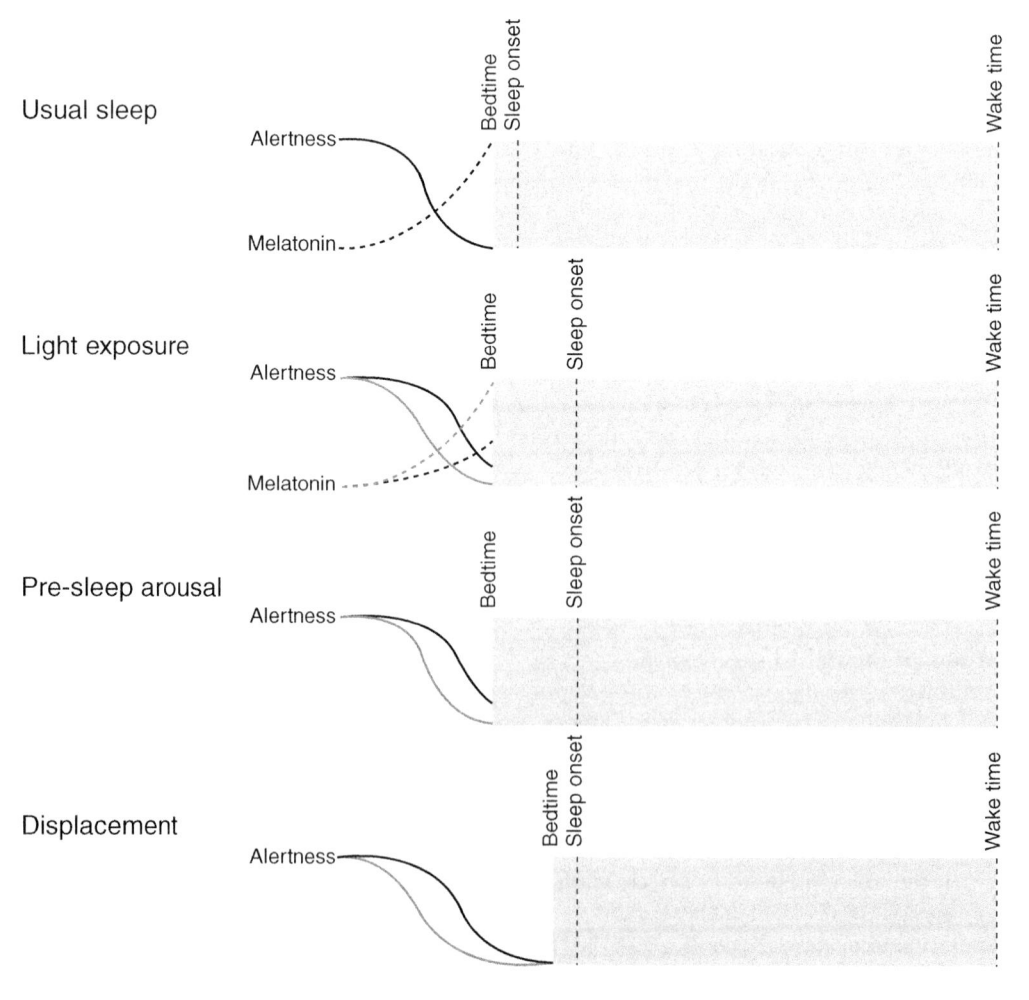

Figure 38.1 Possible mechanisms for disruption to sleep onset from digital media.

Light Exposure

Light from digital media may directly interfere with sleep onset and indirectly affect circadian (body clock) timing in children. The human physiological system has evolved to synchronise with a natural light–dark cycle that is very bright during the day and very dark at night (Smolensky, Sackett-Lundeen, & Portaluppi, 2015). In contrast, the light environment experienced by many children in their homes and bedrooms bears little resemblance to that natural state. Daytime has been effectively extended by the use of ambient artificial lighting, by at least several hours in the wintertime (Stothard et al., 2017), and this extension has likely been exacerbated by the proliferation of light-emitting electronic devices (Gringras, Middleton, Skene, & Revell, 2015). People's non-visual circadian system is particularly sensitive to the *type* of light emitted from these devices, which is rich in short (blue) wavelengths (Cajochen et al., 2011; Lucas et al., 2014; Zeitzer, Dijk, Kronauer, Brown, & Czeisler, 2000). Children also use devices close to their eyes (and therefore light receptors) relative to other ambient sources such as ceiling lights, increasing the relative 'dose' of biologically meaningful light that is received (Gringras et al., 2015).

The effect of evening light exposure from digital devices is twofold. First, bright light is directly alerting and, second, light acts to delay the body's internal clock. The immediate effects of light on alertness and cognitive performance are well-demonstrated in adults (Lok, Smolders, Beersma, & de Kort, 2018; Souman, Tinga, te Pas, van Ee, & Vlaskamp, 2018) and a smaller, but sound, body of evidence demonstrates these same effects in children (e.g., Hartstein, LeBourgeois, & Berthier, 2018). Acute alerting effects can be desirable during the day, however in the evening they directly conflict with sleep initiation which ordinarily requires darkness.

Indirectly, light can influence sleep by delaying the timing of children's internal body clock. The circadian rhythm is a fundamental physiological rhythm that drives daily patterns of rest and activity, as well as many other biological and metabolic processes (Roenneberg, Kantermann, Vetter, & Allebrandt, 2013). Light is the primary input to this body clock and can directly shift the circadian rhythm in and out of synchrony with the outside world (Duffy & Wright, 2005). In both children and adults, the hormone melatonin starts to rise in the hours before bedtime, marking the onset of pre-sleep processes (Benloucif et al., 2005). The release of melatonin also acts to synchronise the central clock with other 'clocks' distributed throughout the body (LeBourgeois et al., 2013). Exposure to light suppresses the normal evening release of melatonin and can delay the timing of the internal clock (Zeitzer et al., 2000). This delay means that children may only feel sleepy later in the evening, resulting in later sleep onset and morning wake-up times. Because wake-up times are often fixed by regular daily commitments such as carer work routines and attendance at childcare or school, delayed sleep onset can result in shorter overall sleep duration (see the second bar in Figure 38.1).

Experimental studies have shown that bright evening light does suppress melatonin production in pre-school-age children (delaying the internal clock and associated sleepiness; Akacem, Wright, & LeBourgeois, 2018), and that a delayed internal clock is associated with later bedtimes in children (Akacem, Wright, & LeBourgeois, 2016). Therefore, light from devices could be similarly disruptive. In adults, reading on a device before bed reduces sleepiness and delays deep sleep onset when compared with reading a physical book (Grønli et al., 2016). Consistent with this, light from a tablet device is sufficient to suppress evening melatonin release in adolescents following an hour of use in the evening, with longer duration linked to increased suppression (Figueiro & Overington, 2016). Duration of screen time after 9 p.m. has also been associated with later melatonin onset in adolescents (Perrault et al., 2019). Available evidence suggests that children and adolescents are *more* sensitive to the effects of light than are adults (Crowley, Cain,

Burns, Acebo, & Carskadon, 2015; Higuchi, Lee, Kozaki, & Harada, 2016), such that light from digital devices may have an even greater effect on their sleep.

This underlying mechanism for sleep disruption has a strong causal evidence base, particularly in adults and adolescents. However, emitted light varies considerably based on device type, brightness settings, and the content on the screen (Gringras et al., 2015). As yet, the meaningful impact of light from habitual device use on children's sleep outcomes is unknown. The effect of light before sleep can be reduced by minimising its intensity (by reducing brightness settings), reducing the amount of short/blue wavelengths emitted, and changing its timing (reducing both overall exposure duration and exposure close to bedtime) (Figueiro & Overington, 2016; Gringras et al., 2015; Nagare, Plitnick, & Figueiro, 2018).

Pre-Sleep Arousal

While light emission from digital devices raises concerns regarding hardware, there are equally plausible effects from device content. Sleep initiation occurs following a complex set of interrelated psychological and physiological transitions that involve a gradual decrease in arousal, and eventually sleep (Ogilvie, 2001). Recommendations around bedtime routines and 'sleep hygiene' (principles of good sleep habits) generally target the pre-bed period, in which children should be withdrawing from the emotional and cognitive attachments and demands of the outside world (Mindell & Williamson, 2018). Sleep hygiene practices aim to block out or limit external and internal stimuli (both physical and psychological). In contrast, some device-mediated activities may induce pre-sleep arousal, a psychologically or physiologically stimulated state that makes it difficult to subsequently initiate sleep (Bootzin & Epstein, 2011). In this case, even if bedtime is not delayed, children may take longer to fall asleep once in bed, reducing overall sleep time (see bar three in Figure 38.1). Higher levels of reported pre-sleep arousal (particularly cognitive arousal) have been associated with sleep disturbance in children aged 8–10 years (Gregory et al., 2008). Changing media content *type* without altering overall screen time has been shown to affect sleep (Garrison & Christakis, 2012). Activities that induce a high level of anxiety or psychological arousal, regardless of their format, are very likely to interfere with a child's ability to fall asleep (Garrison, Liekweg, & Christakis, 2011).

A number of studies have demonstrated connections between social media use and pre-sleep arousal. In a study assessing pre-bed behaviours in adolescents, pre-sleep arousal partially mediated the relationship between social media use and time taken to fall asleep (Harbard, Allen, Trinder, & Bei, 2016). Scott and Woods (2018) reported an association between social media use and increased pre-sleep cognitive arousal, however how this compares with the psychological stimulation provided by other pre-bed activities is unclear. Finally, Reynolds, Meltzer, Dorrian, Centofanti, and Biggs (2019) demonstrated an association between high-frequency online social interactions (email and instant messaging) and perceived insufficient sleep duration, but not reduced time in bed, in children aged 8–16 years. There are also demonstrated relationships between playing violent video games and physiological arousal in adolescent boys, with potential subsequent effects on sleep (Ivarsson, Anderson, Åkerstedt, & Lindblad, 2013). However, children may respond differently to the same content or activity, depending on their temperament or previous exposure (Ivarsson et al., 2013).

Even if pre-sleep activities are not themselves stimulating, the presence of devices in the bedroom provides a *reminder* of connection to an infinitely large social group and stream of information. Experimental evidence in adults demonstrates that the simple presence of one's smartphone can reduce available cognitive resources (Ward, Duke, Gneezy, & Bos, 2017). Lessons from behavioural psychology and the potency of classical conditioning mean that even if device use is restricted to calming or relaxing activities closer to bedtime, it could still induce psychological arousal associated with previous use. These principles underpin the practice of stimulus control therapy, a fundamental component of interventions to address insomnia disorders (Bootzin & Perlis, 2011).

There are other possible pathways via which pre-sleep arousal might affect sleep in children. In addition to interfering with sleep onset, psychologically stimulating activities prior to bed may also reduce sleep maintenance and consolidation (Beyens & Nathanson, 2019). It is also possible that stressful parent–child interactions around limiting or stopping device use could increase physiological arousal prior to the sleep period. Frequent use of media devices throughout the day could also minimise children's ability to self-soothe, such that when there is 'quiet time' prior to bed, they struggle to relax. Although plausible, these possibilities remain to be explored in empirical research.

Sleep Displacement

Finally, undertaking particularly engaging activities in the pre-sleep period may delay children's bedtime. Digital device use may *displace* sleep, such that children spend time that they would otherwise be sleeping using digital technology (see the final row of Figure 38.1). Pre-sleep arousal and sleep displacement may work together to delay sleep onset and therefore reduce sleep duration (Exelmans & Van den Bulck, 2017). Any pre-bed activity has the potential to displace sleep in children. However, there is early evidence that screen-based activities may reduce children's sleep to a greater extent than reading a book prior to bed, although this should be interpreted cautiously due to the observational nature of the research (Hale et al., 2018).

Digital media are most likely to displace sleep when use becomes excessive or unregulated. Children who use digital devices excessively may meet criteria for digital addiction (an emerging but contentious definition of problematic digital media use). Digital addiction has demonstrated relationships with poor sleep in children, although these are better established in adolescents (Chen & Gau, 2016). Even moderate levels of screen time are consistently associated with shorter sleep duration (Cain & Gradisar, 2010; Carter et al., 2016; Harbard et al., 2016; Scott & Woods, 2018), suggesting that it is not only extremely high device use that has the potential to delay sleep onset and displace sleep. While there has been considerable research addressing the personal characteristics of individuals susceptible to online addiction, there is limited empirical scrutiny of the design decisions made by online service providers to drive use and engagement. Design of the online environments in which content is presented and strategies that are used to engage users may be equally as important as the content itself. The next section explores characteristics of digital activity environments that may increase the risk of sleep displacement in children, however these possibilities are speculative and have not been empirically tested.

Online activities rewarding constant connection may result in sleep displacement, and social rewards or punishments can be particularly powerful. Providing likes on social media activates brain circuitry involved in reward processing in teenagers and young adults (Sherman, Hernandez, Greenfield, & Dapretto, 2018), suggesting high potency of online services. Some social networking platforms incorporate reward-based strategies that can induce fear of missing out (FOMO; Scott & Woods, 2018) and pressure to stay connected. Examples of this are messaging applications that quantify 'streaks' of communication between friends, that make content expire after a set time period, require attention at specified times of the day, or require constant 'check-ins' from users for rewards such as points or badges. Massively multiplayer online games (MMOs) have been specifically identified as leading to excessive screen time and interference with sleep (Lam, 2014). These games can also have strong social expectations, where the feeling of 'letting down' team-mates might limit children's willingness to stop play at their usual bedtime, and children may game with older players (who have later bedtimes) or those in different time zones.

These effects are true for both children and adults, but children may have more difficulty self-regulating their engagement, as the executive functions that underpin self-regulation are still developing during childhood (Rothbart, Posner, & Kieras, 2006).

Activities that encourage children to lose track of time or lack clear exit points may also delay bedtime and displace sleep. Games and services can induce a sense of 'flow', where a user feels fully immersed and has a distorted perception of time (Rau, Peng, & Yang, 2006). Children may have less control over stopping an activity if they have reduced awareness of time passing. A number of design features can minimise clear exit points from digital activities. These include auto-play features, which are present in many online video streaming services, games that lack clear save points, and the 'infinite scroll' of many social media feeds, where information is not presented in discrete pages, but instead as a never-ending stream of content. There is large variation in the extent to which digital applications, services, and games utilise compelling reward and control strategies. It is almost certainly the case that some types of digital media activities are more prone to displacing sleep than are others; however, there is scarce evidence examining what specific digital media characteristics are more likely to delay children's sleep.

Potential Benefits of Digital Media

Digital media also has considerable potential to provide information, deliver activities, or promote ambient conditions that encourage and facilitate healthy sleep in children. There are many learning applications used by children that are delivered via digital media and have important benefits for children. There is also great potential for digitally supported relaxation and passive digitally automated strategies to promote sleep, such as programmable lighting, music, storytelling, or relaxation sounds. Further, there are many existing apps and devices to track and support sleep in children, and this increased availability presents opportunities for greater awareness of children's sleep behaviour and needs in families. However, there is no current evidence base for these strategies in children, despite the current proliferation of health management apps (Byambasuren, Sanders, Beller, & Glasziou, 2018). Indeed, there is evidence that the information provided by commercially available sleep apps and devices can be misleading (Meltzer, Hiruma, Avis, Montgomery-Downs, & Valentin, 2015), if not counterproductive. Even if individual applications *are* beneficial for creating a sleep-supportive environment, the fact that they are embedded in a device that is also highly connected and can still deliver other cognitively arousing content means that they should be used with some care.

Limitations of Existing Research

The existing research base is almost exclusively observational in nature and should be interpreted with some caution. It is not possible to determine with much certainty whether technology use contributes to sleep difficulties or whether children with sleep difficulties turn to digital media as a coping or mitigation strategy for their sleep difficulties. Children's health, social, and environmental context are also confounding factors associated with both sleep difficulties and increased screen use. For example, overall screen time seems to be higher in lower-income families with less educated caregivers (Przybylski, 2019; Tandon et al., 2012). Families that allow their children more screen time report both increased sleep latency (time to fall asleep) and a more negative family environment (Bartel et al., 2015). These family and home-life factors may explain both the increased screen use and poor sleep observed in current studies. Digital media could also impact sleep indirectly via other aspects of well-being. Sleep duration is related to other health outcomes such as dietary habits and obesity (Tambalis, Panagiotakos, Psarra, & Sidossis, 2018). Increased screen time could displace daytime physical activity, quality social time and relationships, and increase obesity, all of which have their own associations with sleep. These relationships are not yet sufficiently examined, and this limits the ability to attribute changes in sleep to digital media use

Most studies have relied on parental report or self-report of both digital media use and sleep in children, which is likely to introduce considerable error, particularly where all data come from a single observer (e.g., the problem of common method variance and other sources of bias; Exelmans & Van den Bulck, 2019; Hale et al., 2018). Studies that incorporate objective sleep measurement techniques are needed. There is also immense variation in the measurement of 'digital media use', which is often operationalised poorly or simplistically (e.g., high versus low screen time) (Hale & Guan, 2015). 'Screen time' today runs the full gamut of the human cognitive and emotional experience, and it is increasingly difficult to disentangle digital activities from one another. Children can task-switch frequently, both between and within devices, encouraged by notifications and application cross-integration. Devices can provide *both* calming and alerting experiences, sometimes closely juxtaposed. This introduces challenges for researchers and, thus far, the field has not effectively characterised screen-based activities to establish what types may be problematic for children's well-being, and for sleep in particular (Exelmans & Van den Bulck, 2019).

There has been broader analysis of multiple large-scale cross-sectional social datasets to examine the relationship between digital technology use and psychological well-being in adolescents, in a way that accounts for the pitfalls inherent in analysing data from large observational studies. These analyses show that even if a causal relationship between digital technology and well-being does exist, current data suggest that the size of this relationship is likely very small, with minimal meaningful impact on day-to-day well-being (Orben & Przybylski, 2019). Most of the available research reported here rates poorly on schema designed to rate the certainty of an evidence base (Carter et al., 2016). Together, this means that a causative relationship cannot be currently established. In order to improve the quality of evidence, strongly controlled trials in the field are needed. Existing reviews have already called for future research that adopts experimental designs to supplement the predominantly observational research base (Carter et al., 2016; Hale et al., 2018). A clearer and more nuanced description of the causal mechanisms involved will allow better identification of what specific digital media features may be problematic (or beneficial) for sleep.

Practice Points

The American Academy of Pediatrics (AAP) has guidelines regarding screen use in children, suggesting that screens should not be used for one hour prior to bedtime, and that bedrooms remain screen-free, particularly before bed (AAP, 2016). Because there is limited evidence about the *types* of activities that cause sleep problems, the blanket advice (i.e., no screen time) is likely reasonable, but would ideally be refined to be more activity-specific in the future as the evidence base evolves. Existing research and knowledge of the pre-sleep processes outlined in this chapter suggest a number of practice points. These recommendations relate specifically to sleep, and sit within broader advice regarding healthy management of digital media use in children (see Hill et al., 2016). The following considerations and practical strategies may be of use to parents and carers for managing devices in the hours prior to bedtime:

- Light from devices should be minimised in the hours before bed, as longer periods of exposure have larger effects on the body clock. Melatonin onset occurs several hours before habitual sleep onset, so the potential for suppression of melatonin by light from light-emitting devices extends over at least that period;

- Brightness of screens should be dimmed as much as possible when used near to bedtime;
- The use of 'Night-mode' on many devices to change the colour and brightness of screens may help to reduce the proportion of blue light emitted;
- The effect of light upon sleep–wake regulation is time-specific, so there is no reason to be concerned about the effects of increased morning or daytime light exposure on children's sleep. In fact, bright light may be beneficial during the day;
- To minimise the potential for dysfunctional associations and pre-sleep arousal, avoid allowing children to use devices in the bedroom, and do not allow use of devices in the bed itself at any point during the day;
- Consider the potential emotional and arousal content of activities completed on devices in the lead up to bedtime. Avoid content that has the potential to increase psychological and physiological arousal;
- Establish clear expectations with social networks regarding 'off-time' that starts well prior to the sleep period;
- Limit activities that have reward structures designed to encourage persistent and ongoing use (e.g., 'streaks') in the hours prior to bedtime, and substitute for activities that have clear time limits or clear 'break points';
- Disable auto-play features where possible, to limit children losing track of time and delaying sleep preparation.

Summary

Sleep is critical for children, and current evidence suggests that increased digital media use is associated with a range of negative sleep outcomes, particularly later bedtimes and reduced sleep duration. There are multiple plausible pathways underpinning this relationship, with some support but limited rigorous evidence to support these mechanisms as causal, particularly in children. The rate of technological change means that evaluation of the impact of digital media lags well behind adoption. Given the embeddedness of digital devices in modern childhood, there is a great need for high-quality field research around this issue. Well-controlled field trials will be required to establish whether digital media use has a meaningful impact on children's sleep. Future research also needs to be re-framed around activity characteristics and online environments such as reward structures and sense of connection to broader networks rather than differences in device type, which is becoming an increasingly immaterial distinction as portable devices mediate all aspects of life.

References

AAP. (2016). Media and young minds. *Pediatrics*, *138*(5), e20162591. doi:10.1542/peds.2016-2591.

Akacem, L. D., Wright, K. P., & LeBourgeois, M. K. (2018). Sensitivity of the circadian system to evening bright light in preschool-age children. *Physiological Reports*, *6*(5), 1–10. doi:10.14814/phy2.13617.

Akacem, L. D., Wright, K. P., & LeBourgeois, M. K. (2016). Bedtime and evening light exposure influence circadian timing in preschool-age children: A field study. *Neurobiology of Sleep and Circadian Rhythms*, *1*(2), 27–31. doi:10.1016/j.nbscr.2016.11.002.

Bartel, K. A., Gradisar, M., & Williamson, P. (2015). Protective and risk factors for adolescent sleep: A meta-analytic review. *Sleep Medicine Reviews*, *21*, 72–85. doi:10.1016/j.smrv.2014.08.002.

Benloucif, S., Guico, M. J., Reid, K. J., Wolfe, L. F., L'Hermite-Balériaux, M., & Zee, P. C. (2005). Stability of melatonin and temperature as circadian phase markers and their relation to sleep times in humans. *Journal of Biological Rhythms*, *20*(2), 178–188. doi:10.1177/0748730404273983.

Beyens, I., & Nathanson, A. I. (2019). Electronic media use and sleep among preschoolers: Evidence for time-shifted and less consolidated sleep. *Health Communication*, *34*(5), 537–544. doi:10.1080/10410236.2017.1422102.

Bootzin, R. R., & Epstein, D. R. (2011). Understanding and treating insomnia. *Annual Review of Clinical Psychology*, 7(1), 435–458. doi:10.1146/annurev.clinpsy.3.022806.091516.

Bootzin, R. R., & Perlis, M. L. (2011). Stimulus control therapy. *Behavioral treatments for sleep disorders*. Elsevier Inc. doi:10.1016/B978-0-12-381522-4.00002-X.

Byambasuren, O., Sanders, S., Beller, E., & Glasziou, P. (2018). Prescribable mHealth apps identified from an overview of systematic reviews. *Npj Digital Medicine*, 1(1), 1–12. doi:10.1038/s41746-018-0021-9.

Cain, N., & Gradisar, M. (2010). Electronic media use and sleep in school-aged children and adolescents: A review. *Sleep Medicine*, 11(8), 735–742. doi:10.1016/j.sleep.2010.02.006.

Cajochen, C., Frey, S., Anders, D., Späti, J., Bues, M., Pross, A., ... Stefani, O. (2011). Evening exposure to a light-emitting diodes (LED)-backlit computer screen affects circadian physiology and cognitive performance. *Journal of Applied Physiology*, 110(5), 1432–1438. doi:10.1152/japplphysiol.00165.2011.

Carter, B., Rees, P., Hale, L., Bhattacharjee, D., & Paradkar, M. S. (2016). Media use and sleep. *JAMA Pediatrics*, 170(12), 1236. doi:10.1001/jamapediatrics.2016.2341.

Chaput, J., Gray, C. E., Poitras, V. J., Carson, V., Gruber, R., Olds, T., ... Tremblay, M. S. (2016). Systematic review of the relationships between sleep duration and health indicators in school-aged children and youth. *Applied Physiology, Nutrition, and Metabolism*, 41(6 (Supplement 3)), S266–S282. doi:10.1139/apnm-2015-0627.

Chen, Y. L., & Gau, S. S. F. (2016). Sleep problems and internet addiction among children and adolescents: A longitudinal study. *Journal of Sleep Research*, 25(4), 458–465. doi:10.1111/jsr.12388.

Crowley, S. J., Cain, S. W., Burns, A. C., Acebo, C., & Carskadon, M. A. (2015). Increased sensitivity of the circadian system to light in early/mid-puberty. *Journal of Clinical Endocrinology and Metabolism*, 100(November), 4067–4073. doi:10.1210/jc.2015-2775.

Duffy, J. F., & Wright, K. P. (2005). Entrainment of the human circadian system by light. *Journal of Biological Rhythms*, 20(4), 326–338. doi:10.1177/0748730405277983.

Exelmans, L., & Van den Bulck, J. (2017). Bedtime, shuteye time and electronic media: Sleep displacement is a two-step process. *Journal of Sleep Research*, 26(3), 364–370. doi:10.1111/jsr.12510.

Exelmans, L., & Van den Bulck, J. (2019). Sleep research: A primer for media scholars. *Health Communication*, 34(5), 519–528. doi:10.1080/10410236.2017.1422100.

Figueiro, M., & Overington, D. (2016). Self-luminous devices and melatonin suppression in adolescents. *Lighting Research and Technology*, 48(8), 966–975. doi:10.1177/1477153515584979.

Galland, B. C., Taylor, B. J., Elder, D. E., & Herbison, P. (2012). Normal sleep patterns in infants and children: A systematic review of observational studies. *Sleep Medicine Reviews*, 16(3), 213–222. doi:10.1016/j.smrv.2011.06.001.

Garrison, M. M., & Christakis, D. A. (2012). The impact of a healthy media use intervention on sleep in preschool children. *Pediatrics*, 130(3), 492–499. doi:10.1542/peds.2011-3153.

Garrison, M. M., Liekweg, K., & Christakis, D. A. (2011). Media use and child sleep: The impact of content, timing, and environment. *Pediatrics*, 128(1), 29–35. doi:10.1542/peds.2010-3304.

Gómez, R. L., & Edgin, J. O. (2015). Sleep as a window into early neural development: Shifts in sleep-dependent learning effects across early childhood. *Child Development Perspectives*, 9(3), 183–189. doi:10.1111/cdep.12130.

Gregory, A. M., Willis, T. A., Wiggs, L., Harvey, A. G., Eley, T. C., Buttery, R., ... Nicholson, R. (2008). Presleep arousal and sleep disturbances in children. *Sleep*, 31(12), 1745–1747. doi:10.1093/sleep/31.12.1745.

Gringras, P., Middleton, B., Skene, D. J., & Revell, V. L. (2015). Bigger, brighter, bluer-better? Current light-emitting devices – Adverse sleep properties and preventative strategies. *Frontiers in Public Health*, 3 (October), 1–6. doi:10.3389/fpubh.2015.00233.

Grønli, J., Byrkjedal, I. K., Bjorvatn, B., Nødtvedt, O., Hamre, B., & Pallesen, S. (2016). Reading from an iPad or from a book in bed: The impact on human sleep. A randomized controlled crossover trial. *Sleep Medicine*, 21, 86–92. doi:10.1016/j.sleep.2016.02.006.

Hale, L., & Guan, S. (2015). Screen time and sleep among school-aged children and adolescents: A systematic literature review. *Sleep Medicine Reviews*, 21, 50–58. doi:10.1016/j.smrv.2014.07.007.

Hale, L., Kirschen, G. W., LeBourgeois, M. K., Gradisar, M., Garrison, M. M., Montgomery-Downs, H., ... Buxton, O. (2018). Youth screen media habits and sleep. *Child and Adolescent Psychiatric Clinics of North America*, 27(2), 229–245. doi:10.1016/j.chc.2017.11.014.

Harbard, E., Allen, N. B., Trinder, J., & Bei, B. (2016). What's keeping teenagers up? Prebedtime behaviors and actigraphy-assessed sleep over school and vacation. *Journal of Adolescent Health*, 58(4), 426–432. doi:10.1016/j.jadohealth.2015.12.011.

Hartstein, L. E., LeBourgeois, M. K., & Berthier, N. E. (2018). Light correlated color temperature and task switching performance in preschool-age children: Preliminary insights. *PLoS ONE*, *13*(8), 1–14. doi:10.1371/journal.pone.0202973.

Higuchi, S., Lee, S., Kozaki, T., & Harada, T. (2016). Late circadian phase in adults and children is correlated with use of high color temperature light at home at night. *Chronobiology International*, *33*(4), 448–452. doi:10.3109/07420528.2016.1152978.

Hill, D., Ameenuddin, N., Chassiakos, Y. R., Cross, C., Radesky, J., Hutchinson, J., ... Swanson, W. S. (2016). Media use in school-aged children and adolescents. *Pediatrics*, *138*, 5. doi:10.1542/peds.2016-2592.

Ivarsson, M., Anderson, M., Åkerstedt, T., & Lindblad, F. (2013). The effect of violent and nonviolent video games on heart rate variability, sleep, and emotions in adolescents with different violent gaming habits. *Psychosomatic Medicine*, *75*(4), 390–396. doi:10.1097/PSY.0b013e3182906a4c.

Lam, L. T. (2014). Internet gaming addiction, problematic use of the Internet, and sleep problems: A systematic review. *Current Psychiatry Reports*, *16*, 4. doi:10.1007/s11920-014-0444-1.

LeBourgeois, M. K., Carskadon, M. A., Akacem, L. D., Simpkin, C. T., Wright, K. P., Achermann, P., & Jenni, O. G. (2013). Circadian phase and its relationship to nighttime sleep in toddlers. *Journal of Biological Rhythms*, *28*(5), 322–331. doi:10.1177/0748730413506543.

LeBourgeois, M. K., Hale, L., Chang, A.-M., Akacem, L. D., Montgomery-Downs, H. E., & Buxton, O. M. (2017). Digital media and sleep in childhood and adolescence. *Pediatrics*, *140*(Supplement 2), S92–S96. doi:10.1542/peds.2016-1758J.

Lok, R., Smolders, K. C. H. J., Beersma, D. G. M., & de Kort, Y. A. W. (2018). Light, alertness, and alerting effects of white light: A literature overview. *Journal of Biological Rhythms*, *33*(6), 589–601. doi:10.1177/0748730418796443.

Lucas, R. J., Peirson, S. N., Berson, D. M., Brown, T. M., Cooper, H. M., Czeisler, C. A., ... Brainard, G. C. (2014). Measuring and using light in the melanopsin age. *Trends in Neurosciences*, *37*(1), 1–9. doi:10.1016/j.tins.2013.10.004.

Meltzer, L. J., Hiruma, L. S., Avis, K., Montgomery-Downs, H., & Valentin, J. (2015). Comparison of a commercial accelerometer with polysomnography and actigraphy in children and adolescents. *Sleep*, *38*(8), 1323–1330. doi:10.5665/sleep.4918.

Miller, M. A., Kruisbrink, M., Wallace, J., Ji, C., & Cappuccio, F. P. (2018). Sleep duration and incidence of obesity in infants, children, and adolescents: A systematic review and meta-analysis of prospective studies. *Sleep*, *41*(4), 1–19. doi:10.1093/sleep/zsy018.

Mindell, J. A., & Williamson, A. A. (2018). Benefits of a bedtime routine in young children: Sleep, development, and beyond. *Sleep Medicine Reviews*, *40*, 93–108. doi:10.1016/j.smrv.2017.10.007.

Nagare, R., Plitnick, B., & Figueiro, M. G. (2018). Does the iPad Night Shift mode reduce melatonin suppression? *Lighting Research and Technology*, 1–11. doi:10.1177/1477153517748189.

Ogilvie, R. D. (2001). The process of falling asleep. *Sleep Medicine Reviews*, *5*(3), 247–270. doi:10.1053/smrv.2001.0145.

Orben, A., & Przybylski, A. K. (2019). The association between adolescent well-being and digital technology use. *Nature Human Behaviour*, *3*(February). doi:10.1038/s41562-018-0506-1.

Paruthi, S., Brooks, L. J., D'Ambrosio, C., Hall, W. A., Kotagal, S., Lloyd, R. M., ... Wise, M. S. (2016). Recommended amount of sleep for pediatric populations: A consensus statement of the American Academy of Sleep Medicine. *Journal of Clinical Sleep Medicine*, *12*(6), 785–786. doi:10.5664/jcsm.5866.

Perrault, A. A., Bayer, L., Peuvrier, M., Afyouni, A., Ghisletta, P., Brockmann, C., ... Sterpenich, V. (2019). Reducing the use of screen electronic devices in the evening is associated with improved sleep and daytime vigilance in adolescents. *Sleep*, *42*(9), 1–10. doi:10.1093/sleep/zsz125.

Przybylski, A. K. (2019). Digital screen time and pediatric sleep: Evidence from a preregistered cohort study. *Journal of Pediatrics*, *205*, 218–223.e1. doi:10.1016/j.jpeds.2018.09.054.

Quach, J., Hiscock, H., Canterford, L., & Wake, M. (2009). Outcomes of child sleep problems over the school-transition period: Australian population longitudinal study. *Pediatrics*, *123*(5), 1287–1292. doi:10.1542/peds.2008-1860.

Rau, P. L. P., Peng, S. Y., & Yang, C. C. (2006). Time distortion for expert and novice online game players. *Cyberpsychology and Behavior*, *9*(4), 396–403. doi:10.1089/cpb.2006.9.396.

Reynolds, A. C., Meltzer, L. J., Dorrian, J., Centofanti, S. A., & Biggs, S. N. (2019). Impact of high-frequency email and instant messaging (E/IM) interactions during the hour before bed on self-reported sleep duration and sufficiency in female Australian children and adolescents. *Sleep Health*, *5*(1), 64–67. doi:10.1016/j.sleh.2018.10.008.

Roenneberg, T., Kantermann, T., Vetter, C., & Allebrandt, K. V. (2013). Light and the human circadian clock. *Handbook of Experimental Pharmacology*, *217*. doi:10.1007/978-3-642-25950-0.

Rothbart, M. K., Posner, M. I., & Kieras, J. (2006). Temperament, attention, and the development of self-regulation. In *Blackwell handbook of early childhood development* (pp. 338–357). Oxford, UK: Blackwell Publishing Ltd. doi:10.1002/9780470757703.ch17.

Sadeh, A., Gruber, R., & Raviv, A. (2002). Sleep, neurobehavioral functioning, and behavior problems in school-age children. *Child Development, 73*(2), 405–417. doi:10.1111/1467-8624.00414.

Scott, H., & Woods, H. C. (2018). Fear of missing out and sleep: Cognitive behavioural factors in adolescents' nighttime social media use. *Journal of Adolescence, 68*(February), 61–65. doi:10.1016/j.adolescence.2018.07.009.

Sherman, L. E., Hernandez, L. M., Greenfield, P. M., & Dapretto, M. (2018). What the brain 'likes': Neural correlates of providing feedback on social media. *Social Cognitive and Affective Neuroscience, 13*(7), 699–707. doi:10.1093/scan/nsy051.

Smolensky, M. H., Sackett-Lundeen, L. L., & Portaluppi, F. (2015). Nocturnal light pollution and under-exposure to daytime sunlight: Complementary mechanisms of circadian disruption and related diseases. *Chronobiology International, 32*(8), 1029–1048. doi:10.3109/07420528.2015.1072002.

Souman, J. L., Tinga, A. M., te Pas, S. F., van Ee, R., & Vlaskamp, B. N. S. (2018). Acute alerting effects of light: A systematic literature review. *Behavioural Brain Research, 337*(July 2017), 228–239. doi:10.1016/j.bbr.2017.09.016.

Stothard, E. R., McHill, A. W., Depner, C. M., Birks, B. R., Moehlman, T. M., Ritchie, H. K., ... Wright, K. P. (2017). Circadian entrainment to the natural light-dark cycle across seasons and the weekend. *Current Biology, 27*(4), 508–513. doi:10.1016/j.cub.2016.12.041.

Tambalis, K. D., Panagiotakos, D. B., Psarra, G., & Sidossis, L. S. (2018). Insufficient sleep duration is associated with dietary habits, screen time, and obesity in children. *Journal of Clinical Sleep Medicine, 14*(10), 1689–1696. doi:10.5664/jcsm.7374.

Tandon, P. S., Zhou, C., Sallis, J. F., Cain, K. L., Frank, L. D., & Saelens, B. E. (2012). Home environment relationships with children's physical activity, sedentary time, and screen time by socioeconomic status. *International Journal of Behavioral Nutrition and Physical Activity, 9*(1), 88. doi:10.1186/1479-5868-9-88.

Vriend, J. L., Davidson, F. D., Corkum, P. V., Rusak, B., Chambers, C. T., & McLaughlin, E. N. (2013). Manipulating sleep duration alters emotional functioning and cognitive performance in children. *Journal of Pediatric Psychology, 38*(10), 1058–1069. doi:10.1093/jpepsy/jst033.

Ward, A. F., Duke, K., Gneezy, A., & Bos, M. W. (2017). Brain drain: The mere presence of one's own smartphone reduces available cognitive capacity. *Journal of the Association for Consumer Research, 2*(2), 140–154. doi:10.1086/691462.

Zeitzer, J. M., Dijk, D. J., Kronauer, R. E., Brown, E. N., & Czeisler, C. A. (2000). Sensitivity of the human circadian pacemaker to nocturnal light: Melatonin phase resetting and suppression. *Journal of Physiology, 526*(3), 695–702. doi:10.1111/j.1469-7793.2000.00695.x.

39
SICK CHILDREN AND SOCIAL MEDIA

Ana Jorge, Lidia Marôpo, and Raiana de Carvalho

Introduction

Social media, as a particular form of digital media, occupies a significant role in the everyday life of children and young people across the world for various personal and public purposes (boyd, 2010, 2014; Mascheroni & Ólafsson, 2014). Although research on digital media use by children and youth has long focussed on risks and negative outcomes (Livingstone, Mascheroni, & Staksrud, 2015), recent studies have identified some positive health impacts of digital media upon children's physical, psychological, mental (Goodyear, Armour, & Wood, 2019, p. 674), and emotional well-being, improving their social skills online, developing character, and offering support (Frith, 2017), and also in providing leisure activities, relieving stress, fostering creativity, and facilitating learning (Swist, Collin, McCormack, & Third, 2015). Although social media can be a productive place for health education, delivered by professional health providers and also children's peers, it can also lead to inaccurate information and the normalisation of bad health choices, e.g., regarding food (Holmberg, Chaplin, Hillman, & Berg, 2016). Moreover, young people might wish to avoid being associated with certain health information if it compromises their privacy and the desired self-presentation (Byron, Albury, & Evers, 2013).

This chapter examines social media and children in the context of sickness, offering a literature review that is predominantly drawn from medical sciences, children/youth media, and digital media studies. It also considers the affordances and constraints of social media for children and young people, before discussing a case study of a teenager living with cancer and using YouTube to chart her journey. The chapter finishes by arguing for a perspective that considers intersectionality in combination with a framework of children's (digital) rights, positioning children's well-being within the interaction of online and offline realms.

Networked Illness

While there has been extensive research into children's (aged 0–18), and especially young people's (teenagers') use of social media, few studies have considered the types of health-related information young people come into contact with, create, and share through social media (Goodyear et al., 2019, p. 674). Social media can offer health information both from institutions and from peers via user-generated content (Hausmann, Touloumitz, White, Colbert & Gooding, 2017). Such content is often circulated in a context of entertainment and sociability. As a consequence, health information is increasingly accessible to young people, being "more available, shared and tailored" (Goodyear et al., 2019, p. 674). Indeed, health providers have acknowledged the many positive possibilities offered by digital media for communication with teenage patients with chronic illness (Santos, Tavares, Ferreira, & Pereira, 2015). Two obvious risks posed to younger patients are, however, the threat of encountering inaccuracies and unreliable sources online, and feeling overwhelmed by the amount of information on offer (Frith, 2017).

Young patients and their families may also experience social benefits, such as "increased interaction [and] peer/social/emotional support" (Goodyear et al., 2019, p. 674), empowerment through network building, acceptance, and belonging to society; understanding, and validation and information sharing amongst online community members (Merolli, Gray, & Martin-Sanchez, 2013; Pruulmann-Vengerfeldt, 2018; Stage, 2017). While providing a space to potentially help a child cope with illness, social media resources can also constitute 'networked publics' (boyd, 2010) around 'health-related interests' including chronic and rare diseases (Wittmeier et al., 2014). The notion of a 'networked illness' as supported by social media offers the possibility of co-creating and sharing new knowledge that is shaped by a child's personal experience (Koteyko & Hunt, 2016), shifting the reliance from professionally delivered expert knowledge to positioning the patient as an expert, and in turn challenging the authority of medical practitioners.

For sick children who might need to travel away from their homes and/or schools during treatment, communication technologies and particularly social media play a pivotal role in maintaining a connection with their social circle. Young cancer survivors have reported that during treatment they increase their use of digital media for both entertainment and for contacting their personal networks (Jorge & Marôpo, 2017). These technologies also allow chronically ill children to participate in special or everyday activities at a distance (e.g., through video chat) and to receive updates and encouraging comments (Liu, Inkpen, & Pratt, 2015). Social media use enables children to receive information about their illness from (more experienced) peer patients, and to educate their healthy peers about their experience of the illness (Merolli et al., 2013).

Social media interaction helps constitute the social (e.g., cultural and ethnic membership) and personal identities (e.g., unique attributes) of sick children (Ting-Toomey, 2016). Digital media, especially social media, acquires special importance in the context of suffering or overcoming serious illness and forms part of the child's identity work, helping to define how children view themselves and how they want to be seen by others. Even when young people share a lot of personal information online, however, they remain concerned about maintaining personal privacy and managing their online reputation (Hausmann et al., 2017). These priorities seem a common preoccupation for (teenage) users of social media, in what has been termed the 'privacy paradox' (Van der Velden & El Emam, 2013).

Few studies of teenage patients and social media focus on the topic of privacy. Teenagers with chronic or long-term illness seem to be selective about sharing feelings and thoughts about their diagnosis, treatment, and prognosis as a means of protecting themselves (Van der Velden, 2012), and "to prevent or reduce the likelihood of embarrassment, difficult questions, and feelings of vulnerability" (Van der Velden & El Emam, 2013, p. 19). Such emotional imperatives are not fixed, but evolve over the different stages of the illness. Instead, young people with chronic health conditions may choose to promote themselves as regular teenagers (Van der Velden & El Emam, 2013), and use social media to manage real-time reactions, e.g., by sharing progress pictures or their new appearance before going back to school (Merolli et al., 2013). Thus, social media use provides a degree of choice and control for children and young people over how they might present and assert themselves, as well as regarding how much they disclose about their condition. Even so, young patients' decisions to restrict privacy settings are sometimes made difficult by the user-interface design of social media platforms and apps, which may lead to an illusion of control (Van der Velden, 2012).

Social media also provides an opportunity for children with chronic and serious diseases to narrate their experiences (Gibson et al., 2016; Merolli et al., 2013). Some sick children and young people share their stories, reflections and questions through digital channels such as blogs, YouTube, Instagram, and Facebook. They may be looking for emotional catharsis, audience understanding, sympathy, and support in coping with their disease and, at times, hoping for advocacy (Nesby & Salamonsen, 2016). Potential positive benefits are the prevention of feelings of isolation, softening the mental stress of being seriously ill, promotion of an interactive social life, public self-expression, participation in the construction of young people's community, and the experience of a novel form of social agency in which it is possible to create meaning from distress (Nesby & Salamonsen, 2016). The use of social media to discuss and reflect upon their illness may also provide an opportunity for entrepreneurship (Stage, 2017). Sick children who are active on social media can act as role models by spreading knowledge about how to live proactively with a serious disease, offering exceptional examples of courage and self-assertion while discussing the struggle against stigma. Nevertheless, from a critical perspective, children's use of social media to disclose a personal experience of illness may run the risk of falling into exhibitionism (Nesby & Salamonsen, 2016).

Although there are a range of potential benefits, not all social media interactions are supportive. Some comments may be intrusive, suspicious, critical, or insensitive (Merolli et al., 2013, p. 8), and these responses might be stressful for young people. Given this, some children might prefer comparatively anonymous online spaces where they can discuss sensitive topics at ease (Nesby & Salamonsen, 2016). In addition, some studies of young cancer survivors demonstrate that they avoid dramatisation, victimisation, or heroification by actively protecting their privacy, rather keeping their emotional labour around their illness to the personal sphere of their family and close friends (Carvalho, Sampaio, & Marôpo, 2016).

Sick children can also be represented on social media by others, such as relatives, peers, or advocacy groups. Even if social media provides more agentic opportunities for teenagers, young children can be involved as well, for instance through parent-initiated and parent-led social media campaigns (Jorge & Marôpo, 2017; Wittmeier et al., 2014). Some young cancer survivors express discomfort at the possibility of picturing themselves in this type of digital campaign while others accept it, hoping for the possibility of significant benefits such as bone marrow donors, or funds for treatment, or to build a persona for later activism (Jorge & Marôpo, 2017). Sometimes, peers may share pictures or other information about a sick child through social media. This can be problematic, for example, if a friend tries to give support by sharing a picture of them with the sick child without their consent (Carvalho et al., 2016).

Besides campaigns by sick children's parents, many advocacy and awareness-raising campaigns use social media for a myriad of purposes. For example, to challenge negative stereotypes, to find bone marrow donors, to promote health literacy, to raise funds (individually or institutionally), to support research, and to improve therapeutic options available for a patient, and for others. One such Brazilian campaign was found to have disclosed significant information about individual sick children and to have promoted children as victims in ways that the children resented (Marôpo, Carvalho, & Sampaio, 2015), however. Informed consent and the active participation of children in such campaigns, in ways that consider and uphold children's dignity, comfort, and safety, should be the minimum requirements for best practice in this area.

All these different activities use social media to help construct the social meanings of diseases affecting children while promoting aspects of their identities. Social media use offer benefits as well as a range of risks, while potentially emphasising existing inequalities. Yet, social media can also bring new challenges to children and their families at different stages of an illness, requiring both awareness and a range of competencies.

A Case Study: Lorena Reginato and *CarecaTV*

"Globally, childhood and adolescent cancer is threatening to overtake infectious diseases as one of the highest causes of disease-related mortality in children" (Childhood Cancer International, 2018). While the incidence of child cancer is lower than that in adults, and despite the fact that children tend to respond better to cancer treatment than adults, children are more likely to have side-effects since their bodies are still growing. Moreover, if the treatment causes long-term side effects, this may require children to have careful follow-up for the rest of their lives (American Cancer Society, 2019). The concern with childhood cancer is increased in the case of low- to middle-income countries: not only do 80% of children with cancer live in low- to middle-income countries, but the survival rate in these countries can be as low as 10%, while in developed countries it can be more than 80% (Childhood Cancer International, 2018). In this section the authors analyse the case of YouTube channel *CarecaTV* (BaldTV, with 1.8 million subscribers as of January 2018), created in 2016 by Lorena Reginato, a Brazilian girl then aged 12, who was undergoing treatment for brain cancer (Reginato, n.d.; G1, 2016). Produced by a girl from the Global South, the case also demonstrates the situated nature of these experiences, with Brazil being the second largest user of YouTube in comparative country terms (Dogtiev, 2019). This case study therefore lends itself to a rich discussion about the possibilities and challenges of networked illness among children and youth. This section draws upon a conceptual framework that discusses the emergence of cancer identities and how they are intertwined with the patient's online practices. Further, the case study exemplifies the application of a proposed framework for studying sick children and social media.

The most common post-cancer identities adopted by adults (Park, Zlateva, & Blank, 2009) are 'survivor' (encouraged by advocacy groups and health care professionals and correlated with greater mental well-being, post-traumatic growth, and involvement in advocacy) and the more neutral 'person who has had cancer' (correlated with cancer-related activities and a stronger sense of life purpose, but also with concerns about recurrence). Less frequently, individuals identify as a patient post-treatment, which is a more passive posture, indicating a decision to remain vigilant concerning recurrence, and as a 'victim', which shows passivity and continued vulnerability, related to reduced well-being but also, surprisingly, to a greater involvement in cancer-related activities.

In her inaugural video, Lorena presented herself as someone who had cancer. She had undergone brain surgery and experienced side-effects made evident in the video. She explained:

> I'm bald – look how beautiful this bald head is . . . I have a high-pitched voice and talk a little slowly, but don't you mind about this, OK? Sometimes I shake a little, but don't mind, I am normal . . . I'm not walking yet, but I will walk again.
>
> *(26/03/2016)*

Rather than focussing on a detailed account of her illness trajectory, Lorena emphasised she was 'normal' and wanted her channel to focus on game playing.

However, as *CarecaTV* gained online and traditional media recognition, Lorena's narration of the different stages of her cancer treatment became more prominent and she began to respond to questions and comments from her audience. Adopting the identity of a patient, Lorena described the challenges and inherent suffering as part of her treatment, expressing her uncertainties and the struggle to find meaning in a life-crisis situation: "sometimes in the afternoon I cry with my mum, a lot. Really, I ask 'why with me, what have I done?' But, it's like, crying won't help, it only helps to express my anger" (29/03/2018).

Children's and young people's experiences of cancer are filled with challenges: intense stress post-diagnosis; the side-effects of the treatments; the need to rebuild their imagined life trajectory; and dealing with feelings of vulnerability (Jones, Parker-Raley, & Barczyk, 2011). As with other sick children, Lorena's engagement with social media often worked as a form of distraction from these challenges: "when I'm very sad, what I do often times is going to Instagram, Snapchat, Facebook, Twitter, you know, then I check the messages" (29/03/2018). Crucially, her social media visibility has been a source of support and encouragement:

> when I felt discouraged, I decided to make this channel to distract myself. That was when you all helped me, a lot, by sending me messages of support, by telling me to go on, giving me strength and, because of that, I'm happy.
>
> *(18/01/2017)*

Videos about being a patient also help educate viewers about cancer treatments. Lorena recorded a chemotherapy session in the hospital with her cell phone, explaining the procedures and showing the environment in which it takes place (21/10/2016). She answered questions from followers on the effects of chemotherapy, as well as social side-effects like bullying (29/03/2018). In offering her experiences, Lorena positioned herself as a health-literate young person, symbolically bringing teenage sufferers of cancer into the public sphere and challenging the conception of illness as something private or socially invisible (Stage, 2017).

Nevertheless, Lorena had to deal with offensive and hateful comments, including false information being spread online about her having passed away, the hacking of her channel, and a mocking 'I also have cancer' video by another YouTuber. Some of her videos responded to criticism and invited sympathy. For example, she commented on the suffering and anxiety that young people who have had cancer go through, and condemned the insensitive remarks directed at them (20/07/2018). In this way, Lorena is negotiating a revised awareness of online ethics.

Not only does an individual's background, psychological factors, and different aspects of the experience of the disease affect how cancer survivors form these identities (Park et al., 2009), but they also change over time (Cheung & Delfabbro, 2016). The experience of cancer during childhood, which is an essential time of identity formation, can significantly disrupt a person's self-conceptualisation and identity-construction (Song et al., 2012), and, consequently, their social cognition, affective being, and behavioural tendencies (Ting-Toomey, 2016). In *CarecaTV*, Lorena combined her presentation as a patient with that of a survivor, embracing a process in which overcoming cancer is associated with a battle. She used fighting metaphors infused with optimism and hope. For example, Lorena recalled when she first learned she had cancer: "the first thing I did was to cry a lot. Then I said: 'well, I can die and not try to live, and I can die trying'" (09/05/2016). She also talks about her cancer experience as a means to emphasise that she has completed her treatment. For example, when answering one of her followers about how she felt after she overcame cancer, she said: "I'm glad I won, I am strong, I will always be" (26/06/2016). Lorena also shared her plans for the future and focussed on her good health (Jones et al., 2011): "I hope that 2018, now, can be a year of victories because this year I have a lot of things to do". Her positive activities included equine, occupational, and speech therapies, as well as physiotherapy and swimming. These plans are entwined with her normal life as teenager: "I'm going to start high school in a very cool school … I'm super excited to get to know new people, to study" (09/01/2018).

During recovery, children and young people go through several physical and cognitive changes, psychological experiences (such as poor performance at school, anxiety, depression, and fear of recurrence), and a range of social side-effects (including isolation, poor peer relations, and some limitations associated with their frail physical condition, such as not being allowed to play sports) (Jones et al., 2011). As part of this process, children face a paradoxical identity struggle: they are not sick anymore, but they cannot go back to the life they lived pre-cancer diagnosis (Cantrell & Conte, 2009). Likewise, they must reinvent their identity by articulating their previous 'normal' childhood and adolescence; their cancer experiences; and an early survivorship identity (Jones et al., 2011). Such a process involves engagement with family, peers, and new people, which can be hard as teenagers report a decline of support after treatment, and many express feelings of isolation (Jones et al., 2011). This situation can be particularly challenging since adolescents are "a group that is developmentally focused on identity formation and peer relationships" (Jones et al., 2011, p. 5).

In overcoming her illness, Lorena constructed a new-normal identity (Cantrell & Conte, 2009; Gibson et al., 2016; Liu et al., 2015) by discussing topics that do not revolve around cancer. For example, she created the series "Careca's Adventure", where she plays online games, a peer activity that she can maintain despite her limitations with mobility. She is also shown interacting with friends and family members, as well as enjoying new relationships facilitated by social media, such as with other YouTubers and followers. As she moves into the survivor group and as her hair starts to grow she abandons the salutation "Hello, bald males and bald females" (01/04/2016) (even though the majority of her viewers are not cancer patients) and rather addresses her imagined audience with "Hello bald and hairy people" (01/06/2016). This process is full of ambivalence: Lorena sometimes referred to being bald as inevitable, yet at other times she talked about it as something that profoundly impacted her identity. She discussed in a video whether she will rename her channel *BaldTV* once her hair has grown back, going on to say she will not because that is part of her story and her identity (19/01/2017).

Through adopting a survivor identity, *CarecaTV* functioned as an environment where Lorena could engage in activism while connecting her cancer experiences and emotions with wider social issues, such as being a teenager in the Global South. For example, she selected hats to donate to a hospital that assists children with cancer, and invited viewers to donate pieces of clothing to homeless people (11/01/2016). On another occasion she posted about herself and other peer-patients playing in the children's hospital playground to promote an awareness-raising campaign about the early symptoms of childhood cancer (13/10/2016). The YouTuber is also publicly affiliated with campaigns that donate hair to children with cancer (24/10/2016; 07/11/2016), and with the Ronald McDonald House in her hometown (2017). Crucially, *CarecaTV* is also a platform to engage with wider political issues. For example, Lorena raised the problem of equitable internet access in Brazil and collaborated with another YouTuber, Atila, by asking for a "#fairinternet" (29/04/2016).

Lorena has also used her channel to approach issues related to gender and health, such as when she discussed women's reproductive rights and the Brazilian abortion laws in a video she recorded with her mother (03/12/2016). In this way, YouTube gives Lorena an opportunity to control and manage how she positions herself in society, not only as a patient or a survivor, but also as a citizen. Simultaneously, Lorena's illness is symbolically constructed around private issues and entrepreneurial efforts. As Lorena becomes a microcelebrity (Abidin, 2015), her participation in social media is marked by public recognition as well as financial compensation, from the monetisation of videos on the *CarecaTV* platform. Lorena is also affiliated with brands and products. For example, she has endorsed a brand of hair products by providing an account of their use and a review of their safety for people with serious illness, or for children with allergies. Additionally, she offered a discount code for her viewers to use when purchasing the products online (05/05/2018). Lorena used her social media visibility to fundraise and buy a car, as her family did not have one, and she argued it would help make her travels to treatment more comfortable (01/04/2017). Lorena also launched a book about her story – a practice that has become increasingly common among Brazilian YouTubers – and this was intensely marketed through her videos.

These entrepreneurial attitudes can be interpreted as one way to try to gain control over an otherwise unpredictable future (Stage, 2017), especially in a country where financial conditions for many families are challenging and for what appears to be a lower-middle-income family relying on a precarious public health system and not-for-profit organisations (Dixon-Woods, Young, & Heney, 2005).

Lorena has adopted a status of being 'exceptional', infusing her public visibility with affect, embracing her personal mission "to address social problems, needs, and solutions" (Stage, 2017, p. 47). Through her social media presence, Lorena's transition from cancer treatment to survivorship results in a performance of a range of cancer identities which often coalesce with her promotion of normalcy and a projection of her 'new-normal' identity. While making sense of the paradoxical struggles involved in recovering from a serious illness, Lorena is inevitably influenced by her interactions in this networked environment, as well as by the media attention and public recognition. The next section uses this case study to advance a proposed framework to account for the complexity of the processes described.

A Proposed Framework

In contemporary societies where youth is increasingly mediated, the relationship between children and social media can be seen as both positive and negative, with a special focus on perceiving these as interacting (Livingstone, 2016). As *CarecaTV* has illustrated, this complex perspective also applies to the experience of sick children within these online spaces. Moreover, the experience should be constructed in a comprehensive way, where digital media is not considered a realm that is separate from everyday life. Rather, focus should be "on how new intersections between physical, mobile and digital spaces have the potential to impact children and young people's wellbeing" (Swist et al., 2015, p. 23). This framework thus rejects the 'effects' paradigm (Staksrud & Milojevic, 2017) and adopts a focus on digital rights – an adaptation of the provision, protection, and participation rights of the United Nations Convention on The Rights of the Child in the context of the digital environment (Livingstone, 2016). Besides the right to access digital media, these intersections highlight rights to digital, media, and social literacy as providing a fundamental foundation for accessing, understanding, and participating in digital media creation and, thus, to exercising full communication rights in society. Interestingly, Lorena Reginato also dedicated one of her videos to call for attention to be given to securing a #fairinternet (29/04/2016).

From this perspective, sick children and their families can be empowered through *health media literacy* education (Higgins & Begoray, 2012) regarding their contact with health information shared on social media. Such education would help avoid any misinterpretation of individual circumstances and experiences, prevent an inadequate context in which to investigate the implications of a diagnosis, and assist in guarding against inaccurate or inappropriate medical treatments. Such literacy should also promote coping skills to support children who are faced with unwanted and harmful comments. It is important to review the ethics of sharing information or images of sick children on social media in terms of their rights to privacy, or to allow subsequent removal of content through 'a right to be forgotten', as may happen when a child is the author of his/her own social media visibility, and later regrets these activities when they are old enough to see them in an adult context.

As Lorena's case exemplifies, children's digital experiences across the world are affected by variations in digital environments that reflect "differences in language, geography, culture and power – as defined by the state, commerce or, most locally, family and community" (Livingstone & Third, 2017, p. 664). Therefore, sick children's use of social media should be considered in relation to their multidimensional and fluid identities. Alper, Katz, and Clark (2016) argue for the use of *intersectionality* in children and media scholarship so as to consider the "links between different dimensions of identity, different forms of inequality, and different 'degrees of marginality' (Murdock, 2002, p. 387)" (p. 108). Experiences of children who craft a media presence are diverse in relation to the advantages they might have in one dimension, and the disadvantages in others. In this regard, one could take an 'asset-based' rather than a 'deficit-based' perspective to identify "the abilities, agencies, and aspirations individuals draw on in order to address life challenges and opportunities" (Alper et al., 2016, p. 109), such as illness. Researchers and commentators analysing these instances of children's digital media use should consider not only the impact of social and geographical inequality on the prevalence of disease, but also the different ways in which forms of inequality can affect how children and their families – and their country – cope with illness. These aspects may translate into differences in the use of social media for potential benefits, and to limit possible drawbacks during and after treatment.

Moreover, however transitional, illness can be seen as a challenge that defies the future hopes of the child and his/her family, and imposes feelings of vulnerability. Yet, at the same time, if it can be overcome, the illness can be taken as an opportunity and a journey which can be amplified through social media. *CarecaTV* demonstrates how a teenager used the advantage of her family background to establish herself as an entrepreneur and activist, while appreciating the online social support for her illness as well as facing the perils of unwanted commentary and trolling. While networked illness may counter the stigmatisation and isolation of sick children and contribute to an improvement in their psychological well-being, it may also "reproduce many of the biases that exist in other publics [such as] social inequalities, including … around race, gender, sexuality, and age" (boyd, 2010, p. 54).

References

Abidin, C. (2015). Communicative <3 intimacies: Influencers and perceived interconnectedness. *Ada: A Journal of Gender, New Media, and Technology, 8*. doi:10.7264/N3MW2FFG.

Alper, M., Katz, V. S., & Clark, L. S. (2016). Researching children, intersectionality, and diversity in the digital age. *Journal of Children and Media, 10*(1), 107–114.

American Cancer Society. (2019, October 14). What are the differences between cancers in adults and children? Retrieved from: www.cancer.org/cancer/cancer-in-children/differences-adults-children.html.

boyd, d. (2010). Social network sites as networked publics: Affordances, dynamics, and implications. In Z. Papacharissi (Ed.), *A networked self* (pp. 39–58). London: Routledge.

boyd, d. (2014). *It's complicated: The social lives of networked teens*. New Haven: Yale University Press.

Byron, P., Albury, K., & Evers, C. (2013). 'It would be weird to have that on Facebook': Young people's use of social media and the risk of sharing sexual health information. *Reproductive Health Matters, 21*(41), 35–44.

Cantrell, M. A., & Conte, T. M. (2009). Between being cured and being healed: The paradox of childhood cancer survivorship. *Qualitative Health Research, 19*(3), 312–322.

Carvalho, R., Sampaio, I., & Marôpo, L. (2016). Entre a dor e a superação: adolescentes com câncer discutem sua representação nas notícias [Between pain and overcoming: Adolescents with cancer debate their representation in the news]. *Animus, 15*(30), 224–240.

Cheung, S. Y., & Delfabbro, P. (2016). Are you a cancer survivor? A review on cancer identity. *Journal of Cancer Survivorship, 10*(4), 759–771.

Childhood Cancer International. (2018). International childhood cancer day. Retrieved from: www.internationalchildhoodcancerday.org.

Dixon-Woods, M., Young, B., & Heney, D. (2005). *Rethinking experiences of childhood cancer: A multidisciplinary approach to chronic childhood illness*. Maidenhead, UK: McGraw-Hill.

Dogtiev, A. (2019, January 7). YouTube revenue and usage statistics (2018). *Business of Apps*. Retrieved from: www.businessofapps.com/data/youtube-statistics.

Frith, E. (2017). *Social media and children's mental health: A review of the evidence*. Retrieved from: https://epi.org.uk/publications-and-research/social-media-childrens-mental-health-review-evidence.

G1. (2016, March 13). Após câncer, menina realiza sonho de ter canal de vídeo e comove a web [After cancer, teenage girl fulfills her dream of having a video channel and makes all web feel touched]. *G1*. Retrieved from: http://g1.globo.com/sp/bauru-marilia/noticia/2016/03/apos-cancer-menina-realiza-sonho-de-ter-canal-de-video-e-comove-web.html.

Gibson, F., Hibbins, S., Grew, T., Morgan, S., Pearce, S., Stark, D., & Fern, L. A. (2016). How young people describe the impact of living with and beyond a cancer diagnosis: Feasibility of using social media as a research method: Young people describe their cancer experience using social media. *Psycho-Oncology*, *25*(11), 1317–1323.

Goodyear, V. A., Armour, K. M., & Wood, H. (2019). Young people and their engagement with health-related social media: New perspectives. *Sport, Education and Society*, *24*(7), 673–688.

Hausmann, J. S., Touloumtzis, C., White, M. T., Colbert, J. A., & Gooding, H. C. (2017). Adolescent and young adult use of social media for health and its implications. *Journal of Adolescent Health*, *60*(6), 714–719.

Higgins, J. W., & Begoray, D. (2012). Exploring the borderlands between media and health: Conceptualizing 'critical media health literacy'. *Journal of Media Literacy Education*, *4*(2), 136–148.

Holmberg, C., Chaplin, J. E., Hillman, T., & Berg, C. (2016). Adolescents' presentation of food in social media: An explorative study. *Appetite*, *99*, 121–129.

Jones, B. L., Parker-Raley, J., & Barczyk, A. (2011). Adolescent cancer survivors: Identity paradox and the need to belong. *Qualitative Health Research*, *21*(8), 1033–1040.

Jorge, A., & Marôpo, L. (2017). Meios digitais e direitos: perspetivas de jovens com cancro [Digital media and rights: The perspectives of young people with cancer]. *Comunicação Pública*, *12*(22), 1–12.

Koteyko, N., & Hunt, D. (2016). Performing health identities on social media: An online observation of Facebook profiles. *Discourse, Context & Media*, *12*, 59–67.

Liu, L. S., Inkpen, K., & Pratt, W. (2015). 'I'm not like my friends': Understanding how children with a chronic illness use technology to maintain normalcy. In *Proceedings of the 18th ACM Conference on Computer Supported Cooperative Work & Social Computing* (pp. 1527–1539). Vancouver: ACM. doi:10.1145/2675133.2675201.

Livingstone, S. (2016). Reframing media effects in terms of children's rights in the digital age. *Journal of Children and Media*, *10*(1), 4–12.

Livingstone, S., Mascheroni, G., & Staksrud, E. (2015). *Developing a framework for researching children's online risks and opportunities in Europe*. London: EU Kids Online.

Livingstone, S., & Third, A. (2017). Children and young people's rights in the digital age: An emerging agenda. *New Media & Society*, *19*(5), 657–670.

Marôpo, L., Carvalho, R., & Sampaio, I. V. (2015). A visão de adolescentes com câncer sobre a divulgação da sua imagem: entre a privacidade e a autoafirmação [The views of adolescents with cancer about the disclosure of their image: Between privacy and self-assertion]. In C. Camponez, B. Araújo, F. Pinheiro, I. Godinho, & J. Morais (Eds.), *Comunicação e Transformações Sociais* (Vol. 1, pp. 274–283). Coimbra: SOPCOM.

Mascheroni, G., & Ólafsson, K. (2014). *Net children go mobile: Risks and opportunities*. Milan: Educatt.

Merolli, M., Gray, K., & Martin-Sanchez, F. (2013). Health outcomes and related effects of using social media in chronic disease management: A literature review and analysis of affordances. *Journal of Biomedical Informatics*, *46*(6), 957–969.

Nesby, L., & Salamonsen, A. (2016). Youth blogging and serious illness. *Medical Humanities*, *42*(1), 46–51.

Park, C. L., Zlateva, I., & Blank, T. O. (2009). Self-identity after cancer: 'survivor', 'victim', 'patient', and 'person with cancer'. *Journal of General Internal Medicine*, *24*(2), S430–S435.

Pruulmann-Vengerfeldt, P. (2018). CHARGE on: Digital parenting of a child with rare genetic syndrome with the help of Facebook Group. In G. Mascheroni, C. Ponte, & A. Jorge (Eds.), *Digital Parenting: The challenges for families in the digital age* (pp. 189–198). Gothenburg: Nordicom Clearinghouse.

Reginato, L. (n.d.). *CarecaTV*. Retrieved from: www.youtube.com/channel/UCB10CGoy2ywaODqN3Aefe6Q.

Santos, G. S., Tavares, C., Ferreira, R., & Pereira, C. (2015). Rede social e virtual de apoio ao adolescente que convive com doença crônica: uma revisão integrativa [Social and virtual support network for adolescents living with chronic illness: An integrative review]. *Aquichan*, *15*(1), 60–74.

Song, H., Nam, Y., Gould, J., Sanders, W. S., McLaughlin, M., Fulk, J., & Ruccione, K. S. (2012). Cancer survivor identity shared in a social media intervention. *Journal of Pediatric Oncology Nursing*, *29*(2), 80–91.

Stage, C. (2017). *Networked cancer: Affect, narrative and measurement*. New York: Palgrave Macmillan.

Staksrud, E., & Milojevic, T. (2017). Adolescents and children in global media landscape: From risks to rights. *Annals of the International Communication Association*, *41*(3–4), 235–241.

Swist, T., Collin, P., McCormack, J., & Third, A. (2015). *Social media and the wellbeing of children and young people: A literature review*. Perth: Commissioner for Children and Young People, Western Australia.

Ting-Toomey, S. (2016). Identity negotiation theory. In C. R. Berger & M. E. Roloff (Eds.), *The international encyclopedia of interpersonal communication* (pp. 1–10). Hoboken, NJ: Wiley.

Van der Velden, M. (2012). *Teenage patient privacy: Self-presentation and self-protection in social media.* Paper presented at Amsterdam Privacy Conference (APC), University of Amsterdam, Amsterdam, The Netherlands, 7–10 October, 2012.

Van der Velden, M., & El Emam, K. (2013). 'Not all my friends need to know': A qualitative study of teenage patients, privacy, and social media. *Journal of the American Medical Informatics Association, 20*(1), 16–24.

Wittmeier, K., Holland, C., Hobbs-Murison, K., Crawford, E., Beauchamp, C., Milne, B., ... Keijzer, R. (2014). Analysis of a parent-initiated social media campaign for Hirschsprung's Disease. *Journal of Medical Internet Research, 16*(12), e288. doi:10.2196/jmir.3200.

40
CHILDREN'S SEXUALITY IN THE CONTEXT OF DIGITAL MEDIA

Sexualisation, Sexting, and Experiences with Sexual Content in a Research Perspective

Liza Tsaliki and Despina Chronaki

Introduction

Social concerns about young people's encounters with sexual content or sexual communication have been following every new medium. In the past 20 years these concerns have been exacerbated further because of the broad diffusion of digital culture and online media. Effects and mass communication research have been feeding the public discourse with claims about the potential risks that experiences with sexual content or sexual communication might pose for childhood; especially since the incorporation of online media in young people's lifestyles and everyday communication routines, policy-making, legislation, and political initiatives have been focussing on parental monitoring practices of young people's use of online media. In effect, this becomes an attempt to regulate as much as possible their 'inner' desire to explore representations of sexuality and access or communicate sexual information (Tsaliki, 2016). This chapter provides a critical reading of available research on childhood, sexuality, and digital culture to offer a social constructionist understanding of pertinent theoretical conceptualisations to date. The critical reading positions itself at a safe distance both from alarming voices about children's sexualisation and the pornification of culture, as well as from celebratory voices about children's sexual autonomy and agentic sexual expression. Instead, the chapter argues that a historical and cultural conceptualisation of children's sexuality would provide a more effective analytical framework at both research and policy-making levels (e.g., sex educators, policymakers). In what follows, issues about the sexualisation of childhood as well as young people's engagement with sexting and encounters with sexual content are first discussed within two dominant paradigms, namely the effects research tradition and the 'communication risk' approach (Chronaki, 2014). Then follows a discussion about how these topics are contextualised within constructionist, feminist, and materialist perspectives, where researchers offer more inclusive conceptualisations of childhood and sexuality and less technology-driven accounts. An alternative epistemological framework is then proposed, endorsed by a significant majority of cultural studies researchers since the late 1990s. Given that all three issues entail an exhaustive investigation and regulation of childhood, the topics are discussed through different paradigms, as reflections of social anxieties about childhood sexuality overall; in effect, the discussion is built to underscore the need to contextualise children's sexuality further in contemporary research.

Discourses about Risk and Effects: Assumptions about Children's Problematic or Risky Experiences Online

Experts have been trying to prove a causal relationship between (what was perceived as) sexualised culture and young users' behaviour, attitudes, or development, in pretty much similar ways as they did with mainstream media and adult populations (Buckingham & Bragg, 2004). As a result, a long list of studies, coming mostly from the US, has informed public and policy agendas for some time now, while also attracting constant funding, something which serves to reiterate claims about the existence of effects of sexuality-related information or communication on young people (Chronaki, 2014). In Europe, Peter and Valkenburg's work (2008) or Horvath et al.'s (2013) policy-driven evidence review have fuelled already established concerns about online pornography and children. In Australia, Flood's work (e.g., 2009) has also been consistent in trying to prove that online pornography is harmful to minors, alongside Mitchell, Finkelhor, and Wolak's work in the US (2003, 2007). In research of this kind, sexual content online (the 'catch-all' notion of pornography) is assumed to possibly impact upon young people's attitudes towards women or sex. It is also assumed to potentially lead to unsolicited sexual practices, or early engagement with sex. Not least, there are assumptions that consumption of such content provides sexualising or objectifying representations of the male or female body (e.g., Flood, 2009), and in many cases is examined as an addictive practice (e.g., Tsitsika et al., 2009). In the majority of such studies, usually conducted with college students, participants are assumed to hold individual attitudes towards life, sexuality, and gender, which exposure to online porn changes or distorts. Their cultural, ideological, or life background and experiences do not seem to be of interest for researchers, while the meaning of the vague term 'pornography' or 'sexual content' is taken for granted, as is participants' understanding of (and even perceptions about) 'romance' and 'intimacy' (Chronaki, 2013). The 'otherness' of the young porn consumer (McKee, 2013), as well as the absence of their voice, is evident in the assumptions, phrasing, and results of such studies, leading to an assertion that research takes place about them but without them (Buckingham & Bragg, 2004).

Within the same conceptual framework, effects researchers examine sexual communication (i.e., sexting) as another potentially damaging practice of young people. The issue of sexting emerged as a problem of young people's practices online in 2008, with the spread of a policy-driven report from the US-based National Campaign to Prevent Teen and Unplanned Pregnancy (2008) (Hasinoff, 2012, 2015). While in this case, the adult population seems to be less at risk from the hazardous impact of sexting, researchers of this tradition highlight the potential impact of sexting upon young people's initiation of sexual life. They also express concerns about effects upon girls' sexual identity or self-perception and self-confidence (e.g., Garcia-Gomez, 2017; Subrahmanyam et al., 2004) but also upon audiences' attitudes towards female and (to a lesser degree) male bodies and sexualities. Especially in the Australian context, the issue of young people's sexting has received extensive public and academic attention because of its legal conceptualisation as potential child pornography or molestation (McGovern et al., 2016). In this case, the discourse around sexting raised questions about legal consent as well as about who and under what circumstances are young people allowed to sext without being at risk of practising something illegal (see critical discussions from Albury, 2017; Albury & Byron, 2014; Angelides, 2013). According to Simpson (2013, p. 690), "'sexting' appears to be caught between debates on the sexual rights of children and the role of the state in protecting children from themselves". As expected, policy documents, the media, and public agendas draw upon alarming effects voices underscoring the potentially harmful effects of sexual communication on children. Most effects studies seem to be gender specific, either via victimising girls (Ringrose et al., 2013) or via abstracting masculinities and leaving them out of the picture (Hasinoff, 2015). Overall, this body of studies (not just in Australia but in Europe as well) assumes that children are predominantly heterosexual (see Albury & Byron, 2014; De Ridder & Van Bauwel, 2013 for a critique on the matter), and unable to understand and cope with the paedophile danger that abounds.

Following the same theoretical, methodological, and reporting patterns as in research about online pornography or sexting, studies about the impact of the sexualisation of culture are also gender-specific (in that they mostly discuss girls) (e.g., Du Plooy et al., 2018) or focus on young children's marketisation from consumer culture (Bailey, 2011). They mostly assume that the sexual forces underpinning contemporary mass and popular culture are effectively impacting on the ways young people understand sexuality, sexual life, family, intimacy, and romance, while they fall victim to the fake expectations that online technologies and the market forces create (Bragg & Buckingham, 2013; Tsaliki, 2016). Widely cited reports in the US, Australia, and the UK (see, for example, Bailey (2011) and Rush and La Nauze (2006)) on children's sexualisation raised concerns about childhood innocence, fallen childhood, and the corrupting influence of private-turned-public sexual information, attracting critical responses from feminist, sociology of childhood, and cultural studies scholars. These critical scholars responded to such epistemologically flawed claims via empirical research in a feminist (Ringrose, 2011; Ringrose & Renold, 2012) or cultural feminist (e.g., Egan, 2013; Jackson & Vares, 2015) and cultural studies context (e.g., Tsaliki, 2016), or via contextualising theoretical accounts about the origins of 'sexualisation of childhood' discourses (Bragg & Buckingham, 2013; Egan & Hawkes, 2012; Faulkner, 2010; Lumby & Albury, 2010; Tsaliki, 2015; Vänskä, 2017).

Deriving from a more balanced perspective, one that does not take the figure of the child as the individual to be corrected (Egan & Hawkes, 2010), a mass communication approach is introduced by the extensive empirical and conceptual work of the EU Kids Online Network (EU Kids Online, 2018). Drawing upon an interdisciplinary approach to childhood, combining the work of a large number of researchers representing different fields in media studies and social sciences, this extensive research network established a less alarming way of thinking and talking about children's experiences online, albeit in the context of a risk-averse culture (Buckingham & Chronaki, 2014; Tsaliki, 2016). The empirical and policy work of this network managed to inform policy, public, and academic agendas about children's use of online media, children's rights in the digital age, and to provide the body of research about children and the media with systematically collected rigorous data from 21 European countries (Livingstone et al., 2011). Its influential work led to the development of related country projects and sub-networks outside the EU, where research knowledge and expertise was transferred to researchers who adopted the EU Kids Online model of research to study children's practices with online media (EU Kids Online, 2018).

The innovative epistemological and methodological stance of this network has been the classification of children's experiences online into risks and opportunities (Hasebrink et al., 2009). In this context, sexuality and consequently sexual content online, sexting, and any type of sexuality-related information (except formal sources of sexual education) are considered a risk (Livingstone et al., 2011). Mentions of the risky nature of such experiences are found in most of the EU Kids Online reports, implying that any sexually related experience online is potentially a risk (though not necessarily harmful), unless it comes from a formal educational or regulatory source (Buckingham & Chronaki, 2014). The findings relating to sexual risks online could be summarised as follows (Rovolis & Tsaliki, 2012; Tsaliki et al., 2014):

1 It is mostly boys rather than girls who have such experiences, and older children rather than younger;
2 It is primarily girls and younger children who are likely to report being bothered by such experiences;
3 Girls' and younger children's experiences are mostly accidental in comparison with older children and boys;
4 Experiences with sexual content online are not significantly more than experiences with sexual content in mainstream media like TV;
5 The number of children who report having been bothered by such experiences overall is rather small (4% of the 23% who reported experiencing sexual content). Of the 25,000 children who were interviewed, 5,750 reported experiences with sexual content; of those, 230 reported having been bothered by the experience;
6 Experiences with sexting range from 4% to 22% in different countries, with a tendency to decrease over time.

It is notable that illegal or abusive activities like sexual harassment and sexual abuse ('grooming') also fall within the range of sexual risks online and are invariably blended with experiences like sexual content and sexting and attributed to the 'child as perpetrator' (Livingstone et al., 2011, p. 135). In effect, children's active engagement with sexual communication is by default considered not just problematic, but almost having legal implications. This understanding of children's sexual agency and the construction of their experiences as in need of censoring, regulation, and guidance reflect – as argued later – the anxieties that frame childhood as a status of innocence and as an uncontrolled, monstrous period in one's life (Egan & Hawkes, 2010). As scholars argue, such constructions reflect further anxieties about societies' current state and future (Egan & Hawkes, 2012; Tsaliki, 2016).

Although robust, systematic, representative, and recent, the EU Kids Online methodological and analytical framework points at a polarised understanding of how online experiences are articulated by children out of the binary context of risk and opportunity. The researchers argue that they bring children's voices to research, which is true; nevertheless, in asking children to position themselves towards predetermined and adult-defined categories of practices, EU Kids Online limits children's agency to define what is risky for them online and discursively construct it in ways they choose.

As derived from the data, children have not had so many experiences with sexual content as moralistic, alarming voices have been arguing thus far (Rovolis & Tsaliki, 2012). Yet, by adopting a mass communication approach, the EU Kids Online research reads children's voices within the dominant, hegemonic approach where children are seen facing a variety of risks. For a detailed critique of the EU Kids Online conceptual framework, see Tsaliki (2016) Chapters 3 and 4.

Overall, dominant discourses about childhood and sexuality in academia are overwhelmingly about the sexual risks or effects to which children are exposed in the context of digital culture and about their incapacity to cope or filter them effectively. In this context there are calls about the need for children to be regulated, monitored, and guided by adults, but also the need for their sexual conduct to be governed in some sort of censorious and adult-driven way (Chronaki, 2013). In discussing such research critically, it should be mentioned that the authors do not argue that online experiences are risk-free, nor that there are no children who have probably been harmed or influenced in their online use. However, as discussed later in this chapter, it is the dominant understandings of sexuality and childhood as well as their contemporary constructions (going back to nineteenth-century Europe) that render them epistemologically unstable and in need of further contextualisation.

Critical Approaches to Sexuality: Empowerment or Victimisation?

Partly as a response to increased concerns discussed above, scholars representing critical approaches to sexuality (feminist, materialist, and constructionist) have also discussed children's experiences with sexual content online and sexuality more broadly. Studies within this context conceptualise children's discussions further, offering less empirical data, but better-contextualised accounts. Most of the studies reviewed appear to be concerned with the issue of the sexualisation of culture, a little less with sexting, and even less with online sexual content. They seem to share some common understandings about culture and childhood, raising issues like children's sexual agency, sexual rights, and ethics (Albury, 2017, 2018; Hasinoff, 2015); queer constructions of sexualities and the marginalisation of queer identities in a heteronormative context (Albury & Byron, 2014; De Ridder, 2015; De Ridder & Van Bauwel, 2013); or even class and patriarchal pressures on children's experiences and practices online (e.g., Renold & Ringrose, 2013; Ringrose, 2011). A significant contribution of studies situated within a feminist/postfeminist or materialist context is that in contextualising children's sexuality in broader terms than merely arguing about the media's damaging impact upon them, they make further claims about gender performance, and about gender constructions. In this way, such studies are situated more effectively within the policy discourse about sexuality education and children's sexual rights (e.g., Fox & Bale, 2018). Nevertheless, in building almost political accounts about gender equality and freedom of sexual identity, they do not seem to take into account the cultural, historical, and political complexities of sexualisation as indicated by cultural thinkers (Attwood, 2006). Many studies in this context, especially those drawing upon feminism and postfeminism, attempt to prove either that effects do not exist, or that the prevalence of risk in young people's experiences with mediated sexuality is overstated, and thus potential positive outcomes regarding literacy or agency are largely neglected (e.g., Ringrose et al., 2013). In effect, several feminist accounts engage with the same either/or polarity as studies from the previous paradigm, albeit from a subtly implied effects perspective or a risk/opportunity one (e.g., Renold & Ringrose, 2011; Ringrose & Barajas, 2011; Ringrose et al., 2013). Moreover, in many cases, the discussion revolves around young girls and public concerns about their sexualisation ('the girl at risk' or the 'risky' girl, Ringrose et al., 2013), while boys' perceptions and voice are still missing.

The lack of focus on boys' sexualisation, both in terms of theoretical conceptualisation and empirical work, is highlighted by feminist (Clark & Duschinsky, 2018; Vänskä, 2017) and cultural studies researchers (Bragg & Buckingham, 2013; Tsaliki, 2016). Notable exceptions in this context are Albury's work (2017, 2018) on children's sexual rights via a cultural feminist critique of policy and public discourses about sexting panic, as well as Hasinoff's (2012, 2015) account of young people's agency while sexting. Non-heteronormative sexualities are to be found in a few cases, as in the work of Albury and Byron (2014) and Albury and Crawford (2013), or De Ridder (2015) and De Ridder and Van Bauwel (2013), where LGBTQ youth and their sexting practices or sexual expression through social media is discussed through a cultural studies and queer studies lens. Not least, a focus on people from different racial backgrounds is scarce in the literature. In one of the few studies, Fischel (2016) discusses how black children are constructed in public discourses as deprived, with limited citizenship rights (including technology and sexuality) and therefore victimised within a sexualised culture. They are also seen as being in need of empowerment, reiterating discourses about a racialised and class-based childhood innocence (Bernstein, 2011; Tsaliki, 2016).

A significant number of studies contextualise their accounts and findings within the ethical, pedagogical, or feminist and postfeminist discourses through which children's sexuality is performed and asserted in digital contexts (Albury, 2017; Albury & Crawford, 2013; De Ridder, 2015; De Ridder & Van Bauwel, 2013; Nielsen et al., 2015). In this context they also take into account how policy, public, and academic agendas should consider children's sexual and intimate citizenship more seriously. For example, Scarcelli (2015) discusses gendered performance in online pornography perception, while Attwood et al., (2018) offer a culturally contextualised discussion of young people's accounts of (online) porn in terms of taste and identity. Significant though these constructionist contributions may be for understanding in what terms these young people articulate their experiences with sexual content online, without engaging in a polemical debate about children's sexuality, they seem however to also miss the cultural, cosmopolitan, or political discourses through which children might construct their encounters with sexual content or sexual communication online. What they also seem to miss is how young people make claims about sexual citizenship, sexual literacies, or sexual rights, thus how young people rework the overall concept of sexuality, sexual norms, and practices in an ethical and self-governing context. Hence, it is argued that researchers representing critical approaches need to go further from the political project of children's sexual citizenship and talk more thoroughly about the whole range of cultural and life repertoires that young people deploy in talking about their experiences but also their sexuality more broadly. In so doing, researchers will be able to intervene more effectively in policy and public debates about sexual education and children's sexual rights.

Children's Sexuality in Historical Perspective: What Academic and Public Discourses Show About Our Understanding of Childhood and Sexuality

The authors' aim in this chapter has been to review a representative sample of the available literature on children's experiences with sexual content and sexual communication online. Although some thinkers distinguish between realist, materialist, and constructionist approaches in talking about children's sexuality (e.g., Fox & Bale, 2018), provided here is a classification of risk/effects, critical, and constructionist/poststructuralist approaches. With this it is argued that if researchers wish to address public and policy agendas more effectively, they need to turn towards a broader contextualisation of children's sexuality in historical terms. The significant work of cultural studies scholars like Buckingham and Bragg (2004), Egan and Hawkes (2010, 2012), Jackson (1982), Hunt (2009), and Tsaliki (2015, 2016) conceptualise children's experiences with sexual content and sexual communication (and, further, sexual agency, rights, and citizenship) as reflections of eighteenth- and nineteenth-century anxieties about childhood that emerged and keep evolving hand in hand with anxieties and concerns about sexuality. The aim of this section is to highlight cultural studies' empirical and theoretical work that calls for a need to conceptualise sexuality and childhood more broadly, and, for this reason, sexual content, sexting, and sexualisation are not discussed separately.

Most studies in this context situate their work by drawing upon historical, cultural, and political developments in late modernity to understand how and why young people discuss their experiences with sexuality (offline or online) in the way they do, and how these accounts are being perceived by adults, namely parents, experts, policymakers, and the media. In this context, Allen (2006) adopts a social constructionist approach to consider how sexuality and sex education are socially and culturally understood within the school context. Similarly, Bale (2012) uses a constructionist framework to discuss how young people perceive the impact of sexualised media on their sexual health, drawing on sociological theories of sexuality and risk. Monique Mulholland (2013) draws mainly upon a constructionist perspective and explores how young people engage with 'pornification' discourses through their understanding and engagement with key terms such as the 'normal', the 'perverse', and the 'illicit'. Berg (2007) draws upon social constructionism to consider the ethical and cultural dimensions of girls' accounts of their bodily reactions to pornography, and how girls discursively define the balance between real-life sex and arousal from pornography. Chronaki (2013) analyses the ethical, political, and cosmopolitan dimensions of young people's constructions of sexual content (not focussing on digital culture) and the articulation of porn literacies as indications of intimate citizenships, by putting them in the cultural-historical perspective of Michel Foucault's notion of governmentality (1986/2012). In a similar vein, Tsaliki (2016) explores girls' discursive constructions of sexualisation in digital contexts by focussing not just on gender performance but also on political and ethical articulations of taste, agency, and literacy; her empirical work is contextualised through historical accounts about the discursivity of sexuality and childhood and the question of leisure. Masanet and Buckingham (2015, p. 486) explore the pedagogical possibilities and limitations of online fan forums as a source of informal sex education, "arguing that the presentation of issues to do with sexuality sometimes challenges young people to engage in debate and to move beyond established discourses". Last but not least, Bond (2010, p. 587) explores "the relationship between young people's talk of sexuality and sexual acts in their discussions of mobile phone use, within the wider theoretical debates about risk and self-identity", via a social constructivist perspective.

Through research of the kind mentioned in this section, one may understand the cultural trajectories that young people's articulations of sexuality follow and how they construct childhood, agency, and citizenship outside the context of sexuality. For example, Albury (2018, p. 1331) usefully notes that "apps are not the only digital technologies to be associated with sexual risks. As smartphone ownership has become more widespread among young people, adult anxieties regarding young people's sexual expression have crystallised around digital practices". Along the same lines, De Ridder and Van Bauwel (2013, p. 570) argue that digital literacy merely implies technical skills, "while young people should be trained as late modern ambassadors of intimacy, playing this out in networked publics, sharing openness and plurality, criticising racism, sexism and homophobia". Such anxieties and concerns about children's control or increasing ownership of technological capital reflect for some researchers the socially constructed problem of leisure. Children's leisure in the nineteenth century and particularly the leisure of the working class was constructed as a problem, given that childhood had already been established as a state that needs to be appropriated and guided towards an ethical (self-governed) adulthood. As researchers note, "the notion of 'unstructured leisure' as a cause of juvenile deviance emerged during Victorian times, when the increase in the free time available for young people resulted in young people 'with too much in their hands', ending up intoxicated" (Blackman, 2011; Tsaliki, 2015, p. 503).

Anxieties about how childhood is negotiated by children and how it should be regulated and censored by adults (especially when it comes to the 'masses', or the working class) are one of the main issues upon which cultural scholars draw when talking about childhood and sexuality. Egan and Hawkes (2012, p. 271), among others, argue that the construction of the sexual child has emerged from social purity and hygiene anxieties in the nineteenth century. In talking about sexualisation specifically, they argue that the discourses through which it is articulated draw upon problematic assumptions about the child, reflecting middle-class attempts to secure the boundaries of class, race, and age distinctions. A well-established construction of nineteenth-century urban space as morally depraving, unstable in terms of race and class, enabled calls for specific (censorious, disciplinary, and regulatory) modes of parenting and child rearing that would ensure future self-governed and productive members of the broader social group (see Tsaliki (2016) for a more detailed discussion). As a result, the child figure became a central platform of purity reform and anything outside the context of a healthy, well-regulated, and properly guided childhood (namely the 'morally infectious' poor) posed a threat to white middle-class children (Egan & Hawkes, 2010).

The emergence of childhood into a distinct social category, begging for certain ways of management and carrying specific political, cultural, and ethical connotations, also signifies 'innocence' lost, or nostalgic moments of what an adult is not anymore (Faulkner, 2010). In effect, innocence is synonymised with preciousness and helplessness and is crystallised as the iconic, desirable image of childhood that "potentially supplants concern for *children*. This sort of innocence tends to a 'politics of the ban'" (Fischel, 2016, p. 207, emphasis in original). In the context of the 'purification' and 'naturalness' of the Romantics, sexuality takes from the eighteenth century onwards the form of a discursive construction; as something to be spoken of, cross-cutting and at the same time defining and establishing the boundaries between private and public (Foucault, 1986/2012). The emergence of technologies like medical sciences and confession within the context of Catholicism means that the human body is scrutinised and put in the discursive context of the private, the 'appropriate', and the 'normal' (Chronaki, 2013). The impact of such technologies takes place in the context of the further political and social organisation of modern Western societies, where the notion of citizenship becomes a matter of priority for the well-being of the social group and is articulated through the governing of both the body and the soul (see Rose, 1999 for a more detailed discussion). In effect, sexuality is removed from public space to one which is private, and it only becomes a matter to be spoken of once it asks for regulation, medical, or spiritual (religious) intervention. As a result, sexuality becomes a socially defined category and is constructed as a set of binaries (acceptable/unacceptable; appropriate/inappropriate; ethical/unethical; healthy/unhealthy; private/public) and soon the notion of 'peripheral sexualities' emerges, where – among other things – childhood and same-sex sexuality are included (Rose, 1999).

It is therefore in this historical and socio-cultural context that the authors' work on children's experiences with sexual content and sexual communication online is situated, providing an effective analytical framework within which researchers could possibly get past a polarised debate about the effects and risks (or absence) of anything relevant to sexuality and children. In this respect, Plummer's (1995, p. 151) approach to intimate citizenship is followed, within which "new emerging rights and responsibilities come to the forefront in making decisions about controlling and accessing such intimate self-representations, but also making choices about how to give shape to eroticisms, sexual and gender identities in these specific mediated places".

Hence, if children's sexuality is considered from such perspectives, informed by historical and cultural accounts about childhood, sexuality, and technology, more accurate contributions to policy and public agendas can be made and possibly address public anxieties and panics more effectively.

References

Albury, K. (2017). Just because it's public doesn't mean it's any of your business: Adults' and children's sexual rights in digitally mediated spaces. *New Media & Society*, *19*(5), 713–725.

Albury, K. (2018). Young people, digital media research and counterpublic sexual health. *Sexualities*, *21*(8), 1331–1336.

Albury, K., & Byron, P. (2014). Queering sexting and sexualisation. *Media International Australia*, *153*, 138–147.

Albury, K., & Crawford, K. (2013). Sexting, consent and young people's ethics: Beyond Megan's story. *Continuum: Journal of Media & Cultural Studies*, *26*(3), 463–473.

Allen, L. (2006). "Looking at the real thing": Young men, pornography, and sexuality education. *Discourse: Studies in the Cultural Politics of Education*, *27*(1), 69–83.

Angelides, S. (2013). Technology, hormones, and stupidity: The affective politics of teenage sexting. *Sexualities*, *16*(5/6), 665–689.

Attwood, F. (2006). Sexed up: Theorising the sexualization of culture. *Sexualities*, *9*(1), 77–94.

Attwood, F., Smith, C., & Barker, M. (2018). 'I'm just curious and still exploring myself': Young people and pornography. *New Media and Society*, *20*(10), 3738–3759.

Bailey, R. (2011). *Letting children be children: Report of an independent review of the commercialization and sexualisation of childhood* (Vol. 8078). Retrieved from: www.gov.uk/government/publications/letting-children-be-children-report-of-an-independent-review-of-the-commercialization-and-sexualization-of-childhood.

Bale, C. (2012). Exploring young people's perceptions of the impact of sexualized media on their sexual health: A qualitative study. (Doctoral dissertation). The University of Sheffield, Sheffield, UK. Retrieved from: https://ethos.bl.uk/OrderDetails.do?uin=uk.bl.ethos.574480.

Berg, L. (2007). Turned on by pornography: Still a respectable girl? In S. V. Knudsen, L. Löfgren-Mårtenson, & S.-A. Månsson (Eds.), *Generation P? Youth, gender and pornography* (pp. 293–307). Copenhagen: Danish School of Education Press.

Bernstein, R. (2011). *Racial innocence performing American childhood from slavery to civil rights*. New York: New York University Press.

Blackman, S. (2011). Rituals of intoxication: Young people, drugs, risk and leisure. In P. Bramham and S. Wagg (Eds.), *The New Politics of Leisure and Pleasure* (pp. 97–118). Basingstoke, UK: Palgrave Macmillan.

Bond, E. (2010). Managing mobile relationships: Children's perceptions of the impact of the mobile phone on relationships in their everyday lives. *Childhood*, 17(4), 514–529.

Bragg, S., & Buckingham, D. (2013). Global concerns, local negotiations and moral selves: Contemporary parenting and the 'sexualisation of childhood' debate. *Feminist Media Studies*, 13(4), 643–659.

Buckingham, D., & Bragg, S. (2004). *Young people, sex and the media: The facts of life?* London: Palgrave Macmillan.

Buckingham, D., & Chronaki, D. (2014). Saving the children? Pornography, childhood and the Internet. In S. Wagg & J. Pilcher (Eds.), *Thatcher's grandchildren* (pp. 301–317). Basingstoke: Palgrave Macmillan.

Chronaki, D. (2013). Young people's accounts of experiences with sexual content during childhood and teenage life. *The Communication Review*, 16(1–2), 61–69.

Chronaki, D. (2014). *Young people's accounts of experiences with sexual content during childhood and teenage life*. (Doctoral dissertation). Retrieved from: https://dspace.lboro.ac.uk/dspace-jspui/bitstream/2134/15928/3/Thesis-2014-Chronaki.pdf.

Clark, J., & Duschinsky, R. (2018). Young masculinities, purity and danger: Disparities in framings of boys and girls in policy discourses of sexualisation. *Sexualities*, 0(0), 1–18. doi.org/10.1177/1363460717736718.

De Ridder, S. (2015). Are digital media institutions shaping youth's intimate stories? Strategies and tactics in the social networking site Netlog. *New Media and Society*, 17(3), 356–374.

De Ridder, S., & Van Bauwel, S. (2013). Commenting on pictures: Teens negotiating gender and sexualities on social networking sites. *Sexualities*, 16(5/6), 565–586.

Du Plooy, C., Coetzee, H., & Van Rensburg, E. (2018). Psychological effects of multimedia-induced sexualisation of girls in middle childhood: A systematic literature review. *Journal of Child & Adolescent Mental Health*, 30(2), 67–85.

Egan, D., & Hawkes, G. L. (2010). *Theorising the sexual child in modernity*. New York: Palgrave Macmillan.

Egan, D., & Hawkes, G. L. (2012). Sexuality, youth and the perils of endangered innocence: How history can help us get past the panic. *Gender and Education*, 24(3), 269–284.

Egan, D. R. (2013). *Becoming sexual: A critical appraisal of the sexualization of girls*. Cambridge: Polity Press.

EU Kids Online. (2018). *Enhancing knowledge of European children's online opportunities, risks and safety*. Retrieved from: www.lse.ac.uk/media-and-communications/research/research-projects/eu-kids-online (accessed on 15 June 2019).

Faulkner, J. (2010). The innocence fetish: The commodification and sexualisation of children in the media and popular culture. *Media International Australia*, 135(1), 106–117.

Fischel, J. (2016). Pornographic protections? Itineraries of childhood innocence. *Law, Culture and the Humanities*, 12(2), 206–220.

Flood, M. (2009). The harms of pornography exposure among children and young people. *Child Abuse Review*, 18(6), 384–400.

Foucault, M. (1986/2012). *The history of sexuality, vol. 3: The care of the self*. New York: Vintage.

Fox, N., & Bale, C. (2018). Bodies, pornography and the circumscription of sexuality: A new materialist study of young people's sexual practices. *Sexualities*, 21(3), 393–409.

Garcia-Gomez, A. (2017). Teen girls and sexual agency: Exploring the intrapersonal and intergroup dimensions of sexting. *Media, Culture and Society*, 39(3), 391–407.

Hasebrink, U., Livingstone, S., Haddon, L., & Ólafsson, K. (2009). *Comparing children's online opportunities and risks across Europe: Cross-national comparisons for EU Kids Online* (2nd ed). Deliverable D3.2. Retrieved from: http://eprints.lse.ac.uk/24368/1/D3.2_Report-Cross_national_comparisons-2nd-edition.pdf.

Hasinoff, A. A. (2012). Sexting as media production: Rethinking social media and sexuality. *New Media & Society*, 15(4), 449–465.

Hasinoff, A. A. (2015). *Sexting panic: Rethinking criminalisation, privacy and consent*. Chicago, IL: University of Illinois Press.

Horvath, M. A. H., Alys, L., Massey, K., Pina, A., Scally, M., & Adler, J. R. (2013). *Basically, porn is everywhere: A rapid evidence assessment on the effects that access and exposure to pornography has on children and young people*. London: Office of the Children's Commissioner. Retrieved from: www.childrenscommissioner.gov.uk/wp-content/uploads/2017/07/Basically_-_Porn_is_everywhere_-_The_Appendicies.pdf.

Hunt, P. (2009). Children's literature and childhood. In M. J. Kehily (Ed.), *An introduction to childhood studies* (2nd ed, pp. 50–69). Maidenhead: Open University Press–McGraw-Hill.

Jackson, S. (1982). *Childhood and sexuality*. Oxford: Blackwell.

Jackson, S., & Vares, T. (2015). Too many bad role models for us girls': Girls, female pop celebrities and 'sexualization'. *Sexualities, 18*(4), 480–498.

Livingstone, S., Haddon, L., Görzig, A., & Ólafsson, K. (2011). *Risks and safety on the internet: The perspective of European children: Full findings and policy implications from the EU Kids Online survey of 9-16 year olds and their parents in 25 countries*. EU Kids Online. London. Retrieved from: http://eprints.lse.ac.uk/33731.

Lumby, C., & Albury, K. (2010). Too much? Too young? The sexualisation of children debate in Australia. *Media International Australia, 135*(1), 140–152.

Masanet, M.-J., & Buckingham, D. (2015). Advice on life? Online fan forums as a space for peer-to-peer sex and relationships education. *Sex Education, 15*(5), 486–499.

McGovern, A., Crofts, T., Murray, L., & Milivojevic, S. (2016). Media, legal and young people's discourses around sexting. *Global Studies of Childhood, 6*(4), 428–441.

McKee, A. (2013). Why are children the most important audience for pornography in Australia? In A. Moran & K. Aveyard (Eds.), *Watching films: Perspectives on movie-going, exhibition and reception* (pp. 87–100). Bristol: Intellect.

Mitchell, K., Finkelhor, D., & Wolak, J. (2003). Exposure of youth to unwanted sexual material on the Internet: A national survey of risk, impact, and prevention. *Youth Society, 34*(3), 330–358.

Mulholland, M. (2013). *Young people and pornography: Negotiating pornification*. New York: Palgrave Macmillan.

Nielsen, S., Paasonen, S., & Spisak, S. (2015). "Pervy role-play and such": Girls' experiences of sexual messaging online. *Sex Education, 15*(5), 472–485.

Peter, J., & Valkenburg, P. M. (2008). Adolescents' exposure to sexually explicit Internet material, sexual uncertainty, and attitudes toward uncommitted sexual exploration: Is there a link? *Communication Research, 35*(5), 579–601.

Plummer, K. (1995). *Telling sexual stories: Power, change and social worlds*. London: Routledge.

Renold, E., & Ringrose, J. (2011). Schizoid subjectivities? Re-theorising teen girls' sexual cultures in an era of 'sexualization'. *Journal of Sociology, 47*(4), 389–409.

Renold, E., & Ringrose, J. (2013). Feminisms re-figuring 'sexualisation', sexuality and 'the girl'. *Feminist Theory, 14*(3), 247–254.

Ringrose, J. (2011). Are you sexy, flirty, or a slut? Exploring 'sexualization' and how teen girls perform/negotiate digital sexual identity on social networking sites. In R. Gill & C. Scharff (Eds.), *New Femininities* (pp. 99–116). London: Palgrave Macmillan.

Ringrose, J., & Barajas, K. (2011). Gendered risks and opportunities? Exploring teen girls' digitised sexual identities in postfeminist media contexts. *International Journal of Media and Cultural Politics, 7*(2), 121–138.

Ringrose, J., Harvey, L., Gill, R., & Livingstone, S. (2013). Teen girls, sexual double standards and 'sexting': Gendered value in digital image exchange. *Feminist Theory, 14*(3), 305–323.

Ringrose, J., & Renold, E. (2012). Teen girls, working-class femininity and resistance: Retheorising fantasy and desire in educational contexts of heterosexualised violence. *International Journal of Inclusive Education, 16*(4), 461–477.

Rose, N. (1999). *Governing the soul: The shaping of the private self*. London: Free Association Books.

Rovolis, A., & Tsaliki, L. (2012). Pornography. In S. Livingstone, L. Haddon, & A. Görzig (Eds.), *Children, risk and safety on the Internet: Research and policy challenges in comparative perspective* (pp. 165–176). Bristol: Policy Press.

Rush, E., & La Nauze, A. (2006). *Letting children be children: Stopping the sexualisation of children in Australia*. Canberra: The Australia Institute. Retrieved from: www.tai.org.au/sites/default/files/DP93_8.pdf.

Scarcelli, M. (2015). "It's disgusting, but . . .": Adolescent girls' relationship to Internet pornography as gender performance. *Porn Studies, 2*(2–3), 237–249.

Simpson, B. (2013). Challenging childhood, challenging children: Children's rights and sexting. *Sexualities, 16*(5/6), 690–709.

Subrahmanyam, K., Greenfield, P. M., & Tynes, B. (2004). Constructing sexuality and identity in an online teen chatroom. *Applied Developmental Psychology, 25*, 651–666.

Tsaliki, L. (2015). Popular culture and moral panics about 'children at risk': Revisiting the sexualisation-of-young-girls debate. *Sex Education, 15*(5), 500–514.

Tsaliki, L. (2016). *Children and the politics of sexuality: The sexualization of children debate revisited*. London: Palgrave Macmillan.

Tsaliki, L., Chronaki, D., & Ólafsson, K. (2014). *Experiences with sexual content: What we know from the research so far*. London: EU Kids Online.

Tsitsika, A., Critselis, E., Kormas, G., Konstantoulaki, E., Constantopoulos, A., & Kafetzis, D. (2009). Adolescent pornographic internet site use: A multivariate regression analysis of the predictive factors of use and psychosocial implications. *CyberPsychology & Behavior, 12*(5), 545–550.

Vänskä, A. (2017). "I am Lenni": Boys, sexualisation, and the dangerous colour pink. *Sexualities, 22*(3), 296–309.

Wolak, J., Mitchell, K., & Finkelhor, D. (2007). Unwanted and wanted exposure to online pornography in a national sample of youth Internet users. *Pediatrics, 119*(2), 247–258.

41
DIGITAL INEQUALITIES AMONGST DIGITAL NATIVES

Ellen J. Helsper

Introduction

The idea of young people as digital natives, effortlessly using Information and Communication Technologies (ICTs), has regained traction in the era of easy access and use. While much is written about young people's immersion in digital media, less attention is paid to those who are struggling to participate fully online. That is, extensive research around digital inequalities amongst adults is not mirrored in similar attention to detail in studying inequalities amongst young people. This chapter examines the evidence for the continued existence of different types of digital inequalities amongst young people who grew up around tablets and smartphones.

Prensky famously coined the term digital native to describe individuals whose "brains have physically changed – and are different from ours – as a result of how they grew up. But whether or not this is literally true, we can say with certainty that their thinking patterns have changed" (2001, p. 1). Prensky's digital natives (born after 1980) grew up with non-mobile, PC-based technologies. As they approach middle age, the digital landscape has changed; mobile phone diffusion increased exponentially, tablets and smart objects came onto the scene (Chaudron et al., 2017).

There has been extensive critique of the digital native concept (see Bennett, Maton, & Kervin, 2008; Jones & Czerniewicz, 2010; Ng, 2012). This chapter contributes to this ongoing debate by contesting the idea that *all or most* young people are able to use ICTs on an equal footing. The cross-national evidence presented in this chapter shows that, even with increased accessibility and ease of use, many so-called digital natives are not able to take advantage of the opportunities that ICT access and use can offer.

The general inequalities literature makes a distinction between first-, second-, and third-level digital inequalities (Nie, Sousa-Poza, & Nimrod, 2017; van Deursen & van Dijk, 2015). The first level at which a person might be disadvantaged refers to inequalities in the infrastructure and devices to which individuals have access. A distinction can be made between potential and actual access, that is, between the availability of infrastructure and devices in the neighbourhoods and households that people live in and the actual use of these devices. The second level concerns inequalities in the breadth and depth of ICT skills that people have and the ways in which they use these. There is an extensive literature on the different types of skills that should be considered (Hargittai, 2002; Van Dijk & Van Deursen, 2010) and an agreed-upon distinction between technical-operational, critical information-navigation, social-communicative, and content-creation skills (Van Deursen, Helsper, & Eynon, 2016). For uses there is more variety in classifications but they can be largely grouped into information seeking, entertainment, financial or economic, communication, political or civic engagement, and identity-motivated activities (Eastin, Cicchirillo, & Mabry, 2015; Opgenhaffen & d'Haenens, 2012). Third-level digital inequalities refer to the inequalities in the positive and negatives outcomes of ICT use (Nie et al., 2017; Van Deursen & Helsper, 2015).

Theorisation in the field of digital inequalities argues that historical economic, social, cultural, political, and other vulnerabilities are replicated in digital inequalities (Helsper, 2012; Ignatow & Robinson, 2017). Empirical research confirms that this is indeed the case for adults (Ignatow & Robinson, 2017; Van Deursen, Helsper, Eynon, & Van Dijk, 2017). This approach is often lacking in research with youth and especially absent is the theorisation of different types of inequalities and how these translate into differences in use and outcomes (Brown & Czerniewicz, 2010; Selwyn, 2009). While not as theoretically grounded, there is a growing body of empirical evidence suggesting the existence of systematic inequalities amongst young people who have grown up in more digital environments (i.e., digital natives).

A review of the literature[1] produces 122 articles in the last ten years with evidence for inequalities amongst digital natives based on household *socio-economic status* (e.g., Jara et al., 2015; Katz & Gonzalez, 2016a; Katz, Moran, & Gonzalez, 2018; Ono & Tsai, 2008; Thornham & Cruz, 2017; Tondeur, Sinnaeve, van Houtte, & van Braak, 2011; Vekiri, 2010; Zhang, 2015), and *gender* (e.g., Bilal & Jopeck, 2014; Cotten, Shank, & Anderson, 2014; Hinostroza, Matamala, Labbe, Claro, & Cabello, 2015; Martinez-Cantos, 2017; McQuillan & d'Haenens, 2009; Pagani, Argentin, Gui, & Stanca, 2016; Steeves & Kwami, 2017; Wartberg et al., 2015). Inequalities based on *ethnicity* (e.g., Jackson et al., 2008; Janisse, Li, Bhavnagri, Esposito, & Stanton, 2018; Katz, Gonzalez, & Clark, 2017; Mertens & d'Haenens, 2010; Ono & Tsai, 2008; Oyedemi, 2015) and *rurality* (e.g., Awan & Gauntlett, 2013; Li & Ranieri, 2013; Liao, Chang, Wang, & Sun, 2016; Lichy, 2011; Steeves & Kwami, 2017) are also reported. Research done in the *Global South* (e.g., Arora, 2010; Awuor, Khisa, & Rambi, 2015; Chuma, 2014; Mo et al., 2013; Munyengabe, Zhao, He, & Hitimana, 2017) focusses mostly though not exclusively on *access*-related inequalities and education and civic participation questions. Research in the *Global North* emphasises inequalities in *skills* and frequency of *use* of ICTs for different activities (e.g., d'Haenens & Ogan, 2013; Katz et al., 2017; Martinez-Cantos, 2017; Mascheroni & Olafsson, 2016; Simoes, Ponte, & Jorge, 2013).

There are few studies which directly focus on outcomes or third-level inequalities amongst youth. These mostly examine differences in educational performance between those who have and do not have access or those with higher or lower skills, rather than on different outcomes from the *same uses* of ICTs (Pagani et al., 2016). In addition, negative outcomes have been more broadly studied in internationally comparative studies such as the EU and Global Kids online projects than positive outcomes. More importantly, there is little analysis of datasets as regards inequalities in these negative outcomes experienced by young people. There is some evidence that the psychologically vulnerable and those more likely to have non-dominant positions in society (e.g., girls and ethnic minority youth) are more likely to experience negative outcomes from intense use (Helsper & Smahel, 2019) and that they are more likely to experience cyberbullying and harassment (Beckman, Hagquist, & Hellstrom, 2013; d'Haenens & Ogan, 2013; El Asam & Katz, 2018; Smith, Thompson, & Davidson, 2014) though these are not framed or theorised within an inequalities perspective. It remains to be seen whether the socio-economic and socio-cultural inequalities widely reported in the literature for adults regarding the positive outcomes achieved (e.g., Van Deursen & Helsper, 2017) can be observed amongst young people.

Methodology

This chapter aims to answer the question: *Are there socio-digital inequalities amongst young people at the three levels of access, participation, and outcomes?*

Very few studies exist that allow for empirical testing of the theoretical frameworks that link different types of socio-economic and socio-cultural inequalities to inequalities in access, skills, and use of ICTs and their outcomes. These are even more scarce if these issues are to be studied for youth across a variety of contexts. To overcome this gap this chapter analyses cross-national data with information on a variety of aspects of young people's backgrounds (socio-economic, socio-cultural, and personal well-being) as well as ICT access, skills, use, and positive and negative outcomes of use. Besides not including a range of disadvantage- and outcomes-based measures, most representative studies do not include the most vulnerable. This is a crucial gap if one wants to understand entrenched inequalities. Therefore, this international comparative work is combined with the analysis of a UK dataset which included a sizable sample of youth Not in Employment, Education, or Training (NEETs).

The *Net Children Go Mobile* study (www.netchildrengomobile.eu) allows for cross-national analyses of socio-digital inequalities in access, skills, uses, and negative outcomes amongst European digital natives (9- to 16-year-olds). It surveyed 3,500 internet-using children aged 9–16 and their parents in seven European countries. The fieldwork was conducted in 2013 in Denmark, Ireland, Italy, Romania, and the UK; and in early 2014 in Belgium and Portugal. The samples were nationally representative of internet-using youth.

The *From Digital Skills to Tangible Outcomes (DiSTO) NEETs* study in the UK (www.lse.ac.uk/media-and-communications/research/research-projects/disto/disto-youth) was specifically designed to examine inequalities in access, skills, uses, and beneficial as well as negative outcomes for advantaged and severely disadvantaged youth (14 to 24). *DiSTO NEETs* surveyed a nationally representative sample of 1,026 young internet users with an additional quota sample of 318 internet-using young people Not in Employment, Education, or Training (NEETs) (see Helsper & Smirnova, 2016).

The two datasets included different indicators that have been linked to systematic inequalities in adult research (e.g., Van Deursen et al., 2017). A general distinction is made between household and youth's own *socio-economic* characteristics (i.e., caretaker education level, household socio-economic status, youth's poverty history, and NEET status), as well as between individual *socio-cultural* characteristics (i.e., gender, age) and *personal vulnerability* (i.e., problem-solving capability, social self-esteem). Ideally all these datasets would have included a broader set of social and cultural indicators (e.g., social capital, ethnic minority/majority status) but this was not the case. Indicators are different for access, skills, use, and outcomes in the datasets analysed. Since the purpose of the analysis is to examine broader patterns of digital inequalities in different contexts this was considered acceptable though not ideal.[2]

Linear and logistic regression analyses were conducted related to access, skills, uses, and negative and positive outcomes.[3]

Results

Results of the analyses comparing young people with different socio-economic, socio-cultural, and personal well-being backgrounds are presented in relation to first-, second-, and third-level inequalities.

First-Level Inequalities

Both projects measured potential and actual access in relation to the number of devices, types of connections, and the locations at which young people have access to/have used the internet.

Socio-economic background is related to access in non-public locations in Europe (see Table 41.1). Wealthier youth are more likely to have wi-fi access at school, have access to more devices, and, while they use smartphones less, they use the internet more frequently at home. Youth from lower SES households rely on smartphones for private access. Youth from higher-educated households have access and use it at more locations, in particular at school.

Socio-cultural background. Older children have access to more devices and are more likely to have access at school, they use the internet at more locations, and are more likely to use it frequently at home and at school. However, younger youth are more likely to rely on the smartphone for daily connectivity. There are less strong relationships with gender and girls have access to fewer devices and are more likely to access the internet at school.

Table 41.1 Inequalities in potential and actual access (Europe).

	Potential access		Actualised access (use)		Daily use	
	No wifi at school	Devices	Locations	Smartphone	Home	School
	Exp(B)	β	β	Exp(B)	Exp(B)	Exp(B)
Education	1.06	0.12★★	0.17★★	0.99	1.01	1.29★★
Socio-economic status (SES)	0.80★	0.07★	0.04	0.64★★	1.43★★	1.01
Age	0.92★★	0.27★★	0.38★★	0.60★★	2.19★★	1.80★★
Gender (girls)	1.08	−0.06★★	0.02	1.01	0.81	1.24★
R^2/% correct	.02/74%	0.11	0.31	.13/39%	.17/79%	.11/79%

Note: ★ p<.05, ★★ p<.01.
Source: Net Children Go Mobile – Mascheroni, G., & Cuman, A. (2014). *Net Children Go Mobile: Final Report (with country fact sheets).* Deliverables D6.4 and D5.2. Milano: Educatt. Further information and reports available at: http://netchildrengomobile.eu.

Youth's *socio-economic situation* is clearly linked to first-level inequalities. Those who received school meals (an indicator of poverty) when they were in education used the internet on fewer devices and at fewer locations, though they were just as likely to rely on their mobile phones for internet access (see Table 41.2). Those who stayed in education longer accessed the internet in a broader variety of locations, while those who dropped out of education and were not employed used it in fewer locations. As regards *socio-cultural* differences, girls were more likely to rely on their mobile phones for access while older youth used the internet on fewer devices and at fewer locations. Those who were less *vulnerable* (higher social self-esteem) were also more likely to access it at a variety of locations.

Second-Level Inequalities

Skills

Net Children Go Mobile asked children to indicate whether they knew how to do 12 things on the internet and 11 things on their mobile phone (summarised in Table 41.3).

Socio-economic inequalities in skills were found for internet skills for household SES and for smartphone skills for household education level.

Table 41.2 Actualised access (UK).

	Devices	Locations	Mobile mostly
Age	−0.09*	−0.14**	0.96
Gender	−0.04	0.05	3.30*
Poverty (school meals)	−0.06*	−0.06*	1.12
Education	0.06	0.19**	0.87
NEET status	−0.01	−0.12**	1.09
Problem solving	0.02	0.06	0.95
Emotional problems	0.00	−0.01	0.72*
Social self-esteem	0.00	0.06*	1.15

Note: * p<.05, ** p<.01.
Source: DiSTO NEETs – Helsper, E. J. (2016). *Slipping through the net: Are disadvantaged young people being left further behind in the digital era?* A Prince's Trust report. Further information and reports available at: www.lse.ac.uk/media@lse/research/DiSTO/DiSTO-NEETs.aspx.

Table 41.3 Internet and smartphone skills (Europe).

	Internet skills	Smartphone skills
Education	−0.04	−0.09*
SES	0.09**	0.07
Age	0.60**	0.51**
Gender (girls)	−0.06**	−0.15**
R2	0.37	0.28

Note: * p<.05, ** p<.01.
Source: Net Children Go Mobile – Mascheroni, G., & Cuman, A. (2014). *Net Children Go Mobile: Final Report (with country fact sheets).* Deliverables D6.4 and D5.2. Milano: Educatt. Further information and reports available at: http://netchildrengomobile.eu.

Socio-cultural background. Older children were more skilled and girls indicate having fewer internet and smartphone skills.

The DiSTO studies have a variety of skills measures and, therefore, can give a more detailed picture of differences between vulnerable and more advantaged youth in the UK (Table 41.4).

Socio-economic background. Poverty (i.e., school meals), is related to lower overall skills levels but mostly to lower information navigation skills. Interestingly, level of education and NEET status do not make a difference for any of the skills. Nevertheless, informal literacy as measured by problem-solving skills is related to all the digital skills as well as confidence, indicating that those who are more adept at solving obstacles in everyday life have higher digital skill levels.

Table 41.4 Internet and smartphone skills (UK).

	Level of high skill (number of times scored 5 on scale 0 to 5)					
	Digital self-efficacy	High skills	Operational	Information navigation	Social and communicative	Content creation
Age	-0.06	0.00	-.02	0.11★★	-0.05	0.00
Gender (girls)	-0.04	0.04	.05	-0.03	0.16★★	-0.13★★
Poverty	-0.05	-0.07★	-.05	-0.07★	-0.04	-0.02
Education	-0.01	0.00	-.02	0.01	0.01	-0.03
NEET	0.05	0.03	.03	0.03	0.05	0.00
Problem solving	0.07★	0.20★★	.10★★	0.13★★	0.10★★	0.27★★
Emotional problems	-0.14★★	-0.06★	-.02	-0.05	-0.08★	0.01
Social self-esteem	-0.03	0.05	-.02	0.03	-0.01	0.15★★

Note: ★ $p<.05$, ★★ $p<.01$.
Source: DiSTO NEETs – Helsper, E. J. (2016). *Slipping through the net: Are disadvantaged young people being left further behind in the digital era?* A Prince's Trust report. Further information and reports available at: www.lse.ac.uk/media@lse/research/DiSTO/DiSTO-NEETs.aspx.

Socio-cultural background is related to skills in ways that do not follow the expected patterns: older youth indicate having only higher information navigation skills and girls have higher social and communicative skills but lower content creation skills.

Vulnerability, measured through emotional problems, is echoed in a lack of self-efficacy and lower skill levels, expressed especially in lower social- and communicative-ICT-related skills. However, a greater sense of social self-esteem was related to more content creation skills.

Use

The Net Children Go Online study measured how often in the last month children had undertaken a certain activity. A factor analysis showed that there were four areas in which they could be classified along the lines of traditional domains of resources (e.g., personal, social, economic, and cultural (see Helsper, 2012). It also measured a range of risky experiences composed of having seen violent or other potentially harmful material online, having seen sexual images and/or sexual messages they received[4] (Table 41.5).

Socio-economic background. Those from higher-education households undertake commercial, cultural, and personal activities more often online and encountered fewer risks. Those from lower socio-economic-status households undertake commercial and cultural activities online more frequently, and had more risky experiences online.

Socio-cultural background. Older children undertake more activities in general and undertake commercial, personal, and social activities, but not cultural activities, more frequently. They also come across more risky content or interactions. Girls undertake slightly fewer activities overall, especially commercial and cultural activities, but undertake social activities more often and have more risky experiences.

The DiSTO NEETs study was designed around Helsper's (2012) inequalities framework classifying activities in correspondence with different traditional resources and these thus

Table 41.5 Online opportunities and risks (Europe).

	Number of activities	Commercial[a]	Cultural[a]	Social[a]	Personal[a]	Risky experiences[b]
Education	0.07*	−0.16**	−0.08*	0.01	−0.11**	0.21**
Socio-economic status (SES)	−0.03	0.11**	−0.09*	0.03	0.02	−0.14**
Age	0.45**	−0.15**	0.02	−0.37**	−0.48**	0.29**
Gender (girls)	−0.03	0.09**	0.24**	−0.16**	0.01	0.08**
R2	0.2	0.04	0.06	0.16	0.32	0.16

Note: * p<.05, ** p<.01.
Source: Net Children Go Mobile – Mascheroni, G., & Cuman, A. (2014). *Net Children Go Mobile: Final Report (with country fact sheets)*. Deliverables D6.4 and D5.2. Milano: Educatt. Further information and reports available at: http://netchildrengomobile.eu.

Notes:
a. Higher (factor) scores mean less frequent use (scales from several times per day to never).
b. Risky experiences should be distinguished from actual harm as they can lead to negative *or* positive outcomes and resilience in avoiding future harm.

mapped onto these different domains exactly. Economic and employment/education uses were separated in analysis because of the specific importance of the latter when studying NEETs (Table 41.6).

Socio-economic background. The well off were more involved on a monthly basis with all activities and NEETs were less likely to undertake cultural, social, and personal activities, while being equally engaged with commercial and employment-/education-related activities.

Table 41.6 Number of different activities undertaken monthly (UK).

	Overall	Economic	Employment and education	Cultural	Social	Personal
Age	.03	.06	−.04	−.01	.06	−.01
Gender (girls)	−.10**	−.10**	−.07**	−.15**	−.03	−.02
Poverty	.10**	.11**	.12**	.09**	.06*	.08**
Education	.03	.04	.06	.04	.01	.01
NEET	−.11**	−.02	.00	−.14**	−.12**	−.09**
Problem solving	.19**	.20**	.18**	.12**	.15**	.17**
Emotional problems	.02	.02	.01	.01	.00	.03
Social self-esteem	.15**	.13**	.14**	.14**	.12**	.12**

Note: * p<.05, ** p<.01.
Source: DiSTO NEETs – Helsper, E. J. (2016). *Slipping through the net: Are disadvantaged young people being left further behind in the digital era?* A Prince's Trust report. Further information and reports available at: www.lse.ac.uk/media@lse/research/DiSTO/DiSTO-NEETs.aspx.

Traditional literacy in the form of problem-solving also related positively to the undertaking of all activities.

Socio-cultural background. While age did not relate to the types of activities undertaken, gender did. Girls undertook fewer activities monthly across the board with the exception of social and personal activities, where there was no difference.

Vulnerability. Emotional vulnerability did not, but social belonging did relate to the activities undertaken, with those with a greater social self-esteem more active across the board.

Third-Level Inequalities

The Net Children Go Mobile study only measured negative outcomes and these could be classified as affective negative outcomes (i.e., upset) and concrete negative outcomes from use (e.g., foregoing interaction, unhealthy eating and sleeping habits) (Table 41.7).

Socio-economic background. There were no significant differences in negative outcomes (see Table 41.7), except for youth from households with lower education levels being more likely to have seen upsetting material online.

Table 41.7 Negative outcomes of internet and smartphone use (Europe).

	Seen upsetting material[a]	Highest level upset across negative experiences	Negative outcomes intense internet use	Negative outcomes intense smartphone use
	Exp(B)	β	Exp(B)	Exp(B)
Education	0.78**	0.08	1.14	1.06
Socio-economic status	1.10	−0.08	0.97	1.00
Age	0.74**	−0.19**	1.67**	1.68**
Gender (girls)	0.59**	0.21**	0.98	1.05
R^2/% correct	.04/82%	0.15	.07/79%	.08/60%

Note: * $p<.05$, ** $p<.01$.
Source: Net Children Go Mobile – Mascheroni, G., & Cuman, A. (2014). *Net Children Go Mobile: Final Report (with country fact sheets).* Deliverables D6.4 and D5.2. Milano: Educatt. Further information and reports available at: http://netchildrengomobile.eu.

Notes:

a. Scales reversed, a higher score means less likely to have seen upsetting material.

Socio-cultural background. While older kids are more likely to have seen something that upset them, they are less upset by these experiences and they are also more likely to have negative outcomes from more intensive internet or phone use. Girls are less likely to have seen upsetting material but are more upset by them.

DiSTO NEETs included 23 positive outcome measures that asked not just whether a certain outcome was achieved but also how high their level of satisfaction was with the outcome. It also included a question about whether they came across something that bothered them and whether they had negative interactions with others online; the latter two questions were combined to be able to look at negative outcomes (Table 41.8).

Table 41.8 Negative and positive outcomes of Internet use (UK).

	Negative	Positive	Economic	Employment/ Education	Cultural	Social	Personal
Age	-0.06	0.04	0.07★	-0.04	0.00	0.07★	-0.01
Gender (girls)	0.02	-0.04	-0.03	-0.03	-0.08★★	-0.07★	0.03
Poverty	0.02	-0.07★	-0.07★	-0.03	-0.04	0.02	-0.10★★
Education	0.02	0.16★★	0.19★★	0.22★★	0.01	0.09★★	0.15★★
NEET	0.00	-0.10★★	-0.08★★	-0.12★★	-0.07★	-0.12★★	-0.03
Problem solving	-0.04	0.14★★	0.13★★	0.12★★	0.11★★	0.17★★	0.04
Emotional problems	0.03	0.11★★	0.09★	0.07★	0.06	0.12★★	0.07★
Social self-esteem	0.19★★	0.09★★	0.08★★	0.11★★	0.09★★	0.10★★	0.04

Note: ★ p<.05, ★★ p<.01.
Source: DiSTO NEETs – Helsper, E. J. (2016). *Slipping through the net: Are disadvantaged young people being left further behind in the digital era?* A Prince's Trust report. Further information and reports available at: www.lse.ac.uk/media@lse/research/DiSTO/DiSTO-NEETs.aspx.

Socio-economic background. Those who are less well-off achieve fewer high-quality outcomes, especially fewer economic and personal well-being outcomes, while those with higher education levels achieve higher-quality outcomes across the board with the exception of cultural outcomes. NEETs achieve fewer high-quality outcomes with the exception of personal well-being outcomes and, similarly, higher problem-solving skills are related to better outcomes.

Socio-cultural background. Older youth have more positive economic and social outcomes and girls are less likely to achieve positive social and cultural outcomes.

Vulnerability. Those with emotional problems are more satisfied with the outcomes they achieve from internet use. Social self-esteem is related to more negative outcomes but also to a wide range of more positive outcomes, with the exception of personal outcomes.

Discussion

This chapter reviewed the existing evidence and conducted analyses of internationally comparative datasets on children and a UK dataset with vulnerable youth to answer the question: *Are there socio-digital inequalities amongst the latest generation of digital natives at the three levels of access, participation, and outcomes?* The short answer is yes, at all levels. Digital inequalities echoing traditional inequalities between advantaged and disadvantaged or vulnerable young people were shown to be present amongst the latest generation of digital natives (born after 2000). Socio-economic and socio-demographic factors continue to relate to the uptake of digital opportunities suggesting it is not generation but personal circumstance that determines uptake (Helsper & Eynon, 2010). While socio-economic background diminished in importance as the analyses moved from the first (access) to the second (skill and use) and the third (positive and negative outcomes of use) level of inequalities, socio-cultural and psychological types of marginalisation and vulnerability became more important.

In terms of *access*, it seems that wealth and other types of advantage are related to better access in private locations. Girls and disadvantaged groups are 'forced' into more public use because they have less private or exclusive personal/home access.

Socio-cultural factors such as gender and age played a role in determining *skills*, though more fine-grained analyses of different types of disadvantage and vulnerability in the UK suggest that this might be due to differences in informal literacy (problem solving) and socio-emotional vulnerability. Nevertheless, socio-economic, but especially socio-cultural and psychological factors, related strongly to how young people *engaged* with ICTs in both datasets. This confirms that even amongst digital natives ICT use is gendered and determined by offline identities, individual confidence, and social marginalisation.

There is much emphasis on the negative outcomes of ICT use in the literature for young people and relatively little on the positive outcomes outside of the education literature. Interestingly, socio-economic and socio-cultural statuses make little difference in encountering negative experiences but do make a difference in the achievement of positive outcomes in the UK study. The analyses confirm that psychological vulnerability might be related to more, and socio-economic vulnerability to fewer, positive outcomes (Helsper & Smirnova, 2019). There were surprises in the data on vulnerability; higher social esteem related to more negative outcomes (as well as to more positive outcomes) and negative outcomes were more common amongst older children. This might be because older youth and those who feel more respected use the technology more intensely, which logically leads to more possibilities of encountering risky content and thus negative outcomes (Helsper & Smahel, 2019; Livingstone & Helsper, 2010; Logar, Anzelm, Lazic, & Vujacic, 2016).

Conclusion

Digital inequalities between young people in access to and use of ICTs continue to exist even in an era of relatively low cost and widely diffused mobile media. Inequalities in use and outcomes of this use mean that inequalities will continue into the future. Elsewhere it has been argued that the socio-technical environments young people grow up in, and not the generation that they belong to, shape future digital inequalities (Helsper, 2017; Helsper & Eynon, 2010). These socio-technical ecologies are shaped by inequalities with long histories that are not changed overnight by the rise of a new platform, application, or activity. Whether a young person is able to take up the opportunities and manage the risks that come with living in increasingly digital societies depends on what they experience and power dynamics in their everyday lives.

The analyses presented in this chapter support this idea with limited data. This chapter could not explore compoundness – the interplay between different social, economic, and well-being inequalities and how these relate different types of ICT access, skill levels, and outcomes of engagement (Van Deursen et al., 2017) – privileging broad, multi-level comparisons on comparative datasets. While NEET youth are known to be multiply disadvantaged, the effect of the combination of their different types of disadvantage could not be untangled here. Better data collection is needed because current datasets are insufficient to study compound disadvantage. Future, carefully designed research with sufficiently large samples of severely disadvantaged youth would allow researchers to examine, for example, whether ethnic minority girls growing up in deprived neighbourhoods are more at risk of negative outcomes than other young people who differ from them in one or more of these characteristics.

In summary, it is likely that youth's socio-digital ecologies are composed not just of parents and their parenting styles, which is the focus of much research in the Global North (e.g., Livingstone et al., 2017), but also of the neighbourhoods (Katz & Gonzalez, 2016b) and the national and regional contexts these young people grow up in (Drabowicz, 2014). These ecologies provide not only access and exposure to ICTs but also to value systems about what a young person (with certain characteristics) is supposed to do with ICTs and, as such, shapes the opportunities and the risks that they are aware off and consider appropriate for them (the socio-digital ecology in Helsper's 2017 definition).

However, most youth research is still too regionally or nationally constricted to draw conclusions about the applicability of digital inequalities theory. There is a dearth of data on ICT skills and outcomes of use especially for disadvantaged youth in the Global South. While individual countries have conducted studies (see www.globalkidsonline.net), no datasets are available that allow for comparative, multi-level analysis and thus it is difficult to know which findings presented here are Europe-specific and which are universal.

What is clear is that, to create a more equal future, the everyday lives of disadvantaged young people need to change both socially and technically to prevent the amplification and entrenchment of inequalities in increasingly digital societies.

Notes

1 Using the Boolean search terms in the Web of Science database TS=(youth OR children OR "young people") AND TS= ("digital divide" OR "digital inequalit*" OR "digital exclusion") NOT TS=(elderly OR adult). Deleting those references that talked about children in relation to adults rather than digital inequalities amongst young people. Search conducted in September 2018.
2 There is no space here to discuss the measures created, the websites give detailed descriptions of the studies and the author can be contacted for further detail on how measures were constructed.
3 Unless indicated otherwise the tables depict (standardised) linear regression coefficients (ß-value).
4 Risky experiences should be distinguished from actual harm, they can lead to negative *or* positive outcomes and resilience in avoiding future harm.

References

Arora, P. (2010). Hope-in-the-wall? A digital promise for free learning. *British Journal of Educational Technology*, *41*(5), 689–702.
Awan, F., & Gauntlett, D. (2013). Remote living: Exploring online (and offline) experiences of young people living in rural areas. *European Journal of Cultural Studies*, *16*(1), 3–23.
Awuor, F. M., Khisa, J. W., & Rambi, D. A. (2015). Delivering equitable and quality education to remote Kenya using ICT. In I. S. Sodhi (Ed.), *Emerging issues and prospects in African E-Government* (pp. 108–117). Hershey (PA): IGI Global.
Beckman, L., Hagquist, C., & Hellstrom, L. (2013). Discrepant gender patterns for cyberbullying and traditional bullying – An analysis of Swedish adolescent data. *Computers in Human Behavior*, *29*(5), 1896–1903.
Bennett, S., Maton, K., & Kervin, L. (2008). The 'digital natives' debate: A critical review of the evidence. *British Journal of Educational Technology*, *39*(5), 775–786.
Bilal, D., & Jopeck, V. (2014). Young girls' affective responses to access and use of information and communication technology (ICT) in information-poor societies. In D. Bilal & J. Beheshti (Eds.), *New directions in children's and adolescents' information behavior research* (pp. 107–133). Bingley, UK: Emerald Publishing.
Brown, C., & Czerniewicz, L. (2010). Debunking the 'digital native': Beyond digital apartheid, towards digital democracy. *Journal of Computer Assisted Learning*, *26*(5), 357–369.
Chaudron, S., Di Gioia, R., Gemo, M., Holloway, D., Marsh, J., Mascheroni, G., ... Yamada-Rice, D. (2017). *Kaleidoscope on the internet of toys – Safety, security, privacy and societal insights*. Retrieved from: https://ec.europa.eu/jrc/en/publication/kaleidoscope-internet-toys-safety-security-privacy-and-societal-insights.
Chuma, W. (2014). The social meanings of mobile phones among South Africa's 'digital natives': A case study. *Media Culture & Society*, *36*(3), 398–408.
Cotten, S. R., Shank, D. B., & Anderson, W. A. (2014). Gender, technology use and ownership, and media-based multitasking among middle school students. *Computers in Human Behavior*, *35*, 99–106.
d'Haenens, L., & Ogan, C. (2013). Internet-using children and digital inequality: A comparison between majority and minority Europeans. *Communications-European Journal of Communication Research*, *38*(1), 41–60. doi:10.1515/commun-2013-0003.
Drabowicz, T. (2014). Gender and digital usage inequality among adolescents: A comparative study of 39 countries. *Computers & Education*, *74*, 98–111.

Eastin, M. S., Cicchirillo, V., & Mabry, A. (2015). Extending the digital divide conversation: Examining the knowledge gap through media expectancies. *Journal of Broadcasting & Electronic Media*, 59(3), 416–437.

El Asam, A., & Katz, A. (2018). Vulnerable young people and their experience of online risks. *Human-Computer Interaction*, 33(4), 281–304.

Hargittai, E. (2002). Second level digital divide: Differences in people's online skills. *First Monday*, 7(4). Retrieved from: www.firstmonday.dk/issues/issue7_4/hargittai.

Helsper, E. J. (2012). A corresponding fields model for the links between social and digital exclusion. *Communication Theory*, 22(4), 403–426.

Helsper, E. J. (2017). A socio-digital ecology approach to understanding digital inequalities among young people. *Journal of Children and Media*, 11(2), 256–260.

Helsper, E. J., & Eynon, R. (2010). Digital natives: Where is the evidence? *British Educational Research Journal*, 36(3), 503–520.

Helsper, E. J., & Smahel, D. (2019). Excessive internet use by young Europeans: Psychological vulnerability and digital literacy? *Information, communication & society*, [online first] 1–19. doi.org/10.1080/1369118X.2018.1563203.

Helsper, E. J., & Smirnova, S. (2016). *Methodological report of the study: Socio-digital skills and wellbeing of disadvantaged young people*. Retrieved from London, UK: www.lse.ac.uk/media@lse/research/DiSTO/Pdf/Methodology-report-DiSTO-NEETs.pdf.

Helsper, E. J., & Smirnova, S. (2019). Chapter 9. Youth inequalities in digital interactions and wellbeing In T. Burns & F. Gottschalk (Eds.), *Educating 21st Century Children* (pp. 163–184). Paris: OECD Publishing.

Hinostroza, J. E., Matamala, C., Labbe, C., Claro, M., & Cabello, T. (2015). Factors (not) affecting what students do with computers and internet at home. *Learning Media and Technology*, 40(1), 43–63.

Ignatow, G., & Robinson, L. (2017). Pierre Bourdieu: Theorizing the digital. *Information Communication & Society*, 20(7), 950–966.

Jackson, L. A., Zhao, Y., Kolenic, A., Fitzgerald, H. E., Harold, R., & Von Eye, A. (2008). Race, gender, and information technology use: The new digital divide. *Cyberpsychology & Behavior*, 11(4), 437–442.

Janisse, H. C., Li, X. M., Bhavnagri, N. P., Esposito, C., & Stanton, B. (2018). A Longitudinal study of the effect of computers on the cognitive development of low-income African American preschool children. *Early Education and Development*, 29(2), 229–244.

Jara, I., Claro, M., Hinostroza, J. E., San Martin, E., Rodriguez, P., Cabello, T., . . . Labbe, C. (2015). Understanding factors related to Chilean students' digital skills: A mixed methods analysis. *Computers & Education*, 88, 387–398.

Jones, C., & Czerniewicz, L. (2010). Describing or debunking? The net generation and digital natives. *Journal of Computer Assisted Learning*, 26(5), 317–320.

Katz, V. S., & Gonzalez, C. (2016a). Community variations in low-income Latino Families' technology adoption and integration. *American Behavioral Scientist*, 60(1), 59–80.

Katz, V. S., & Gonzalez, C. (2016b). Toward meaningful connectivity: Using multilevel communication research to reframe digital inequality. *Journal of Communication*, 66(2), 236–249.

Katz, V. S., Gonzalez, C., & Clark, K. (2017). Digital inequality and developmental trajectories of low-income, immigrant, and minority children. *Pediatrics*, 140, S132–S136.

Katz, V. S., Moran, M. B., & Gonzalez, C. (2018). Connecting with technology in lower-income US families. *New Media & Society*, 20(7), 2509–2533.

Li, Y., & Ranieri, M. (2013). Educational and social correlates of the digital divide for rural and urban children: A study on primary school students in a provincial city of China. *Computers & Education*, 60(1), 197–209.

Liao, P. A., Chang, H. H., Wang, J. H., & Sun, L. C. (2016). What are the determinants of rural-urban digital inequality among schoolchildren in Taiwan? Insights from Blinder-Oaxaca decomposition. *Computers & Education*, 95, 123–133.

Lichy, J. (2011). Internet user behaviour in France and Britain: Exploring socio-spatial disparity among adolescents. *International Journal of Consumer Studies*, 35(4), 470–475.

Livingstone, S., & Helsper, E. J. (2010). Balancing opportunities and risks in teenagers' use of the internet: The role of online skills and internet self-efficacy. *New Media & Society*, 12(2), 309–329.

Livingstone, S., Olafsson, K., Helsper, E. J., Lupianez-Villanueva, F., Veltri, G. A., & Folkvord, F. (2017). Maximizing opportunities and minimizing risks for children online: The role of digital skills in emerging strategies of parental mediation. *Journal of Communication*, 67(1), 82–105.

Logar, S., Anzelm, D., Lazic, D., & Vujacic, V. (2016). *Global kids online Montenegro: Opportunities, risks and safety*. Retrieved from: http://globalkidsonline.net/montenegro-report.

Martinez-Cantos, J. L. (2017). Digital skills gaps: A pending subject for gender digital inclusion in the European Union. *European Journal of Communication, 32*(5), 419–438.

Mascheroni, G., & Olafsson, K. (2016). The mobile Internet: Access, use, opportunities and divides among European children. *New Media & Society, 18*(8), 1657–1679.

McQuillan, H., & d'Haenens, L. (2009). Young people online: Gender and age influences. In S. Livingstone & L. Haddon (Eds.), *Kids online opportunities and risks for children* (pp. 95–106). Bristol: The Policy Press.

Mertens, S., & d'Haenens, L. (2010). The digital divide among young people in Brussels: Social and cultural influences on ownership and use of digital technologies. *Communications-European Journal of Communication Research, 35*(2), 187–207.

Mo, D., Swinnen, J., Zhang, L. X., Yi, H. M., Qu, Q. H., Boswell, M., & Rozelle, S. (2013). Can one-to-one computing narrow the digital divide and the educational gap in China? The case of Beijing migrant schools. *World Development, 46*, 14–29.

Munyengabe, S., Zhao, Y. Y., He, H. Y., & Hitimana, S. (2017). Primary teachers' perceptions on ICT integration for enhancing teaching and learning through the implementation of One Laptop per Child Program in primary schools of Rwanda. *Eurasia Journal of Mathematics Science and Technology Education, 13*(11), 7193–7204.

Ng, W. (2012). Can we teach digital natives digital literacy? *Computers & Education, 59*(3), 1065–1078.

Nie, P., Sousa-Poza, A., & Nimrod, G. (2017). Internet use and subjective well-being in China. *Social Indicators Research, 132*(1), 489–516. doi:10.1007/s11205-015-1227-8.

Ono, H., & Tsai, H. J. (2008). Race, parental socioeconomic status, and computer use time outside of school among young American children, 1997 to 2003. *Journal of Family Issues, 29*(12), 1650–1672.

Opgenhaffen, M., & d'Haenens, L. (2012). Heterogeneity within homogeneity: Impact of online skills on the use of online news media and interactive news features. *Communications-European Journal of Communication Research, 37*(3), 297–316.

Oyedemi, T. (2015). Participation, citizenship and internet use among South African youth. *Telematics and Informatics, 32*(1), 11–22.

Pagani, L., Argentin, G., Gui, M., & Stanca, L. (2016). The impact of digital skills on educational outcomes: Evidence from performance tests. *Educational Studies, 42*(2), 137–162.

Prensky, M. (2001). Digital natives, digital immigrants. *On the Horizon, 9*(5), 1–6.

Selwyn, N. (2009). The digital native – Myth and reality. *Aslib Proceedings, 61*(4), 364–379.

Simoes, J. A., Ponte, C., & Jorge, A. (2013). Online experiences of socially disadvantaged children and young people in Portugal. *Communications-European Journal of Communication Research, 38*(1), 85–106.

Smith, P. K., Thompson, F., & Davidson, J. (2014). Cyber safety for adolescent girls: Bullying, harassment, sexting, pornography, and solicitation. *Current Opinion in Obstetrics & Gynecology, 26*(5), 360–365.

Steeves, H. L., & Kwami, J. (2017). Interrogating gender divides in technology for education and development: The case of the One Laptop per Child Project in Ghana. *Studies in Comparative International Development, 52*(2), 174–192.

Thornham, H., & Cruz, E. G. (2017). Im-mobility in the age of im-mobile phones: Young NEETs and digital practices. *New Media & Society, 19*(11), 1794–1809.

Tondeur, J., Sinnaeve, I., van Houtte, M., & van Braak, J. (2011). ICT as cultural capital: The relationship between socioeconomic status and the computer-use profile of young people. *New Media & Society, 13*(1), 151–168.

Van Deursen, A. J. A. M., & Helsper, E. J. (2015). The third level digital divide: Who benefits most from being online? In L. Robinson, S. R. Cotten, J. Schulz, T. M. Hale, & A. Williams (Eds.), *Communication and information technologies annual: Digital distinctions and inequalities* (Vol. 10, pp. 29–52). Bingley, UK: Emerald.

Van Deursen, A. J. A. M., & Helsper, E. J. (2017). Collateral benefits of Internet use: Explaining the diverse outcomes of engaging with the Internet. *New Media & Society, 20*(7), 2333–2351. doi:10.1177/1461444817715282.

Van Deursen, A. J. A. M., Helsper, E. J., & Eynon, R. (2016). Development and validation of the Internet Skills Scale (ISS). *Information Communication & Society, 19*(6), 804–823.

Van Deursen, A. J. A. M., Helsper, E. J., Eynon, R., & Van Dijk, J. A. G. M. (2017). The compoundness and sequentiality of digital inequality. *International Journal of Communication, 11*, 452–473.

van Deursen, A. J. A. M., & van Dijk, J. A. G. M. (2015). Toward a multifaceted model of Internet access for understanding digital divides: An empirical investigation. *Information Society, 31*(5), 379–391.

Van Dijk, J., & Van Deursen, A. (2010). Inequalities of digital skills and how to overcome them. In E. Ferro, Y. K. Dwivedi, R. Gil-Garcia, & M. D. Williams (Eds.), *Handbook of research on overcoming digital divides: Constructing an equitable and competitive information society* (pp. 278–291). Hershey (PA): IGI Global.

Vekiri, I. (2010). Socioeconomic differences in elementary students' ICT beliefs and out-of-school experiences. *Computers & Education, 54*(4), 941–950.

Wartberg, L., Kammerl, R., Broning, S., Hauenschild, M., Petersen, K. U., & Thomasius, R. (2015). Gender-related consequences of Internet use perceived by parents in a representative quota sample of adolescents. *Behaviour & Information Technology, 34*(4), 341–348.

Zhang, M. L. (2015). Internet use that reproduces educational inequalities: Evidence from big data. *Computers & Education, 86*, 212–223.

42
STREET CHILDREN AND SOCIAL MEDIA
Identity Construction in the Digital Age

Marcela Losantos Velasco, Lien Mostmans, and Guadalupe Peres-Cajías

Introduction: The Rise of Facebook Use Among Street Children

This contribution aims to generate knowledge on how street children's[1] digital identity is shaped by social media. By conducting a study on the Facebook profiles and posts of 20 street children[2] we show how street children's Facebook interactions are shaped by the audiences they aimed to reach and by their capacity to deal with this social media platform's affordances.

In Bolivia, the most recent Nation Census of people living on the street revealed that there were 3,768 persons of which 43% are between 10 and 24 years old (Viceministerio de Defensa Social y Sustancias Controladas, 2015). A significant proportion of Bolivians living on the street are children and young people due to an essential failure of care intervention models (Huang & Huang, 2008) and weak family reunification programmes that led most of these children to grow up in the streets (Losantos Velasco, 2017).

In line with other research about children and social media (boyd, 2014; Guardia & Zegada, 2018; Livingstone, 2003; Livingstone & Helsper, 2007), Bolivian street children are actively using social media platforms, especially WhatsApp and Facebook. In line with previous research (Losantos Velasco, 2017), this study found Facebook profiles of 40 street children living in the city of La Paz and 23 profiles of children living in the streets of the city of El Alto. Forty-eight of these children were using Facebook daily.

Street children and youth are keen users of Facebook, although their use patterns have been poorly studied around the globe. Several reasons can explain their invisibility in this area of research. First, there is a common belief that their living conditions do not allow them to access anything more than the essential assets such as food and clothing. Second, research on education has demonstrated that most of the Bolivian street children and youth have not finished primary school, hence it is generally assumed that many of them are illiterate (Huang & Huang, 2008).

Both of these widespread assumptions need to be nuanced. Related to the first point, the country's largest research study on digital use showed that internet services became cheaper in recent years, internet cafes are trendy for youngsters to get online and there are few legal requirements when buying mobile phone SIM cards, enabling street children to buy them in most street shops to 'upload' data[3] (Vicepresidencia del Estado Plurinacional de Bolivia, 2016). Moreover, new smartphones have become available at a relatively low cost and nowadays second-hand or stolen mobile phones can be easily found in Bolivia's underground markets. Furthermore, even though there is practically no information on precisely how street children and youth have access to smartphones, a previous research project by the first author indicated that nearly everyone from the two street groups had one and was using it on a daily basis, at least for some months during a year. Moreover, they invest a significant part of their daily earnings in order to acquire cell phones and they tend to change mobile phones regularly, because such hardware is used as a exchangeable tool to get easy and quick money.[4]

Regarding the second argument, even though street children have hardly finished primary school, the census shows that 94% can read and write with a certain degree of difficulty (Viceministerio de Defensa Social y Sustancias Controladas, 2015), but well enough to interact on social media.

Social media has therefore become a powerful connection tool between street children and different audiences, with whom it was difficult to stay in touch in the past, including international aid organisations, volunteers, and professionals that work with street children, and street educators with whom they are in contact in their daily lives on the street. This 'virtual sociability' (Cáceres, Señán, & Ruiz San Román, 2017; Delgado & Felice, 2013) has had a great impact on the expansion of the children's social network.

Furthermore, social media also changed the way that street children relate to media in general. Only a few years ago, the only relationship these children had with the media was when TV or radio networks decided to report about them, depicting them at the extreme of two poles: a) as 'victims' in constant need of help, which corresponded with the social construction of them as poor and disadvantaged (Bar-On, 1997); and b) as criminals, with feral and untamed characteristics that demand forced interventions to take them off the street (e.g., Losantos Velasco, & Loots, 2015). Street children have shifted from being objects of news and passive media consumers by virtue of watching TV on the street or in public restaurants and hiding in movie theatres, to becoming active producers of content in social media, as will be discussed in the following paragraphs.

This chapter aims to expand the knowledge and research evidence in the field of street children's use of social media by answering these research questions:

1 How do street children deal with Facebook affordances?
2 Are their Facebook profiles and posts influenced by the audience they are aiming to reach?
3 How do their Facebook interactions shape their digital identity?

The next section will describe the research methodology in which Facebook profiles and posts were selected and then analysed by using a visual and an audience perspective. Subsequently, there is a discussion about how street children's interaction with social media is mediated by their capacity to understand and deal with social media affordances and by the audience to whom they target their posts. The final section examines how this interaction shapes the way street children construct their digital identity.

Methodology

Selection of Participants and Facebook Sample

To select Bolivian street children's Facebook profiles there was first an exploratory search to see which of the first author's street-connected friends had an active profile.[5] The initial selection ended with a list of 63 Facebook accounts.

The first author had had daily contact with all the participants from the selected group up until one year earlier. Therefore, to make sure they were still part of the same street group, a street educator was invited to confirm the children's status at the time of the research. The information provided narrowed the sample down to a total of 54 Facebook accounts of children living on the streets of the cities of La Paz and El Alto, of whom 48 were last connected to Facebook during the previous week.

The second selection criterion was based on the first author's regular Facebook interactions with the selected children during the previous year. This allowed the researchers to follow their updates. Furthermore, it enabled more in-depth study of how their posts related to their personal history.

The final sample consisted of 20 Facebook accounts of children – 13 boys and 7 girls, aged 12- to 16-years-old – that were followed daily for seven months.

Data Collection and Analysis

The first step was to gather together the profile information of the 20 participants. This covered information such as names, photos, addresses, school information, work information, relationship status, and other relevant information that was stored in each of the participant's files.

Second, the children's weekly updates were followed for seven months. Every week all posts from the selected profiles were printed off. The content of each post was checked, setting apart what the children published as a 'shared' post from what they uploaded themselves. The most repeated topics and those posts that had more comments and likes were highlighted and a separate file for each participant was created to compare posts over time.

Once all the materials were gathered, a preliminary analysis compared profile information with data provided by the street educator and by the first author. Next, images and texts of the highlighted posts were first read separately and then compared with the profile information to search for similarities and differences.

Furthermore, to conduct a more in-depth visual and audience-oriented analysis, the understanding of the street children's Facebook profiles and posts was based on the conceptualisation of Mitchell, De Lange, and Moletsane (2017). This states that visual content cannot be assumed as a transparent window into its author's mind, but rather it shows the author's agency when producing meaning with the particular intention to narrate a 'small story'.

Second, the analysis used the concept of 'text–image' proposed by Mitchell (1995) and Rose (2007). This refers to images accompanied by some text or testimony that explains them. Thus, texts and images together provide more information than single images or independent texts and, therefore, are to be analysed as a whole.

Finally, the audience perspective and influence suggested by Fiske (1994) and more recently by Livingstone (2019) was used to reflect upon how the – imaginary or tagged – audience could shape the content posted by each of the participants.

The focus on how and for whom Facebook's profile information and posts were visually and verbally constructed made it possible to identify (a) risks face by and opportunities for street children related to social media affordances, and (b) the relevance of audience when posting. Moreover, it shed light on how their social media interaction shaped the children's digital identity.

Ethical Issues

Considering the research context (street children) and design (visual and audience analysis in a digital environment), we anticipated several ethical issues:

1 Confidentiality. Names were erased from Facebook profiles and changed in the document to guarantee anonymity. Moreover, all identifiable pictures were only for the use of the researchers.
2 Consultation and consent. Because they were street children – without any adult family to give consent for them – these profile owners were asked through Facebook Messenger to

give their consent for the researchers to conduct an investigation of their public posts and to publish findings in academic journals.
3   Protection against social stigma. To deal with social stigma, the focus was not on *typical* street images such as the ones showing the use of glue, or the use of masks. All posts from the last five months of the analysis were included, broadening the scope of the review to cover a variety of posted messages.
4   Respect. The dignity and autonomy of the participants were taken into consideration when requesting their consent to conduct the narrative analysis of the visual material they had publicly posted.

Findings

Street Children's and Social Media Affordances: Risks and Opportunities

Social media technologies, website designs, and interfaces have been described as the 'affordances' (Gibson, 1979) that potentially drive the formation and enactment of social identities, as they influence and prompt users to share, present themselves, and behave in certain ways (Papacharissi, 2010). Specifically, scholars have described five social media affordances that affect what happens to personal information: *persistence, scalability, replicability, spreadability,* and *searchability* (boyd, 2008, 2014; Papacharissi & Yuan, 2011), meaning that recorded and archived data can easily be multiplied, shared, and accessed through an internet search. This fact has created a new stream of information that leads to what Monika Taddicken (2014, p. 250) has called "a recontextualisation of self-disclosure": self-disclosed personal information remains available beyond the moment of its creation. It also means that even if deleted, the data may have been disseminated, stored, and potentially modified by others, possibly reaching an audience far beyond the intended one. Moreover, information can also resurface when it matches search terms by other users, at any point in time.

The topic of children's data and privacy online is one of the most sensitive, and it has been on the table of scholarly debate from some time now (e.g., DiMaggio, Hargittai, Celeste, & Shafer, 2004; Livingstone & Haddon, 2009). Issues such as children's digital literacy (Buckingham, 2015) and cognitive and social competencies to understand and to deal with social media risks are currently under discussion and actions have been taken to raise awareness of the topic. However, as argued by Livingstone, Stoilova, and Nandagiri (2018), privacy protection has a parent-centred approach, which immediately increases the digital divide for street children.

Unsupervised street children's use of social media can be risky in many ways. First of all, they may have a less critical understanding of present and future risks of Facebook posting. Loss of control over their personal information can lead, for example, to the 'spreadability' of their street condition, which can reduce their chances of social reintegration. In this respect, previous research has shown that possibilities of reintegration become limited when their street situation becomes public (Losantos Velasco, 2017). Indeed, some street youth decide to migrate to another city or even another country in order to leave the street definitively.

Moreover, girls face a higher risk because they can become easily traced by trafficking networks. Sixteen-year-old Joana posts: "in a relationship I give more sex than problems" (see Figure 42.1), which can pose a direct threat to her in the near future, depending on who is reading it.

Livingstone, Stoilova, and Nandagiri (2018) report that non-street 12-to-17-year-olds are aware of the privacy risks they take in social media. However, in spite of recognising disclosure threats, it appears to be that their decision on what to publish is somewhat "influenced by the immediacy of and desire for benefits" (p. 19) rather than by possible danger. Street children seem to act on the same basis, but run a more significant risk because there is neither parental nor social control.

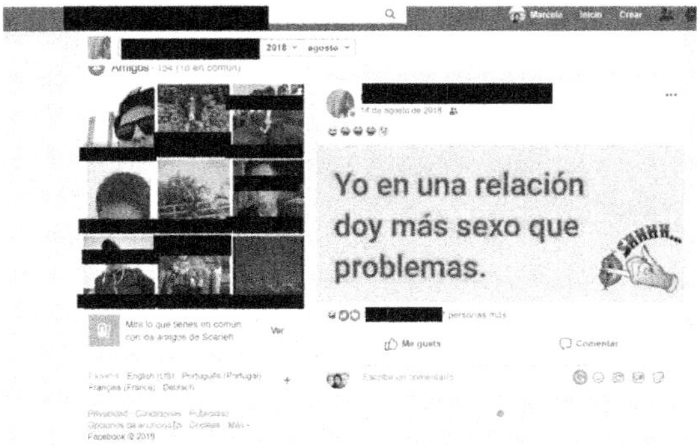

Figure 42.1 Joanna's Facebook post, 14 August 2018.

While social media affordances add risks to their safety, at the same time they can also provide both new, potentially empowering ways and tools for the formation and enactment of the children's social identities and enlargement of their social network.

On 2 March 2018, Leonor (16) denounced the disappearance of her friend Jane (16) on Facebook (Figure 42.2). She tagged some street friends and other Facebook contacts she believed could help her spread the news. To make a stronger statement, she shared her missing girlfriend's partner photo (Leonor's Facebook post, 21 March 2018).

Responses appeared immediately. Former workers of the NGO that used to work with them on the street, old street children, and foreign volunteers that knew them personally responded by offering help, proposing to go to the police or sharing the post. Three days later Jane appeared, explaining that her phone was stolen.

Social media has enabled street children to set up their own connections, bypassing adult mediation as illustrated in the previous example. Moreover, it reveals that although street children face significant digital inequalities, they manage to shape online social contexts and networks actively.

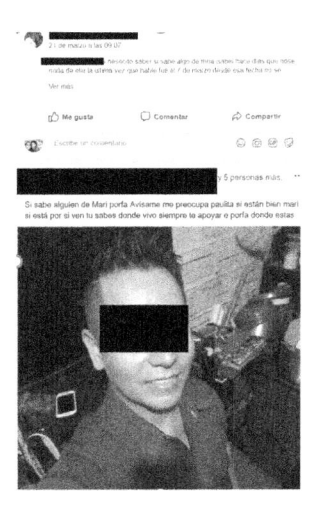

Figure 42.2 Leonor's Facebook post, 21 March 2018.

The Audience Matters: For Whom are Street Children Posting?

María (16) tags Juan (15?) and posts:

> A mature man knows that the secret of making a woman fall in love is to hold her without her asking to, to take care of her without her demanding it and, to love her without her saying it. I love you, my love.
>
> *(Maria's post, 24 June 2018)*

The post presents a message of love directed to her street partner. However, a contradiction appears evident: even though the message seems to state that to make a girl fall in love men have to act and respond in certain ways without being asked to do so, the simple fact of her tagging him can be interpreted as a request for him to behave in the manner she suggests.

A second girl, Natalia (14), takes a selfie (Figure 42.3) and writes:

> I am sorry I am not the person you want me to be. If you knew that I was trying everything for you. I am sorry, love, if when I kiss you, you don't feel butterflies anymore. If you don't love me in the way I love you. I am sorry, love, I don't own your heart. I don't regret hanging around with you. I am sorry love, but it is the moment to take another road. Cupid isn't guilty.

Nonetheless, even if the message seems to be directed to someone she is affectionate with, she tags 21 other street friends. Some of her friends lately reply: "forget him, you don't need him" or "You look nice, Loquita".

The message fulfils two purposes. On the one hand it let the (ex-) partner knows she is suffering from the break-up. On the other, it allows her to receive consolation responses from her street social network.

Both posts target a street audience intentionally. Moreover, both posts follow street norms of female submission and calling for street social support in times of suffering, reproducing what Costa (2018) calls "codes of behaviour existing in the social contexts of the offline world" (p. 3642). Such is the case in the following post (Figure 42.4), where a street boy calls for help when he says he is in a new city, with no money, no place to stay, no hope, and that it is about to rain.

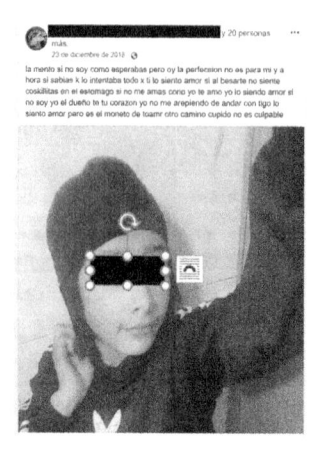

Figure 42.3 Natalia's Facebook post, 23 December 2018.

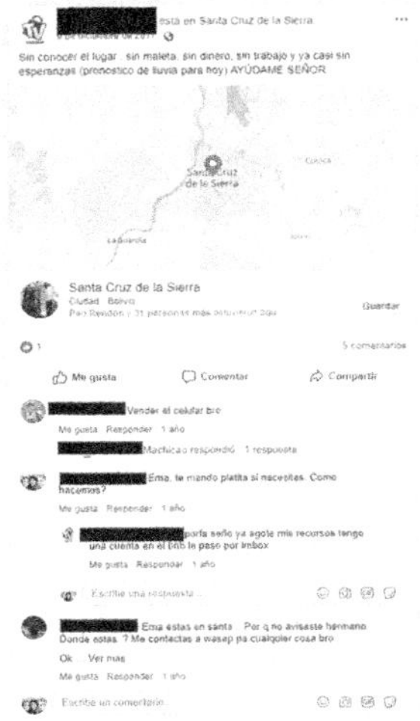

Figure 42.4 A call for help. Facebook post, 9 December 2017.

In contrast to the previous two posts, Diego doesn't tag anyone. However, virtual social support emerges from different audiences. The first comment is from a street friend who immediately suggests selling his mobile phone. The second one comes from a former street educator who offers to send him some money. The third one comes from an old street boy who now lives in Santa Cruz and offers him support if needed.

Each of the online replies concurs with the offline role of the respondents. Moreover, even when there is an evident *collapsed context* (boyd, 2002) in the post, each audience responds accordingly to the social code of the offline world.

Digital Identity Construction on Facebook: Much More Than Street Children Online

The social stigma of being labelled a street child carries a great identity burden that accompanies the person, sometimes even into their adult life. Few stigmas are so permanent. It is not unusual that when a street child decides to leave the street, institutions and professionals continue to identify them as part of the street children's group.

However, the study of their Facebook profiles reveals different identities being developed. The social media digital environment enables the emergence of different – more individual – features of their identities to bubble up. In fact, some profiles were not immediately linked to street life. More than once, the first author felt the need to double-check whether the Facebook profile belonged to a child living on the street.

Figure 42.5 presents a street adolescent Facebook profile and cover photo of him wearing ordinary adolescent clothes. In the information section three sentences stand out: force, #ManythanksGod, and "I didn't give up then ... I won't do it now".

This Facebook profile is one of many in which children and adolescents post typical teenage content such as songs, jokes, memes, and drawings. However, such mainstream adolescent posts are sometimes mixed with other typical '*street publications*' on their Facebook storyline, where they are lying on the street, wearing masks, or sniffing glue.[6] The next post presents a *street-type* Facebook profile photo (Figure 42.6).

Facebook profiles enable them to share both street and non-street aspects of their lives and identities that are more difficult to show in offline social contexts. Dominant identity

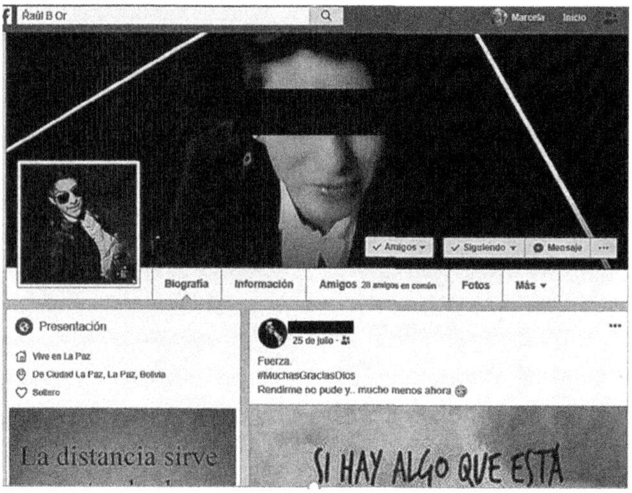

Figure 42.5 Street adolescent Facebook profile photo.

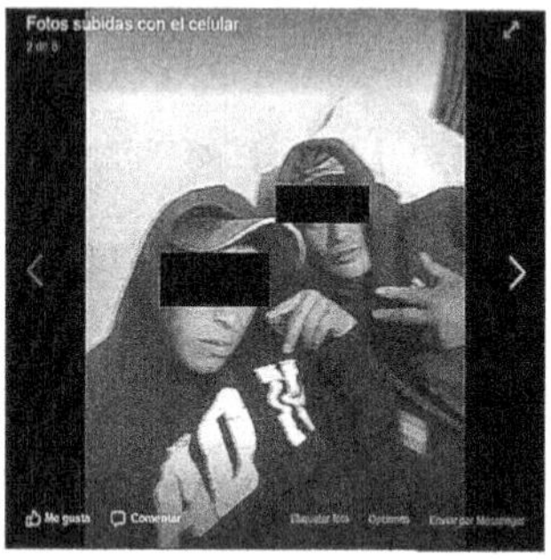

Figure 42.6 Street adolescent Facebook profile photo.

characteristics such as *being a street person* tend to become so relevant that they overshadow alternative identities. However, as observed in this study, social media offers an alternative space for different digital identity construction and for other stories to be told.

The Opportunity for Vindication through Social Media: The Possibility to Tell One's 'Truth'

In July 2018 Carlota (15) posted:

> Here is my truth: at the age of six I was raped by my stepfather. I felt so bad ... traumatised that I became mute. I couldn't speak anymore. My mother took me to an institution because she thought I was sick. After some months the director of the place took me to a psychiatric hospital for adults. I was terrified. I was the only kid. Everybody else was very sick grown-ups. At the hospital, I saw many things that scared me. I started to act like crazy. I heard other people scream and I used to do the same. I copied them: I don't know why.
>
> One day a nurse who was good to me, opened up the door for me and told me I could go: "I am going to leave the gate open for you and if you want you can leave". And I did.

I went onto the street. I was never on the street before, so when other children saw me, they came to offer to take me to their 'torrante'.[7] Sometimes I used to scream for hours for no reason. And they [the other street children] just let me scream and used to say: "she must have nerve problems".

One of them offered me a pill to calm down. I took it. I took them a lot. After a while I started to feel OK. For the first time in my life, I began to feel happy. I am now OK, thanks to many people. I have the strength to stand up and say I am OK because of my effort and the help of some very good people.

(Carlota's post, 16 July 2018)

She tags some street friends, educators, and foreign volunteers in this poignant post. Carlota's audience is therefore defined by those she tags but also by the Facebook friends of the tagged people. Did she want these other publics to read her story? That is difficult to know. What is clear is that she wants to make sure some specific people know her story and that her story reaches a broader audience of Facebook friends. Carlota decided to share a very intimate part of her life with a clear purpose: to vindicate the reasons for her street condition.

The posted story makes it clear why she lives on the street and why she is happier there than in any other place before. A serious violation of rights, together with a considerable amount of violence, is described in the post.

Indeed, Facebook is used as a democratic space in the story of Carlota, a virtual space where she decides what to communicate to whom, which rarely happens for street children in other social spaces. Even though there have been enormous efforts to give street children a voice through participatory research, interventions, and political movements, all of them have always been conducted or at least initiated from someone living outside the street.

Social media allow children living on the street free virtual participation to vindicate, to amplify, and to edit their story so that their strength and capacity for self-improvement can be acknowledged by a broader audience than they can reach through their offline interactions.

Attempts to make Facebook audiences think that they are more than street children were widespread. Other smaller examples of vindication of the street label could be found on the presentation section of nearly all Facebook profiles researched. All of them mentioned the school they went to, even if it was for a few days or months. They also included other references, such as working places, educational programmes where they participated in small training courses, and so on. In some cases there were also references or tags to their family relatives. Finally, some of the street children tagged street educators as family members.

As Morduchowicz, Marcon, Sylvestre, and Ballestrini (2012) observed, social media are one of the few spaces where street (and non-street) children can reinvent who they are, how they are defined socially, and how the society in which they live perceives them. Interaction with social media and technology shapes their individual and collective identity and gives them a digital space to talk about themselves to others.

Conclusions

This chapter aimed to expand the knowledge and evidence in the field of street children's use of social media by conducting a study on their Facebook profiles and posts. First, Facebook's affordances comprise both risks and opportunities for them. Street children's rights continue to be at risk in the digital environment and, therefore, awareness of their social media participation is fundamental. Nonetheless, it is also evident that social media affordances provide new, potentially empowering ways and tools for the formation and enactment of their social identities. Their Facebook posts revealed they were re-thinking and re-orienting ways of behaving and protecting personal information online, sometimes resourcefully and sometimes ambiguously.

Second, street children interact with social media and share information and messages to an intended audience and to an 'imagined' audience – as they are physically absent or 'invisible' (Litt & Hargittai, 2016). Street children – as perhaps all social media users – try to reach a specific audience by tagging them in particular posts and/or producing specific publications to raise concern, empathy, and solidarity to improve their offline conditions. In this respect, Kolko, Nakamura, and Rodman (2000) state that cultural biases that configure unmediated aspects of every-day social interactions also shape what they call 'the mediated experiences' that people have online. Such is the case of street children's Facebook posts where street children tend to follow different offline social codes to address different online tagged or imagined audiences.

Finally, social media are used to vindicate their offline street children identity. Through Facebook, street children present themselves not only within the confines of their street identity but show different aspects of their lives that are rarely known when there is a dominant street discourse surrounding them. The study indicates that street children are using Facebook not only to stay connected to their street friends and peers but to reach other audiences with whom direct communication was almost impossible, apart from through welfare institutions that used to mediate between them and other publics.

The research findings show that street children have taken an active role in social media that counters the passive one they used to have on 'traditional' broadcast media. Moreover, their interaction on social media, specifically on Facebook, has enabled an enlargement of their online connections both with other street children as well as with home-based people. However, a question remains unanswered: what transformation is possible in the lives of street children through social media? The impact of social media in the lives of street children is hard to determine. What can change in their 'real world' as a product of the enlargement of their online social network is not at all clear. But it is clear that street children's online social inclusion may give the false impression of their exclusion in the offline social world.

Notes

1 Although we prefer the term 'street-connected' children or 'children in street situations' (Consortium for Street Children, 2018) we will use the term 'street children' for reading purposes.
2 Marcela Losantos Velasco, henceforth referred to as the first author, had personal contact with these children in various previous research projects and continued to have regular interactions on Facebook afterwards.
3 For more information, the online report can be found at www.cis.gob.bo/wp–content/uploads/2017/03/Bolivia–digital–sello.pdf.
4 The Nation Census of Bolivian street children showed that all children, aged 11 to 18, had a cell phone at some point during the year. However, as it is second hand or stolen, it stops working, or they trade it or sell it when they are in need of money.
5 By active profile we mean those who had performed an activity such posting, commenting, or liking within a week.
6 Street children sniff glue because its psychotropic effects help them deal with hunger and cold.
7 Torrante is the street slang to name the place where street groups sleep. It is usually located under a bridge or under the stairs of some downtown street.

References

Bar–On, A. (1997). Criminalizing survival: Images and reality of street children. *Journal of Social Policy*, 26(1), 63–78.
boyd, d. (2002). Faceted identity: Managing representation in a digital world (Unpublished master's thesis). Massachusetts Institute of Technology, Cambridge, MA.
boyd, d. (2008). Taken out of context: American teen sociality in networked publics (Unpublished doctoral thesis). University of California, Berkeley.
boyd, d. (2014). *It's complicated: The social lives of networked teens*. New Haven: Yale University Press.

Buckingham, D. (2015). Defining digital literacy: What do young people need to know about digital media? *Nordic Journal of Digital Literacy*, 10, 21–35.

Cáceres Zapatero, M. D., Brändle Señán, G., & Ruiz San Román, J. A. (2017). Sociabilidad virtual: la interacción social en el ecosistema digital. *Historia y comunicación social*, 22(1), 233–247.

Consortium for Street Children (2018). Tackling modern slavery on the street. Retrieved from: www.streetchildren.org/wp-content/uploads/2018/08/APPG-Modern-Slavery-Briefing.pdf.

Costa, E. (2018). Affordances-in-practice: An ethnographic critique of social media logic and context collapse. *New Media and Society*, 20(10), 3641–3656.

Delgado, M., & Felice, M. (2013). Sociabilidad virtual en Facebook: Los usos y la construcción de relaciones entre los jóvenes de la ciudad de Buenos Aires. *Question*, 1(39), 29–38.

DiMaggio, P., Hargittai, E., Celeste, C., & Shafer, S. (2004). Digital inequality: From unequal access to differentiated use. In D. B. Grusky & S. Szelényi (Eds.), *The inequality reader: Contemporary and foundational readings in race, class and gender* (pp. 355–400). Cambridge, MA: Westview Press.

Fiske, J. (1994). Audiencing: Cultural practices cultural and cultural studies. In N. K. Denzin & Y. S. Lincoln (Eds.), *The Sage handbook of qualitative methods* (pp. 189–198). Thousand Oaks: Sage.

Gibson, J. J. (1979). *The ecological approach to visual perception*. Boston: Houghton Mifflin.

Guardia, M., & Zegada, M. T. (2018). *La vida política del meme. Interacciones digitales en Facebook en una coyuntura crítica*. La Paz: Plural editores.

Huang, C. C., & Huang, K. (2008). Caring for abandoned street children in La Paz, Bolivia. *Archives of Disease in Childhood*, 93(7), 626–627.

Kolko, B., Nakamura, L., & Rodman, G. (2000). *Race in cyberspace*. London: Routledge.

Litt, E., & Hargittai, E. (2016). The imagined audience on social network sites. *Social Media + Society*, 2, 1–12.

Livingstone, S. (2003). Children's use of the internet: Reflections on the emerging research agenda. *New Media and Society*, 5(2), 147–166.

Livingstone, S. (2019). Audiences in an age of datafication: Critical questions for media research. *Television & New Media*, 20(2), 170–183.

Livingstone, S., & Haddon, L. (2009). *EU Kids Online: Final report*. London School of Economics and Political Science: EU Kids Online.

Livingstone, S., & Helsper, E. (2007). Gradations in digital inclusion: Children, young people and the digital divide. *New Media and Society*, 9(4), 671–696.

Livingstone, S., Stoilova, M., & Nandagiri, R. (2018). *Children's data and privacy online: Reviewing the existing evidence*. London: London School of Economics and Political Science.

Losantos Velasco, M. (2017). *Podemos dejar la calle pero la calle nos dejará a nosotros? Voces de niños, niñas y adolescentes sobre su permanencia en situación de calle*. La Paz: Universidad Católica Boliviana 'San Pablo'.

Losantos Velasco, M. & Loots G. (2015). Protección y participación: la desafiante situación de derechos de los niños y adolescentes que viven en la calle. *Familia, niños y adolescentes en situación de Vulnerabilidad: Aportes para la política pública* (pp. 34–55). La Paz: Universidad Católica Boliviana "San Pablo".

Mitchell, C., De Lange, N., & Moletsane, R. (2017). *Participatory visual methodologies: Social change, community and policy*. South Africa: Sage.

Mitchell, W. T. (1995). *Picture theory: Essays on verbal and visual representation*. Chicago: University of Chicago Press.

Morduchowicz, R., Marcon, A., Sylvestre, V., & Ballestrini, F. (2012). *Los adolescentes y las redes sociales*. Buenos Aires: FCE.

Papacharissi, Z. (Ed.). (2010). *A networked self: Identity, community, and culture on social network sites*. New York: Routledge.

Papacharissi, Z., & Yuan, E. (2011). What if the internet did not speak English? New and old language for studying newer media technologies. In N. Jankowski, S. Jones, & D. Park (Eds.), *The long history of new media* (pp. 89–108). New York: Peter Lang.

Rose, G. (2007). *Visual methodologies: An introduction to the interpretation of visual materials* (2nd ed.). Los Angeles: Sage.

Taddicken, M. (2014). The 'privacy paradox' in the social web: The impact of privacy concerns, individual characteristics, and the perceived social relevance of different forms of self-disclosure. *Journal of Computer-Mediated Communication*, 19(2), 248–273.

Viceministerio de Defensa Social y Sustancias Controladas. (2015). *Censo de personas en situación de calle, 2014: Estudio realizado en niñas, niños, adolescentes y adultos de diez ciudades de Bolivia*. La Paz: Viceministerio de Defensa Social y Sustancias Controladas.

Vicepresidencia del Estado Plurinacional de Bolivia. (2016). *Bolivia Digital. 15 miradas acerca del internet y la sociedad en Bolivia*. La Paz: Vicepresidencia del Estado Plurinacional de Bolivia.

43
PERSPECTIVES ON CYBERBULLYING AND TRADITIONAL BULLYING
Same or Different?

Robin M. Kowalski and Annie McCord

Introduction

"Someone told me to kill myself. Someone told me to hang myself". These words, spoken by a 13-year-old boy, describe how he had been cyberbullied. When asked his reaction, the boy said he was "getting extremely depressed" (Toth, Kowalski, & Webb, 2016). Whether it is communication with classmates, unknown social media users, or online gaming partners, cyberbullying is a part of life for young internet users today, and an important area for research and intervention. This chapter examines both the conceptualisations of and prevalence rates for traditional bullying and cyberbullying with a view to identifying the specific features of cyberbullying. It then discusses the extent to which cyberbullying is distinct from traditional bullying or merely an extension of it. Importantly, although traditional bullying and cyberbullying can occur at any age, this chapter focusses on adolescent-aged youth. However, to understand the context in which cyberbullying occurs, it is important to first examine the pervasive use of digital media among youth today.

Digital Media Use Among Youth

Near current information indicates that, among teens 13 to 17 years of age in the Global North, 95% report having a smartphone, with 45% indicating that they are online almost constantly (Anderson & Jiang, 2018). Social media use predominates among teens with YouTube (85%), Instagram (72%), Snapchat (69%), and Facebook (51%) being used most often (Anderson & Jiang, 2018). As beneficial as digital media can be, however, it is often the means by which maladaptive behaviours, such as cyberbullying, occur. Indeed, research has indicated a relationship between time spent online and involvement in cyberbullying (e.g., Çelik, Atak, & Erguzen, 2012). In addition, the most common venue by which cyberbullying occurs for a particular age group reflects the most common form of digital media in use by that same age group (Katzer, Fetchenhauer, & Belschak, 2009; Kowalski, Giumetti, Schroeder, & Lattanner, 2014). For example, whereas online gaming is prevalent among elementary-school-aged youth, social media dominates among middle- and high-school-aged teens (Kowalski, Giumetti, & Cox, 2019; Kowalski, Limber, & McCord, 2019).

Traditional Bullying and Cyberbullying Defined

The Centers for Disease Control and Prevention (2018) defines traditional bullying as

> any unwanted aggressive behaviour(s) by another youth or group of youths who are not siblings or current dating partners that involves an observed or perceived power imbalance and is repeated multiple times or is highly likely to be repeated. Bullying may inflict harm or distress on the targeted youth including physical, psychological, social, or educational harm.

This definition is generally supported in the literature (Olweus, 1993, 2013), and highlights the three important characteristics of bullying as (1) harmful or unwanted behaviours, (2) involving a power imbalance, and (3) repeatedly occurring over time. For example, a 14-year-old, describing how he was traditionally bullied said, "names, verbal from peers when I was young. Fatty, stuff like that. Followed me and almost led me to my death" (Toth et al., 2016).

Building on this definition of traditional bullying, cyberbullying is defined as "an aggressive, intentional act carried out by a group or individual, using electronic forms of contact, repeatedly and over time against a victim who cannot easily defend him or herself" (Smith et al., 2008, p. 376). Cyberbullying includes the three primary characteristics of traditional bullying with the addition of the contextual features of technology or online communication. These contextual features (i.e., [some] anonymity, 24/7 access, etc.) ultimately have a significant impact on the behaviours and outcomes for victims and perpetrators. A 14-year-old, reflecting on his cyberbullying victimisation stated, "I felt like I wasn't supposed to be on Earth" (Toth et al., 2016).

Prevalence Rates of Traditional Bullying and Cyberbullying

In examining the prevalence of both traditional bullying and cyberbullying, one question that frequently arises is whether such rates are on the rise. An examination of prevalence suggests that, while rates may not be changing markedly over time, awareness of the behaviours is growing (Pontes, Ayres, Lewandowski, & Pontes, 2018). In addition, some scholars suggest that trends in bullying prevalence depend on the particular type of bullying being examined, with rates of traditional bullying showing a steady decrease in recent years, whereas rates of cyberbullying have shown a rather sharp increase (Finkelhor, 2013). This latter finding hints at differences between traditional bullying and cyberbullying, although it may also indicate some substitution in the early days of teen use of mobile digital media.

Traditional Bullying

Traditional bullying and peer victimisation appear to be most frequent during middle school and then to slightly decrease as students move into high school (Olweus, 1993). Though intervention is more frequent and accepted in the school setting, the prevalence of bullying does not appear to be decreasing over time among this age group within educational contexts (Olweus, 2013). A comprehensive report on traditional bullying in the United States in 2011 showed that about 28% of students aged 12 to 18 years reported being bullied at school during the academic year (Robers, Kemp, Rathbun, & Morgan, 2014). Fourteen per cent of youth in the United States in grades 3 through 12 reported being bullied with a high degree of frequency (two to three times a month or more; Luxenberg, Limber, & Olweus 2015, cited in Limber, Olweus, Wang, Masiello, & Breivik, 2018). The most common forms of traditional bullying included being insulted or called names (17.6%) and being the subject of rumours (18.3%). Further, among those who reported being bullied at school, the majority of bullying events happened in the hallway at school (45.6%) or inside the classroom (32.6%; Robers et al., 2014). Perpetration rates of traditional bullying are also high. In a sample of 7,182 youth in grades 6 through 10 in the United States, Wang, Iannotti, and Nansel (2009) found that 13.3% had perpetrated physical bullying at least once in the previous two months, 37.4% verbal bullying, and 27.2% social bullying.

Chester and colleagues (2015) found that almost one third of children aged 11 to 15 years reported at least occasional victimisation from bullying in North America and Europe. This varied from country to country, however, with Italy (4.8% of boys and 2.9% of girls) having the lowest prevalence, while Lithuania (28.5% of girls and 23.4% of boys) reported the highest prevalence rates of bullying. This suggests that, although bullying is common among adolescents, it may vary geographically and there could potentially be a cultural influence on prevalence rates. Additionally, individual factors may increase the frequency of bullying such as the presence of disabilities (Rose et al., 2015) or physical factors such as obesity (DeSmet et al., 2014).

Cyberbullying

As with traditional bullying, one of the vexing issues about cyberbullying has been resolving disparate prevalence rates across studies (Kowalski et al., 2014; Olweus & Limber, 2018). Different researchers have adopted slightly different conceptualisations, leading to slightly different behaviours being measured and, hence, varying prevalence rates (Kofoed & Staksred, 2018; Selkie, Fales, & Moreno, 2016). Additionally, prevalence rates vary with the time frame within which the cyberbullying must have occurred (e.g., previous month, past six months, within the year, over a lifetime) (Olweus, 2016); as well as with the criteria used to determine frequency (the behaviour occurred at least once, versus the behaviour must have occurred two to three times or more during the time frame). In a scoping review of 159 prevalence studies on adolescent cyberbullying across countries, Brochado, Soares, and Fraga (2017) observed wide variability in cyberbullying prevalence rates. Examined just in terms of the time frame involved, and depending on the study, between 4.9% and 65.0% of respondents indicated they had been cyberbullied in their lifetime; between 1.0% and 61.1% had been cyberbullied within the past year; between 1.6% and 56.9% reported being victimised within the preceding six months; and between 5.3% and 31.3% were victimised within the previous month.

Cyberbullying perpetration rates show similar variability across studies: between 1.2% and 44.1% had cyberbullied others in their lifetime; between 3.0% and 39.9% had done so in the prior year; between 1.9% and 79.3% during the past six months; and between 4.9% and 31.5% during the past month (Brochado et al., 2017). A recent survey by the Pew Center (Anderson, 2018) of teens aged 13 to 17 years in the United States found that 59% reported having experienced at least one of six forms of cyberbullying. The most common form of victimisation was name-calling (42%), followed by spreading of false rumours (32%), receiving unwanted explicit images (25%), cyberstalking (21%), physical threats (16%), and the dissemination of explicit images without consent (7%).

Prevalence rates of cyberbullying also vary with the age of the participants in a particular study and the venue by which the cyberbullying occurs. Cyberbullying modality is correlated with the technology and platform most commonly used by individuals of a particular age group. Thus, among middle- and high-school students, social media is currently the most common digital media used and the most common venue by which cyberbullying occurs (Kowalski et al., 2019). A decade ago among the same age group, instant messaging prevailed, reflecting the speed with which technology changes.

Narrative accounts of adolescent cyberbullying victimisation illustrate some of the various methods of online communication, as well as conveying the effects that cyberbullying can have on the victim. Three examples are illustrated below:

> We were in middle school and two of my best friends decided to stab me in the back for no apparent reason. Using instant messenger they talked bad about me and spread mean things about me. Once I received an insult directly from the leader of the two. I kept all of this inside until I got so overwhelmed I could not do anything but stay in the house with my family. My parents called theirs and they claimed to have apologised but they never did. It was never really resolved. I went to the same school as them for the next six years though it was difficult. I stopped playing sports with them and other after-school activities. I went to a psychologist and still do from this time forward as well as take medicine for clinical depression and anxiety. It all started with this emotional trauma and although I am over that mostly, I cannot get rid of the depression and anxiety I now feel stuck with.
> *(Isgett, Kowalski, Lattanner, Schroeder, & Senn, 2012)*

> The worst time I was cyber bullied was when a girl from my classroom pretended to be a popular boy on AIM. She had acted rude to me on AIM and when I responded defensively, she made a fake AIM screenname for a boy from my classroom. She then "asked me out" on AIM acting as this boy. I responded with a hesitant yes and went to school the next day extremely nervous. She went up to me at school and asked me if we were dating and I responded yes. I was then confronted by the boy and asked why I was telling people we were dating. I realised what had happened and responded that I had no idea what he was talking about and tried to forget the whole incident.
> *(Isgett, Kowalski, Lattanner, Schroeder, & Senn, 2012)*

> There was an anonymous joke facebook account going around and all of our friends friended it (on facebook) including myself. I was unfriended/blocked for no reason whatsoever, even though the account grew up to having about 2,000 facebook friends. Before so, the anonymous user was rude to me without any prompt as well. I felt extremely excluded considering it was the talk of the town at the time.
> *(Isgett, Kowalski, Lattanner, Schroeder, & Senn, 2012)*

Perspectives on the Relationship Between Traditional Bullying and Cyberbullying

For over a decade, researchers have debated the nature of this relationship between traditional bullying and cyberbullying. Two perspectives have been advanced to conceptualise the relationship between the two types of bullying (Olweus & Limber, 2018). The 'differences perspective' suggests that cyberbullying and traditional bullying, while sharing certain features in common, are different phenomena, with each contributing unique variance to the negative outcomes associated with bullying victimisation. The 'extension perspective', on the other hand, suggests that cyberbullying is a new form of bullying but not one that is qualitatively different. Researchers who endorse this perspective suggest that individuals who are involved in one type of bullying tend to be the same individuals who are involved in another type of bullying. Olweus (2013; see also Olweus & Limber, 2018), for example, suggests that only 10% of individuals are involved in cyberbullying independently of also being involved in traditional bullying. Mehari, Farrell, and Le (2014) suggest that traditional bullying and cyberbullying merely reflect two ways of classifying aggressive behaviour. Which perspective is adopted becomes important because it determines perspectives on, for example, outcomes of cyberbullying. People who adopt the differences perspective suggest that cyberbullying accounts for unique variance in negative outcomes over and above those accounted for by traditional bullying (e.g., Cole et al., 2016; Menesini, Calussi, & Nocentini, 2012; see, however, Machmutow, Perren, Sticca, & Alsaker, 2012; Salmivalli, Sainio, & Hodges, 2013). Those who endorse the extension perspective argue that it is often difficult to discern outcomes that are uniquely associated with cyberbullying compared with traditional bullying.

Each of these perspectives will be examined in turn. Across the two perspectives, researchers agree that involvement in the two types of bullying is related (e.g., Gradinger, Strohmeier, & Spiel, 2009; Kowalski, Morgan, & Limber, 2012; Menesini et al., 2012). However, simply obtaining positive correlations between traditional bullying and cyberbullying does not support one perspective over another.

Differences Perspective

Using the Olweus (1993, 2013) definition of traditional bullying as a foundation, cyberbullying and traditional bullying share key features in common (Smith, del Barrio, & Tokunaga, 2013). As outlined earlier in this chapter, both are acts of aggression that are intended to cause harm or distress; they are typically repeated over time, although the form of the repetition varies depending on the type of bullying; and they occur among individuals whose relationship is characterised by a power imbalance. Repetition in cyberbullying could mean a single electronic communication being read multiple times by a single victim or a single digital communication being disseminated to hundreds or thousands of individuals (Kowalski, Limber, & Agatston, 2012). Similarly, the power imbalance endemic to traditional bullying is often reflected in differences in physical stature or social status. With cyberbullying, on the other hand, power imbalances may be created by differences in technological expertise or by the perpetrator's anonymity.

In spite of the features that cyberbullying and traditional bullying share in common, they differ in critical ways. First, whereas most traditional bullying occurs at school during the school day, cyberbullying can occur anywhere that technology is available, and at any time. In addition, whereas the perpetrator of traditional bullying is most often known to the victim, perpetrators of cyberbullying can hide behind screen names. Among young people, the punitive fears attached to reporting bullying victimisation also vary with traditional bullying and cyberbullying. Victims of traditional bullying often do not report their victimisation because they fear the perpetrator getting wind of the disclosure and retaliating. Cyberbullying victims, on the other hand, fear that adults will remove their technology upon learning of the victimisation.

Support for the differences perspective has been found across several studies. As noted earlier in the chapter, studies showing decreases in prevalence rates of traditional bullying over time and increases in rates of cyberbullying in recent years (e.g., Finkelhor, 2013) would suggest that the behaviours are distinct from one another. In addition, Giumetti and Kowalski (2016) found that cyberbullying victimisation contributed between 1% and 4% of unique variance in negative outcomes above and beyond that accounted for by traditional bullying. Similarly, Menesini and colleagues (2012) found that traditional bullying and cyberbullying additively accounted for variance in internalising and externalising problems (see also, Bonanno & Hymel, 2013; Kim, Colwell, Kata, Boyle, & Georgiades, 2017; Wigderson & Lynch, 2013). Fredstrom, Adams, and Gilman (2011) found unique contributions of cyber victimisation to self-esteem, stress, anxiety, and depression after controlling for traditional bullying. It is important to note, however, that, among the growing list of studies providing support for the differences perspective, additional percentages of variance in outcomes accounted for by cyberbullying above and beyond traditional bullying tend to be small in magnitude and dependent on the particular outcome being assessed.

Extension Perspective

On the other hand, many researchers argue that cyberbullying is not itself an independent or significantly different construct from traditional bullying, but rather an extension of traditional or school bullying. Proponents of the extension approach often begin their argument in much the same way as proponents of the differences approach – by detailing features that cyberbullying and traditional bullying share in common. They are quick to point out that few researchers define cyberbullying without using the terminology of traditional bullying (National Institute of Justice, 2016). Olweus (2013) specifically cites that the power imbalance that characterises traditional bullying can be applied to cyberbullying by including traditional social power imbalance as well as technological know-how differences between the perpetrator and the victim. Mehari et al. (2014) conceptualised cyberbullying "as a new dimension on which aggression can be classified, rather than cyberbullying as a distinct counterpart to existing forms of aggression" (p. 1). In support of their position, they cited the fact that cyberbullying has in common many of the same antecedents as other forms of aggression (e.g., previous victimisation, somatic symptoms, social anxiety). Similarly, Olweus (2013) stated that

> to be cyber bullied or to cyber bully other students seems to a large extent to be part of a general pattern of bullying, where use of the electronic media is only one possible form and, in addition, is a form with a quite low prevalence.
>
> (p. 767)

Indeed, in their recent article, Olweus and Limber (2018) suggest that studies showing that cyberbullying accounts for small percentages of variance in outcome measures above and beyond that accounted for by traditional bullying do not provide evidence for the differences perspective. Additionally, Olweus (2013) showed that there is a high degree of overlap between victims of cyberbullying and victims of traditional bullying (88% of those cyberbullied had also been bullied traditionally in the United States). This suggests that cyberbullying does not create a great number of new victims, supporting the assertion that cyberbullying is but an extension of traditional bullying.

The meta-analysis by Kowalski et al. (2014) supports the extension approach but not to the extent proposed by Olweus (2013). Rather, Kowalski et al. found a correlation of 0.40 between traditional and cyberbullying victimisation and a correlation of 0.45 between traditional and cyberbullying perpetration (2014). These correlations are significant and suggest there is great similarity between the two concepts and challenges those who argue the differences perspective. Additionally, Olweus (2013) argues that cyberbullying and traditional bullying have similar effects on potential outcomes. For example, those who report being cyberbullied have self-esteem outcomes that are indistinguishable from those who report being traditionally bullied (Olweus, 2013). Ultimately, if schools and parents are concerned with both traditional and cyberbullying, and if the outcomes and experiences are indistinguishable, it can be argued that there is enough similarity to constitute the extension perspective. In resolving these two perspectives, research by Moreno found that "cyberbullying is best understood in the broader context of bullying, but that stakeholder perceptions about the uniqueness of cyberbullying are strong" (National Institute of Justice, 2016).

Conclusion

Ultimately, asking whether cyberbullying is an extension of traditional bullying or a phenomenon distinct from it is, perhaps, focussing on the wrong issue. While conceptually it is important to be able to distinguish the two types of behaviour with their concomitant risk and protective factors and outcomes, in an applied sense, both types of bullying warrant attention. As noted by Modecki, Minchin, Harbaugh, Guerra, and Runions (2014), "findings suggest that cyber and traditional measures may reflect different methods of enacting a similar behaviour (being mean to others) and the form (online vs. offline) of bullying may be less important than the conduct" (p. 607). The fact that youth involved in one type of bullying may also be involved in the other type of bullying, as so many studies have suggested (e.g., Kowalski et al., 2012; Smith, 2015), while supporting the extension perspective, may, more importantly, be supporting the fact that certain individuals are at particular risk for victimisation. The form of the victimisation matters less than the intervention strategies implemented on behalf of those involved in the bullying situation, including bystanders.

In addition, the voices of those involved (as reflected in the narratives included within this chapter) are important to consider when implementing prevention and intervention strategies for any type of bullying. Focus groups conducted with adolescents who had been both victims and perpetrators of cyberbullying, as well as with some who had never been involved with cyberbullying, yielded some interesting perspectives on dealing with youth online activities. Among the comments offered in the focus groups were that parents should: set age-appropriate guidelines; teach their children how to deal with conflict (including online conflict): monitor adolescent use of the internet: and exercise "supervision not snoopervision" (Agatston, Kowalski, & Limber, 2011). In other words, adolescents were satisfied with parents searching their local online histories but not with installing key-stroke software on their computers. They also wanted their parents to watch for warning signs of possible cyberbullying victimisation, such as anxiety, depression, and a drop in school grades. Finally, they asked that their parents not blame them should they be a victim of cyberbullying activity. These suggestions are not only reasonable but also reflect an understanding on the part of the adolescents in the focus groups of the potential for cyberbullying to occur and the need for at least some adult supervision and support.

References

Agatston, P. W., Kowalski, R. M., & Limber, S. E. (2011). Youth views on cyberbullying. In J. Patchin & S. Hinduja (Eds.), *Cyberbullying prevention and response: Expert perspectives* (pp. 57–71). New York, NY: Routledge.

Anderson, M. (2018). *A majority of teens have experienced some form of cyberbullying*. Retrieved from: www.pewinternet.org/2018/09/27/a-majority-of-teens-have-experienced-some-form-of-cyberbullying.

Anderson, M., & Jiang, J. (2018). *Teens, social media & technology 2018*. Retrieved from: www.pewinternet.org/2018/05/31/teens-social-media-technology-2018.

Bonanno, R. A., & Hymel, S. (2013). Cyber bullying and internalizing difficulties: Above and beyond the impact of traditional forms of bullying. *Journal of Youth & Adolescence*, 42(5), 685–697. doi:10.1007/s10964-013-9937-1.

Brochado, S., Soares, S., & Fraga, S. (2017). A scoping review on studies of cyberbullying prevalence among adolescents. *Trauma, Violence, & Abuse*, 18(5), 523–531. doi:10.1177/1524838016641668.

Çelik, S., Atak, H., & Erguzen, A. (2012). The effect of personality on cyberbullying among university students in Turkey. *Eurasian Journal of Educational Research*, 49, 129–150.

Centers for Disease Control and Prevention. (2018). *Preventing bullying* [Fact sheet]. Retrieved from: www.cdc.gov/violenceprevention/pdf/bullying-factsheet508.pdf.

Chester, K. L., Callaghan, M., Cosma, A., Donnelly, P., Craig, W., Walsh, S., & Molcho, M. (2015). Cross-national time trends in bullying victimization in 33 countries among children aged 11, 13 and 15 from 2002 to 2010. *European Journal of Public Health*, 25(supplement 2), 61–64. doi:10.1093/eurpub/ckv029.

Cole, D. A., Zelkowitz, R. I., Nick, E., Martin, N. C., Roeder, K. M., Sinclair-McBride, K., & Spinelli, T. (2016). Longitudinal and incremental relation of cybervictimization to negative self-cognitions and depressive symptoms in young adolescents. *Journal of Abnormal Psychology*, *44*(7), 1321–1332. doi:10.1007/s10802-015-0123-7.

DeSmet, A., Deforche, B., Hublet, A., Tanghe, A., Stremersch, E., & De Bourdeaudhuij, I. (2014). Traditional and cyberbullying victimization as correlates of psychosocial distress and barriers to a healthy lifestyle among severely obese adolescents – A matched case–control study on prevalence and results from a cross-sectional study. *BMC Public Health*, *14*(1), 1–23. doi:10.1186/1471-2458-14-224.

Finkelhor, D. (2013). *Trends in bullying and peer victimization*. Durham, NH: Crimes against Children Research Center. Updated August, 2014.

Fredstrom, B. K., Adams, R. E., & Gilman, R. (2011). Electronic and school-based victimization: Unique contexts for adjustment difficulties during adolescence. *Journal of Youth & Adolescence*, *40*(4), 405–415. doi:10.1007/s10964-010-9569-7.

Giumetti, G. W., & Kowalski, R. M. (2016). Cyberbullying matters: Examining the incremental impact of cyberbullying on outcomes above and beyond traditional bullying in North America. In R. Navarro, S. Yubero, & E. Larrañaga (Eds.), *Cyberbullying across the globe: Gender, family, and mental health* (pp. 117–130). New York, NY: Springer.

Gradinger, P., Strohmeier, D., & Spiel, C. (2009). Traditional bullying and cyberbullying: Identification of risk groups for adjustment problems. *Zeitschrift Für Psychologie/Journal of Psychology*, *217*(4), 205–213. doi:10.1027/0044-3409.217.4.205.

Isgett, S., Kowalski, R. M., Lattanner, M., Schroeder, A., Giumetti, G., & Senn, W. (2012). Cyberbullying among college students. Paper presented at the annual meeting of the *Southeastern Psychological Association*, New Orleans, LA.

Katzer, C., Fetchenhauer, D., & Belschak, F. (2009). Cyberbullying: Who are the victims? A comparison of victimization in internet chatrooms and victimization in school. *Journal of Media Psychology: Theories, Methods, and Applications*, *21*(1), 25–36. doi:10.1027/1864-1105.21.1.25.

Kim, S., Colwell, S. R., Kata, A., Boyle, M. H., & Georgiades, K. (2017). Cyberbullying victimization and adolescent mental health: Evidence of differential effects by sex and mental health problem type. *Journal of Youth and Adolescence*, *47*(3), 661–672. doi:10.1007/s10964-017-0678-4.

Kofoed, J., & Staksrud, E. (2018). 'We always torment different people, so by definition we are no bullies': The problem of definitions in cyberbullying research. *New Media & Society*, *21*, 1006–1020. doi:10.1177/1461444818810026.

Kowalski, R. M., Giumetti, G., & Cox, H. (2019). Differences in technology use among demographic groups: Implications for cyberbullying research. In G. Giumetti & R. Kowalski (Eds.), *Cyberbullying in schools, workplaces, and romantic relationships: The many lenses and perspectives of electronic mistreatment* (pp. 15–31). New York, NY: Routledge.

Kowalski, R. M., Giumetti, G. W., Schroeder, A. N., & Lattanner, M. R. (2014). Bullying in the digital age: A critical review and meta-analysis of cyberbullying research among youth. *Psychological Bulletin*, *140*(4), 1073–1137. doi:10.1037/a0035618.

Kowalski, R. M., Limber, S., & McCord, A. (2019). A developmental approach to cyberbullying: Prevalence and protective factors. *Journal of Aggression and Violent Behavior*, *45*, 20–32. doi:10.1016/j.avb.2018.02.009.

Kowalski, R. M., Limber, S. E., & Agatston, P. W. (2012). *Cyberbullying: Bullying in the digital age* (2nd ed.). Malden, MA: Wiley-Blackwell.

Kowalski, R. M., Morgan, C. A., & Limber, S. E. (2012). Traditional bullying as a potential warning sign of cyberbullying. *School Psychology International*, *33*(5), 505–519. doi:10.1177/0143034312445244.

Limber, S. P., Olweus, D. A., Wang, W., Masiello, M., & Breivik, K. (2018). Evaluation of the Olweus Bullying Prevention Program: A large scale study of U.S. students in grades 3–11. *Journal of School Psychology*, *69*, 56–72. doi:10.1016/j.jsp.2018.04.004.

Machmutow, K., Perren, S., Sticca, F., & Alsaker, F. D. (2012). Peer victimisation and depressive symptoms: Can specific coping strategies buffer the negative impact of cybervictimisation? *Emotional and Behavioral Difficulties*, *17*(3–4), 403–420. doi:10.1080/13632752.2012.704310.

Mehari, K. R., Farrell, A. D., & Le, A. H. (2014). Cyberbullying among adolescents: Measures in search of a construct. *Psychology of Violence*, *4*(4), 399–415. doi:10.1037/a0037521.

Menesini, E., Calussi, P., & Nocentini, A. (2012). Cyberbullying and traditional bullying: Unique, additive, and synergistic effects on psychological health symptoms. In Q. Li, D. Cross, & P. K. Smith (Eds.), *Cyberbullying in the global playground: Research on international perspectives* (pp. 245–262). Malden, MA: Wiley-Blackwell.

Modecki, K. L., Minchin, J., Harbaugh, A. G., Guerra, N. G., & Runions, K. C. (2014). Bullying prevalence across contexts: A meta-analysis measuring cyber and traditional bullying. *Journal of Adolescent Health*, *55*(5), 602–611. doi:10.1016/j.jadohealth.2014.06.007.

National Institute of Justice. (2016, September 9). *Understanding cyberbullying: Developing an evidence-based definition*. Retrieved from: http://nij.gov/topics/crime/pages/understanding-cyberbullying.aspx.

Olweus, D. (1993). *Bullying at school: What we know and what we can do*. New York, NY: Blackwell.

Olweus, D. (2013). School bullying: Development and some important challenges. *Annual Review of Clinical Psychology*, *9*(1), 751–780. doi:10.1146/annurev-clinpsy-050212-185516.

Olweus, D. (2016). Cyberbullying: A critical overview. In B. Bushman (Ed.), *Aggression and violence: A social psychological perspective* (pp. 225–240). New York, NY: Routledge.

Olweus, D., & Limber, S. P. (2018). Some problems with cyberbullying research. *Current Opinion in Psychology*, *19*, 139–143. doi:10.1016/j.copsyc.2017.04.012.

Pontes, N. H., Ayres, C. G., Lewandowski, C., & Pontes, M. F. (2018). Trends in bullying victimization by gender among U.S high school students. *Research in Nursing & Health*, *41*(3), 243–251. doi:10.1002/nur.21868.

Robers, S., Kemp, J., Rathbun, A., & Morgan, R. E. (2014). *Indicators of school crime and safety: 2013* (NCES 2014-042/NCJ 243299). Washington, DC: National Center for Education Statistics, U.S. Department of Education, and Bureau of Justice Statistics, Office of Justice Programs, U.S. Department of Justice.

Rose, C. A., Stormont, M., Wang, Z., Simpson, C. G., Preast, J. L., & Green, A. L. (2015). Bullying and students with disabilities: Examination of disability status and educational placement. *School Psychology Review*, *44*(4), 425–444. doi:10.17105/spr-15-0080.1.

Salmivalli, C., Sainio, M., & Hodges, E. (2013). Electronic victimization: Correlates, antecedents, and consequences among elementary and middle school students. *Journal of Clinical Child & Adolescent Psychology*, *42*(4), 442–453. doi:10.1080/15374416.2012.759228.

Selkie, E. M., Fales, J. L., & Moreno, M. A. (2016). Cyberbullying prevalence among US middle and high school-aged adolescents: A systematic review and quality assessment. *Journal of Adolescent Health*, *58*, 125–133. doi:10.1016/j.jadohealth.2015.09.026.

Smith, P. K. (2015). The nature of cyberbullying and what we can do about it. *Journal of Research in Special Education Needs*, *15*(3), 176–184. doi:10.1111/1471-3802.12114.

Smith, P. K., del Barrio, C., & Tokunaga, R. (2013). Definitions of bullying and cyberbullying: How useful are the terms? In S. Bauman, J. Walker, & D. Cross (Eds.), *Principles of cyberbullying research: Definitions, measures, and methods* (pp. 26–40). New York, NY: Routledge.

Smith, P. K., Mahdavi, J., Carvalho, M., Fisher, S., Russell, S., & Tippett, N. (2008). Cyberbullying: Its nature and impact in secondary school pupils. *Journal of Child Psychology and Psychiatry*, *49*(4), 376–385. doi:10.1111/j.1469-7610.2007.01846.x.

Toth, A., Kowalski, R. M., & Webb, M. (2016). Bullying among boys with disabilities. *Psychology and Education Journal*, *53*(1–2), 34–39.

Wang, J., Iannotti, R. J., & Nansel, T. R. (2009). School bullying among adolescents in the United States: Physical, verbal, relational, and cyber. *Journal of Adolescent Health*, *45*(4), 368–375. doi:10.1016/j.jadohealth.2009.03.021.

Wigderson, S., & Lynch, M. (2013). Cyber- and traditional peer victimization: Unique relationships with adolescent well-being. *Psychology of Violence*, *3*(4), 297–309. doi:10.1037/a0033657.

44

DIGITAL STORYTELLING

Opportunities for Identity Investment for Youth from Refugee Backgrounds

Lauren Johnson and Maureen Kendrick

Introduction

Many youth from refugee backgrounds, especially those with interrupted schooling, are at risk of underachievement unless the reproduction of social disadvantage is altered through more equitable educational opportunities (Cummins, 2014; Dooley & Thangaperumal, 2011). Although there is a consensus among researchers and educators that diminishing social disadvantage involves extending students' knowledge of academic language, scaffolding meaning, and activating background knowledge, the role of literacy engagement and identity affirmation have been largely ignored in recent debates on closing the achievement gap of social groups defined on the basis of language, income, and racialised status (Cummins, 2014, p. 146). There is an urgent need for school cultures to better understand how to design language and literacy learning experiences that respond to the identities and background experiences of this vulnerable population. In this chapter we examine how digital storytelling as a pedagogical tool can provide more equitable opportunities for literacy engagement and identity affirmation for refugee-background youth. This chapter presents Abdullahi's digital story as an "instance of practice" (Cummins & Early, 2011) that demonstrates possibilities for powerfully engaging refugee-background learners intellectually, affectively, and agentively in telling stories of accomplishment and depicting future aspirations in meaningful ways (Appadurai, 2004; Cummins, 2014). It addresses how engaging with the affordances of different modes such as audial, visual, and linguistic through digital storytelling can offer individualised entry points into self-expression and help students from refugee backgrounds become more aware of their skills, knowledge, strengths, and capacities, ultimately promoting positive identities as students imagine their futures and a place of belonging within their new social environments.

Interrupting Educational Disadvantage: Identity Investment and Multimodal Pedagogies

Tracking studies show that an unacceptably high percentage of English Language Learners (ELLs), and in particular those who entered as refugees, do not graduate from high school (Garnett, 2010; Gunderson, 2004, 2007; Toohey & Derwing, 2008). Gunderson (2004, 2007) reports that refugee-background youth, especially those from socio-economically disadvantaged circumstances, disappear from academic courses (between grades 8 and 12) at an alarming rate. A contributing factor is that many educators in secondary schools struggle to identify, understand, and meet the language and literacy needs of learners with limited or interrupted schooling, and experiences of trauma (Cummins, 2014). Moreover, there has been little success among educators to make visible "who refugees are as individuals, what literacy skills they possess, and their experiences navigating a new and unfamiliar culture and language" (Saleh, 2018).

'Disadvantage', however, is not a fixed construct socially determined by what takes place outside of schools; rather, it is a dynamic process enabled or disrupted through the structures of schooling, including the patterns of interaction between teachers and students (Cummins, 2014). In other words, "significant components of the background experiences of [at-risk] groups ... are transformed into actual educational disadvantages only when the school fails to respond appropriately to these background experiences" (Cummins, 2014, pp. 147–8). Dooley and Thangaperumal (2011) argue that educators need to interrupt the reproduction of social disadvantage through literacy education and educational opportunities that "capitalise on students' affective and identity investment" (p. 386). This chapter focusses on how digital storytelling as a multimodal pedagogy can nurture educational opportunities for refugee-background youth by prioritising their lived experience and background knowledge, affirming their identities, and engaging them in imagining possibilities for the future (Cummins, 2014). This ability to 'write a map of a journey into the future' has been referred to by Appadurai (2004) as the "capacity to aspire" (p. 76). A map of the future, he argues, needs to be made "more real, available, and powerful" for all members of a society, including those belonging to marginalised populations who may have more limited access to the kinds of diverse experiences that manifest into personal wishes and wants, enabling individuals to produce their own narratives and pathways linked to larger social contexts and more abstract norms and beliefs (Appadurai, 2004, p. 70).

We take a multimodal approach to designing learning experiences. This approach recognises that language alone only partially reflects how people make meaning in the world (Kress & van Leeuwen, 1996). Digital storytelling as a multimodal pedagogy offers opportunities for youth to use images, sound, and language. This broad array of semiotic resources taps into how cultures and individuals select from and choose to develop particular possibilities to "produce and communicate meanings in specific social settings" (Kress & van Leeuwen, 1996, p. 264). In this study, these semiotic resources are understood as having the ability to simultaneously communicate the here and now of a social context while representing the resources youth from refugee backgrounds have 'to hand' from the world around them (Kress, 1997).

The study focusses on pedagogic possibilities for students from refugee backgrounds, aligning with an innovative area of research that examines the dialogic process of multimodal meaning making (Campano & Low, 2011; Early, Kendrick, & Potts, 2015). Historically, devaluation of the linguistic and cultural knowledge that refugee-background students bring to school has reinforced societal power structures that exclude certain minority groups from social participation and advancement (Cummins, 2014). Digital storytelling, because it capitalises on learners' communicative resources, identities, and ways of being, has the potential to shift the power relations in classroom settings. As a pedagogy, it is rooted in collaborative and interactive relations of power that enable students to draw on their own life experiences and communicative and intellectual resources to tell their own stories in their own voice, empowering them to achieve much more than what might be possible through more traditional print-based pedagogies alone (Cummins, 2014).

Digital storytelling as a multimodal pedagogy can provide enhanced opportunities and intellectually engaging ways for students to tell stories about their lives, experiences, and preferred ways of knowing. Kress (1997) insists that it is necessary to uncouple the assumed link between language and cognition and to instead adopt the proposition that cognition is accomplished in all modes. Different modes give rise to different ways of thinking, and digital storytelling provides opportunities to constantly translate meaning from one mode to another (e.g., from visual/images to audial/musical). According to Kress (1997), this transmediation is essential for humans to understand the world (see also Kendrick, 2016). This process of engaging with and across different modes can provide students with a heightened awareness of their own knowledge, skills, and accomplishments; in essence, digital storytelling provides an experimental and highly productive space for combining ideas, experiences, imaginings, and modes for meaning-making.

Digital Storytelling Pedagogies

Digital storytelling as a narrative form first emerged in the 1990s. It was originally developed by Lambert (2013) and his colleagues at StoryCenter in California and took the form of a two-to-three minute film that used digital media such as photographs, video clips, music or sound, and voiceover to tell the story of the author's lived experience. Research has foregrounded how digital storytelling can provide a compelling way to share rich life lessons and experiences (Lenette, Cox, & Brough, 2015). Digital storytelling has also been advanced as pedagogical innovation. Vinogradova, Linville, and Bickel (2011) illustrate how using photos, voice, and music can enhance the development of multimodal design, especially for English language learners (ELLs), as they learn the affordance of different modes as integral to the storytelling process. Similarly, Hull and Katz (2006) emphasise that digital storytelling's integration of personally chosen resources and artifacts enables authors to express important moments in their lives from a reflective position of strength. For refugee background learners, Emert (2013) argues that digital storytelling can foreground rich learning resources over academic challenges, enabling them to advance their abilities as multimodal meaning-makers.

The digital storytelling composing process has most often been described as a collective linear one that engages learners in a series of steps beginning with script writing. Because this pedagogic design begins with writing, it typically positions nonlinguistic modes as supplementary to the linguistic (Shin & Cimasko, 2008). Research shows, however, that when the composing process is open and flexible with no predetermined sequence, learners will bring their communicative resources together dialogically (Yang, 2012), simultaneously reflecting, thinking, and designing in different modes (Nelson & Hull, 2008).

We opted for a non-sequential pedagogical design to maximise students' understanding of the communicative potential of each mode (e.g., visual, audial, gestural) as integral to the storytelling process. This design was critical for the participants, many with limited English or first-language (L1) literacy abilities, because of its "empowering and agentic potential" to enable students who "are low-performing in ... traditional written assignments ... the opportunity to express themselves in new ways ... other than the written text" (Erstad & Silseth, 2008, p. 221).

Context and Methodology

As a means of showcasing how digital storytelling can open up identity options for diverse students, Abdullahi's process is traced as he shares a personal accomplishment. The research was conducted in a school district's transitional class that provides specialised support for refugee and immigrant background senior-high-level students. The class was located in the Metro Vancouver area in an English language learner welcome centre. Pseudonyms for all project participants are used throughout this chapter.

Of Somali background, Abdullahi was born in Yemen. At the time of the study, he was 20 years of age and had no formal schooling in his country of origin. He arrived in Canada at age 17.5 and had been enrolled at the welcome centre for approximately two years. He is the eldest child in a single-parent home and carries considerable family responsibilities. For this reason, he was often absent from class.

At the beginning of the digital storytelling project, the students completed a handout which involved filling in sentence stems related to their identities (e.g., I am a _____; I enjoy _____) and circling images representing their preferred ways of expressing and learning information (e.g., singing, watching television). On this handout, Abdullahi describes himself as 'happy' and a 'nice guy'. Activities that he enjoys include reading, dancing, and playing on the computer. He defines himself as a 'student' and a 'brother'. He identified his countries of origin as both Somalia and Yemen and wrote that he speaks Indian, Somali, English, and Arabic. He explained in an interview (25 February 2014) that he likes to communicate or learn information through 'writing' and indicated that he prefers the visual mode, emphasising that he likes "to look at the movie".

The 'instance of practice' example comes from an ethnographic, qualitative case study focussing on the possibilities of digital storytelling for meaning-making and identity-affirmation among youth from immigrant and refugee backgrounds. Abdullahi's story represents one example of an accomplishment story that the students in the study were able to communicate through digital storytelling. His story was selected because it included clearly defined future aspirations. (Even though students were not instructed to describe future goals in their digital stories, a number of students chose to include more general ambitions, such as graduating from high school and helping their families; for other examples see also Johnson & Kendrick, 2017.) Although, as Hull and Katz (2006) note, human lives can rarely be reduced to simple cause and effect, this analysis here aligns with Cummins and Early (2011) who stress that "actuality implies possibility" (p. 19). That is, "if a particular intervention has happened, and if particular effects have been observed, then this intervention and its impact can happen" (p. 18). Such cases "have immense power to effect change both in the instructional choices made by teachers, administrators and policy-makers, and in the identity options opened up to diverse students" (p. 19).

The methods of data generation included classroom observations, field notes, informal in-class conversations with participants, semi-structured interviews following the project to gain understanding of the students' composing processes and the effects of participation in the project on their identities, student-created artifacts (e.g., storyboards, writing), and the digital stories.

The study used a multiliteracies framework (see New London Group, 1996) in collaboratively designing the digital storytelling project with the classroom teacher. The need for a "pedagogy of multiliteracies" (New London Group, 1996) is premised on a two-pronged argument: the salience of cultural and linguistic diversity amidst a rapidly changing multimodal communication landscape. Fundamental to the framework is the concept of Design, which includes six major modes of communication: linguistic, visual, audio, gestural, and spatial, plus "multimodal" that relates the five modes to each other. The data were coded categorising modes of communication and common themes (e.g., accomplishments, aspirations).

Rose's (2011) sites of visual meaning making are used as the organisational structure for presenting the findings. Rose describes three sites through which meaning is made in visual (or in this study, multimodal) texts: "the site(s) of the **production** of an image, the site of the **image** itself, and the site(s) where it is seen by various **audiences**" (p. 19; emphasis in the original). These three sites refer to the circumstances surrounding the production of an image (site of production), the compositional nature of an image (site of the image), and how it is viewed (site of audience). Working across the sites of production, image, and audience, the findings showcase Abdullahi's digital storytelling process and the slides he created, drawing attention to how he was thinking visually, musically, and linguistically to realise a fuller range of affective expression.

Participants

The students in the study had all been in Canada for a maximum of three years. The centre had identified them as 'at-risk' because of critical barriers to successful participation in the mainstream education system including significant gaps in literacy learning in English, social and communication barriers, and mental health challenges stemming from trauma or grief (programme information sheet, prepared 21 September 2012).

The Digital Storytelling Project

The digital storytelling project took place on Friday mornings over five consecutive weeks. The pedagogic design included the following overlapping stages: gathering artifacts, designing a storyboard, and using digital storytelling software to assemble the story. First, the teachers defined 'digital storytelling' as a short, personal video containing visual and audial layers (Lambert, 2013). A few examples of digital stories were presented (from StoryCenter's YouTube channel: www.youtube.com/channel/UCKLPPDaG0bCj1Yqy6PlcouQ). Afterwards, the students were asked which elements made the stories powerful and effective (e.g., music, colours), and they grouped them on the Smartboard according to mode (e.g., hearing, seeing). The class discussed how each mode had distinct potentials and limitations for communication, and explained how the authors had been intentional in their design choices. The teachers told the class that each student would be creating an accomplishment story (Lambert, 2013), which described a past experience of achieving a goal. The authors explained to the students that their digital stories would be shared at a screening event held at the centre for their classmates, teachers, staff members, and parents. Students were given free time to create or locate images and music and prepare a script in whichever language(s) they felt most comfortable using. Because of the project's limited timeframe, many students chose to use photographs and recorded songs. Most of the students either had few personal photos or felt uncomfortable sharing photos of family and friends. For this reason, the photographs mainly came from various online sources. Finally, the students were presented with a number of options for organising the elements of their digital stories on a storyboard (e.g., paper-based templates or computer software such as PowerPoint). Students assembled their stories using Photo Story 3, a digital storytelling software that was selected because it was free, user-friendly, and compatible with the centre's PC laptops.

Abdullahi's Digital Story of Accomplishment and Aspiration

Site of Production

Abdullahi completed his digital story in class in January 2014. First, he began searching for visuals from his Facebook account and Google images that connected to his life (e.g., photos of Yemen and interests such as Middle Eastern dancing). He saved them to a flash drive. He also began searching for music on YouTube. Abdullahi then selected a paper storyboard. He chose one of his saved images and wrote a description in English. The authors asked Abdullahi which specific accomplishment he had decided to share, and gave him examples from his classmates. He remembered how his uncle had taught him mechanics, a skill he acknowledged that his classmates did not know about him. Following this, Abdullahi began to write a script in English on his storyboard. A discussion followed with him about how he could expand his story with more detail ("What skills did your uncle teach you?" "How did you feel when you were learning these skills?").

Then he completed his storyboard by searching for visuals in Google images. He used keywords such as 'Yemen people', 'Somalian young man', 'Somalian woman', and 'Somalian mechanic'. After this, he continued his search for music on YouTube. He specified that he wanted "relax music" because "if you put loud music, it won't be comfortable with the story". He decided to search for music from Yemen, and selected "the music dancing Arabic … because it connect with my story". He explained the beginning of his story was "sad" and the ending was "happy" (excerpts from interview, 25 February 2014).

Abdullahi was asked about the approach he had taken to gathering ideas for his digital story. He explained,

> I tried to research my family information including my mom in the Facebook and elsewhere but then I figure out the easiest was to do my uncle's mechanic because at that time I was ten years old and he taught me a lot. I did not have a picture that time that I could write about. But I had all the story in my head and I said if I start writing then I will be able to tell.
> *(interview, 25 February 2014, translated from Somali by a welcome centre settlement worker)*

When Abdullahi was asked which modes he used in his story, he recalled "picture" and "writing", which reflect what he had expressed to be his preferred ways of communicating information (excerpts from interview, 25 February 2014).

Site of Image

Abdullahi's digital story begins, "Hello. My name is Abdullahi [last name]. I'm from Yemen". We see a photo of Sanaa, a town in Yemen. He explained in an interview (25 February 2014), "This is where I grow up. You need some picture to show the people … where you come from" (interview, 25 February 2014). The words "Learning about Mechanics/By Abdullahi" are centred at the bottom of the page in distinctive white font. We hear a fast-paced Arabic song.

In the following slide, Abdullahi narrates, "When I was ten years old, my mom and I we went to visit my uncle in Sanaa". The image is a school-aged boy holding a long, narrow wooden board with Arabic script written on it (see Figure 44.1). Abdullahi shared that he did not have a photo of himself as a ten-year-old boy, so he searched Google images and found this picture of a boy who looked approximately that age and was of a similar ethnic background. He also pointed out that he chose this image "because he's writing Hadith" (referring to literature reporting the deeds and sayings of Muhammad) in the Arabic language (interview, 25 February 2014).

The story continues, "I stay with my uncle six month. He was teaching me how to be a mechanic". We see the image of a Somali man wearing a polo shirt, standing in a yellow room. He looks at the camera with a serious expression. This man is not Abdullahi's real uncle (he found this picture by searching 'Somalian young man' in Google images), but he selected this image because of their physical similarities: "my uncle and him they're same, almost same" (interview, 25 February 2014).

Abdullahi continues, "First, it was too difficult for me because I did not have more experience". The black and white image is of a Somali man sitting cross-legged on the ground (see Figure 44.2). He has an expression of concentration as he focusses on the small mechanical tools he is holding in his hands. Abdullahi explained in the interview, "This picture I chose 'cause it's a man confused and he have a hard time fixing cars, and that's why I used this one" (interview, 25 February 2014).

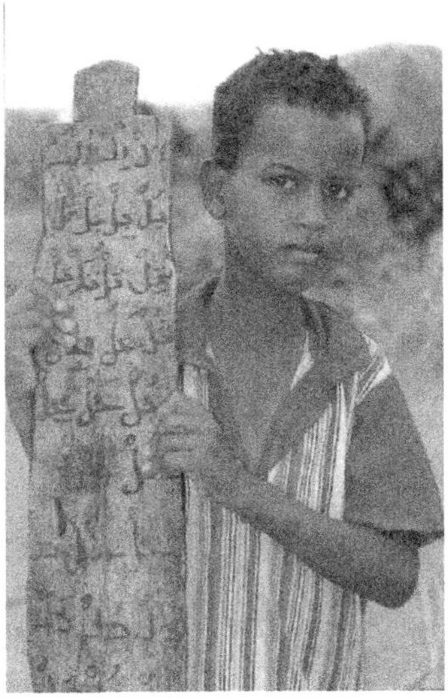

Digure 44.1 Somali refugee camp run by UNHCR. Young boy attending Koranic school holding a piece of wood inscribed with Koranic script. Moslem United Nations High Commissioner for Refugees.
Source: © Crispin Hughes (Hughes, 2006).

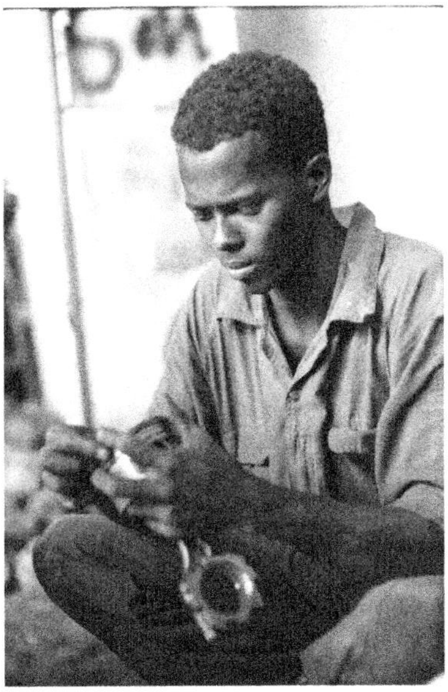

Figure 44.2 Mechanic in Hargeisa, Somaliland.
Source: © Alfred Weidinger (Weidinger, 2011).

Abdullahi then narrates, "He was teaching me how to use oil and wrench". We see the image of a large yellow can with the word 'oil' written on its centre against a white backdrop. This image is followed by that of a silver wrench, also against a simple white backdrop.

In the next slide, Abdullahi shares, "Now I know how to fix my bike and a car". It shows a man kneeling down to fix the gears on the back tyre of his bike. He specified that he wanted a picture of a man fixing a bike to represent that he had learned this skill.

The narrative continues, "My uncle always he told me, Abdullahi, you are a good person". For this slide, Abdullahi repeats the image of the man who resembles his uncle, used on the third slide of his digital story. In the next slide, he narrates, "My auntie always she believe in me to do the right thing". This image shows the faces of two African women smiling at the camera and wearing black headscarves. He found this image through a Google search and selected it because the women's friendliness reminded him of his aunt.

The following slide continues: "my mom she came back from the vacation. After I went with my mom in Sanaa". The picture is an African woman wearing a bright blue head-covering with stars. She is sitting on a chair as part of an audience and smiles as she claps her hands. He thought this woman looked "almost same" as his mom – "like the smile and her face" (excerpts from interview, 25 February 2014).

Abdullahi's voiceover says, "My uncle were not happy about me leaving him alone". Again, there is the image of the man who looks like his uncle ("Because I still talk about him, and me lefting [leaving] him in Sanaa … so we need [his] picture" (interview, 25 February 2014).

The slide that follows is an image of the exterior of the Canadian Parliament Buildings in Ottawa, Ontario. Abdullahi narrates, "The government sent me and my family to Canada". The final picture shows a stone university with a well-groomed lawn (see Figure 44.3). His voiceover expresses, "My goal is to be a mechanic when I finish school". He explained that he selected this image because "it's big college and there's [so] many people, so I say when I finish college, so I wanna be a mechanic you know" (interview, 25 February 2014).

Abdullahi concludes his narrative, "As you can see, this is what I wanna be for my life. Thank you very much for your attention and I appreciate" (video cuts out). (He believes the final words are "for your attention", interview, 25 February 2014.) The slide shows the words "Thank you very much for your attention!!!" in red font against a blue background.

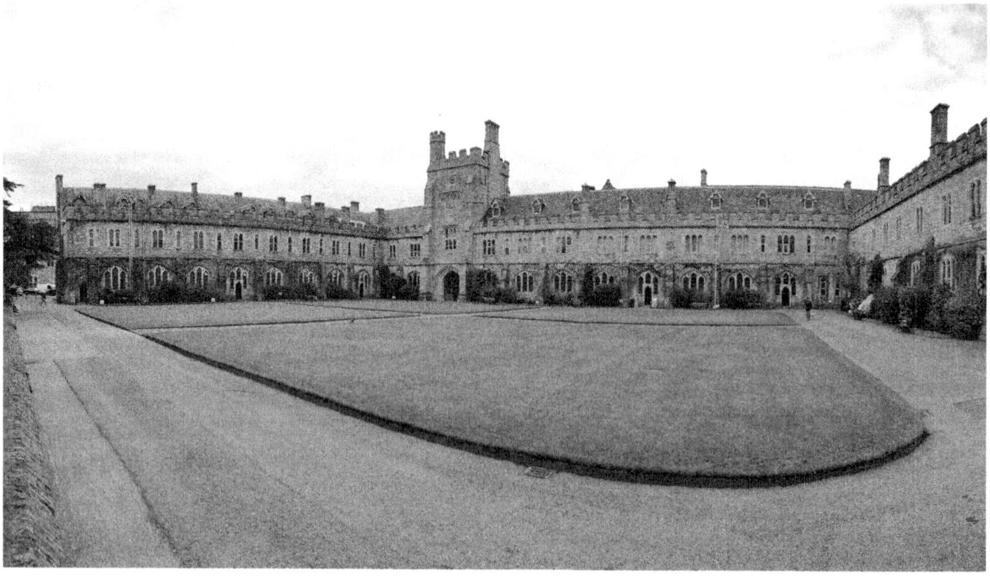

Figure 44.3 The long hall and the clock tower of the UCC quadrangle.
Source: © Bjørn Christian Tørrissen, https://bjornfree.com/CC BY-SA 3.0 (Tørrissen, 2012).

Site of Audience

Abdullahi knew that his digital story would be shown on a Smartboard to a 'safe' audience of his classmates, teachers, parents, and staff members at the welcome centre. His awareness of audience is evident within his story through the narration of his opening and closing slides in which he introduces himself ("Hello. My name is Abdullahi") and thanks his audience for watching his film ("As you can see, this is what I wanna be for my life. Thank you very much for your attention and I appreciate [for your attention]"). It is also revealed through his decision to include a photograph of Sanaa, Yemen "You need some picture to show the people … where you come from" (interview, 25 February 2014).

Pride and Affirmation in Accomplishments

Abdullahi's digital story conveys his pride in learning mechanics. He expresses, "Now I know how to fix my bike and a car", and follows this with several statements revealing the affirmation he felt from his aunt and uncle: "'Abdullahi, you are a good person.'" "My auntie always she believe in me to do the right thing."

Additionally, Abdullahi communicates his future aspirations through stating twice that he plans to be a mechanic in the future. He narrates, "My goal is to be a mechanic when I finish school" and emphasises, "As you can see, this is what I wanna be for my life". His use of visuals gives us insight into his feelings of pride and positive construction of self. He uses the image of a "big college" (Figure 44.3) when he expresses his future aspiration. Arguably, this image is reflective of his imagined sense of achievement upon completing his goal. He also uses the image of a boy 'writing Hadith' to represent himself as a child (Figure 44.1). Abdullahi had not completed formal education prior to attending the welcome centre programme; he explained in the interview, "when I was [in Yemen], I wasn't know how to write and research, but here I learned" (interview, 25 February 2014). He expressed that through participating in the project, "I felt I'm … student learning about everything" (interview, 25 February 2014). This image reveals how he now sees himself in this light.

Upon completion of his digital story, Abdullahi expressed a sense of pride at having created a "movie". As earlier mentioned, he stated how he likes "to look at the movie" and was pleased that "after I could do it [make a movie himself]" (interview, 25 February 2014). He furthermore demonstrated pride in his accomplishment through expressing in the interview "in future I could teach more people" (interview, 25 February 2014). He explained his plans to share his story on Facebook: "and maybe after two years or three my brother if he wanted to do story by his country, so he could see example from his brother" (interview, 25 February 2014).

Abdullahi was also asked about his participation in the screening event at the welcome centre. He said that sharing his digital story "was scary" at first, and he felt "nervous". He thought that it might have been an "embarrassment" to watch the stories on the big screen. However, he added, "after it was excellent. I felt very happy that time". The audience, he expressed, were his "fans"; he described their reactions to his digital story as being "Like a fan, you know, the many people. Like when people watching football and that stuff" (excerpts from interview, 25 February 2014).

Final Thoughts

The lived experiences and knowledge that refugee background learners bring to formal education contexts are rich learning resources that offer possibilities rather than disadvantages. Educators need to design learning experiences that help all students meaningfully communicate their knowledge and identities, and facilitate their "capacities to aspire" (Appadurai, 2004). A multimodal approach to learning enables students to feel capable of self-expression in spite of any gaps in formal education. It also encourages them to think more deeply about themselves and their experiences through engaging with the intellectual and communicative possibilities of different modes. This process can ultimately act as a powerful navigational tool for students, accentuating positive identities for them (i.e., their strengths, knowledge, capacities) and guiding them to capitalise on their own life experiences and ways of knowing and being.

Abdullahi's digital story, as a multimodal pedagogy, is a window on his identity. In the absence of family photos, he searched for Google images to help reconstruct his memory and remembered his uncle teaching him mechanics when he was ten years old. His process of selecting images and music for his story invited him to think visually, musically, as well as linguistically, and through the process, he was able to consider his experiences in different ways. For example, selecting an image that represented the personally challenging experience of learning mechanics involved contemplating how this experience made him feel (i.e., proud). In order to choose music that "connect[ed]", Abdullahi reflected on the trajectory of his story as a whole.

The process of identifying the skills and knowledge he gained through past experiences, and remembering affirmations from loved ones, opened up imagined future possibilities such as attending a "big college" where he envisioned himself as part of a learning community with "[so] many people". His pride in his accomplishment, as evident in the exit interview, revealed other imagined future identities that involve teaching others how to create digital stories. A StoryCenter facilitator, Daniel Weinshenker, comments on personal growth as part of the storytelling experience. He insightfully notes that "oftentimes the stories we tell are the stories we don't understand" because "digital storytelling is about getting underneath of that surface"; it creates "a space where people feel listened to" as individuals (Nurstory: a documentary).

Multimodal pedagogies such as digital storytelling can be powerful tools through which students can become more aware of their strengths and skill sets, recognising them as important resources that can be harnessed to build positive identities in their new social contexts. Digital storytelling also has the potential to make visible to educators the literacy knowledge and individual identities of a population of students that educators so often struggle to understand and engage intellectually, affectively, and agentively.

References

Appadurai, A. (2004). The capacity to aspire: Culture and the terms of recognition. In V. Rao & M. Walton (Eds.), *Culture and public action* (pp. 59–84). Stanford, CA: Stanford University Press.

Campano, G., & Low, D. (2011). Multimodality and immigrant children. *Contemporary Issues in Early Childhood*, 12(4), 381–384. doi:10.2304/ciec.2011.12.4.381.

Cummins, J. (2014). Beyond language: Academic communication and student success. *Linguistics and Education*, 26, 145–154.

Cummins, J., & Early, M. (2011). *Identity texts: The collaborative creation of power in multilingual schools*. Stoke-on-Trent, Staffordshire, UK: Trentham Books.

Dooley, K. T., & Thangaperumal, P. (2011). Pedagogy and participation: Literacy education for low-literate refugee students of African origin in a western school system. *Language and Education*, 25(5), 385–397.

Early, M., Kendrick, M., & Potts, D. (2015). Multimodality: Out from the margins of English language teaching. *TESOL Quarterly*, 49(3), 447–460. doi:10.1002/tesq.246.

Emert, T. (2013). 'The transpoemations project': Digital storytelling, contemporary poetry, and refugee boys. *Intercultural Education*, 24(4), 355–365. doi:10.1080/14675986.2013.809245.

Erstad, O., & Silseth, K. (2008). Agency in digital storytelling: Challenging the educational context. In K. Lundby (Ed.), *Digital storytelling, mediatized stories: Self-representations in new media* (pp. 213–232). New York, NY: Peter Lang.

Garnett, B. (2010). Toward understanding the academic trajectories of ESL youth. *The Canadian Modern Language Review/La revue canadienne des langues vivantes*, 66(5), 677–710.

Gunderson, L. (2004). The language, literacy, achievement, and social consequences of English only programs for immigrant students. In J. Hoffman, D. Schallert, B. Maloch, J. Worth, & C. Fairbanks (Eds.), *The 53rd yearbook of the National Reading Conference* (pp. 1–33). Milwaukee, MI: National Reading Conference.

Gunderson, L. (2007). *English-only instruction and immigrant students in secondary school: A critical examination.* New York, NY: Lawrence Erlbaum.

Hughes, C. (2006). Somali refugee camp run by UNHCR. Young boy attending Koranic school holding piece of wood inscribed with Koranic script. Moslem United Nations High Commissioner for Refugees. [Photograph]. Retrieved from: www.eyeubiquitous.com/stock-photo/20076555/search/detail-0_00014972.html.

Hull, G. A., & Katz, M. (2006). Crafting an agentive self: Case studies of digital storytelling. *Research in the Teaching of English*, *41*(1), 43–81.

Johnson, L., & Kendrick, M. (2017). 'Impossible is nothing': Expressing difficult knowledge through digital storytelling. *Journal of Adolescent and Adult Literacy*, *60*(6), 667–675.

Kendrick, M. (2016). *Literacy and multimodality in global sites.* New York, NY: Routledge.

Kress, G. (1997). *Before writing: Rethinking the paths to literacy.* London, UK: Routledge.

Kress, G., & van Leeuwen, T. (1996). *Reading images: The grammar of visual design.* New York, NY: Routledge.

Lambert, J. (2013). *Digital storytelling: Capturing lives, creating community.* New York, NY: Routledge.

Lenette, C., Cox, L., & Brough, M. (2015). Digital storytelling as a social work tool: Learning from ethnographic research with women from refugee backgrounds. *The British Journal of Social Work*, *45*(3), 988–1005. doi:10.1093/bjsw/bct184.

Nelson, M. A., & Hull, G. A. (2008). Self-presentation through multimedia: A Bakhtinian perspective on digital storytelling. In K. Lundby (Ed.), *Digital storytelling, mediatized stories: Self-representations in new media* (pp. 123–141). New York, NY: Peter Lang.

New London Group. (1996). A pedagogy of multiliteracies: Designing social futures. *Harvard Educational Review*, *66*(1), 60–92. Retrieved from: http://hepg.org/her-home/home.

Nurstory: A documentary. *Small moments, Big stories.* Retrieved from: www.storycenter.org/nurstory.

Rose, G. (2011). *Visual methodologies: An introduction to the interpretation of visual materials* (3rd ed.). London, UK: Sage.

Saleh, A. (2018). Who am I? Refugee adolescents' transformation and negotiation of identities at the cultural borders (Unpublished doctoral dissertation). Clemson University, Clemson, SC.

Shin, D., & Cimasko, T. (2008). Multimodal composition in a college ESL class: New tools, traditional norms. *Computers and Composition*, *25*(4), 376–395. doi:10.1016/j.compcom.2008.07.001.

Toohey, K., & Derwing, T. (2008). ESL students and secondary school achievement in BC. *Alberta Journal of Educational Research*, *54*(2), 178–193.

Tørrissen, B. C. (2012). The long hall and the clock tower of the UCC quadrangle. [Photograph]. Retrieved from: http://commons.wikimedia.org/wiki/File:University-College-Cork-Panorama-2012.JPG.

Vinogradova, P., Linville, H. A., & Bickel, B. (2011). 'Listen to my story and you will know me': Digital stories as student-centered collaborative projects. *TESOL Journal*, *2*(2), 173–202. doi:10.5054/tj.2011.250380.

Weidinger, A. (2011). Mechanic in Hargeisa, Somaliland. [Photograph]. Retrieved from: www.flickr.com/photos/a-weidinger/6452863879.

Yang, Y. F. D. (2012). Multimodal composing in digital storytelling. *Computers and Composition*, *29*(3), 221–238. doi:10.1016/j.compcom.2012.07.001.

45
CHILDREN, DEATH, AND DIGITAL MEDIA

Kathleen M. Cumiskey

Introduction

The integration of digital media into everyday life challenges traditions and beliefs surrounding death and afterlife (Graham, Gibbs, & Aceti, 2013). Funereal rituals become remediated through digital media use. Intimate virtual spaces generate a kind of public grieving, including for child audiences (Cumiskey & Hjorth, 2017). Online communities have become important to individuals and families in the care of the dead and the dying (DeGroot, 2012; Gibbs, Meese, Arnold, Nansen, & Carter, 2015). This chapter focusses on digital media in child and adolescent experiences related to death. It uses two case studies to demonstrate the complexities related to the use of digital media in the amelioration of traumatic experiences and the processing of loss. Digital media will be understood in this chapter as a means through which children facilitate the continuation of bonds with lost loved ones. Understanding children's use of digital media in times of grief illuminates how relationships are maintained and losses validated through the storing, saving, and sharing of affective digital content.

Digital media are used to both engage with emotional content and to distract users from overwhelming emotion (Cumiskey & Hjorth, 2017). Most children in wealthier countries access digital media of their own volition (Haddon, 2013; Livingstone et al., 2017). They control when they want to approach their feelings of grief, and when they want to avoid them. Virtual connections generate a sense of presence of others which can relieve the user of feelings of isolation (Hampton, Sessions, & Her, 2011; Katz & Aakus, 2002). Users of digital technology often move through all life experiences with their digital devices as companions and witnesses (Papailias, 2016). People's most private and intimate moments are shared with the public through social and mobile media (often without their consent) (Hjorth & Lim, 2012). As a consequence, mobile devices and digital media change how users think about death and cope with traumatic experiences (Brubaker, Kivran-Swaine, Taber, & Hayes, 2012).

Communicating death to children can become complicated by technology (Wandel, 2019). Indirect means of communicating information makes it more difficult for the child to comprehend what has happened. Children are often present in crisis situations. They overhear communication between adults. They receive bits and pieces of the facts of the circumstances. Adults often fail to communicate directly with children and, in the context of traumatic loss, this lack of direct communication can have long-term consequences (Ellis, Dowrick, & Lloyd-Williams, 2013). The indirectness of digital communication adds to children's misunderstandings by blurring details related to death. For example, children may become confused by posts that say 'Rest in Peace', mistaking death with sleep. Such references can reinforce that erroneous belief (National Institute of Mental Health, 1979) if the real situation is not clarified by the adults in children's lives. On the other hand, digital media complicate matters with their directness when children are exposed to traumatising details surrounding a death without being provided with a context of support. How a child engages (or not) with digital media in the immediate aftermath of loss differs from how they might use it later in the grieving process (Cupit & Kuchta, 2017).

As digital media users begin to transition from childhood to adolescence, they become contributors to growing *digital affective cultures*: the digital spaces within which users conceive, mediate, represent, and co-construct their social, emotional, and spiritual lives (Döveling, Harju, & Sommer, 2018; Hjorth & Arnold, 2013; Hjorth & Cumiskey, 2018). The porous nature of digital affective cultures means that the co-presence, non-presence, and virtual presence of others online, and the intimacy with which children connect to personal digital devices, allows death to become elusive and perplexing. Developmentally, children begin to comprehend the finality of death between the ages of five to nine, although they believe that it only happens to other people. After age ten, the finality and causes of death are understood as inevitable (Osterweis, Solomon, & Green, 1984). How children use digital media during their time of grief reflects their individual psychological and social development.

Children's needs are often overlooked or avoided when a loss occurs (Blin & Jonas-Simpson, 2018), and adults tend not to recognise the need for children to grieve. Interestingly, on the YouTube Kids app, which supports parental control over YouTube content accessible to children, if a kid searches 'my dad died' no results are shown. This app allows for searches of the term 'grief', although results are not curated extensively for kid-related content. Many bereaved children are mourning the loss of a grandparent or parent (Silverman & Nickman, 1996). Some also experience grief related to sibling loss and the loss of peers (as well as mentors and adored celebrities). Ensuring that children and adolescents have safe venues for expressing grief is important for their healing (Buxton & Vest, 2018), as coping with the grief of adults often dominates children's loss experiences and results in the child feeling isolated, neglected, and ignored in their own grief (Blin & Jonas-Simpson, 2018).

Digital Evidence of How Children Cope with Death

Adults dominate defining how (and even whether) children grieve (Arnold, 2018). As a consequence, adults have created dedicated online spaces for children to express their grief. For example, in the United States, the National Alliance for Grieving Children (n.d.) states that they are a "nationwide network comprised of professionals, institutions and volunteers who promote best practices, educational programming and critical resources to facilitate the mental, emotional and physical health of grieving children and their families". None of their board members are children. Child Bereavement UK (n.d.) has the goal "for all families to have the support they need to rebuild their lives, when a child grieves or when a child dies". Even though their website was created and run by adults, their royal patron is HRH The Duke of Cambridge, who experienced the loss of a parent as a child. Their website features the voices of children, but the site and the resources do not seem to be curated by bereaved children. This renders sites like these unwelcoming and difficult for children to access. YouTube provides ample evidence that children respond to digital material created and communicated by peers (Berg, 2019).

Meeting bereaved children in the spaces and places they occupy within digital media motivated game developers in the United Kingdom to create a game called Apart of Me. This game helps young people who have experienced loss to increase their emotional literacy and wisdom around death ("The mobile game created to help grieving children", 2018). The game begins with the player encountering a 'Guide', a figure who has not only experienced loss, but also learned about managing loss with the help of wise others. The Guide assists children in mastering knowledge about grief and using that wisdom to become a guide themselves. The game encourages players to access external UK-based resources and other players' recorded stories of loss. Characters within the game challenge the player to complete quests in the real world, including building emotional supports and strengthening relationships. This hybridisation of experience, utilising digital media's capacity to support a narrative, interactive approach to processing loss, offers significant potential for supporting bereaved children.

Children's engagement with digital media is integral to how they process life experiences. Like adults, children use the digital platform they are most comfortable with to access people with whom they want to share their grief experiences (Sofka, Cupit, & Gilbert, 2012). Döveling (2017) argues that children are not sharing their experiences online to be judgemental or to make themselves seem exceptional despite their exceptional circumstances. Instead, children engage in emotional expression on social media platforms to generate a sense of intimacy between themselves and their online community and to strengthen the bonds they have with their followers, whether they know them in real life or not (Cumiskey & Hjorth, 2017). Children often express gratitude for those that have offered them support online and address their audiences as though they know each individual. Their willingness to share intimate moments of grief online happens in the context of the poster not knowing who is accessing their digital content. Contact happens when a viewer makes themselves known by either responding with a posted comment or by sending the user a direct message. Grief-related posts are viewed by those known to the poster, with secondary impacts on those with whom they have close ties. Video-sharing platforms like YouTube are used in this way. A simple search of 'My dad died' or 'My mom died' yields examples of expressions of childhood grief. As the following case study demonstrates, these videos are made by users that have followers for non-grief-related content (i.e., playing video games, singing, comedy, general vlogging).

Case Study 1: James Playz (Age 9)
James Playz, a YouTuber with 126,000 subscribers, has posted over 130 videos. The majority of those videos are scenes from his Fortnite gameplay with his recorded voiceover as an accompaniment. On 20 December 2016, James posted a video entitled "About My Dad" (James Playz, 2016). This video has been viewed more than 150,000 times since being posted and was a complete departure from his usual videos in both style and content. James was alone in the video with a close-up head shot of him in front of a plain white wall. He starts the video, which is 2 minutes and 33 seconds long, by saying:

> Hey guys, welcome to a new video, it is James Playz here with a video and I'm here to say, that I have not really told you about my mom or dad so about my dad, this is about my dad this video.
>
> *(James Playz, 2016, 0:01)*

James' introduction of "Hey guys ... it is James Playz here" characterises him as a YouTuber since he uses a video opening style that has come to be understood as the 'YouTube voice'. It indicates his intention of being known on the platform, that he has subscribers to his channel, and that he broadcasts to his audience (Hagi, 2017). James continues:

> Um, if it looks like I have cried it is because I have and I will tell you why I have been crying, it's because my dad, he has brain cancer and he's been through a lot of surgeries

and stuff in his life so he had an MRI today and we thought it was going to be good but it didn't turn out so good so I will try to keep you guys posted on what's going on with my life and my family but just if I don't just upload I just probably won't feel like uploading any videos because of what's going on ... so hopefully you've enjoyed ...

(James Playz, 2016, 0:16)

James' motivation for making this video was to bring his audience and his community into his life, for them to better understand his circumstances and why his participation on YouTube and in the gaming community may be limited in the near future. He apologises to his viewers but also requests understanding. At 1 minute and 17 seconds into the video, it appears James was about to end his video with "hopefully you've enjoyed", which again indicates his knowledge of how the most popular YouTubers' videos begin and end. The sad and unusual circumstance of his dad's terminal illness did not shift him away from meeting viewers' expectations around typical video opening and closing sequences. This mismatch of format versus the emotional content of his video could indicate James Playz' own conflict around the role YouTube plays in his life. He appears to be struggling with his desire to maintain his channel and subscribers alongside the demands of his family life. He also wants to use the YouTube platform as a source of support during this difficult time. This is indicated by James' decision at the 1 minute and 17 second mark to not end the video but to continue to talk about facing his father's terminal illness. James continues from this point for another minute to discuss details related to his father's cancer treatment.

Just over five weeks later, on 28 January 2017, James published his next video, titled "MY DAD DIED!!!! TODAY FOR REAL!!!" (James Playz, 2017). This video is 7 minutes and 42 seconds long and has been viewed close to 7.5 million times. The setting for this video is similar to the previous one. James is the only person in the video, shot as a close-up head shot with a white wall in the background. James appears to be visibly shaken based on his facial expression and hand gestures:

Hey guys, James is back with a video [hides face with left hand]. I haven't made a video in such a long time, and I have a really, really bad reason [face starts to flush, eyes teary] ... So this morning, I got up at 1:30 and my mom had to wake me up and we had to go somewhere. So this morning ... it is like 8:51 at night now! ... I went to bed for only two hours [puts two fingers up], right ... I woke up at 1:30 [covers face with left hand] and we got a call from my uncle, well a text, and [covers face] so you know how my dad has brain cancer? Well [covers mouth with hand and puts head down, pauses for five seconds then lifts head] ... the nurses knew by his breathing that he was going to pass. Ok? [rests left hand on his temple].

(James Playz, 2017, 0:01)

It is evident in this video that James has adults around him that are honest with him and choose to share the details surrounding his father's death. James explains how unexpected news disrupted his usual routine and his sleep pattern, causing him to feel disoriented. By emphasising the details of this disruption for him and his family, and his loss of continuity, he indicates the enormity of this loss and a source of his grief (Ellis et al., 2013):

So I went at 1:30 at night. My mom picked my mom and I up at 1:30. I stayed until 7 AM [emphasises the time] and I left at 7 AM, I didn't get any sleep, only those two hours and I got only three hours once I got back until like 11 ... [speaking emphatically] and then I didn't go to sleep since. So this is really bad, like but then ... [face flushes and eyes tear up, pauses, covers face with left hand] ... um ... [covers mouth with left hand, pauses for 13 seconds] so around 12:35, that was the exact time, everyone, like everyone in my family, close friends to him, were circling around him, and they were like just talking and he was in his bed and then like he was taking like 50 secs [stares into camera intensely] like that was the highest like minute breath like he would only breathe like in one minute he would only breathe like twice in one minute. And so, everyone was around him at 12:35 and then it just happened like his last breath [4 second pause, he looks to the right away from the camera and then stares back into the camera] ... he ... he ... he passed. [pause] Today! ... [holds head in his hands] I don't know ... [shakes head as he looks into camera for six seconds]. It all happened so fast, it's like three hours [holds three fingers up to the camera. then four fingers] no, four hours after I got home, it happened and it was all over like. So it's Saturday now ... my whole family got no sleep at all ... and I only got five hours [of sleep] and to me I keep on thinking that it's a different day than Saturday but it's Saturday ... I don't know if I am going to school on Monday and Tuesday, my mom said I don't know if I wanted to or not [then hides face in hands] I just don't know. [holds head, appears distressed, shaking head for seven seconds] ... I don't know].

(James Playz, 2017, 1:24)

James' video, made on the very day his dad died, demonstrates how James is already actively engaged in processing the loss. He narrates how the experience of the loss is difficult to comprehend and disorienting. He also bravely faces this loss (and the camera), accepting its reality and expressing emotional distress (Mannarino & Cohen, 2011). James continues at the 5 minute and 46 second mark:

But we all knew that it was coming, we knew it and it happened [said emphatically] that day so ... [pauses and starts to tear up for nine seconds and hangs head]. This is really so crazy, I am only nine years old and this is happening to me ... almost 10? He was 46! His birthday was January 8th and it's like January 28th – 20 days ago [said incredulously] that is freaky! ... and if I look disgusting with this sweatshirt on, I know that I probably do, I don't really care how I look anymore because I don't, I don't care [gets emotional] I can't believe this is happening to me [pauses for ten seconds]. Well that's pretty much it. I don't know what else I am going to say so ... [covers face with hands, pauses for 12 seconds, visibly sad]. Ok, I am going to end the video then, so ... hopefully you enjoyed the video guys, and see you in the next one – buh bye.

(James Playz, 2017, 5:46)

James' use of YouTube during the acute phase of his grief is not to ask his subscribers for help or advice. Indeed, James disabled the comment facility for all the posts relating to his dad. Instead, James turns to his subscribers at this time to provide information about a major event in his life; to intensify the connection he has with the community he has created. This intensification of his identity as part of the YouTube community is ritualistic, but also affirming. By posting a video, he is reinforcing his identity as a YouTuber and staying connected to his sense of self as "James Playz" despite the dissociative aspects of losing his father (Wheeler-Roy & Amyot, 2004).

The 7.5 million views of James' post on the day of his dad's death, in the context of a 123,000 subscriber base and the 130,000 views of the video about his father's terminal diagnosis, indicates the need and demand for authentic materials that engage with children's experiences of loss and bereavement.

Case Study 2: Farah (16 Years Old at Time of Loss)

Adolescents use social media for socialising and leisure. These platforms also play a critical role in identity development, relationship enhancement, ego validation, and emotional regulation (Throuvala, Griffiths, Rennoldson, & Kuss, 2019). Adolescent development includes challenges around emotional regulation and confusion around behavioural limitations and consequences, with adolescents particularly vulnerable to the emotional impact of loss (Dahl, 2004). Adolescent deaths are highlighted via digital media platforms. These deaths are often sudden or violent (Malone, 2007). The sensational aspects of a tragic death are provocative and at times alluring, and especially when promoted via viral news stories and blog posts (Green, 2019).

Teens use the private spaces on mobile devices to store content never shared with others (Cumiskey & Hjorth, 2017). In the following case study, mobile content is shown to be emotionally charged and capable of impacting the psychological well-being of the young person. This case study emerged from data collected and included in the book *Haunting Hands: Mobile Media Practices and Loss* (Cumiskey & Hjorth, 2017).

When Farah (pseudonym used) was 16 years old, her best friend was killed in an automobile accident. Farah believed she was responsible for her friend's death because the authorities believed the accident occurred when her friend was reading a text message that Farah sent her. After the accident, Farah ceased texting anyone, other than her deceased friend. Farah's use of her mobile phone shifted from typical use to a vehicle for her to communicate with her friend from beyond the grave. Farah described how she suspended her disbelief in order to make communicating with her friend real:

> [She] is the [only] person that I felt OK to text, even after her death. Other than that, because in that year and a half [after her death], I used to talk to her like she was around. Like she is not gone yet, so I would text her, "Hi, how are you, what are we doing today?" Stuff like that. [I would text her] in the morning, in the afternoon, sometimes between the morning and the afternoon. [It started] after the forty days [significant in Arab Orthodox funereal tradition]. So only her [the deceased], I would text, and not as often as we used to, *we* would text, uh, *I* would text, but not as often [as when she was alive]. (*Interviewer: did you anticipate her responding?*) Yeah, all the time. I remember I texted her one time [after she died] about the joke we had, I used to call her [wild] and she would say [when she was alive], "Of course, I am [wild], that is what you love". One time I texted her that [after she died], "[Wild]?" And *she's* like, well *I* anticipated her, "Yeah of course I'm [wild], that is what you love". So I texted back, I said, "Of course that's what I love, how could I not love you!" Stuff like that … I was having a conversation in my head and the texts were in the phone … I mean for most of the times, back then I could have sworn she was answering back. But now, I don't know, was she answering? Was she not answering?
>
> (Cumiskey & Hjorth, 2017, pp. 168–9)

The personal and private nature of her mobile phone allowed Farah to construct an intimate space only shared between herself and her dead friend. The open, continuous, never-ceasing nature of most text messaging applications provides a perfect vehicle for cultivating a sense of presence with a loved one beyond death. The continuation of bonds with the deceased is a critical component in the integration of loss into the life of the bereaved (Klass, Silverman, & Nickman, 1996). Farah's life was shattered by her loss. She reported withdrawing from life, deepening her guilt related to the accident and mistrusting both her peers and her parents. Out of loyalty to her deceased friend, no one could ever match their bond. The mobile phone became a safe private space through which Farah could strengthen her connection to the deceased and keep it secret from the rest of the world. Farah continued:

> At that time [of her death], I wasn't on Facebook all that much. My phone was really only for texting *her*. I feel like this stuff is mine. There, and not sharable with everyone. I feel like, maybe everyone forgot about her but I didn't. I can't.
> *(Cumiskey & Hjorth, 2017, p. 170)*

Grief work for children and adolescents comes in the form of meaning-making, reconnecting with others, building support networks and developing resources, rituals, and collective activities (Papadatou, Bellali, Tselepi, & Giannopoulou, 2018). Engagement with digital media, whether it be via popular social media platforms or private mobile phone, enhances these processes.

Conclusion

For children born today, digital media, as a companion from before birth, becomes an integral part of their existence. As a consequence, digital media shapes their encounters with death, loss, grief, and coping while expanding their notions of existence, continuity, self-reflection, and connection. Maintaining a presence on social media is an investment in symbolic immortality: a protection against being forgotten. The on-going narration and companionship of social networks emphasises the importance of connection while also reducing the users' ability to tolerate isolation and disconnection (Hoge, Bickham, & Cantor, 2017).

The power of digital media can be harnessed to improve mental health outcomes for children and adolescents. The impetus for memorialising the deceased is now built into some social media platforms like Facebook. These platforms serve as a fertile medium for the continuation of bonds and to guarantee that every person will have an eternal presence beyond death (DeGroot, 2012; Wandel, 2019). Experts predict dead users will surpass living users on Facebook by 2098 (Hiscock, 2019). As users come face to face with death on a daily basis through digital media, the focus shifts to how to control the distribution of disturbing content and questioning the motivations for such posts. Children now bear witness to tragic events and the pain of others and, due to the nature of the media, they can revisit these events over and over again (Papailias, 2016). These events go on to have personal significance for the young person and can become a part of how they come to understand the meaning of life (and death) (Hjorth & Cumiskey, 2018).

References

Arnold, C. (2018). Developmental considerations for grieving youth. In C. Arnold (Ed.), *Understanding child and adolescent grief: Supporting loss and facilitating growth* (pp. 7–18). New York, NY: Routledge.

Berg, M. (2019). The highest-paid YouTube stars of 2019: The kids are killing it. *Forbes*. Retrieved December 18, 2019 from: www.forbes.com/sites/maddieberg/2019/12/18/the-highest-paid-youtube-stars-of-2019-the-kids-are-killing-it/#4dd5b5b338cd.

Blin, C., & Jonas-Simpson, C. (2018). Disenfranchised grief among bereaved youth. In C. Arnold (Ed.), *Understanding child and adolescent grief: Supporting loss and facilitating growth* (pp. 34–46). New York, NY: Routledge.

Brubaker, J. R., Kivran-Swaine, F., Taber, L., & Hayes, G. R. (2012). *Grief-stricken in a crowd: The language of bereavement and distress in social media*. Paper presented at ICWSM-12, Dublin, Ireland. 4 June, 2012.

Buxton, D., & Vest, T. R. (2018). Social media consequences of pediatric death. *Child and Adolescent Psychiatric Clinics of North America*, 27(4), 599–605. doi:10.1016/j.chc.2018.05.008.

Child Bereavement UK. (n.d.). *Home page*. Retrieved from: www.childbereavementuk.org.

Cumiskey, K. M., & Hjorth, L. (2017). *Haunting hands: Mobile media practices and loss*. New York, NY: Oxford University Press.

Cupit, I. N., & Kuchta, O. (2017). Death version 2016: How children adolescents are learning and grieving in cyberspace. In R. G. Stevenson & G. R. Cox (Eds.), *Children, adolescents and death: Questions and answers* (pp. 25–36). New York, NY: Routledge.

Dahl, R. E. (2004). Adolescent brain development: A period of vulnerabilities and opportunities. Keynote address. *Annals of the New York Academy of Sciences*, *1021*(1), 1–22. doi:10.1196/annals.1308.001.

DeGroot, J. M. (2012). Maintaining relational continuity with the deceased on Facebook. *Omega: Journal of Death & Dying*, *65*(3), 195–212.

Döveling, K. (2017). Online emotion regulation in digitally mediated bereavement. Why age and kind of loss matter in grieving online. *Journal of Broadcasting & Electronic Media*, *61*(1), 41–57.

Döveling, K., Harju, A. A., & Sommer, D. (2018). From mediatized emotion to digital affect cultures: New technologies and global flows of emotion. *Social Media + Society*, *4*(1). doi:10.1177/2056305117743141.

Ellis, J., Dowrick, C., & Lloyd-Williams, M. (2013). The long-term impact of early parental death: Lessons from a narrative study. *Journal of the Royal Society of Medicine*, *106*(2), 57–67. doi:10.1177/0141076812472623.

Gibbs, M., Meese, J., Arnold, M., Nansen, B., & Carter, M. (2015). #Funeral and Instagram: Death, social media, and platform vernacular. *Information, Communication & Society*, *18*(3), 255–268.

Graham, C., Gibbs, M., & Aceti, L. (2013). Introduction to the special issue on the death, afterlife, and immortality of bodies and data. *The Information Society*, *29*(3), 133–141.

Green, L. (2019). "Judge me, or be there for me": How can narratives be used to encourage action and intervention by parents, schools, the police, policymakers, and other children? In H. Vanderbosch & L. Green (Eds.), *Narratives in research and interventions on cyberbullying among young people* (pp. 213–228). Dordrecht, The Netherlands: Springer Netherlands.

Haddon, L. (2013). Mobile media and children. *Mobile Media & Communication*, *1*(1), 89–95.

Hagi, S. (2017, March 27). The rise of 'YouTube Voice' and why vloggers want it to stop—VICE. *Vice*. Retrieved from: www.vice.com/en_ca/article/aepn94/the-rise-of-youtube-voice-and-why-vloggers-want-it-to-stop.

Hampton, K. N., Sessions, L. F., & Her, E. J. (2011). Core networks, social isolation and new media: How Internet and mobile phone use is related to network size and diversity. *Information, Communication & Society*, *14*(1), 130–155.

Hiscock, M. (2019, June 26). Dead Facebook users will soon outnumber the living. *Loop*. Retrieved from: www.theloop.ca/dead-facebook-users-will-soon-outnumber-the-living.

Hjorth, L., & Arnold, M. (2013). *Online@AsiaPacific: Mobile, social and locative media in the Asia-Pacific*. Abingdon, Oxon: Routledge.

Hjorth, L., & Cumiskey, K. (2018). Affective mobile spectres: Understanding the lives of mobile media images of the dead. In Z. Papacharissi (Ed.), *A networked self and platforms, stories, connections* (pp. 111–124). New York, NY: Routledge and Taylor & Francis Group.

Hjorth, L., & Lim, S. S. (2012). Mobile intimacy in the age of affective mobile media. *Feminist Media Studies*, *12*(4), 477–484.

Hoge, E., Bickham, D., & Cantor, J. (2017). Digital media, anxiety, and depression in children. *Pediatrics*, *140*(Supplement 2), S76–S80. doi:10.1542/peds.2016-1758G.

James Playz. (2016, December 20). About my dad [Video File]. Retrieved from: www.youtube.com/watch?v=k9eh3gWWBP4.

James Playz (2017, January 28). MY DAD DIED!!!! TODAY FOR REAL!!! [Video File]. Retrieved from: www.youtube.com/watch?v=DuH3C1s87ag.

Katz, J. E., & Aakus, M. (Eds.). (2002). *Perpetual contact: Mobile communication, private talk, public performance*. Cambridge, MA: Cambridge University Press.

Klass, D., Silverman, P. R., & Nickman, S. L. (Eds.). (1996). *Continuing bonds: New understandings of grief*. New York, NY: Taylor & Francis.

Livingstone, S., Lemish, D., Lim, S. S., Bulger, M., Cabello, P., Claro, M., … Wei, B. (2017). Global perspectives on children's digital opportunities: An emerging research and policy agenda. *Pediatrics*, *140*(Supplement 2), S137–S141. doi:10.1542/peds.2016-1758S.

Malone, P. A. (2007). The impact of peer death on adolescent girls: A task-oriented group intervention. *Journal of Social Work in End-of-Life & Palliative Care*, *3*(3), 23–27.

Mannarino, A. P., & Cohen, J. A. (2011). Traumatic loss in children and adolescents. *Journal of Child & Adolescent Trauma*, *4*(1), 22–33. doi:10.1080/19361521.2011.545048.

National Alliance for Grieving Children. (n.d.). *About the NAGC*. Retrieved from: https://childrengrieve.org/about-us/about-the-nagc.

National Institute of Mental Health. (1979). *Caring about kids: Talking to children about death*. Bethesda, MD: National Institute of Mental Health.

Osterweis, M., Solomon, F., & Green, M. (1984). Bereavement during childhood and adolescence. In M. Osterwei, F. Solomon., & M. Green, (Eds.), *Bereavement: Reactions, consequences, and care* (pp. 97–141). Washington, DC: National Academy Press.

Papadatou, D., Bellali, T., Tselepi, K., & Giannopoulou, I. (2018). Adolescents' trajectory through peer loss after a road traffic accident. *Death Studies*, *42*(6), 383–391.

Papailias, P. (2016). Witnessing in the age of the database: Viral memorials, affective publics, and the assemblage of mourning. *Memory Studies*, *9*(4), 437–454. doi:10.1177/1750698015622058.

Silverman, P. R., & Nickman, S. L. (1996). Children's construction of their dead parents. In D. Klass, P. R. Silverman, & S. L. Nickman (Eds.), *Continuing bonds: New understanding of grief* (pp. 73–86). Philadelphia, PA: Taylor & Francis.

Sofka, C. J., Cupit, I. N., & Gilbert, K. R. (Eds.). (2012). *Dying, death and grief in an online universe: For counselors and educators*. New York, NY: Springer New York.

The mobile game created to help grieving children. (2018, November). *ITV News*. Retrieved from: www.itv.com/news/london/2018-11-16/the-mobile-game-created-to-help-grieving-children.

Throuvala, M. A., Griffiths, M. D., Rennoldson, M., & Kuss, D. J. (2019). Motivational processes and dysfunctional mechanisms of social media use among adolescents: A qualitative focus group study. *Computers in Human Behavior*, *93*, 164–175. doi:10.1016/j.chb.2018.12.012.

Wandel, T. L. (2019). Losing a friend: Social media's impact on child and adolescent grief. In G. San (Ed.), *Handbook of research on children's consumption of digital media* (pp. 24–40). Hershey, PA: IGI Global.

Wheeler-Roy, S., & Amyot, B. A. (2004). *Grief counseling resource guide: A field manual*. Albany, NY: New York State Office of Mental Health.

PART VI

Local Complexities in a Global Context

46

VERY YOUNG CHILDREN'S DIGITAL LITERACY

Engagement, Practices, Learning, and Home–School–Community Knowledge Exchange in Lisbon, Portugal

Vítor Tomé and Maria José Brites

Children, Media, and Social Participation

Despite the continued existence of digital divides, most children live nowadays within rich digital environments, even those from underprivileged families (Chaudron, 2016), enabling them to engage with the internet and digital technologies from an increasingly early age, often starting when they are infants (Kotilainen & Suoninen, 2013) and rapidly increasing their use and practices over the following years (Danby, Fleer, Davidson, & Hatzigianni, 2018; Hooft Graafland, 2018; Marsh, 2014; Palaiologou, 2016; Sefton-Green, Marsh, Erstad, & Flewitt, 2016). Children gradually become more independent in their use, consumption, production, and sharing of media content within digital environments, having a greater opportunity to participate as they grow older (Marsh, 2014). These activities do not mean, however, that children are increasing their social participation. As Livingstone, Kardefelt Winther, Kanchev, Cabello, Claro, Burton, and Phyfer (2019, p. 6) purport, even if children "are already enjoying some online opportunities in sizeable proportions", they do not climb the "ladder of participation" in that "most children do not reach the point where they commonly undertake many of the civic, informational and creative activities online that are heralded as the opportunities of the digital age".

This chapter will demonstrate that a community-based action research project aimed to develop very young children's digital literacy competencies was successful when developed through a model proposed by Sefton-Green et al. (2016), enriched with in-service teacher training, and by employing a deep characterisation of the community in order to model and adapt the project to specific contexts.

Very young children's online practices have been largely ignored by policy-makers in many countries (Holloway, Green, & Livingstone, 2013). Only 12% of approximately 1,200 research projects identified included children under the age of seven, while only 20% included the perspectives of teachers and 13% of parents (O'Neill & Staksrud, 2014). The scenario has considerably changed in recent years, namely through relevant projects such as EU Kids Online and Global Kids Online. However, data on young children's digital use and practices

> does not tell us what such engagement means in terms of the child's learning especially their developing literacy ... their understanding of the world, their understanding of social relationships and indeed what implications such use might have for their education as a whole.
>
> (Sefton-Green et al., 2016, p. 9)

Thus, it is a key task for educators and researchers "to understand how young learners make sense of multimodal texts in digital environments, and how they impose order on the juxtaposition of different modes" (*idem*, p. 20). Young children "learn watching others, especially parents and other family members" (Chaudron, 2015, p. 14). There is a need to articulate formal and non-formal learning contexts, i.e., to embed core skills in the school curriculum, such as flexibility, innovation, creativity, and problem solving, as well as helping children's families evolve from family literacy to family digital literacy (Marsh, Hannon, Lewis & Ritchie, 2015). Digital literacy is "a social practice that involves reading, writing and multimodal meaning-making through the use of a range of digital technologies" as well as traditional technologies that "can involve accessing, using and analysing texts [in a broader sense: text, sound, moving and still image], in addition to their production and dissemination", which implies "the acquisition of skills, including traditional skills related to alphabetic print, but also skills related to accessing and using digital technologies" (Sefton-Green et al., 2016, p. 15), such as "create, work, share, socialise, investigate, play, work, communicate and learn" (Meyers, Erickson, & Small, 2013, p. 356).

Regarding digital literacy and children, the leading themes are "parental mediation of children's digital literacy practices in homes, children's media engagement and literacy learning in homes, and home–school knowledge exchange of children's digital literacy practices" (Kumpulainen & Gillen, 2017, p. 3). This chapter focusses on the third theme, i.e., on the interconnected and interrelated connections between home and school, taking into consideration the non-formal places of action, such as where children act daily and where the home is established. This context can blur the boundaries of the different geographies (*idem*, 2017).

Recognising the need to develop children's digital literacy through the implementation of multidimensional projects that aim to create 'digital citizens' who can fully exert their "digital participation in society" (Ribble, 2011), the community project 'Digital Citizenship Education for Democratic Participation' (2016–2018) was developed in Portugal between 2015 and 2018. The project aimed to foster the social participation of children (aged 3–8 years) through their media use, and to involve teachers, parents, and the local community of Caneças, a district in Portugal's capital of Lisbon.

A Project Adapted to the Specific Context

Caneças is a small community of 12,000 inhabitants, situated within the county of Odivelas in the northern part of Lisbon. The neighbourhood has the second highest population density in the country, with around half (51%) having only completed basic education (to grade nine) and a quarter having only completed the first cycle of schooling (four years). The school-age population of Caneças is 11% (although the total youth population is 15%), and 16% of the total population are immigrants.

The research project aimed to answer the following question: to what extent can a local (and replicable) project, teachers, and out-of-school contexts including families, empower pre-school and primary-school-aged children to become active and effective citizens in the digital era? The main hypothesis was that a concerted approach within the family, school, and out-of-school contexts can empower pre-school and primary-school children to exercise an active and effective citizenship in the digital era. The project was organised in five stages: i) production and validation of data collection instruments (March–December 2015); ii) in-service teacher training course (January–February 2016); iii) characterising the context through data collection from parents, children, and the community (April–June 2016); iv) sharing results with participants and setting up a digital literacy intervention plan (September 2016); v) longitudinal study with teachers who volunteered after the training course (September 2016–February 2018).

The methodological approach of this exploratory project was founded on action research. The study has undergone frequent improvements as the authors followed a research model proposed by Sefton-Green et al. (2016), which was inspired by authors such as Carrington (2013), Colvert (2015), and Green (1988). According to the model, there are three interrelated areas that form the basis of how the individual produces and receives media messages, whether in formal settings or in an informal context:

1 Operational – capacities and skills needed to read, write, and interpret messages from different media and its various platforms;
2 Critical – interaction with texts and digital products, seeking to answer questions related to power and agency, representation and voice, authenticity and veracity;
3 Cultural – concerns interpretations and actions that develop according to its involvement in digital literacy practices in specific social and cultural contexts.

When a citizen wants, for example, to communicate a message, he/she draws on these three areas and makes decisions within the context of the following four levels: design (if the message is multimodal or not); production (creation of the text); distribution (which are the channels); and implementation (imagine how the receivers will interpret the message, depending on the background). All these processes take place within the frameworks that influence the digital literacy practices of children, including: micro (with the child), meso (formal and informal learning contexts, family, friends, and the local community), and macro (the nation state). Following a model keeps balance and consistency, but the use of technology is much more eclectic, as it is multidimensional and changing rapidly (Carrington, 2013, quoted by Sefton-Green et al., 2016). Without disregarding balance and consistency, the research design was tailored to the local context, i.e., the project was very dynamic and subject to frequent rebalancing and reconfigurations in order to overcome tensions, incompatibilities, and to maintain the participants' active involvement.

The context was based on four data collection processes:

1 A questionnaire sent to the 25 teachers that attended the training (10 pre-school and 15 primary-school teachers), which focussed on digital media uses and practices, the perception of the pupils' media use, and their perceptions on learning potential, risks, and opportunities;
2 A questionnaire sent to 38 parents (some questions were adapted from Mathen, Fastrez, & De Smedt, 2015), which focussed on digital media uses and practices, perception of children's media use, perceptions on risks and opportunities, on learning, as well as on parental mediation;
3 An interview script (adapted from Chaudron, 2015) answered by 38 children (22 aged 4–6 years and 16 aged 7–10 years) which focussed on media use and practices, skills, parental mediation, and family rules;
4 Field notes. The data was processed using the *Statistical Package for Social Sciences* (quantitative data) and *Atlas.ti* (qualitative data).

Results from 1), 2) and 3) allowed us to characterise this multidimensional context, a crucial task in order to adapt the intervention model accordingly. Regarding media use, most teachers (22 out of 24) and parents (30 of the 38) used the internet daily, while all children consumed the same amount of television (36 of the 38 every day) and YouTube (although with different weekly frequency). However, this was not the case with digital games (3 of the 38 children did not play them) even though five of them did not have access to the internet at home. These reported practices were in line with the observation by Edwards, Nolan, Henderson, Mantilla, Plowman, and Skouteris (2016) that children consider three categories related to their everyday life and the internet: "1. Family: Use of the internet by and for family members/2. Information: To access and/or produce information/3. Entertainment: Enjoy movies/games for fun and/or relaxation" (p. 6).

The research also observed that parents used the internet via their smartphone the most (28 out of 38), followed by the children (18 of the 38) and the teachers (8 of the 24). Among the adults, the most used means to access the internet was through their personal laptops. Among the children, tablet devices were the most popular (33 of the 38), with 17 also using the internet through console devices. There was also clear evidence that the time children spent using digital equipment increased on the weekend. If, from Monday to Friday, three children did not use any digital device and 19 only used them up to an hour per day, they all used them on the weekend, with 12 using them up to one hour, 10 (instead of four during the week) using them for two to four hours and seven (instead of one during the week) for more than four hours.

According to the guardians, children had learned to use and access digital media from their mother (26 of the 38) and/or father (20), with other family members (12), or friends (2). Only one parent stated that his son had learned how to use the computer at school and nine stated that the child had learned on his/her own, which is consistent with learning through imitating adult practices, through trial and error, or learning through the games' interactive tutorials (Edwards et al., 2016). All guardians stated they watched television with their children and 34 stated that they went with them to the cinema (30 on the weekend). However, only 16 read books with their children and only 15 read newspapers or magazines with them. Parent mediation was lower when it came to the children's use of mobile digital media. While 31 stated they researched online with the children (26 solely on the weekend), only 14 played video games with them (13 solely on the weekend). When considering the parent's perception, parent mediation practices included restrictive (implying usage restraints) and active (implying debate with children) and joint use mediation (implying the use of both parents and children). Even so, it is important to exclude no mediation in some cases or distance mediation (use of media as a baby-sitter). However, there is no clear evidence of mediation through participatory learning, in which parents and children debate use, learn together, and define use strategies (Zaman, Nouwen, Vanattenhoven, de Ferrerre, & Van Looy, 2016).

All the teachers considered that digital media has pedagogical potential, yet it was in these teachers' classrooms that media content was used sporadically. Around three out of four of the teacher respondents stated that they used media content in their teaching practices, especially printed newspapers (79%), magazines (83%), and films (83%), while two out of three stated that they used videos (67%), and one out of two used digital games (50%). Other media formats such as televisions, smartphones, or tablets were absent from their classrooms. Furthermore, if and when media content was used, the children's direct interaction with digital technology in the classroom was either weak or entirely absent. In this respect, the use of digital equipment that is most preferred by European children under eight years of age is not made largely available in schools (Chaudron, 2016). The reasons for this infrequent use were explained by the teacher respondents as being due to the lack of time available for children to be able to use media and technology in the classroom (22 out of 24) (92%), the pressure to prepare students for exams, the lack of resources available to be used by students, and the lack of technical support in schools (22 out of 24 for all issues identified) (92%), the latter being the reason why most teachers said they totally agree (11 out of 24) (46%). Most parents agreed that children learn school content (30 of the 38) and non-school content (35 of the 38) through media, highlighting the importance of digital technologies in helping their children do their homework (especially parents of children attending primary school).

Nevertheless, even if 33 out of the 38 parent respondents admitted to talking with their children about digital media, the conversations focussed more on limiting usage time and risk and less on encouraging information-search practices, including homework, and the advantages of online gaming. In brief, "even when holding negative attitudes towards digital media penetrating the home environment, parents seem to acknowledge beneficial uses" (Zaman et al., 2016, p. 15). This suggests that the "'digital generation' keep on being recalibrated" and the familiar context is "now entering a period where the parents of children born today might themselves very much come from a generation that itself had been labelled, digital" (Sefton-Green et al., 2016, p. 3). Even if parents are moving from beyond "the debate whether their children should or not use digital devices … there are still some concerns on the use of digital devices that parents are finding themselves being 'confused' and 'without clear guidance'" (Palaiologou, 2017).

Finally, the results showed a lack of dialogue between teachers and parents regarding children's digital media use and practices (16 teachers admitted to having these conversations, while only seven parents answered similarly). When they communicated with each other, digital media was always negatively referred to (that it was used for too long, the potential for video game addiction, and the dangers of the internet). Even the dialogue between teachers and students (referred to by 15 teachers but not confirmed by the children) allegedly occurred occasionally ('some days'), with teachers admitting to discussing these issues with children 'many days' or 'everyday'. This lack of dialogue may explain why teachers' perceptions of media practices and uses by children clearly differed from the perspectives of the parents.

Training Teachers on Digital Literacy

Nowadays, "classrooms have become more diverse by virtue of students' differing social roles, gender and ethnic differences, identity politics, life experiences and cultural settings" (Kulju et al., 2018, p. 81). Taking into consideration this above statement and the results presented, teacher training was the next step in the research project. An in-service teacher training programme (25 hours) was provided to teachers, taking place in January and February of 2016. The programme focussed on technical, operational, critical, and cultural competencies (such as critical analysis, reflexive and creative production of media messages), intercultural issues, human rights, and children's rights. Teachers organised themselves in ten groups and developed digital literacy activities with 366 of their students (147 pre-schoolers and 219 primary-school students). The activities were embedded in the work that had been previously planned, and they were to use media (traditional and/or digital) as a resource and/or a study object. Each group established a duly justified topic, its objectives, and the development of the activity. Participants always had the support of the trainer (researcher and journalist) and had access to resources available through a course blog.

The activities covered diverse topics and objectives and were related with the operational area of the intervention model they followed, such as organising a book or creating a collective text from image exploitation. Concerning the critical area, teachers and students discussed the role of newspapers, internet safety, learning with and through the media, as well as critically analysing media messages (print and online newspapers, YouTube videos, comics) including advertising. The cultural competency aspect of the programme, especially related with social intervention through media, was covered less than the others, as only one group organised an activity aimed at tackling bullying in a school setting.

During the training assessment, teachers highlighted four aspects resulting from both the training course and the subsequent activities developed:

1 Knowledge about children's media practices ("From the work done by the students, we reached the conclusion that we had not even considered initially, for example, that students from pre-school watch little television, but use the tablet more than an hour a day" – T24);
2 New resources ("It has enabled me, with the knowledge acquired, to lead students and to reflect on the different resources you can use to learn" – T1);
3 New pedagogical practices ("Students' involvement allowed carrying out activities in the classroom for the first time. There was freedom to approach the classroom themes/resources according to each class/school" – T13);
4 Knowledge sharing among colleagues ("The presentation of the work was very enriching and allowed me to do some learning and put it into practice in my teaching activity" – T23).

Intervention Plan and Strategies

By the end of the training course, teachers were challenged to organise an intervention plan in partnership with the research team (including the trainer), but only eight teachers, who worked at the same school, accepted the proposal. The school had three pre-school and five primary-school classes, totalling 170 children aged from 3 to 9 years. Those eight teachers helped the research team during the data collection phase, aimed at characterising the context (April–June 2016) and developing digital literacy activities with children, as well as benefiting from the trainer support. The intervention plan was discussed and approved in September 2016. Its main aims were to develop digital literacy activities involving the children's teachers, families, and their broader community, focussing on the operational, critical, and cultural areas when designing, producing, distributing, and implementing media messages. It was decided to start the publication of a printed school newspaper with four main objectives:

1 To reinforce the link between the school, the families, and the community;
2 To ensure that the children have the opportunity to express their opinion through the media;
3 To reinforce children's critical thinking on the media and on social issues through the production of media messages;
4 To promote democracy at school and in the community, to advocate for human rights in general and children's rights in particular.

Although aware of the contradiction of having a project on digital citizenship based on traditional printed media, the team decided to start this way as a means of overcoming the limitations of the context, namely the lack of technological and trained human resources at the school, and the fact that some families had no internet access at home.

The newspaper's name ("*O Cusco*", the busybody) and logo were chosen through a contest open to all the pupils. The design project was made for free by a company in collaboration with the research team, and the printing of the newspaper (250 copies per edition) was sponsored by the Odivelas Municipality. Each edition was designed at the beginning of the term in collaboration with the eight teachers (three from pre-school and five from primary school). The school coordinator collected all the stories and information and coordinated the layout of the newspaper. The draft layout was analysed by the team, who suggested alterations, after which it was printed. The newspaper was first distributed within the school and among the families. From the second issue onwards, the newspaper was also distributed on the last day of class of each term within the broader community.

The headline of the first edition was "Being a digital citizen" (December 2016) and involved pre-school children interviewing their parents and grandparents about what toys they had when they were little and what they played with. First- and second-year pupils asked their parents and grandparents what the media was like when they were children, while third- and fourth-year pupils organised debates on the development of the media. One of these debates was marked by a pupil's question: "teacher, what was the internet like when you were a child?". The intergenerational activity contributed to the pupils' better understanding of how the media, toys, and games have developed over the years. It also allowed for dialogue and reflection at school, within the families, and in the community. Children produced media messages, participated and intervened socially and, in this respect, the intervention model was being applied.

In March 2017 the children debated on human rights and children's rights. One of the pre-school teachers took a rabbit to school inside a wooden box and asked children to think about the animal's needs, imagining that it was alone in the world. The children named the rabbit "Pantufa" (translated to Slipper, which was the most-voted-for name) and listed all its necessities, including its need for a home, family, and food. Next, they were asked to think that, instead of a rabbit, they were considering a child. Although many children confused rights and duties, the activity allowed, through drawing, to stress that the interests of children come before those of adults (Article 3), that their right to life is inalienable (Article 6), as is the right to express their opinions, and, furthermore, that their opinions should be considered regarding any matter that concerns them (Article 12). These ideas were reinforced in the school newspaper for the adults to read.

In June 2017, in compliance with new legislation which decreed that recreation time in the school yard was pedagogical time, pupils were invited to submit proposals to change their school yard (which consisted of a football field and areas surrounding the primary school, where there was no equipment at all). Given the opportunity to express their opinions and wishes through the school newspaper, either through text or drawing, the pre-schoolers drew a yard with wooden houses in trees, swings, and slides, whereas the primary-school children expressed their desire for a swimming pool, a disco, and even a circus. Second-year pupils wrote to the local authorities and concluded their letter saying: "we would just like to be heard and that our requests are taken into consideration when you consider and are able to renovate the school, which belongs to everyone but is mostly the children's". Both the drawings and the letters were published in the school newspaper. In 2018 the children again needed to rethink both the school yard and the school itself by building a scale model with the help of one of the children's mother (an architect) and the husband of one of the kindergarten teachers. The photo of the model would be the headline of the June edition.

In December 2017 they wrote a letter to the Minister of Education (headline of the fourth edition). Among their several requests, children focussed on the renovation of the school yard and the changes to course contents: "we have analysed course contents and consider them too long. We do not have time to practice what we are taught! We suggest that the contents are revised and improved and take us, six to ten-year-old pupils, into consideration".

In March 2018 children expressed their interest in creating audio-visual content, so the team designed a proposal that linked the pupils' interests in terms of current affairs and critical analysis of the news through the production of a news broadcast, hosted by the children and video-recorded. On a Friday, all the children were asked to choose a news story that interested them, a task they could carry out with the help of their family or someone within the broader community. On Monday, the topics of the news were listed on the board of all the classrooms and the pupils voted on the news they considered most relevant. The 16 most-voted-for pieces of news were selected for Cusco TV's first news broadcast, which they called "Telecusco". The images were recorded with a mobile phone and edited using *Movie Maker*. The pupils debated current affairs and involved their families and members of their community. The video was watched by the children as well as by the parents, to whom the need to talk about current affairs with their children was reiterated, as many of the pupils found it difficult to understand what was being said, as the intended audience for the news is adults.

Although the project officially ended in February 2018, teachers and pupils have continued to produce content for the school newspaper with the help of the researchers and local authorities. In February 2019 they recorded their first 'professional' news service at the Autonoma University of Lisbon studios.

Summary and Analysis

The project and its results showed that the intervention model is suitable to develop a community-based action research project aimed to develop very young children's citizenship and digital literacy competencies. Starting with an in-service teacher training programme (and to continue supporting teachers through planning and assessment meetings), to then characterising the community context, and adapting the model on a regular basis, it is possible to continuously develop adequate digital literacy activities involving teachers, children, parents, and other community members.

The school's voluntary adoption of the project enabled its continued sustainability, with the school newspaper progressively becoming the community newspaper. According to the teachers' perceptions, the activities have helped children to mobilise their operational, critical, and cultural areas, as well as increasing the children's social participation both in and outside the school and shaping their practices as citizens. Results also showed that children are "digitally fluent from a very young age", suggesting the need for "a re-conceptualisation of young children's learning in early years pedagogy" as well as a re-examination of "the way children learn and the way in which the early years workforce organise their learning environments" (Palaiologou, 2016). As the project showed, children participating largely through traditional printed media are slowly converting across to digital media, as exemplified by the production of the news broadcast. This situation must evolve rapidly to overcome the gap between high digital use at home versus low digital use at school.

This project is however limited by a set of factors. First, it has been developed in a local context and its results cannot be extrapolated. Second, the results are also based on teachers' and parents' perceptions, and on data collected by the researchers through tools adapted or designed by them and not validated for the Portuguese population. Third, study participants were those who voluntarily accepted and/or those authorised to participate, which means that the results may have been different even if they involved individuals in the same context.

Acknowledgement

This chapter is an output from two research projects funded by Science and Technology Portuguese Foundation: SFRH/BPD/77874/2011 e SFRH/BPD/92204/2013.

References

Carrington, V. (2013). An argument for assemblage theory: Integrated spaces, mobility and polycentricity. In A. Burke & J. Marsh (Eds.), *Children's virtual play worlds: Culture, learning and participation* (pp. 200–216). New York, NY: Peter Lang.

Chaudron, S. (2015). *Young children & digital technology: A qualitative exploratory study across seven countries*. Luxembourg: Publications Office of the European Union.

Chaudron, S. (2016). *Young children, parents and digital technology in the home context across Europe: The findings of the extension of the young children (0–8) and digital technology pilot study to 17 European countries*. DigiLitEY Project Meeting, 3., Lordos Hotel, Larnaca, Chipre, 17–18 May.

Colvert, A. (2015). Ludic authorship: Reframing literacies through peer-to-peer alternate reality game design in the primary classroom. Unpublished PhD, Institute of Education, University College of London.

Danby, S., Fleer, M., Davidson, C., & Hatzigianni, M. (Eds.). (2018). *Digital childhoods: Technologies and children's everyday lives*. Singapore: Springer.

Edwards, S., Nolan, A, Henderson, M., Mantilla, A, Plowman, L., & Skouteris, H. (2016). Young children's everyday concepts of the internet: A platform for cyber-safety education in the early years. *British Journal of Educational Technology, 49*(1), 45–55. doi.org/10.1111/bjet.12529.

Green, B. (1988). Subject-specific literacy and school learning: A focus on writing. *Australian Journal of Education, 32*(2), 156–179.

Holloway, D., Green, L., & Livingstone, S. (2013). Zero to eight: Young children and their Internet use. LSE, London: EU Kids Online. Retrieved from: http://eprints.lse.ac.uk/52630.

Hooft Graafland, J. (2018). *New technologies and 21st century children: Recent trends and outcomes*. OECD Education Working Papers, No. 179, OECD Publishing, Paris. doi: 10.1787/e071a505-en.

Kotilainen, S., & Suoninen, A. (2013). Cultures of media and information literacies among the young: South-North viewpoints. In U. Carlsson e S. H. Culver (Eds.), *Media and information literacy and intercultural dialogue* (pp. 141–162). Goteborg: Nordicom.

Kulju, P., Kupiainen, R., Wiseman, A., Jyrkiäinen, A., Koskinen-Sinisalo, K.-L., & Mäkinen, M. (2018). A review of multiliteracies pedagogy in primary classrooms. *Language and Literacy, 20*(2), 80–101. doi:10.20360/langandlit29333.

Kumpulainen, K., & Gillen, J. (2017). *Young children's digital literacy practices in the home: A review of the Literature*. COST ACTION IS1410 DigiLitEY. ISBN: 9780902831469. Retrieved from: http://digilitey.eu.

Livingstone, S., Kardefelt Winther, D., Kanchev, P., Cabello, P., Claro, M., Burton, P., & Phyfer, J. (2019). *Is there a ladder of children's online participation? Findings from three Global Kids Online countries*. Innocenti Research Briefs no. 2019–02, UNICEF Office of Research – Innocenti, Florence.

Marsh, J. (2014) Young children's online practices: Past, present and future. *Literacy Research Association Conference*, Marco Island, USA. Retrieved from: www.academia.edu/9799081/Young_Childrens_Online_Practices_Past_Present_and_Future.

Marsh, J., Hannon, P., Lewis, M., & Ritchie, L. (2015, June 18). Young children's initiation into family literacy practices in the digital age. *Journal of Early Childhood Research*. Published online before print. doi: 10.1177/1476718X15582095.

Mathen, M., Fastrez, P., & De Smedt, T. (2015) Les enfants et les écrans – Usages des enfants de 0 à 6 ans, représentations et attitudes de leurs parents et des professionnels de la petite enfance. Louvain-la-Neuve: UCL-Institut Langage et Communication. Retrieved from: http://dial.uclouvain.be/handle/boreal:165802 [last accessed: 29 June 2016].

Meyers, E. M., Erickson, I., & Small, R. V. (2013). Digital literacy and informal learning environments: An introduction. *Learning, Media and Technology, 38*(4), 355–367.

O'Neill, B., & Staksrud, E. (2014). *Final recommendations for policy*. London: EU Kids Online, LSE.

Palaiologou, I. (2016). Children under five and digital technologies: Implications for early years pedagogy. *European Early Childhood Education Research Journal*, Birmingham (UK), 24(1), 5–24.

Palaiologou, I. (2017). Digital violence and children under five: The phantom menace within digital homes of the 21st century? *Education Sciences & Society*, 1, 123–136.

Ribble, M. (2011). *Digital citizenship in schools* (2nd ed.). Eugen, OR: International Society for Technology in Education (ISTE).

Sefton-Green, J., Marsh, J., Erstad, O., & Flewitt, R. (2016). *Establishing a research agenda for the digital literacy practices of young children*. A White Paper for COST Action IS1410. Retrieved from: http://digilitey.eu.

Zaman, B., Nouwen, M., Vanattenhoven, J., de Ferrerre, E., & Van Looy, J. (2016). A qualitative inquiry into the contextualized parental mediation practices of young children's digital media use at home. *Journal of Broadcasting & Electronic Media*, 60(1), 1–22.

47

THE VOICES OF AFRICAN CHILDREN

Chika Anyanwu

Introduction

Children's use and engagement with information communication technology (ICT) is informed by a myriad of different stakeholders, including, on a grand scale, national and multinational telecommunication corporations, and, on a local level, governments, communities, schools, and parents. Cost of access set by telecommunication service providers, the terrestrial access set by governments, and the device usage at both home and at school as set by parents and teachers, all inform the way in which children adopt and use ICT. Yet the major stakeholders themselves, the children, can be at the receiving end of the negotiations or at times completely absent. In an African context specifically, cultural hierarchy plays an important role in absenting the voice of the child in these negotiations. For example, in the Igbo culture of Nigeria, age plays a pivotal role in the dynamics of social power, with children needing to be subservient to adults and parents. It is therefore important to identify a cultural context through which children can be empowered by elders to represent their communal interests in online environments.

This chapter examines in detail the sociocultural, technological, and economic challenges that African children face in engaging with ICT and in forging their own digital identities. As Third, Bellerose, Diniz De Oliveira, Lala, and Theakstone identified in their report for *The State of the World's Children 2017 Companion Report*, there were three key barriers to connectivity among those from the Global South: quality of internet connection, cost of access, access to power supply and battery capacity (2017, p. 40). Furthermore, age, socioeconomic status, geophysical location, gender, and level of literacy all impact the degree to which people not only have access to, but also the extent to which they engage in, ICT.

Discussion in this chapter will first consider how the sociocultural principles of Ubuntu and Asuwada influence children's participation in an online environment. It will then consider the technological challenges that limit children's participation, identifying that slow mobile technology and a lack of reliable power supply are the primary prohibiting factors. Consideration will also be given to the socioeconomic limitations that African children face, recognising that, for both economic and cultural purposes, the concept of individual mobile phone access does not exist among African families, but rather within a shared mentality. This discussion will be supported throughout by data collected from *The State of the World's Children 2017 Companion Report* (Third et al., 2017) and the South African Kids Online report (Phyfer, Burton, & Leoschut, 2016), as well as a number of United Nations Children's Fund (UNICEF) Country

Office reports from recent years. This chapter will conclude with a range of suggestions to support African children's digital agency.

Recent Investigations into African Children's Engagement with ICT

Africa is a continent of 54 countries with different cultural, linguistic, economic, and geopolitical systems. Although the research samples analysed in this chapter are mere snapshots of a complex continent, the global and transgressive nature of digital platforms arguably cross geocultural and political landscapes, therefore making it necessary to analyse the voices of African children in relation to their international peers. In this respect, analysis in this chapter is localised through an African sociocultural lens. However, it is important to note that ICT adoption and access in African countries is not homogeneous. Rather, there are different levels of adoption and access among the 54 countries themselves, and also between those living in urban, regional, or rural communities within those countries.

The data examined in this chapter are drawn from a number of international research studies that investigated children's online activities. Third et al. (2017), for example, carried out a 26-country survey of 490 children's perspectives in the online environment and, while it does not focus exclusively on African children, the African sample population within the report covered six African countries (Burundi, Central African Republic, Democratic Republic of Congo, Tunisia, Senegal, and Nigeria) and thus covered three of the five regional zones of Africa: North Africa, West Africa, and Central African Republic.

Another study, South African Kids Online (Phyfer et al., 2016), provided data for a fourth regional zone: Southern Africa. These research projects were facilitated through the UNICEF Country Offices, who used their network to coordinate the workshops and run focus group sessions of 13 participants each. The project of Third et al. (2017) is also aligned with the UNICEF report, *State of the World's Children 2017: Children in a Digital World* (2017), which offered a comparative analysis of children's experiences, especially through a socioeconomic and cultural lens.

Sociocultural Challenges Faced by African Children

Many communal societies in Africa can be understood from Akiwowo's (1986) sociological theory of Asuwada: the myth of creation. Within this theoretical framework, individuals are composite units of a family and indivisible from its familial unit. In Southern Africa specifically, communities are also understood from the Zulu concept of Ubuntu. In Ubuntu "each individual's humanity is ideally expressed in relationship with others" (Mabovula, 2011, p. 40). These close communal societies leverage their existence through collective resilience and competitive practice, where people collaborate in order to collectively compete against common threats.

Asuwada emphasises contextual relationships between social beings who make valuable contributions to societal survival, community integration, and development (Omobowale & Akanle, 2017). Within Asuwada, there is a social expectation from all to associate or co-exist by internalising and rightly exhibiting values which enable community survival and development. Similarly, Ubuntu espouses a fundamental respect of the rights of others, as well as a deep allegiance to the collective.

In this context of collective responsibility and fundamental rights, concerns regarding children's online safety and cyberbullying take on a new level of importance. African children's engagement with cyberbullying was considered in a South-African focus group (Byrne, Kardefelt-Winther, Livingstone, & Stoilova, 2016) made up of girls aged between 11 and 12. The girls maintained that there was little difference between their online social interactions with other girls and their physical ones. One girl remarked "girls gossip about each other" but in an online environment "you don't put your names there" (Byrne et al., 2016, p. 61). These comments are in line with the concept of what Nigerian youths call yabis. Yabis is a form of competitive performance where young people make fun of and ridicule each other publicly while bystanders voyeuristically enjoy and urge the contestants on. Although far from the principles espoused in Ubuntu, this form of bullying existed before African children could engage with ICT and, in this sense, the evidence of cyberbullying could be seen as an online extension of physical actions.

In Ubuntu, according to Omobowale and Akanle, "there exists a symbiotic relationship between the individual and their community. Without the contribution and participation of constituent individuals, the community becomes void, and likewise, the community gives meaning to an individual's being" (2017, p. 45). This interdependent relationship between the individual and its community is similar to the social network perspective of Qun, Jiming, and Juan (2009, p. 326), who used the work of Tönnies and Loomis (1957) to argue that individuals who share values and beliefs are linked by social ties. Such social ties in the African perspective become important economic assets which yield network success (Kadushin, 2012). It could be argued that under Ubuntu, children begin to look after each other once they understand their interconnectedness.

As the online environment is still predominantly Western-dominated by content and structure, the social relationships fostered within it have limited cultural signifiers for African children. This can make some African parents develop anxiety over the impact such a medium can have on their children's cultural and moral education. This fear is compounded by the ubiquity of ICT, which has many unintended consequences. For example, in a focus group survey undertaken in 2016, South African parents stated that they had "lost our culture … our culture is lost" as a result of their children's engagement with ICT (Le Mottee, Leoschut, Leoschut, & Burton, 2016, p. 39). In a Pew Research report, parents also complained about how their children were losing the ability to communicate face-to-face with their families or peers (Silver et al., 2019, p. 12). If these concerns are analysed using the lens of Asuwada and Ubuntu, it could be argued that African parents and elders fear their children are losing a physical connection with community. This would be concerning because community enables cultural transmission, and losing community could threaten cultural survival.

Concerns were also raised about the security and safety of children's online participation. A 2017 UNICEF report in Ghana found that the children maintained security consciousness in an online environment. For example, a 14-year-old girl from Upper West claimed: "I don't accept friend requests from everyone … ignoring unofficial messages … I always want to chat with only people I know" (UNICEF, 2017, p. 61). She continued: "I blocked somebody who started sending me pornographic pictures" (UNICEF, 2017, p. 61). Interestingly, and in line with Ubuntu principles, the report also showed evidence of altruism and care among the children interviewed. One 14-year-old girl said: "I helped a friend to accept friend request … I also helped a friend to block a bad friend … I helped my friend to post a picture on facebook … my sister helped me to block someone" (UNICEF, 2017, p. 96). These interdependent relationships demonstrate that the key principles of Ubuntu, collective responsibility and respect, can be developed and encouraged within an online environment.

Furthermore, from a social capital analysis, Adams and Hess (2010) point out that social capital is directly related to personal and collective well-being. This collective wellbeing includes "physical and mental health; educational achievement; lower crime rates; and increased capacity for a community to respond to threats and intervention" (Adams & Hess, 2010, p. 141). As communal societies, African people have built strong social capital through reciprocal relationships espoused in Ubuntu and Asuwada. This form of embedded capital has sustained the people through different human and environmental challenges. It is an intangible asset built through the reciprocity of its constituent memberships. Therefore, the use of ICT within close-knit African communities is often received ambivalently.

With African children facing these sociocultural limitations, the task therefore is how to negotiate and implement ICT policies in Africa in a way that ensures children's ICT development is taken into consideration, but not at the cost of losing their cultural identity and capital.

Technological Challenges Faced by African Children

According to the GSM Association (GSMA), Africa is predicted to have the fastest mobile technology economy by 2025, with almost 50% penetration (GSMA, 2019). This forecast is important, as internet access in many African countries is, due to topographical challenges, through mobile telephony. While this implies that there is more untapped economic potential in Africa, which is the world's most youthful and fastest-growing population (Kemp, 2019), GSMA in fact represents the commercial interests of mobile telecommunication companies. In this context, their prediction should be read just as much as a commercial opportunity for telecommunication businesses than an affirmation of Africa's technological development.

Exploring this idea further, as of June 2019, Africa accounted for only 11.5% of global internet usage, North America accounted for 7%, and Europe accounted for 16%. Yet, these statistics change dramatically when they are placed against population ratio. For example, the 2019 United Nations population estimate put North America's population at 367.4 million, and that of Europe at 747.3 million, making a combined total of 1.1 billion, while that of Africa was 1.3 billion. In this respect, Europe and North America commanded twice that of Africa's usage. Similarly, internet penetration in Europe sat at 88% while North America was 89%. This is in comparison to Africa, which had an average of 40%, and this varied largely across different regions. For example, 51% in Southern Africa, 49% in Northern Africa, 49% in Western Africa, and 27% in Eastern Africa (Kemp, 2019).

However, as Oyedemi contends, in the case of Southern Africa specifically, "black Africans ... are generally the least positioned to benefit from [the] internet's potentials for enhancing participation and citizenship" (2015, p. 20), suggesting that generic data can obscure the more nuanced internal dynamics, whether it be in Africa or in Western countries. This obfuscation has occurred more often between ICT-connected urban areas and disconnected rural areas in Western countries, leading to what Park considers "as an eternal dependent relationship between the centre and periphery" (1999, p. 85). In African countries, however, it is often socio-economically determined between the wealthy few who can afford to send their children to well-equipped private schools with internet access, and the poor who depend on public schools with limited infrastructure.

Another important consideration is the state of ICT infrastructure within African countries. The Rwandan private media outlet *The New Times* ("Sub-Saharan Africa's", 2019) reported that many countries were operating on 2G networks and were in the process of moving to 3G and 4G networks. This indicates that African children relying on GSM mobile connectivity have the download speed capability of between 64 Kilobytes per second to 2Mbps. This is in comparison to their Western peers who are already transitioning from 4G network connectivity, which offers up to 100 Mbps, to 5G networks which promise an internet speed 100 times faster than its predecessor.

These challenges relating to internet quality, cost of internet access, and power supply were considered by a number of African children in Third et al. (2017, p. 68): "when you connect there is the network issue and it cuts out and when you are connected the battery runs out and there is the problem of credit". The children also acknowledged that they depended on their parents' phone to connect. A 15-year-old boy from Greater Accra stated that the phone is not mine. It is for my mom … when you want something fast and the network is slow … I waited for long … sometimes during some periods from 6am to 12pm. I don't have the money to buy the bundle … paying for the internet bills.

(UNICEF, 2018, p. 41)

Research by Byrne et al. (2016, p. 34) also came across similar challenges to access, with a 12-year-old girl from the Western Cape claiming that "if you don't have airtime…. then you can't chat … then you get mad … And then you don't have any pocket-money" (Byrne et al., 2016, p. 34). From these examples it is evident that while African children are keen to participate in online environments, they are hindered by technical challenges.

Socioeconomic Challenges Faced by African Children

There is also a need to consider an alternative communication model which enables wider access to affordable and high speed connectivity for African children. For many African families, the cost of a data subscription for basic internet access is beyond their reach, and the cost of owning a smartphone is equivalent to more than 10% of a high-income earner's monthly salary (Okeleke & Suardi, 2019; Radcliffe, 2018). This is reinforced in the UNICEF (2018, p. 41) research study on Ghanaian children's online participation, with an 11-year-old girl from East Ghana stating that her primary issue in engaging with ICT was "when you have no money to go to the café (cybercafé)". According to Mutsvairo and Ragnedda (2019, p. 14), the

digital divide … remains a major problem in Africa. Mobile phones are too expensive for many and accessing mobile internet is even worse. Therefore, unless affordable smartphones are made available to people with low socioeconomic status, the digital divide will persist

(Mutsvairo & Ragnedda, 2019, p. 14)

Furthermore, research suggests that from an economic and cultural perspective, African children do not require individualised smartphones or computers to connect or interact online. Rather, what they require is access to affordable and reliable bandwidth, power supply, and to be equipped with technical skills. For example, the research carried out by Joyce-Gibbons et al. (2018, p. 18) found that four out of ten adults in Tanzania shared a mobile phone. This observation is consistent with the analysis of Anyanwu (2019), who used the Pareto principle to examine ICT penetration in African countries. The Pareto principle is often regarded as the 80/20 rule or that of the 20% making 80% of the decisions. An understanding of the family structure in African communities would indicate that often a single mobile phone would serve as a gateway for family members to the rest of the world. As Yang and Laroche (2011, p. 980) observe, communal societies emphasise collaboration, openness, and sharing. In this respect, such prohibitive costs and economic limitations can be, to a certain degree, leveraged through collective ownership, which, while enabling cultural cohesion, can also leverage the cost of participation.

The Voices of African Children

Despite the challenges discussed above, there is a growing number of successful young Africans whose entrepreneurial spirit and creativity have transcended sociocultural and socioeconomic barriers. The 2018 *Forbes* list (Nsehe, 2018), for example, lists a number of promising young African entrepreneurs who have used those challenges to enable creativity. Many of them have used their childhood experiences to find creative solutions to increase other African children's participation in the online world. These entrepreneurs have established co-creative spaces, affordable power sources, educational platforms, sustainable farming support applications, and a host of other innovative products. For example, in Nigeria, Temitope Ogunsemo's MySkool Portal (https://myskoolportal.com.ng), a web-based application for a school information management system, has been adopted by many high schools in Nigeria to help track students' progress. In South Africa, Nthabiseng Mosia's Easy Solar (www.easysolar.sl) aims to provide access to reliable cost-effective energy to rural communities through renewable sources. Mosia's Easy Solar is an important example of how Africans can address the issue of unreliable power supply and battery life, which was a key barrier in *The State of the World's Children 2017 Companion Report* (Third et al., 2017, p. 40).

As part of the 2019 Children's Day celebration, Nzekwe Henry (2019) also compiled a list of African children who made global impact through their brilliant and innovative efforts. Among them is Kelvin Doe from Sierra Leone who, at the age of 13, became a self-taught engineer who had built his own radio station, transmitters, generators, and batteries from scrap metals. He was later invited to MIT and subsequently signed a solar project pact with Canadian high-speed service provider Sierra WiFi. Betelhem Dessie from Ethiopia started working, at the age of nine, in her father's electronic shop in order to get some pocket money. She began to develop an interest in computing and coding and within one year was able to code in HTML. She combined this work with her studies and was able to teach her classmates basic computer skills. At the age of 12 she was employed as a developer by the Ethiopian Information Network Security Agency (INSA), and at the age of 20 she was founder and CEO of Anyone Can Code (ACC), with four patented projects as well as others in collaboration. Finally, in 2017, a group of five Kenyan school girls aged 15 to 17 developed an app called i-Cut, which was aimed at tackling the issue of female genital mutilation. The app was designed to alert authorities and provide support for victims. These students won the African entry in the finals of the Technovation Challenge, which took place in California of that year.

These examples demonstrate that African children can engage in ICT in innovative, and in turn successful, ways. There can be more of these success stories if the sociocultural, socioeconomic, and technical limitations considered in this chapter are addressed. Education is an important tool to foster and encourage such empowerment. African parents send their children to school to empower them and to accomplish what they, as parents, were unable to accomplish. Digital literacy and participation could be extended to play a similar role. This is reinforced by the voices of the African children themselves. A 14-year-old child from the Central African Republic summarised: "digital technology allows me to search and learn anything I am interested in and use it for my academic work" (Third et al., 2017, p. 68). A 14-year-old boy from Ghana also claimed that he uses "Google to answer questions and do my homework" (UNICEF, 2018, p. 53).

So too does ICT assist in fulfilling their basic social needs, including being identified as part of the online community. As a 14-year-old Ghanaian girl stated: "I feel happy when I chat with my friends … when I read jokes, I am happy" (UNICEF, 2018, p. 51). For these African children, technology and ICT were not viewed as inhibitors to expanding their education, but rather as a facilitator. For example, a 12-year-old girl from the Central African Republic remarked that "technology never got in the way of learning or caused problems at school: with technology we get information for our lessons" (Third et al., 2017, p. 53). A 14-year-old girl from Ghana continues this idea, stating that "I learnt how to type fast … and use shortcuts of words … I learnt a lot about current affairs, and this helped in my academic work" (UNICEF, 2018, p. 51).

Conclusion and Suggestions

From the various examples and data used in this chapter it is fair to conclude that ICT is a global disruptive technology which challenges political, sociocultural, and economic boundaries. Its impacts permeate every society and therefore it is not a question of if, but when, governments and communities can take strategic initiatives to ensure that their children are adequately prepared to embrace it. It is also evident that while African children do not have the same level of access and opportunities as their Western counterparts, they are very creative and innovative with the few resources at their disposal.

While this chapter has acknowledged the challenges and difficulties facing African children and institutions, it is also important to understand that playing the dependency card will no longer enable African leaders to assert their authority and political independence before their global counterparts. Therefore, it is time that African leaders started investing in a strategic developmental agenda without expecting handouts from foreign countries. Investment in ICT should be regarded as an integral part of children's education, and national and continental development. In this regard, African governments should consider opening up more spectrum allocation and to have competitive tender processes to ensure that more stakeholders can compete to provide affordable services to the people.

While the emphasis of this chapter is on children, it is suggested that the education of parents on the uses and implications of ICT would enable them to understand and empower their children to take more control in the online environment. It is also recommended that community-based co-creative spaces be established to enable children to balance their creativity with cultural integration. Such creative space could serve as locations for professional development, as well as adult training grounds. It is also suggested that such training should consider using children as facilitators and trainers. This approach would enable families to share their cultural and digital experiences together, and indirectly recognise the need to transfer digital powers to their children.

Governments should also consider mandating telecommunication service providers to fund co-creative spaces in their communities of operation, either as joint initiatives or as part of their corporate social responsibility. Educational institutions should consider professional development opportunities for their teachers to enable them to improve their technical skills so as to support children in this digital environment. They should also review their curriculum to include coding and programming as an integral part of children's education. It is expected that these small steps will enable the continent to prepare for the digital revolution which has already started.

References

Adams, D., & Hess, M. (2010). Social innovation and why it has policy significance. *The Economic and Labour Relations Review*, *21*(2), 139–155. doi:10.1177/103530461002100209.

Akiwowo, A. A. (1986). Contributions to the sociology of knowledge from an African oral poetry. *International Sociology*, *1*(4), 343–358. doi:10.1177/026858098600100401.

Anyanwu, C. (2019). Digital divide or information divide: Interrogating telecommunication penetration measurements in communal African societies. In B. Mutsvairo & M. Ragnedda (Eds.), *Mapping the digital divide in Africa: A mediated analysis* (pp. 173–194). Amsterdam: Amsterdam University Press.

Byrne, J., Kardefelt-Winther, D., Livingstone, S., & Stoilova, M. (2016). *Global kids online research synthesis, 2015–2016*. Florence: UNICEF Office of Research Innocenti and London School of Economics and Political Science. Retrieved from: www.unicef-irc.org/publications/869.

GSMA. (2019) *The mobile economy sub Saharan Africa 2019*. Retrieved from: www.gsma.com/r/mobileeconomy/sub-saharan-africa.

Henry, N. (2019, May 27). *To mark this year's children's day; 10 African kids who rocked the world with their brilliant innovative efforts* [online publication]. Retrieved from: https://weetracker.com/2019/05/27/african-children-innovation-entrepreneurs.

Joyce-Gibbons, A., Galloway, D., Mollel, A., Mgoma, S., Pima, M., & Deogratias, E. (2018). Mobile phone use in two secondary schools in Tanzania. *Education and Information Technologies*, *23*(1), 73–92. doi:10.1007/s10639-017-9586-1.

Kadushin, C. (2012). *Understanding social networks: Concepts, theories, and findings.* New York, NY: Oxford University Press.

Kemp, S. (2019, July 17). *Digital 2019: Global social media users pass 3.5 billion.* We Are Social. Retrieved from: https://wearesocial.com/blog/2019/07/global-social-media-users-pass-3-5-billion.

Khosravi, S. (2011). *'Illegal' traveller: An auto-ethnography of borders.* London, UK: Palgrave Macmillan.

Le Mottee, C., Leoschut, L. T., Leoschut, L. C., & Burton, P. (2016). *Digital parenting in South Africa: Understanding parental mediation in the digital age.* Cape Town: The Centre for Justice and Crime Prevention. Retrieved from: www.cjcp.org.za/uploads/2/7/8/4/27845461/digital_parenting_info_booklet.pdf.

Mabovula, N. N. (2011). The erosion of African communal values: A reappraisal of the African Ubuntu philosophy. *Inkanyiso: Journal of Humanities and Social Sciences, 3*(1), 38–47. doi:10.4314/ijhss.v3i1.69506.

Mazrui, A. A. (2013). Cultural amnesia, cultural nostalgia and false memory: Africa's identity crisis revisited. *African and Asian Studies, 12*(1–2), 13–29. doi:10.1163/15692108-12341249.

Mutsvairo, B., & Ragnedda, M. (Eds.). (2019). *Mapping the digital divide in Africa: A mediated analysis.* Amsterdam: Amsterdam University Press.

Nsehe, M. (2018, April 18). 30 Most promising young entrepreneurs in Africa 2018. *Forbes Magazine.* Retrieved from: www.forbes.com/sites/mfonobongnsehe/2018/04/18/30-most-promising-young-entrepreneurs-in-africa-2018/#52a8a2757474.

Okeleke, K., & Suardi, S. (2019, July 16). *The mobile economy sub-Saharan Africa 2019.* Retrieved from: www.gsmaintelligence.com/research/2019/07/the-mobile-economy-sub-saharan-africa-2019/786.

Omobowale, A. O., & Akanle, O. (2017). Asuwada epistemology and globalised sociology: Challenges of the south. *Sociology, 5*(1), 43–59. doi:10.1177/0038038516656994.

Oyedemi, T. (2015). Participation, citizenship and internet use among South African youth. *Telematics and Informatics, 32*(1), 11–22. doi:10.1016/j.tele.2014.08.002 0736-5853/2014.

Park, H. W. (1999). *The press, the state and hegemony: A theoretical exploration* (Doctoral dissertation, University of Minnesota, Ann Arbor). Retrieved from: http://search.proquest.com/docview/304522127?accountid=10344.

Phyfer, J., Burton, P., & Leoschut, L. (2016). *South African kids online: Barriers, opportunities and risks. A glimpse into South African children's Internet use and online activities.* Technical Report. Cape Town: Centre for Justice and Crime Prevention. Retrieved from: www.cjcp.org.za/publications.html.

Qun, W., Jiming, W., & Juan, L. (2009). Applying social network theory to the effects of information technology implementation. In Y. Diwedi, B. Lal, M. Williams, S. Schneberger, & M. Wade (Eds.), *Handbook of research on contemporary theoretical models in information systems* (pp. 325–335). Hershey, PA: IGI Global.

Radcliffe, D. (2018, October 16). *Mobile in Sub-Saharan Africa: Can world's fastest-growing mobile region keep it up?* ZDNet. Retrieved from: www.zdnet.com/article/mobile-in-sub-saharan-africa-can-worlds-fastest-growing-mobile-region-keep-it-up.

Silver, L., Smith, A., Johnson, C., Taylor, K., Jiang, J., Anderson, M., & Rainie, L. (2019, March 7). *Mobile connectivity in emerging economies.* Pew Research Center. Retrieved from: www.pewinternet.org/2019/03/07/mobile-connectivity-in-emerging-economies.

Sub-Saharan Africa's mobile economy valued at over $150 billion in 2018. (2019, July 17). *The New Times.* Retrieved from: www.newtimes.co.rw/business/sub-saharan-africas-mobile-economy-valued-over-150-billion-2018.

Third, A., Bellerose, D., Diniz de Oliveira, J., Lala, G., & Theakstone, G. (2017). *Young and online: Children's perspectives on life in the digital age* (The state of the world's children 2017 companion report). Sydney: Western Sydney University. doi:10.4225/35/5a1b885f6d4db.

Tonnies, F., & Loomis, C. P. (1957). *Community and society.* East Lansing, MI: Michigan State University Press.

United Nations Children's Fund (UNICEF). (2017). *The state of the world's children 2017: Children in a digital world.* Retrieved from: www.unicef.org/publications/index_101992.html.

United Nations Children's Fund (UNICEF). (2018). *Risks and opportunities related to children's online practices: Ghana country report – December 2017.* Retrieved from: http://globalkidsonline.net/findings-ghana.

Yang, Z., & Laroche, M. (2011). Parental responsiveness and adolescent susceptibility to peer influence: A cross-cultural investigation. *Journal of Business Research, 64*(9), 979–987. doi:10.1016/j.jbusres.2010.11.021.

48
LIMITING THE DIGITAL IN BRAZILIAN SCHOOLS
Structural Difficulties and School Culture

Daniela Costa and Juliana Doretto

Introduction

This chapter presents data that demonstrates the difficulties and contradictions of working with digital technologies in Brazilian schools. Two research surveys will be discussed, both conducted by the Regional Center for Studies on the Development of the Information Society (Cetic.br) in Brazil: ICT in Education and ICT Kids Online Brazil. ICT in Education investigated 1,106 schools in urban areas in Brazil in 2016, interviewing 11,069 students and 1,854 teachers. The second survey interviewed 2,999 children and young people (aged 9 to 17 years) from 2016–2017. The data collected is compared with Brazil's public policies on the educational use of digital technologies. The objective is to show contradictions between the data, which reveal schools do not have adequate internet connections or basic supplies, and government policies in a developing country. In this case, governmental decisions reflect social discourses that understand children's digital technology skills as being key to addressing education problems (Livingstone, 2017), even though the capacity to support widespread digital engagement is lacking.

Technology in Brazil's Educational Policies

On 6 November 2017, Geraldo Alckmin, governor of the State of São Paulo, approved Law No. 16567, allowing the use of mobile phones by elementary- and high-school students for 'educational purposes' in the classrooms of schools in the state education system. Before this law, their use was not permitted under any circumstances in classrooms during school hours. The governor argued at the time that "internet on mobile phones opens up countless possibilities for activities and research. It will therefore be a major leap forward for the benefit of students", ("Alckmin libera celular", 2017). The government also announced that, by October 2018, all 5,000 state schools would be equipped with wi-fi and broadband systems ("Alckmin libera celular", 2017). Although there is no national law in Brazil that regulates the adoption of mobile phones in schools, in most of the 27 Brazilian states their use within classrooms remains forbidden. Importantly, São Paulo is one of the wealthiest states in the country, although the majority of students in the state education system are from low-income families as middle- and upper-income earners prefer private education (Moraes & Belluzzo, 2014; INEP, 2018).

In January 2018, *Folha de S. Paulo* published an article that examined the impact of the law (Caldeira, 2018), stating that "all it takes is a quick visit to a school to realise that the law means almost nothing in relation to what is a conspicuous and, especially, tense reality" (2018). The article argued that even when classroom mobile use was prohibited, teachers working on the outskirts of São Paulo claimed they used mobile phones for educational activities since the students already brought them to school. Although the mobiles' primary purpose was for children's communication with parents, the students also used their devices for entertainment, even during classes.

Teachers were trying to reverse this situation by attracting their students' attention through mobile phone use and introducing educational elements. For example, they created WhatsApp groups to send educational content, used audio recorders on students' devices for school projects, treated the phones as stimuli for playing logic-based games, and listened to music and discussed the lyrics (Caldeira, 2018). English teacher Katia Josefa told the journalist "It was irritating to do this when there was a sign in the classroom saying that their use was prohibited" (Caldeira, 2018). Daniela Cacure, a history teacher, also noted that "the school network is not open to students; you can only ask them to do research on their own mobile phones, but not all of them have an internet plan, which gives rise to 'discrimination'" (Caldeira, 2018). A quote by chemistry teacher Rodrigo Matos ended the article, stating that "It is difficult to use mobile phones as a pedagogical tool ... but this is a battle that must be won" (Caldeira, 2018).

The sentiments of the teachers echo what Livingstone (2017) argued in an ethnographic study that monitored the technological habits, both inside and outside the classroom, of a class of young students aged 13 and 14 in a suburban high school in London:

> Now that digital networks underpin and enable social networks, it seems that the logic of the digital age dictates that connection is good and, therefore, disconnection is bad ... Many hope that the affordances of digital, networked technologies can be harnessed to connect disaffected or "underperforming" young people with exciting learning opportunities, or disillusioned teachers with innovative ways of engaging their students, or marginalised families with knowledge traditionally accessible only to the privileged. But how many connections do people need or want?
>
> *(pp. 63–4)*

Livingstone clearly outlines the social expectations regarding technology, expressing also the inherent contradictions within that hope. The digital realm emerges as a way of creating a closer bond between schools and the 'connected' youth. Common sense says that educators will attract more students' attention if they stop using traditional learning methods and adopt digital devices to structure their lessons.

According to Livingstone (2017, p. 64), these technologies are hoped to be something of a 'cure' for uninspired teachers (who feel distant from their students) and unmotivated students (who are far from achieving the expectations socially imposed upon them). Digital technologies would be even more important in critical cases, since they could serve as a path for providing more opportunities for disadvantaged young people or those with learning or behavioural difficulties. However, as Livingstone (2017, p. 56) contends, it is important to overcome technological determinism, since it is not the technologies that produce change in schools, but the use that people make of them. It is necessary to look at contextual and multidimensional variables, which are beyond the technology itself, such as access to quality education, family structure, and the equalisation of income gaps.

Reflecting upon these social expectations in Brazil, as exemplified by the news article cited above, school capabilities are considered out of sync in relation to the technological consumption of younger students. As one teacher noted, "Our school model is not technology-ready" (Caldeira, 2018). Although the new law in São Paulo, which allows cell phone use in schools, is considered an advance in terms of public strategies, it does not discuss important issues such as internet quality, open wi-fi access in schools, or the doubts teachers may have in using the devices as a pedagogical tool. Rather, the law only states that the network cannot be closed to students, while also acknowledging a lack of available computer monitors within the schools.

Buckingham (2006) has noted that the term "a 'digital' generation – a generation defined through its relationship with a particular technology or medium – goes beyond education and clearly runs the risk of attributing an all-powerful role to technology". He explained that there are children who have access to digital devices and use them in an advanced way. Yet there is a social narrative that circulates the idea that there is a generation capable of transforming its reality through technology, something that schools are not able to facilitate and, for lack of this, may fail to support young people in the digital realm. This narrative, however, does not deal with a real scenario, since young people have different degrees of access and skills in relation to information and communication technologies (ICT). It does, rather, reproduce a hegemonic social discourse that establishes "a set of imperatives" about what young people "should be or what they need to become" regarding digital technologies (Buckingham, 2006). That is, the terminology of a 'digital generation' contemplates the idea that if children and young people have access to technology – which is, of course, important and can even be considered a right, according to Livingstone (2014) – they can solve any problem they encounter during their lives. In this respect, the community needs only to provide them with access to devices, and this would be sufficient. Livingstone (2017) argues for caution, noting that:

> The competitive individualism of the aspiring middle-classes [is] now spreading also to encompass the diversity of families including many poor ones. This [has] often led to enthusiastic adoption of digital media goods along with the latest digital skills; but the vision is not necessarily that of connected learning, and it certainly doesn't promote social justice.
>
> *(p. 64)*

Therefore, solely providing young people with access to digital media runs the risk of being a panacea for surmounting obstacles on both national and individual levels, as well as an immediate path for families to climb socially. Yet, the quality and end goal of their technology use is not questioned, nor the lack of criticality associated with it. As the *Net Children Go Mobile* project claims: "it is not sufficient to know how to use the equipment technology, it is essential to be able to use in the rational way the enormous quantity and diversity of information and interactions available in the digital networks" (Simões et al., 2014, pp. 60–1).

boyd (2014) compiled a series of observations of young people's digital media use in various American states between 2005 and 2012. She conducted formal and semi-structured interviews with teens, conversing with them in their homes, at school, and in public places. She also interviewed parents, teachers, librarians, church staff, and other adults who worked with young people in a wide range of socioeconomic and ethnic communities. She observed social networking websites, blogs, and other media resources that were part of youth culture. Among the various themes addressed in her study is the denial of the idea that there is a naturally hyperconnected, homogeneous digital generation. In her study, boyd had contact with adolescents with very different characteristics. Some programmed complex websites, whereas others did not know what an internet browser was. There were adolescents who disseminated content through the internet and had many followers, while others were unable to recognise spam mail. In fact, boyd establishes that to assume that young people are naturally gifted in digital technologies may put them at risk, since they stop receiving support from adults who would have much to offer them in terms of experience (p. 197). Apart from this, assuming equitable access conceals serious social differences.

The article in *Folha de S.Paulo* clearly demonstrates the struggles that teachers have in following this narrative of obligatory technological inclusion – in their words "this is a battle that must be won" – as well as the struggles of children to use these technologies in a balanced (and profitable) way (Caldeira, 2018). In contrast with the seven educators who were interviewed, Caldeira (2018) also interviewed and published the views of two students. Student Lorhaynne Xavier said she used to use her mobile phone constantly, but it got better when her mother "imposed limits" on the amount of time she could use it (Caldeira, 2018). Kaio Miranda, despite having a mobile phone for reading about matters of interest, had problems in several subjects, saying that the school "has a very limited repertoire" and he wanted to "greatly expand [his knowledge]" (Caldeira, 2018). This student seemed unable to take advantage of his online skills for school activities, blaming the school for not facilitating this and not supporting the development of his mobile phone use as a means of addressing the school's limitations.

Although the article only published the opinions of two students, their views call attention to some of Brazil's problems regarding internet access. Lorhaynne Xavier said that she and her friends had problems connecting their devices to the internet, because they cannot use their school's wi-fi. The students, however, needed money to purchase prepaid 'credits' (a data package) in order to access the online elements of their school lessons. This theme is explored further in the following section of this chapter.

Young People's ICT Use and Skills in Numbers

The results of the ICT Kids Online Brazil 2016 survey (Brazilian Internet Steering Committee [CGI.br], 2017b) corroborated the reality described by boyd and exemplified by Lorhaynne. Conducted by Cetic.br in Brazil, the survey interviewed 2,999 children and young people (aged 9 to 17 years) in 2016 and 2017. A rigorous statistical methodology was used, including face-to-face research and the application of structured questionnaires in households according to census enumeration sectors developed by the Brazilian Institute of Geography and Statistics. This methodology allowed the results to be extended to the national population of this age group, taking into account sampling errors. The survey showed that around eight out of ten Brazilian children (9–17) use the internet. This statistic could bolster the idea of a digital generation, if the data is not examined more closely. This is due to children's usage not being the same throughout the country, or equivalent across cultural contexts.

In urban areas, 86% of the population in this age group used the internet, compared with 65% in rural areas. In the Southeast region, the richest area in the country, which includes the state of São Paulo, 91% of those between the ages of 9 and 17 had internet access. In the poorer regions of Brazil – the North and Northeast – the numbers dropped to 69% and 73%, respectively. There was greater inequality among social classes. Within the highest group (classified in the survey as AB), almost all the children (98%) accessed the internet, while in the lowest (DE), this was only 66%. Parents' education also impacted internet usage, with 92% of children whose parents had completed at least high school accessing the internet, but only 71% of children where parents had only studied for around four years. In relation to gender, however, no relevant differences were found (CGI.br, 2017b, p. 212).

It is important to note that an internet user was defined as someone who had accessed the internet in the three months prior to the survey, as defined by International Telecommunication Union (2014). In other words, it did not necessarily correspond to frequent use (9% of those who used the internet did so "at least once a week", 4% "at least once a month", and 69% reported "more than once a day") (CGI.br, 2017b, p. 254). The findings underline Buckingham's

(2006) caution that, "the meanings and uses of technology are so variable, that we need some quite fine distinctions in order to capture what is happening here".

The Brazilian findings illustrate the inequality of access to digital technologies in Brazil, the so-called 'digital divide' described by van Dijk and Hacker as something that extends beyond the possibility of accessing new technologies. Rather, the divide is represented by a:

> *usage gap* between parts of the population systematically using and benefiting from advanced digital technology and the more difficult applications for work and education, and other parts only using basic digital technologies for simple applications with a relatively large part being entertainment.
>
> *(2003, p. 316)*

These differences in use are not only due to personal choices (the decision to connect or not to connect), but are also generated by structural factors that are difficult to overcome (such as being unable to afford to connect).

It is important to remember that in a networked society, competent use of technology affords greater opportunities for professional and social mobility, associated with other social factors such as gender and social class. This generates a vicious cycle, where non-users (or less frequent users, or those whose use is less sophisticated) remain in a condition where

> Inequalities become structural when they "solidify", that is, when [the] positions people occupy in society, in social networks, and in media networks, or other media, become lasting and determine to a large degree whether they have any influence on decisions made in several fields of society.
>
> *(van Dijk & Hacker, 2003, p. 324)*

Hargittai (2010) also argued that those who have more and better opportunities to use these technologies also receive more stimuli for the development of certain ICT skills. These perspectives are reinforced by data from the ICT Kids Online Brazil survey series (CGI.br, 2017b), which show the persistence of these inequalities over the course of several years of research, starting in 2012.

In the 2016 Kids Online Brazil survey, more differences between social groups were noted regarding children's digital media activities. For internet use by mobile phone, for example, the inequalities observed in relation to access reappeared: 61% of children in classes DE who used the internet accessed it solely by mobile phone (in classes AB it was 12%, implying access to a range of internet-connected technologies). In rural areas this was observed in 54% of cases, compared with 34% in urban areas. In the Southeast, 27% of children who used the internet did so solely by mobile phone, as opposed to 52% in the North and 49% in the Northeast (CGI.br, 2017b, p. 251). The survey of children conducted by Cetic.br draws attention to these differences by affirming that "despite the inclusive potential of mobile devices, quality of access has important implications for the profile of online activities actually carried out, and consequently, can serve as a factor that maintains inequalities" (CGI.br, 2017b, p. 105). Bearing in mind that mobile phones permit less complex digital activities than computers, children's development of computer-based skills is still crucial for equitable access to the labour market.

This differential profile of internet access has also been found in other Latin-American countries, according to data collected by Global Kids Online (of which Cetic.br is part). Global Kids Online conducted quantitative surveys with the same methodology used in the European research network, from which the initiative arose. The Uruguayan report said that as indicated in the country context section, Uruguay has significantly reduced connectivity gaps; however, disparities in this aspect persist. In terms of socioeconomic level, 78% of children in higher classes accessed the internet from home daily, as opposed to 55% of those from the middle class and 37% from lower classes.

(Kids Online Uruguay, 2018, p. 54)

The results from Chile showed that 40% of children in classes DE who used the internet accessed it "every day, several times a day", compared with 60.5% of those who belonged to higher socioeconomic classes (Global Kids Online, 2019, p. 15). Likewise, 67% of young people whose families had lower incomes used the internet on portable computers and, among children whose families had higher incomes, 96% used these devices (Global Kids Online, 2019, p. 14).

Within this context of structural inequalities, schools represent a venue for addressing disadvantage related to connectivity deficiencies. The next section discusses some aspects of internet use in Brazilian schools in regards to the country's public policies.

Brazil's Public Policies on Internet Use in Schools

Brazil has around 48 million basic education students enrolled in public schools, according to data from the 2017 Basic Education School Census, conducted by the Anísio Teixeira National Institute for Educational Studies and Research (INEP, 2018). In rural areas, public schools have more than a pedagogical function; they also perform an important role in social inclusion. Most of the national public policies on digital inclusion and skills development focus on schools.

The first public policies that encouraged the use of ICT in schools were developed in the 1980s, when the economic value of having computer skills first became apparent. The need to train a contingent of people who were skilled in the use of these new devices and languages led the Brazilian government to draft a national informatics policy. This involved actions by various public entities connected to fields such as science and research, health, agriculture, culture, national defence, and, above all, education. The focus of public policies for digital inclusion and professional training for the use of these technologies in schools was to be the trademark of all government programmes in the sector from that point on (Almeida & Valente, 2016).

The National Program for Informatics in Education (ProInfo) (Ordinance No. 522, 1997) has been the longest-lasting public policy for the development of strategies to integrate technology within children's learning and teaching in Brazil. Launched in April 1997, ProInfo's main initiatives were primarily dedicated to installing computer labs in schools. When the programme was relaunched in 2007 under the name of ProInfo Integrado, in addition to providing computer and internet access, other initiatives included the creation and dissemination of digital educational resources, the distribution of mobile devices, lower taxes for equipment purchases by educators, and teacher training.

In 2017, the Brazilian Ministry of Education launched a new programme to expand the use of ICT in schools (Ordinance No. 9204, 2017). Its main dimensions relate to improving internet access in schools, supplying training for teachers and public managers, and providing open educational resource repositories for teachers and students. The primary objective of the programme is to enhance the quality of public education.

According to Barbosa and Fernandes (2017), these programmes occur in the context of a demand for basic education that meets the economic needs of the country and develops a skilled workforce for the increasingly complex contemporary labour market. Schools also have a responsibility to create conditions for students that enable them to develop their digital skills and learn the necessary content to understand and participate in economic, social, and cultural relationships. Combining the use of technologies and the development of education gives ICTs much more relevance than merely serving as a tool for pedagogical use. In this context, technologies are understood as a language through which people take ownership of culture, while the school is seen as a means of accessing this culture, especially for children in conditions of social vulnerability. This imperative to develop a digitally competent labour force also assigns teachers responsibility for supporting student learning with and through the use of these technologies.

However, as van Dijk and Hacker (2003) contend, reducing digital inequalities requires more than simply providing connectivity and training for labour tasks. It also involves quality access, in terms of the use of technological resources to enhance the freedom of individuals to express themselves, gain knowledge, participate, interact, and join others. As seen above, when addressing the inequalities faced by children, the mere fact of having access to a cell phone may not be sufficient for them to benefit from the opportunities offered by the technologies. This is an issue that has not yet been resolved by Brazilian public policies.

The next section uses data from another survey developed by Cetic.br to help demonstrate other consequences of the most recent governmental policies and the struggles Brazilian system education must face in improving the use of digital technologies in school students' learning and teaching processes.

ICT in Brazilian Schools

ICT in Education (CGI.br, 2017a) is a sampling survey, conducted face to face in public and private schools in urban and rural areas in all Brazilian states, with students from the 5th and 9th year of Elementary Education and/or the 2nd year of Secondary Education. Every year since 2010, researchers have visited selected schools to collect data, via structured questionnaires, from students aged 11 to 17 years. Teachers, directors of studies, and principals are also surveyed about educational access to ICT opportunities, including the use and appropriation of these resources in their daily lives, as well as the conditions of access and use of ICT in the school for administrative and pedagogical activities. For the ICT in Education 2016 survey, 1,106 urban schools were visited and 935 principals, 894 directors of studies, 1,854 teachers, and 11,069 students answered the questionnaires.

The survey reveals contradictions in use between children and teachers inside and outside of school. Reflecting the data collected from children in the ICT Kids Online Brazil survey, the students interviewed for the ICT in Education 2016 (CGI.br, 2017a, p. 199) survey also said that mobile phones were the main device they used for internet access, and 51% of public-school students reported using their mobile phones in school-related activities. Eight out of ten children cited research for their school work as being among the activities for which they used the internet – a percentage very close to that for sending instant messages. Most of these young people used their own mobile phones, but only 5% said they had permission to use mobile phones in classrooms (CGI.br, 2017a, p. 209), which is consistent with Caldeira's *Folha de S.Paulo* article (2018). Although it is arguably forbidden to many children, 30% reported using the internet via mobile phones at school (CGI.br, 2017a, p. 210).

Apart from prohibitions concerning mobile phone use in schools, wi-fi network restrictions are another challenge for school students. In 2016, more than 90% of public schools in urban areas had wi-fi access, but for 61% this use was restricted to administrative staff and educators. A password was required and not disseminated to the students. Because of such restrictions, many students did not consider school to be a place where they could access the internet, with only 39% of students saying they had used their school's internet.

The conditions for using ICTs in Brazilian public schools are still closely linked to the actions taken during the ProInfo period. The ICT in Education 2016 survey indicates that 96% of urban schools and 45% of rural schools had internet access, i.e., at least one computer (desktop, portable, or tablet) with internet access for student use. However, in the case of urban public schools, which serve most of the school population, especially from lower social classes, only 55% had internet access in classrooms, while 47% had access in libraries or study rooms for students. The 2016 survey indicated that internet access for students was mainly concentrated in computer labs (73%), a practice still linked to early public policies such as ProInfo. However, these labs were available to students in less than 60% of these schools, due to infrastructure problems and also because managers often feared that the equipment would be damaged or stolen. Even so, there was internet access in the offices of principals and directors of studies in 92% of schools.

Connection speed was another main reason for inequalities in internet use in schools. Around 45% of public schools located in urban areas had speeds of up to 4 Mbps; in rural public schools this percentage was 55% and, in 47% of these, speeds did not exceed 2 Mbps. Under these conditions, it is very difficult to share internet access among teachers and, especially, among students. Low speeds also inhibit use of the internet in areas outside computer labs, as the computers cannot easily open video files, good quality images, or websites. In such disadvantaged schools, managers prioritised internet access in the offices of principals and directors of studies in order to use school management systems and carry out the school's administrative activities. Consequently, these conditions increased the digital divide among students, and between students and their teachers. Notably, whereas only 25% of public schools had connection speeds exceeding 5 Mbps, this speed was available in 58% of private schools (CGI.br, 2017a, p. 202).

There were also regional inequalities among teachers. Almost all of them had internet access at home, and even the lowest percentage for this (91%, for teachers in the Northern region) was comparatively high. However, when teachers were asked if they accessed the internet at school, greater differences emerged. In the country's more economically developed Southeast regions, more than 90% of teachers could access the internet at work. In the North and Northeast regions, these percentages dropped to 72% and 75%, respectively (CGI.br, 2017a, p. 244).

To a certain extent, the public policies implemented by the government have had a positive effect on teachers using these technologies in teaching and learning processes. After more than 20 years of teacher training activities, many involving partnerships with public and private universities, teachers conduct at least a few activities with students using computers and the internet (CGI.br, 2017a, p. 214). The focus remains on more instrumental and centralised activities of teachers demonstrating use, however, rather than encouraging hands-on student-based skill development. Teachers often said they circumvented their school's technology deficiencies by using their own devices and internet access networks in educational activities. One in ten teachers said they used their own portable computers or tablets every day for activities with students, and 12% reported using the internet at least once a week (CGI.br, 2017a, p. 295).

As with students, there has been an upward curve in teachers' use of mobile phones for internet access. Between 2011 and 2016, the number of teachers who used their mobile to access the internet rose from 15% to 91%. Public school teachers' use of personal mobile phones for supporting digital activities with students rose from 36% to 46% between 2015 and 2016. Interestingly, although differences still exist between the country's regions, results across Brazil are very similar in this respect. This finding complements the information published in Caldeira's article (*Folha de S. Paulo*, 2018) relating to the use of mobile phones by teachers as a means of gaining students' attention during class, demonstrating that portable devices, with their own network connections, serve as a means for navigating difficulties encountered by teachers and students in accessing digital content in schools.

Conclusion

In Brazil, digital inclusion in schools reflects the social inequality that marks the country. The schools in the poorest areas are the least connected, although the public educational system as a whole presents systemic problems such as wi-fi networks that are closed to students, low internet speeds, and a lack of adequate equipment. However, there are advances in school connectivity, albeit slowly.

Although most Brazilian children and young people have access to the internet out of school, this digital inclusion is made possible through access to mobile phones, with internet usage restrictions such as high network access costs. Teachers are using their own, and students' own, access to the internet in order to incorporate technology within the curriculum.

The liberation of the use of cell phones in schools is a step towards recognising students' and teachers' existing practices. It is necessary, however, to take into account that, more than just encouraging the use of digital devices, which is strongly stimulated by social expectations in the country, public policies on education should make technologies a part of the whole educational process, including time spent outside school. This requires changes in the way digital media curricula and education are understood: as being more than just training for the labour market.

According to the line of thought adopted by van Dijk and Hacker (2003), today's society understands technologies as languages through which individuals construct their identities, interact with each other, and appropriate reality. Technologies permeate cultural, economic, and social dynamics. Thus the use of technologies in schools relates to the equalisation of access to cultural, economic, and social assets. The purpose of the technology-driven curriculum is to provide incentives for school community members to develop a critical vision, to find ways of expressing themselves, and spaces for affirming identity. It is thus not the technologies that produce the change, but the use that individuals make of them.

This line of thinking about the relation between technologies and education also takes into account the fact that students have an active voice and should participate in democratic processes within their educational contexts and in the formulation of public policies.

References

Alckmin libera celular em escolas estaduais para fins pedagógicos [Alckmin releases cell phone in state schools for educational purposes]. (2017, November 17). *Exame*. Retrieved from: https://exame.abril.com.br/brasil/alckmin-libera-celular-em-escolas-estaduais-para-fins-pedagogicos.

Almeida, E., & Valente, J. A. (2016). *Políticas de tecnologia na educação brasileira: Histórico, lições aprendidas e recomendações [Technology policies in Brazilian education: History, learned lessons and recommendations]*. Retrieved from: http://cieb.net.br/wp-content/uploads/2019/04/CIEB-Estudos-4-Politicas-de-Tecnologia-na-Educacao-Brasileira-v.-22dez2016.pdf.

Barbosa, M., & Fernandes, N. (2017). Public policies for teacher training and its impacts on basic education. *Em Aberto*, 1(1), 23–39.

boyd, d. (2014). *It's complicated: The social lives of networked teens*. New Haven, CT and London: Yale University Press.

Brazilian Internet Steering Committee. (2017a). *Survey on the use of information and communication technologies in Brazilian schools: ICT in education 2016*. São Paulo: CGI.br. Retrieved from: http://cetic.br/media/docs/publicacoes/2/TIC_EDU_2016_LivroEletronico.pdf.

Brazilian Internet Steering Committee. (2017b). *Survey on Internet use by children in Brazil: ICT kids online Brazil 2016*. São Paulo: CGI.br. Retrieved from: http://cetic.br/media/docs/publicacoes/2/TIC_KIDS_ONLINE_2016_LivroEletronico.pdf.

Buckingham, D. (2006). Is there a digital generation? In D. Buckingham & R. Willett (Eds.), *Digital generations: Children, young people and new media* (pp. 1–13). Mahwah, NJ: Lawrence Erlbaum Associates Publishers.

Caldeira, J. (2018, January 12). Lei que permite celular em aula dá 'trégua' para professores e alunos [Law that allows cell phones in class gives 'truce' to teachers and students]. *Folha de S.Paulo*. Retrieved from: www1.

folha.uol.com.br/educacao/2018/01/1949859-lei-que-permite-celular-em-aula-da-tregua-para-professores-e-alunos.shtml.

Global Kids Online. (2019). *Chilean children's internet use and online activities: A brief report*. Retrieved from: http://globalkidsonline.net/wp-content/uploads/2017/07/Chile-findings-report-FINAL.pdf.

Hargittai, E. (2010). Digital na(t)ives? Variation in Internet skills and uses among members of the 'net generation'. *Sociological Inquiry*, 80(1), 92–113.

International Telecommunication Union. (2014). *Manual for measuring ICT access and use by households and individuals 2014*. Retrieved from: www.itu.int/dms_pub/itu-d/opb/ind/D-IND-ITCMEAS-2014-PDF-E.pdf.

Kids Online Uruguay. (2018). *Informe: Niños, niñas y adolescentes conectados [Report: Connected children and teenagers]*. Montevideo: UNICEF Uruguay. Retrieved from: www.bibliotecaunicef.uy/doc_num.php?explnum_id=188.

Livingstone, S. (2014). Children's digital rights: A priority. *Intermedia*, 42(4/5), 20–24. Retrieved from: http://eprints.lse.ac.uk/60727.

Livingstone, S. (2017). The class: Living and learning in the digital age. In S. Tosoni, N. Carpentier, M. F. Murru, R. Kilborn, L. Kramp, R. Kunelius, A. McNicholas, T. Olsson, and P. Pruulmann-Vengerfeldt (Eds.), *Present scenarios of media production and engagement* (pp. 55–66). Bremen: Edition Lumière.

Moraes, A. G. E. de, & Belluzzo, W. (2014). O diferencial de desempenho escolar entre escolas públicas e privadas no Brasil [The school performance differential between public and private schools in Brazil]. *Nova Economia*, 24(2), 409–430.

National Institute for Educational Studies and Research (INEP). (2018) Anísio Teixeira. *Censo escolar 2017 (School census 2017)*. Retrieved from: http://portal.inep.gov.br/microdados.

Ordinance No. 522, April 9, 1997. (1997). Retrieved from: www.fnde.gov.br/fndelegis/action/UrlPublicasAction.php?acao=getAtoPublico&sgl_tipo=POR&num_ato=00000522&seq_ato=000&vlr_ano=1997&sgl_orgao=MED.

Ordinance No. 9204, November 23, 2017. (2017). Retrieved from: http://portal.mec.gov.br/docman/novembro-2017-pdf/77511-decreto-n9-204-de-23-de-nobembro-de-2017-pdf/file.

Simões, J. A., Ponte, C., Ferreira, E., Doretto, J., & Azevedo, C. (2014). *Crianças e meios digitais móveis em Portugal: Resultados nacionais do projeto Net Children Go Mobile* [Children and mobile digital media in Portugal: National results of the Net Children Go Mobile Project]. Lisbon: Cesnova. Retrieved from: http://netchildrengomobile.eu/ncgm/wpcontent/uploads/2013/07/ncgm_pt_relatorio1.pdf.

van Dijk, J., & Hacker, K. (2003). The digital divide as a complex and dynamic phenomenon. *The Information Society*, 19(4), 315–326.

49
AUSTRALIA AND CONSENSUAL SEXTING

The Creation of Child Pornography or Exploitation Materials?

Amy Shields Dobson

The Emergence of 'Sexting': Digital Cameras, Digital Cultures, Bodies

In Australia and elsewhere around the world, there are laws in place designed to protect children from possible harms and abuse relating to the creation, viewing, and distribution of child pornography and exploitation materials. Child pornography is loosely defined in federal law as images of people under 18 years old, or who appear to be under 18 years old, "showing their private parts (genitals, anus, or breasts) for a sexual purpose; posing in a sexual way; doing a sexual act; or in the presence of someone who is doing a sexual act or pose" (Youth Law Australia, 2019). The Youth Law Australia website, designed to inform young people in Australia of their legal rights and laws effecting them, notes that child pornography is defined as such based on notions of what is 'offensive to the average person', so that photos of babies in bathtubs are generally not judged as such, while "a picture of a naked teenager in a bed could be in some circumstances" (Youth Law Australia, 2019). Images that are considered child pornography can be images of real bodies, photoshopped images, cartoons, or moving images. In the context of federal child pornography laws, it is illegal to create such images, to ask for such images, to send, distribute, or upload such images digitally, to receive and keep them, or to pass them around. The laws in Australia around this category of visual material labelled 'child pornography' were designed and put in place before the internet and the world wide web became widely accessible and used in everyday life in the way it is today. However, they have been recently strengthened directly in response to the increased ubiquity of the web and the possibilities for the intensified spread of child exploitation materials it enables.

The internet no longer functions as, or is seen as, just a 'useful tool'. Rather, society now relies on "global digital networks for its very infrastructure" (Livingstone & Third, 2017, p. 658), and thus the internet is a key part of social and cultural infrastructure and life for many people. Further, the use of digitally connected smartphones with cameras in them has dramatically increased in recent years, among the general population and among young people in particular (Hand, 2012; ACMA, 2013). The prevalence of digitally connected cameraphones has changed the place of photography in everyday lives. New photographic cultural practices, new meanings and significations, and novel uses for photos and other digital images emerge in relation to cameraphones and the relatively easy sharing of images enabled via digitally networked devices, social media platform apps, and digital messaging platform apps. As Hand notes, "contemporary Western cultures involve unprecedented levels of *visual mediation*", and as cameraphones have become prevalent in everyday lives and places, "digital imaging has shifted from a professional or specialised process to a routine and unavoidable aspect of everyday life" (Hand, 2012, p. 3). In short, taking photographs and viewing them or sharing them with others via digital networks is now an everyday practice or part of mundane life for many people: it is near-ubiquitous, albeit in very different ways in places around the world, rather than something reserved for special occasions such as family get-togethers or social celebrations (Hand, 2012). Digital images now commonly function as a form of *social and cultural communication*, and, as Couldry has identified, in the digital era people engage socially with each other via practices of "showing and being shown" (Couldry, 2012, p. 47) things on digitally connected devices. Taking images of bodies via cameraphones can be seen as part of broader cultural and technological shifts in the era of global digital networks and the common presence of smartphones in public and private places and spaces.

'Sexting' is a recent phenomenon that has sparked much debate and concern about the new affordances of digitally networked devices and media platforms, and the potential for new technologies to contribute to, increase, or intensify bullying, harassment, and sexual abuse and exploitation. However, as Hasinoff and Shepherd (2014) remind us, sexting can be seen as "the latest incarnation of a long history of personal sexual media production, including love letters, diary entries, and Polaroid photos" (2014, p. 2935). A portmanteau first used widely in news media in the late 2000s, sexting combines the words 'sex' and 'texting'. But 'sexting' has come to be used mainly in relation to digitally self-produced bodily images, while also being a somewhat vague and indistinct term that, as several researchers have now pointed out, is not used commonly by young people themselves (Albury et al., 2013; Ringrose et al., 2013; Crofts et al., 2015; SWGFL/Safer Internet Centre, 2017). The term could potentially refer to or encompass a wide range of media practices involving the production, exchange, and circulation of texts and images involving sexuality or bodies via digital networks and connected devices. Different kinds of images featuring bodies and faces have emerged with the social, cultural, and technological pervasiveness of cameraphones, such as selfies, nudes, dick pics, sneaky-hat images, and frexts. Selfies and sexy selfies, for instance, are generally considered to be images of one's own face, or face and upper torso, taken by the self in question, at arms' length, with a digital camera or phone (Albury, 2015; Senft & Baym, 2015). Nudes is a term many young people use to describe nude or semi-nude self-produced images of bodies (Albury et al., 2013; Crofts et al., 2015; SWGFL Safer Internet Centre, 2017). Sneaky-hat images describe a humorous genre of nudes where a cap or hat is deployed to cover the genitals (Albury, 2015). Dick pics refer to the increasingly common practice of sharing images of penises in various digital contexts and platforms such as via hook-up apps like Tinder or Grindr, via messaging platforms and apps, or ephemeral media platforms such as Snapchat (Paasonen, Light, & Jarrett, 2019; Waling & Pym, 2019). Frexting refers to the practice of sending nude or sexy self-produced images of one's body to platonic friends, often for the purpose of obtaining bodily or aesthetic advice, support, or just bonding and connection (Waling & Pym, 2019). These are all various types of self-produced images of bodies that could potentially be classified as child pornography under Australian laws, even if created, shared, and received consensually, if depicting the bodies of young people or people who are, or appear, under the age of 18, and even if created by the subjects of the images themselves.

As Crofts et al. (2015) outline, laws surrounding child pornography have been strengthened in Australia in recent years, along with those in other developed nations, in response to growing concerns about the accessibility of child pornographic and exploitation materials in the digital era, as well as increased understanding of the harms associated with such material. The United Nations Convention of the Rights of the Child specifically addresses the need to protect children from sexual exploitation and abuse in relation to pornography (Crofts et al., 2015, pp. 47–9). As such, 'children' are now defined in relation to federal laws as those under 18. The definition of what may reasonably be interpreted as pornographic material featuring 'children' has been broadened to include a range of representational material "that might be sexualised by an adult with a sexual interest in children", as Crofts et al. outline (2015, p. 48). The possession of such material is now criminalised in Australia and many jurisdictions internationally, rather than only the creation and distribution of such (Crofts et al., 2015, p. 49). It is in relation to the heightened criminalisation of child pornography that, in several jurisdictions across Australia and elsewhere around the world, the age of sexual consent is out of line with the age at which a young person is considered a 'child' in relation to child pornography laws. In short, in several states across Australia, 16- and 17-year-olds can lawfully consent to sexual activities "but not to the recording of the same activity" (Crofts et al., 2015, p. 49), nor to a range of other 'potentially sexualised' digitally produced self-images (Albury et al., 2013).

'Consent' is a complex concept in youth and adult sexual cultures alike, and in relation to young people's sexual media practices. Ringrose et al. (2012, p. 7) suggest it is unhelpful to describe sexting in "absolute terms – wanted vs. unwanted sexual activity, deliberate vs. accidental exposure" (2012, p. 7), because such terms fail to capture the complexities of young people's participation in digital and mediated sexual interactions. Similarly, Drouin, Ross, & Tobin's (2015) research with young adults suggests that simplistic distinctions between 'consensual' and 'non-consensual' sexting practices are complicated in a social context where sexual harassment and violence against women is prevalent. They found that 12% of the young men and 22% of young women they surveyed in a US university said they had participated in sexting when they did not want to. The authors suggest that, in social landscapes characterised by normative gendered and heterosexualised pressures, sexting, like sex, can be "unwanted but consensual" (2015, p. 200). The circulation of dick pics among young people has been noted as an increasingly prevalent phenomenon, where such images are produced by young men in a variety of contexts and can be received in ways that are consensual and wanted or non-consensual and harassing, as well as collected, archived, and shared in ways that may or may not be consensual or intended on the part of the creators (Ringrose & Lawrence, 2018; Paasonen, Light, & Jarrett, 2019; Waling & Pym, 2019). As Wolak and Finkelhor note,

> Sexting episodes are very diverse and complex and cannot be categorised or generalised very easily. In some cases a youth takes pictures and sends them to an adult in what is an exploitative sexual relationship. In other cases, the taking and sending appears to be a feature of a developmentally appropriate adolescent romantic relationship. In still others, it may be hard to determine whether youth who exchange images are agreed about to what use the images may be put.
>
> *(Wolak & Finkelhor, 2011, p. 9)*

However, available research on youth sexting, conducted mostly with older teenagers and young adults in the Anglophone West, tends to indicate that, much of the time, various sexual media practices involving self-produced sexual and bodily images do occur privately and consensually between peers and romantically or sexually involved partners (Wolak & Finkelhor, 2011; Mitchell et al., 2014).

Why Young People Remain Vulnerable under Child Pornography Laws

Child pornography laws have been particularly contentious in relation to youth sexting practices because the wide scope of these laws means they could potentially be applied to images taken of one's own body, stored on one's own phone, or to young people's private sexual explorations and flirtations stored on digital devices, if brought to the attention of adult authorities with an interest in punishing such. Hasinoff (2015) outlines cases in the USA where clearly consensual sexting between young people has been the subject of legal punishment. She suggests that, as with the criminalisation of youth more broadly, it is socially and economically marginalised youth, and particularly racially and sexually diverse young people, who are most vulnerable to such criminalisation of their social and sexual lives (2015). Via such laws, young people are continuously (re)constituted as inherent victims of sexual exploitation just by virtue of their youthful bodies, contributing to cultural semiotic feedback loops whereby youthful bodies are (re)read as either innocent or dangerously sexualised and provocative (Lumby & Albury, 2010; Egan, 2013; Renold, Ringrose, & Egan, 2015). It has been argued that the bodies of girls, particularly black and brown girls, and queer youth are overdetermined as sexual (Egan, 2013; Hasinoff, 2015; Pitcan, Marwick, & boyd, 2018), meaning that complex social inequalities and long-standing gendered dynamics of 'sexualisation' play into such cultural feedback loops concerning what kinds *and whose* images are seen as sexual and dangerous in nature.

Criminologists and legal scholars have argued that the use of child pornography laws is generally inappropriate in relation to youth sexting practices, especially in cases of clearly consensual or private sexual exploration or flirtation; this is not what laws against child exploitation materials were meant to guard against, and there is growing recognition that youth sexting practices generally involve different scenarios and power dynamics to the creation and sharing of images of young people by adults for sexual gratification or exploitation (Crofts et al., 2015; Hasinoff, 2015). In brief, key suggestions are that the law needs to: find ways of distinguishing between sexting and child pornography and exploitation materials; to instigate more legal protections and defences for young people around this issue; and to more consistently apply other relevant existing offences in contexts where harms such as peer harassment and abuse have occurred in relation to young people's digital self-produced images, such as those around indecency and offensive materials (see Crofts et al., 2015, pp. 181–92). Other relevant laws, such as those around indecency and the age of consent, vary in Australia from state to state. The state of Victoria, for example, has led the way with addressing the place of youth sexting practices under the law and has put in place some legal defences to child pornography charges for young people, as well as a requirement that special permission is needed to press federal charges around child pornography for youth under 18 (Youth Law Australia, 2019). However, local police can still press charges of this kind in relation to state-based laws, so the threat, even if rarely enacted, of prosecution for child pornography material in relation to youth sexting practices remains. From criminological research in this area, it appears that the police and courts can and often are using their discretion in applying child pornography laws to youth sexting incidents that come to the attention of authorities, and often opt for less serious charges around indecency, or the use of cautions instead (Crofts et al., 2015). Nevertheless, there is no nationally consistent approach to this issue, meaning that laws around child pornography offences can be applied quite differently and inconsistently in different states in cases relating to youth sexting practices. The existence of federal child pornography laws with such a wide scope of capture in the digital era means that both young people under 18 and those who are close to people under 18 – including friends, family members, parents, care givers, and teachers who may be privy to, involved, or enmeshed in the mediation of youth lives in various ways – are particularly vulnerable to the potential legal consequences of self-produced images of youthful bodies. There are several unintended possible negative impacts of this legal, cultural, and social framing of the digital mediation of youthful sexuality as inherently dangerous. These include:

- Encouraging young people to view their own mediated bodies as inherently exploited and exploitable rather than as pleasurable, joyful, creative, and capacious;

- The possibility of frightening young people away from talking to adults about problematic, confusing, or abusive instances involving digital images of youthful bodies;
- Resultant confused and contradictory messages about the severity of youth sexting practices from adult authorities charged with protecting young people.

These interrelated negative impacts have shaped, produced, and reproduced the ways in which youth sexting is addressed materially and discursively in legal, cultural, and pedagogical discourses, representations, and practices. In co-constitutive feedback loops, the laws and material-discursive pedagogical responses to youth sexting can be seen as shaping and re-shaping youth sexuality and digital media practices and cultures. The remainder of this chapter will outline these impacts in some further detail.

Impacts of Child Pornography Material-Discursive Constitutions: Confused Messages to Young People about the Risks of 'Sexting'

The legal framing of sexting as 'child pornography' that has emerged as dominant over the past decade has caused some serious dilemmas and contradictions in relation to how sexting is discussed with young people and addressed in educational contexts. A significant unintended consequence of these measures, understandably designed as they are to protect children and young people from sexual exploitation in the era of networked communication, is the way such measures contribute to a framing and a material-discursive constitution of youthful bodies as inherently sexualised, inherently exploitable, and thus risky and dangerous. This unintended consequence of laws designed to protect children comes much more obviously into focus (to use a photographic metaphor), is more pronounced, and more intensely relevant in relation to the increased cultural prevalence of self and social photography practices in the digital era. To educate youth about the meaning of child pornography laws in relation to their digital cultural practices is to ask young people to view images of their bodies through a frame of possibilities for sexual exploitation, rather than through more joyful, pleasurable, experimental, and creative frames of perception and understanding. Feminist scholars have explicated the value of pleasure and capacity-oriented framings of youthful bodies in terms of violence prevention, evidencing how foregrounding pleasure and bodily capacity provides a solid basis for sexual ethics and empowerment, and is thus key to gendered and sexual violence prevention strategies (Tolman, 2002; Carmody, 2009; Allen, Rasmussen, & Quinlivan, 2013; Ringrose, 2013).

The crux of the problem is that the law currently pathologises and potentially criminalises everything to do with children's and teen's sexuality as experienced and co-constituted through digital media communication technologies (Angelides, 2013; Simpson, 2013). The sexuality of those under 18 becomes surveilled and pathologised in ways that do not apply, for example, to the older adult siblings or parents of teens under 18, who may regularly use digital media and communication technologies to flirt, connect in romantic or sexual ways, and consensually share sexual or bodily images and texts. Because of these strengthened laws criminalising child pornography and its possession, as well as its creation and distribution, a mediated representation of a youthful body engaged in any kind of sexual act or pose, or that could be *construed as sexualised* by a viewer with an interest in doing so, becomes risky, and is materially and discursively constituted as more potentially dangerous, contentious, or stigmatised, than 'unmediated' sexual acts or behaviours engaged in by youth. For example, young people in the author's research in rural Victoria, Australia, expressed much consternation over why other young people might take any kind of sexual self-images which they articulated as much worse, more shameful, and more risky than 'the real thing'. However, one group of teens, when pressed on why images depicting sexuality or sexual interest were more shameful than (unmediated) sex or bodies, and equated with 'putting yourself down', replied that they didn't know and "couldn't find the right words" (Dobson, 2015, p. 90). Similarly, UK researchers found that the young people with whom they spoke about sexting understood that self-image production was illegal for minors, but could state little about why: "they are told either by teachers or external speakers that it is illegal and if they do it they 'could be in a lot of trouble.' And there the message ends" (SWGFL, 2017, p. 7). The young people with whom they spoke speculated that they did not think peers considered the law much in relation to sexual media practices (SWGFL, 2017, p. 7). The frame of 'child pornography', 'exploitation', and 'self-exploitation' as sexting has been discursively framed in Canadian law (Karaian, 2015), may seem far from young people's experiences, making this framing hard to affectively comprehend, keep in mind, or hold on to in relation to their own bodies and digital cultures. A 'child pornography' framing of youth bodily images allows little room for pleasure, fun, and creativity, and thus may feel over-threatening and irrelevant to young people (Albury & Crawford, 2012). In sum, a notion that the *digital mediation of sexuality is bad* and constitutes a kind of self-exploitation for young people appears to be culturally pervasive. However, a deeper understanding of the legal context of this message often appears to elude young people.

Stakeholders and governments internationally have had to respond quickly to the highly publicised possibilities of extreme legal, social, and psychological consequences for youth involved in sexting, and have been highly proactive in Australia, developing several educational films, campaigns, and fact sheets to address youth sexting. In many schools in Australia, the UK, Canada, and the US, it currently appears that youth sexting is addressed in one-off, single-issue assemblies, with the inclusion of external speakers and/or narrative film resources (Davidson, 2014; Crofts et al., 2015; Dobson & Ringrose, 2016; SWGFL, 2017). Several narrative resources have been produced to address sexting with high-school students including *Tagged*, *Megan's Story*, and *Keep it Tame* in Australia, *Exposed* in the UK, and *I Shared a Photo* and *Respect Yourself* in Canada. (For further analysis and discussion of these, see Dobson & Ringrose, 2016; Dobson, 2019.) The predominant approach taken internationally in educational resources and government campaigns has been to promote youth abstinence from sexting by emphasising social sexual shaming, rather than the legal risks associated with sexting, particularly for girls. These narratives draw on and reinforce a typically heteronormative matrix of gender and sexual stereotypes of active male versus passive female desire, boys as sexual pursuers and predators, and girls as *either* sexual gatekeepers *or* sluts. Widely circulated sext education narratives such as *Megan's Story*, *Tagged*, and *Exposed* commonly narrate stories in which girls have been asked by boys for images, and are thus framed as the ones responsible for preventing sexting by 'saying no' to boys in the first place (Albury & Crawford, 2012; Karaian, 2014; Dobson & Ringrose, 2016). This is despite the ongoing prevalence of dick pics (Ringrose & Lawrence, 2018; Paasonen, Light, & Jarrett, 2019) and other kinds of sexual and bodily images and image-sharing dynamics in digital sexual cultures, such as those briefly mentioned above. In these stories, the girls who have 'given in' to a boy's requests then have their trust betrayed when a boy shares these images with other peers (either widely and maliciously, or in confidence with other male friends who then spread them further). The girls in question are then relentlessly harassed and slut-shamed by their peers at school, often to the point where they are depicted as needing to leave the school to start afresh, as in the ending of *Tagged*.

The laws concerning child pornography are not mentioned in any detail in such resources, although the involvement of police is often depicted or alluded to as a possible consequence for the young people involved. Nor are laws or ethics concerning sexual harassment, abuse, and the perpetration of such via digital technologies mentioned, which is essentially what these sext education narrative resources often depict (Salter, Crofts, & Lee, 2013; Dobson, 2019). As Albury and Crawford argue of *Megan's Story*, the individualising admonishment to 'think again' offers no sense of the broader legal and political environment in which sexting might occur, or any critique of a culture that requires young women to preserve their 'reputations' by avoiding overt demonstrations of sexual knowingness and desire

(2012, p. 465)

Many scholars are critical of taking an abstinence approach to sexting, which can serve to simply reinforce heterosexist notions of young women as sexual gatekeepers, and as the ones ultimately responsible for (often their own) abuse and harassment (Albury & Crawford, 2012; Angelides, 2013; Ringrose et al., 2013; Salter, Crofts, & Lee, 2013; Karaian, 2014; Dobson & Ringrose, 2016). They have called instead for more 'harm minimisation' approaches, while noting, in the current legal context, the situation where young people must still be adequately informed that *any kind of sexual self-image production is legally risky*. This leaves those charged with caring for and protecting young people in a difficult position. Understanding their own bodies through the legal framework of child pornography is a complex and somewhat violent ask of young people, and it is understandable that adult educators, care-givers, and even police are not keen to really emphasise the details of this framing.

To emphasise child porn laws as a key deterrent is also risky in terms of young people's wellbeing. When large numbers of children, young people, and adults close to them can potentially be prosecuted for offences designed to address paedophilia and the digital sexual exploitation of children by adults, this can have the unintended consequence of scaring young people away from confiding in adults about problems or instances of harassment and abuse that have occurred in relation to youth digital practices (SWGFL, 2017). While, as mentioned above, young people often express some confusion around precisely *why* mediated sexuality is bad and illegal, despite knowing it is, they are often clear that the effect of this is that the adults in their lives may well panic over youth digital images, and take these images way too seriously or out of context (Albury et al., 2013; SWGFL, 2017). Researchers in the UK found that, as a result of the sext education involving a talk by police that they had received at school, the young people with whom they spoke said that "there was no way they would ever tell an adult if a friend was experiencing abuse, coercion or exploitation as a result of sharing a nude" (SWGFL, 2017, p. 7). As they note, "If the message given to young people is no more complex than 'if you do this you are breaking the law', the victim is already concerned to disclose" (p. 7). As such, many sext education narrative films convey an awkward message of dire social consequences and slut-shaming, the threat of *potentially* dire-yet-obscure legal consequences, and some kind of consolatory ending, whereby a resolution is suggested as possible after/despite the violent and disruptive involvement of teachers, parents, and police. The young people in our Australian research picked up on the awkward contradictions of the message of *Tagged*, noting that the consolatory ending of *Tagged* did not make much sense given the extreme social and legal consequences suggested in the film for the group of teens involved (Dobson & Ringrose, 2016, p. 18).

Conclusion

For children and teens under 18 in Australia, there is no such thing as 'safe sexting' from a legal standpoint, and yet for many young people the taking and sharing of sexual and bodily images is a part of everyday life and peer digital cultures. Whether actually utilised much in practice by police and prosecutors, the legal and cultural framing of youth sexting practices as potentially 'child pornography' or exploitation materials has some significant unintended negative impacts on young people and those who care for them. As outlined here, to emphasise the meaning and intent of child pornography laws and their relationship to youth digital cultures is to ask young people to view their own bodies as inherently exploited and exploitable. Pleasure, joy, fun, creativity, and capacity is eluded in the process, despite the clear import of such for young people's sexual safety, rights, and empowerment. As suggested, it is understandable that those who care about young people might thus be hesitant to meaningfully emphasise how youthful bodies are actually constructed via child pornography laws. This has resulted in some confusing and evasive messages to young people about sexting. Extreme sexual shaming by peers is often threatened in sex education narratives aimed at young people in a bid to emphasise total abstinence, rather than providing details of laws regarding child pornography, or digital abuse and harassment (as less explicitly didactic websites such as Youth Law Australia do). As a result, young people often associate sexual self-mediation of any kind with shame and illegality, whilst being uncertain or confused as to precisely why this is so. Within the current legal landscape, a very difficult balance must be struck between informing young people about laws relevant to their lives and scaring them away from ever confiding in adults about issues or problems that arise in relation to their sexual or bodily images or communications.

Youth sexting is a complex and multi-faceted phenomenon that will likely challenge legal and social policy for some time. As suggested in this chapter, the strengthening of child pornography laws in the digital era is understandable in the historical and cultural context of concerns about the protection and rights of children in the digital era. At the same time, the bluntness of these laws, and their emergence over the last decade in legal and pedagogical discourses as explicitly related to youth sexting practices, is not ideal. The challenge to address, in overcoming the failures of current legal responses to sexting, is in acknowledging young people as sexual citizens for whom sexual rights and pleasure are important, and de-pathologising young people's sexuality. At the same time, this challenge requires finding ways to address the harms for young people that can result from heteronormative gendered cultural contexts of which sexting practices may be a part.

References

ACMA (Australian Communications and Media Authority) (2013). *Communications report* 2011–12. Pyrmont, NSW: Australian Communications and Media Authority, Commonwealth of Australia. Available at: www.acma.gov.au/Home/theACMA/Library/researchacma.

Albury, K. (2015). Selfies, sexts and sneaky hats: Young people's understandings of gendered practices of self-representation. *International Journal of Communication*, 9(12), 1734–1745.

Albury, K., & Crawford, K. (2012). Sexting, consent and young people's ethics: Beyond Megan's story. *Continuum: Journal of Media & Cultural Studies*, 3(26), 1–11.

Albury, K., Crawford, K., Byron, P., & Mathews, B. (2013). Young people and sexting in Australia: Ethics, representation and the law. *ARC Centre for Creative Industries and Innovation/Journalism and Media Research Centre*, University of New South Wales, Australia. Retrieved from: http://jmrc.arts.unsw.edu.au/media/File/Young_People_And_Sexting_Final.pdf.

Allen, L., Rasmussen, M. L., & Quinlivan, K. (2013). *The politics of pleasure in sexuality education: Pleasure bound*. New York, NY: Routledge.

Angelides, S. (2013). 'Technology, hormones, and stupidity': The affective politics of teenage sexting. *Sexualities*, 16(5–6), 665–689. doi:10.1177/1363460713487289.

Carmody, M. (2009). *Sex and ethics: Young people and ethical sex*. South Yarra: Palgrave-Macmillan.

Couldry, N. (2012). *Media, society, world: Social theory and digital media practice*. Cambridge, UK: Polity Press.

Crofts, T., Lee, M., McGovern, A., & Milivojevic, S. (2015). *Sexting and young people*. New York, NY: Palgrave Macmillan.

Davidson, J. (2014). *Sexting: Gender and teens*. Rotterdam, The Netherlands: Sense Publishers.

Dobson, A. S. (2015). *Postfeminist digital cultures: Femininity, social media, and self-representation*. New York, NY: Palgrave Macmillan.

Dobson, A. S. (2019). 'The things you didn't do': Gender, slut-shaming, and the need to address sexual harassment in narrative resources responding to sexting and cyberbullying. In H. Vandebosch & L. Green (Eds.), *Narratives in research and interventions on cyberbullying among young people* (pp. 147–160). Cham, Switzerland: Springer Nature.

Dobson, A. S., & Ringrose, J. (2016). Sext education: Pedagogies of sex, gender and shame in the schoolyards of Tagged and Exposed. *Sex Education*, *16*(1), 8–21.

Drouin, M., Ross, J., & Tobin, E. (2015). Sexting: A new, digital vehicle for intimate partner aggression? *Computers in Human Behavior*, *50*, 197–204.

Egan, R. D. (2013). *Becoming sexual: A critical appraisal of girls and sexualization*. Malden, MA: Polity Press.

Hand, M. (2012). *Ubiquitous photography*. Malden, MA: Polity Press.

Hasinoff, A. A. (2015). *Sexting panic: Rethinking criminalization, privacy, and consent*. Urbana: University of Illinois Press.

Hasinoff, A. A., & Shepherd, T. (2014). Sexting in context: Privacy norms and expectations. *International Journal of Communication*, *8*, 2932–2955.

Karaian, L. (2014). Policing 'sexting': Responsibilization, respectability and sexual subjectivity in child protection/crime prevention responses to teenagers' digital sexual expression. *Theoretical Criminology*, *18*(3), 282–299. doi:10.1177/1362480613504331.

Karaian, L. (2015). What is self-exploitation? Rethinking the relationship between sexualization and sexting in law and order times. In E. Renold, J. Ringrose, & R. D. Egan (Eds.), *Children, sexuality and sexualization* (pp. 337–351). New York, NY: Palgrave Macmillan.

Livingstone, S., & Third, A. (2017). Children and young people's rights in the digital age: An emerging agenda. *New Media & Society*, *19*(5), 657–670.

Lumby, C., & Albury, K. (2010). Too much? Too young? The sexualisation of children debate in Australia. *Media International Australia*, *135*, 141–152.

Mitchell, A., Kent, P., Heywood, W., Blackman, P., & Pitts, M. (2014). *National survey of Australian secondary students and sexual heath 2013*. La Trobe University, Melbourne: Australian Research Centre in Sex, Health and Society.

Paasonen, S., Light, B., & Jarrett, K. (2019). The dick pic: Harassment, curation, and desire. *Social Media + Society*, *5*(2), 1–10.

Pitcan, M., Marwick, A. E., & boyd, D. (2018). Performing a vanilla self: Respectability politics, social class, and the digital world. *Journal of Computer-Mediated Communication*, *23*(3), 163–179.

Renold, E., Ringrose, J., & Egan, R. D. (Eds.). (2015). *Children, sexuality and sexualization*. New York, NY: Palgrave Macmillan.

Ringrose, J. (2013). *Postfeminist education? Girls and the sexual politics of schooling*. New York, NY: Routledge.

Ringrose, J., Gill, R., Livingstone, S., & Harvey, L. (2012). *A qualitative study of children, young people and 'sexting': A report prepared for the NSPCC*. Retrieved from London: www.nspcc.org.uk/Inform/resourcesforprofessionals/sexualabuse/sexting-research-report_wdf89269.pdf.

Ringrose, J., Harvey, L., Gill, R., & Livingstone, S. (2013). Teen girls, sexual double standards and 'sexting': Gendered value in digital image exchange. *Feminist Theory*, *14*(3), 305–323. doi:10.1177/1464700113499853.

Ringrose, J., & Lawrence, E. (2018). Remixing misandry, manspreading, and dick pics: Networked feminist humour on Tumblr. *Feminist Media Studies*, *18*, 686–704.

Salter, M., Crofts, T., & Lee, M. (2013). Beyond criminalisation and responsibilisation: Sexting, gender and young people. *Current Issues in Criminal Justice*, *24*(3), 301–316.

Senft, T. M., & Baym, N. K. (2015). What does the selfie say? Investigating a global phenomenon. *International Journal of Communication*, *9*, 1588–1606.

Simpson, B. (2013). Challenging childhood, challenging children: Children's rights and sexting. *Sexualities*, *16*(5–6), 690–709.

SWGFL/UK Safer Internet Centre. (2017). *Young people and sexting – Attitudes and behaviours*. A report published by SWGFL/UK Safer Internet Centre, University of Plymouth, Netsafe New Zealand, Office of the ESafety Commissioner Australia. Retrieved from: view.officeapps.live.com/op/view.aspx?src=https%3A%2F%2Fwww.esafety.gov.au%2F-%2Fmedia%2Fcesc%2Fdocuments%2Fcorporate-office%2Fyoung_people_and_sexting_attitudes_and_behaviours_doc.docx.

Tolman, D. L. (2002). *Dilemmas of desire: Teenage girls talk about sexuality*. Cambridge, MA and London: Harvard University Press.

Waling, A., & Pym, T. (2019). 'C'mon, no one wants a dick pic': Exploring the cultural framings of the 'dick pic' in contemporary online publics. *Journal of Gender Studies*, *28*(1), 70–85.

Wolak, J., & Finkelhor, D. (2011). *Sexting: A typology*. Crimes Against Children Research Center. Retrieved from: www.unh.edu/ccrc/pdf/CV231_Sexting%20Typology%20Bulletin_4-6-11_revised.pdf.

Youth Law Australia. (2019). *Photos and videos on your phone*. Retrieved from: https://yla.org.au/vic/topics/internet-phones-and-technology/photos-and-videos-on-your-phone.

50
REVISITING CHILDREN'S PARTICIPATION IN TELEVISION
Implications for Digital Media Rights in Bangladesh

S M Shameem Reza and Ashfara Haque

Introduction

In the contemporary discussions on children and media, participation is central to any understanding of materialising children's communication rights. An obvious reference in this regard is the UN Convention on the Rights of the Child (CRC) that strongly suggests the centrality of the child's participation in media, as well as non-negotiable child rights to mass media and appropriate information. The Convention also enunciates the responsibilities of the State parties to recognise the right, and, in spirit, calls for facilitating child participation in the media. In legacy media, children in general are recipients of media outputs, but not active participants in broadcasting processes. In most parts of the world they are not consulted in decision-making or production process of television programmes that are designed, produced, and disseminated *for* children or in the name of children. The setting of the study reported here is Bangladesh, a South-Asian country where, in spite of some infrequent attempts to promote active child participation in broadcasting, TV programming *by* children or *with* their active participation is not yet a regular practice.

This chapter analyses the current state of and challenges to children's participation in TV programming, referring to UNCRC articles (UN, 1989) on children's media rights, such as Article 12 (on the child's opinion) and 13 (on freedom of expression) that together underscore children's rights to participate in the media, and Article 17 which is related to their access to mass media. This is an outcome of a qualitative study that examines the degree of children's participation in TV shows that are produced for children. From the perspective of the UNCRC, this analysis has identified the challenges to children's access to and participation in TV channels. This involves a reference to the provisions in the Convention that are related to 'participation' and 'media', which, in addition to the above-mentioned aspects, aim to protect the right to privacy and enable access to appropriate media and information.

The programmes were chosen from four TV channels including the state-run national TV, Bangladesh Television (BTV). While the chapter identifies the challenges to implementing the active participation of children in television as legacy media, subsequently it discusses the relevance of access and participation, that is, implications of the UNCRC articles for children's digital media rights. Considering the temporal value and evolving characteristics, the terms 'traditional' and 'legacy' have been used interchangeably for television.

Context of Children's Participation in Television

In spite of recent proliferation of the internet and digital technologies, traditional TV broadcasting still plays significant roles in the shaping of lived culture and setting socio-political agendas. Historically, the state-owned BTV has produced numerous programmes *for* children, but mostly without direct participation of children. Recently, with the support of UN organisations and international non-governmental organisations (INGO), a few TV channels are producing children's shows incorporating some aspects of participation. However, both the government and private TV channels demonstrate the non-participatory characteristics of legacy media. At the same time, they carry patterns of traditional media that provide limited and occasional scope for children to participate in some form.

An Overview of Children's TV Programmes

Broadly, children's TV programmes on Bangladeshi channels can be categorised as news, educational, cultural, and entertainment-oriented. In addition, there are programmes focussing on child rights. News bulletins include items like field reporting and interviews. Other programmes include drama and puppet shows, music tutorials, children's magazines, *Moncho Natok* (stage drama), campus shows, quizzes, specialised shows for pre-schoolers, etc. Rights-based shows include issues of child development, education, safety and protection, and adolescent health. Usually, such programmes are supported by UN agencies and INGOs. Except for a very few programmes, they are planned and produced by adults for children. Children merely appear in the scripted shows or take part as performers or presenters. Only four programmes over the last half a decade could be identified that enabled a greater level of participation of children, in which they were involved in major stages of planning and production, as well as broadcasting.

Concerning the content, an editor and producer of children's participatory video and TV programmes, Fahmidul Shantanu, says:

> Overall content of the children's programmes on Bangladeshi TV channels do not reflect the necessary standards. In addition, producers in general are not familiar with the standards, varieties and elements of children's programmes. This has resulted in the confinement of children's programmes within a few typical categories.
>
> *(Interview, 2018)*

The programmes are usually scheduled for broadcasting as weekly, fortnightly, or monthly. Over the last five years some shows for children were short-lived, while the remainder were discontinued due to funding constraints. Commenting on the down side of the externally funded children's programmes, a retired senior member of staff (the person wishes to remain anonymous) of BTV says:

> In the case of most of the externally funded children's programmes, when the funding period is over, the shows become irregular and are eventually discontinued. Both the state and private broadcasters should have an obligation to produce quality programmes for children and also to broadcast them regularly.
>
> *(Interview, 2018)*

This former BTV official also thinks that the state TV should aim more at serving children's media needs than simply increasing the number of programmes. BTV used to broadcast an interview-based show, *Amader Kotha* (Our Story), in which renowned personalities including politicians appeared and children questioned them about their life and work. Another show, *Shishur Chokhe* (Through the Eyes of the Child), a one-minute news bite, was broadcast by a private TV channel, ATN Bangla. The show was discontinued in 2017. *Shishur Chokhe* was a children-led programme that allowed children to participate actively in the programming processes. United Nations Children's Fund (UNICEF) Bangladesh signed a Memorandum of Understanding (MoU) with four TV channels first in 2011("4 TVs to air", 2011) and again with five channels in 2017 ("Five more", 2017) agreeing to broadcast a one-minute segment for children at prime time on any topic related to children's welfare and development.

Roles of UN Organisations and INGOs

Few UN organisations and INGOs have been supporting and partnering with both the state broadcaster and private TV channels to promote children's TV programmes in order to encourage active participation of children. In 2018, BTV along with two private TV channels launched a show, *Icche Dana* (Wings of Wishes), targeting adolescents. It is a joint effort of the Bangladesh Government's Ministry of Women and Children Affairs, the Ministry of Information, UNICEF, and the United Nations Population Fund (UNFPA). In the late 1990s, UNICEF and Save the Children Sweden–Denmark supported a fully-fledged child-led TV show, *Mukto Khobor* (Free News), on Ekushey TV (ETV), the country's first private TV with terrestrial coverage. The programme involved children in all stages of planning, production, and dissemination. Children as reporters collected information from the field, conducted interviews, and wrote news scripts. They were also consulted by the video editor before final editing of news footage.

ETV's terrestrial broadcasting was shut down in 2002 as it lost a court battle over its license. After the channel had lost its terrestrial facility, it continued operation through satellite broadcasting. However, the country's first child-led and participatory news bulletin *Mukto Khobor* went off air in December 2017. A producer of the show, who does not wish to disclose their name, tells us:

> It was one of the most popular shows on our channel. As our contract with UNICEF ended, we received no other funding for running the programme. The channel authority decided to discontinue the bulletin as they were unable to fund it from their own source.
>
> *(Interview, 2018)*

In contrast, ATN Bangla, the first private satellite TV channel of the country, has been financing on its own a child-led news bulletin (similar to *Mukto Khobor*) called *Amra Korbo Joy* (We Shall Overcome) since 2003. In addition, the private TV channel is running five other shows for children.

Children's Right to Participate in Media

According to Thorfinn (2002), the relationship between children and media is, in an international and legal context, "revolving around three Ps, namely Protection, Provision and Participation. Or expressed differently, in the Convention on the Rights of the Child, CRC articles 12, 13, 16 and 17" (p. 7). According to Article 12, it is expected that:

States Parties shall assure to the child who is capable of forming his or her own views the right to express those views freely in all matters affecting the child, the views of the child being given due weight in accordance with the age and maturity of the child.

(UN, 1989)

Article 13 is somewhat linked to Article 12. It emphasises freedom of expression, as it states that the child shall have (subject to certain restrictions if deemed to be necessary) the right to:

freedom of expression; this right shall include freedom to seek, receive and impart information and ideas of all kinds, regardless of frontiers, either orally, in writing or in print, in the form of art, or through any other media of the child's choice.

(UN, 1989)

UNICEF summarises the entire Article 13 as follows:

Children have the right to get and share information, as long as the information is not damaging to them or others. In exercising the right to freedom of expression, children have the responsibility to also respect the rights, freedom and reputations of others. The freedom of expression includes the right to share information in any way they choose, including by talking, drawing or writing.

(UNICEF, n.d.)

Article 17, according to Thorfinn (2002), is "perhaps the most central but also the most open ended article" (p. 8), regulating children's access to information and media which are most appropriate to them, calls the State Parties to recognise the:

important function performed by the mass media and shall ensure that the child has access to information and material from a diversity of national and international sources, especially those aimed at the promotion of his or her social, spiritual and moral well-being and physical and mental health.

(UN, 1989)

Through this article, the Convention also aims that States Parties shall "encourage the mass media to disseminate information and material of social and cultural benefit to the child and in accordance with the spirit of article 29" (UN, 1989), as well as "encourage the development of appropriate guidelines for the protection of the child from information and material injurious to his or her well-being, bearing in mind the provisions of articles 13 and 18" (UN, 1989). Article 29 refers to Goals of Education and Article 18 refers to Parental Responsibilities and State Assistance.

'Participation'- and 'media'-related CRC articles referred to thus far are interconnected and have threads to some other articles. Arguably, Articles 12, 13, and 17 along with Articles 8 (Protection and Preservation of Identity) and 16 (Right to Privacy), and Article 31 (Leisure, Play, and Culture), are also relevant to an understanding of children's right to mass media, and, in particular, their right to participation in both legacy media and the new media.

Methodology

Focus group discussions were conducted with the children who were involved in children's TV programmes in any capacity. Altogether, 70 children aged between 8 and 12 and 14 to 16 years old took part in separately held focus group discussions. Sixty per cent of the participants were girls. The children who participated in the child-led shows were interviewed as were those who attended TV shows for children as presenters or performers. In total, 22 children were interviewed individually. Interviews were also conducted with parents of the children, media and communication experts, producers, and anchors of children's programmes, and a few programme managers from child rights organisations. The focus groups and interviews were conducted during the period June–November 2018.

Primarily, the outcomes of the focus groups and interviews with the children were useful for comprehending the level and qualitative aspects of participation. Simultaneously, interviews with people like producers or senior managers from the stations were useful as well to identify the challenges to children's TV programming. The contents of the selected children's TV programmes were analysed. Instead of formulating a critical analysis of the shows, the contents were examined in order to identify the gaps or missing dimensions of participation. In this respect, there was also an analysis of the parts that demonstrate the active participation of children. For content analysis, two episodes broadcast in 2018 from each of the three selected children's programmes on individual TV channels were selected.

Selection of TV Channels

In selecting the TV channels, preference was given to the ones which have been consistently delivering significant numbers of programmes for children. Since the channels were selected purposively, this process also took into account credibility, reach, and coverage of the channels. Bangladesh Television (BTV), ATN Bangla, Channel *i*, and Duronto TV were chosen for the study.

State TV network BTV started in 1964. Besides being the network's terrestrial service, it launched an international satellite channel named BTV World in 2004. BTV's terrestrial broadcasting covers around 95% of the country. Among other segments, its audiences consist of huge numbers of children. According to the BBC World Service Trust survey report "Understanding BTV's audiences" (BBC, 2011), BTV is more popular with people from rural areas. The survey results show that BTV is leading in making health-, agriculture-, and child-related programmes. It finds that 33% of the respondents think BTV is best at producing programmes for children, 62% of BTV viewers watch "Programmes for Children", and 69% of respondents also believe that BTV is covering wide-ranging topics for children's programming. BTV broadcasts the highest number of children's programmes. Currently it airs 16 programmes for children. Although the programmes on BTV do not always include elements of direct child participation, in recent years the state TV channel seems to have been keen on promoting children's agendas as a way of participation. For example, a show named *Amader Kotha* (Our Story) (that began in 2009 and was discontinued in 2014) provided children with an opportunity, as well as a (media) space, to question policy makers and the government ministers on issues related to their rights and development.

Currently ATN Bangla is broadcasting the greatest number of children's programmes among the commercial broadcasters. It was the first TV channel to have broadcast a weekly one-minute news segment, *Shishur Chokhe* (In the Eye of the Child) made by children. The channel's programmes for children have received national and international recognition. An ATN Bangla production, *Amrao Pari* (We Too Can), won the International Children's Day of Broadcasting Award at the 32nd International Emmy Awards Gala in 2004. The documentary was shot and directed by a group of 18 children. It focusses on the true story of Abul Khaer, a nine-year-old boy, who prevented an accident by helping to stop a passenger train from approaching a disjointed rail track. According to a BBC Audience Survey Report, ATN Bangla was top among the private satellite channels. Twenty-three per cent of the survey respondents thought ATN was one of the best channels to produce programmes on children (while 34% thought BTV was good at producing similar programmes) (BBC, 2011).

Channel *i* is one of the oldest private TV channels of the country. The channel has been producing programmes for children since its inception in 1999. Children's shows on the channel involve child performers and it encourages outdoor activities. Currently Channel *i* is broadcasting a campus-based school magazine and a children's musical reality show. It has been airing *Shorno Kishoree* (Golden Girl), a programme targeting adolescent health issues, for the last few years. It also jointly organises national conventions with the Shorno Kishoree Network Foundation (SKNF) for promoting an ongoing campaign to ensure the physical and mental health education and conducive environment for adolescents.

Duronto TV, producing programmes specifically for children, began operation in 2017. Among other programmes, the channel broadcasts dubbed internationally popular cartoons, kids sport shows, and films. The channel has its own productions for children, some of which are inspired by local traditions, while others are adapted from foreign shows.

An Analysis of Children's Participation

There was no complete list of children's programmes aired by Bangladeshi TV channels. Part of the programme schedules are available in newspapers and on the channels' websites. But the information is not sufficient to provide a holistic understanding of the child's role in the shows. Therefore, a comprehensive list of children's programmes (currently on air) on the selected four channels (BTV, ATN Bangla, Channel *i*, and Duronto TV), was first prepared, from which two episodes of the following shows were selected (Table 50.1):

Generally, children are involved either as presenters (of news bulletins or magazine shows, for example) or performers (in drama, music, etc.) in children's shows. They are guided and directed by adult producers or directors, and the children follow their instructions. Sometimes children find it difficult to understand their roles in the shows. Most of the children's shows are produced by adults, in which children participate partially in selected aspects. In the interviews with children, one question was whether they are unsatisfied because they cannot do what they wanted to do, or are they happy with their roles? Nehal, Shabbir, Othoi, and Lalin, aged between 8 and 10 years, have taken part in children's magazine shows on private channels. Recently they have been inspired by a child-led news programme and started to think they too can become reporters, as Nehal says:

> We were lucky to have performed on TV shows. Our music teacher helped us to establish contacts with the channels. Among other children's programmes, these days we watch *Amra Korbo Joy*. We find it very inspiring. We want to work as child journalists, but do not how to go about it.
>
> *(Interview, 2018)*

Fareen, a 13-year-old girl who participated in children's magazine shows as a dancer and singer, said that she was happy to be on the TV shows, but wanted to do something else:

> I told the producers that I am good at playing the violin and want to perform in a show. First they did not respond to this. Later one of them told me that the violin is not quite popular in our country and it hard for them to find me an opportunity for playing the instrument. After that, with the help of our parents, I and my twin sister recorded our performance and uploaded it onto YouTube.
>
> *(Interview, 2018)*

Table 50.1 Children's shows for analysis.

TV channel	Programme/show	Brief description/children's role
BTV (Bangladesh Television)	*Moner Kotha* (Voice of Heart)	A puppet show conducted by an adult with an edutainment approach. Children participate in the show as performers.
	123 Sisimpur	An edutainment programme adapted from *Sesame Street*. Children are not part of programme planning, but they take part in all episodes of the show.
	Icchae Dana (Wings of Wishes)	This is a drama show highlighting stories of girl children facing obstacles in life and having to overcome the challenges as adolescents. The programme is a joint effort of the Ministry of Women and Children Affairs, Ministry of Information, UNICEF, and UNFPA. It is also aired by private channels, ATN Bangla and Duranto TV.
ATN Bangla	*Amra Korbo Joy* (We Shall Overcome)	A children-led news bulletin with active participation of children. They perform as presenters of the bulletin, work in the production process, and undertake journalistic assignments.
	Chotoder Prithibi (Children's World)	An edutainment show in which children are engaged in singing, recitation, etc. A child presenter attempts to educate children through storytelling.
	Aha Ki Ananda (Eh What a Joy)	An entertainment-oriented show in which children can sing and dance. They also take part in fashion shows, recitations, quizzes, etc. In a quiz show, children can participate through mobile texting.
Channel i	*Tifin-Tifin*	A campus-oriented TV magazine, organised in different school campuses. Students perform as singers, actors, reciters, and dancers. The show also includes interviews with celebrities.
	Shera Kontho (Best Voice)	This is a musical reality show. The programme searches for talented singers.
	Shorno Kishoree (Golden Girl)	This programme covers issues related to leadership, early marriage, personal hygiene, and the mental health of adolescents. School children attend training sessions with experts and take part in activities such as debates and discussions.
Duronto TV	*B Tae Bondhu* (B for *Bondhu*/Friend)	A family-situation drama show with an edutainment approach.
	Duronto Shomoy (Speed and Time)	Children's health-related show aiming to educate children about food, heath, and exercise.
	Golpo Sheshe Ghumer Deshe (Stories Before Sleep)	Prominent actors and actresses read out or tell stories to children.

Fareen and her sister also told us that they no longer feel sad that they are not able to play the violin on a TV show. They are now happy as finally they could play the musical instrument and that now people can watch it online. There are, however, a few adult-led programmes, such as *Moner Kotha* (Voice of Heart), a puppet show on BTV. This has gained a reputation for providing quality programmes for children. Conducted by a renowned artist and puppeteer, Mostafa Monwar, the show has been on air for around three decades.

Continuity of children's programmes is an outstanding issue in TV programming. As was noted earlier, the country's first fully-fledged child-led show *Mukto Khobor* was discontinued on ETV due to funding constraints. Another private broadcaster, ATN Bangla, also discontinued a child-led news segment, *Shishur Chokhe* (In the Eyes of the Child). Similar things happened to many other children's programmes. As the donor funding was discontinued or the contract period was over, TV channels failed, or, in some cases, were unwilling, to continue to finance children's shows. A number of producers and senior personnel of the TV stations tell us that the commercial sponsors and channel management do not find children's programmes profitable. Referring to TV operators' unwillingness to run children's programmes, Tanzina, a producer of *Amra Korbo Joy*, gives her opinion:

> Channel operators are usually reluctant to produce children's programmes although often they relate this to lack of funding. I don't think funding is the main issue. I see this as a lack of willingness. I think specific provisions need to be included in "National Broadcast Policy" to ensure the TV channels are obliged to allocate certain hours of airtime to children.
>
> *(Interview, 2018)*

In 2018, only one show allowed children to participate in the pre-production and post-production levels. In *Amra Korbo Joy* (We Shall Overcome) on ATN Bangla, children are involved in idea generation, the direction of the camera (but not operating the camera), and in the editing process. An editor consults children to finalise themes or topics for the show. Children collect information from the field, prepare news, and do the editing. In the final stage they present the news. In the editing process children are assisted by adults, although the children have the final say about choosing clips. On receiving help from adult staff from the channel, a child reporter of the news bulletin says, "If we face any difficulty, we ask for advice from the editor. In the absence of the editor, we ask other senior reporters for assistance" (interview, 2018). Parents were asked about their perceptions of the scope of active participation of children in TV: do they want their children to ask for more roles, or are they content with the present level of participation? One parent, Koushik Bhattachariya, thinks that children perform on the media the way producers want them to. He does not see any additional scope for children to propose any further options (interview, 2018). Another parent, Sabita Ghosh, comments:

> My daughter's extracurricular teacher sent her (my daughter) to TV stations to perform. Every time the producers decided what to do and how to do it. I do not think there is any scope here for children to express their wishes.
>
> *(Interview, 2018)*

Except for *Amra Korbo Joy*, children are not involved in content development, neither do they play any role in finalising themes or deciding the treatment of the news. Overall, there is very little scope for children to participate as producers in legacy media. A former Deputy Director General of BTV (the person prefers to remain anonymous) said, "Unless effective guidelines are in place, it will be difficult for us to convince the TV stations to engage children as content generators and producers of children's programmes".

Compared with cultural and educational programmes, child-led news bulletins provide a better opportunity for children to participate actively in key stages of programming. However, participation in news-oriented programmes appears to be more relevant to older children or adolescents. The participation of elementary- or middle-school students, for example, in children's TV programming, is another issue that requires a special focus. With regard to awareness of the right to participate in the media, children in general are either unaware or do not have clear understanding of their rights to participate as makers and disseminators of media content. The children's TV experts are of the view that the government, media and NGOs, and parents have a duty to help children to secure knowledge of their right to participation in media. Tanima, a producer of children's programmes, thinks:

> Informative TV programmes on child rights may be useful for informing audiences of the importance of child rights in general, but not particularly of the right to "participation". For me, there is a need to develop a mechanism so that both children and their parents are aware of the child's right to participation. The government, NGOs and INGOs should play active roles to facilitate the application of this right.
>
> *(Interview, 2018)*

Lack of awareness among the stakeholders on children's media rights has a bearing on the realisation and implementation of children's active participation in TV. In fact, the children who were engaged with the child rights organisations' media projects have a partial understanding about the CRC 'media-articles' and their right to participation. Hence, there is a need to 'develop a mechanism', as well as a media culture, to promote children's active engagement, as much as it is necessary to formulate policy guidelines so that children's shows are incorporated in the programming of legacy media.

Digital Media Rights and Participation

The percentage of Bangladeshi children using mobile phones or smartphones and digital devices is not known, neither is there any official data specifically on the patterns of children's internet use. However, *The State of the World's Children 2017* report informs us that fewer than 5% of Bangladeshi children aged under 15 use the internet (UNICEF, 2017, p. 43). In Bangladesh rapid technological changes, the development of online networks, and the adoption of digital devices have simultaneously posed challenges and opportunities. Digital media also "pose new and broad-ranging challenges for states in meeting their responsibilities to secure children's rights to provision, protection and participation in society" (Livingstone, Lansdown, & Third, 2017, p. 6). While digital media show the potential to facilitate children's expression, access, and active participation, the question is whether the UNCRC articles could still be relevant to ensure protection and participation in the digital age. More specifically, could the CRC 'media articles' still be relevant to children's access to and participation in digital media?

In addressing the above question, it is worth noting that internet facilities and digital devices are not evenly distributed across the globe (Nielson, 2013, n.p.). The situation is affecting children's access to digital media, particularly in the Global South where quality of access is an issue. This is also crucial in "shaping their capacity to leverage digital media and connectivity to enhance their rights" (Third et al., 2014, p. 32). Quality of access is both a prerequisite and integral part of children's digital media rights. UNICEF Young Australia Ambassador Philip Chan perceives access and participation in digital media as:

> a powerful way for children to realise their rights, from accessing information, playing games, to expressing themselves freely and even anonymously. Technology has a crucial role in empowering children by facilitating communication, education and activism.
>
> *(Third et al., 2014, p. 10)*

Children's use of digital media focusses on the right, as well as barriers, to accessing digital media devices, content, and services. Children's rights in digital environments aim at "enhancing ways in which children can enact their rights in online spaces, and overcoming the ways in which their rights are infringed or violated in a host of digital, networked and online spaces" (Livingstone, Lansdown, & Third, 2017, p. 23). This leads to the question of whether there will be a need for another convention like the UNCRC to promote, ensure, and facilitate the right of the child to digital media; or if the existing Convention will do for digital media platform, device, content, and service.

Participation Right in the Digital Future

Given the status quo, implementing child participation in the emerging digital environment looks challenging. The policy responses to children's exposure to digital media are expressed from a protectionist perspective, which does not focus adequately on the opportunities for children to use digital media. The findings of a study, "Online Safety of Children in Bangladesh" (UNICEF, 2019), warns of dangers as it identifies the threats to children posed by online violence, cyberbullying, and digital harassment. According to the study, 32% of children aged 10–17 years who are online are at risk of or victims of bullying or some kind of harassment. On launching the report, Edouard Beigbeder, UNICEF Bangladesh Representative, calls for safeguarding children, as he says:

> Thirty years after the adoption of the Convention on the Rights of the Child and creation of the World Wide Web, it's time for the government, families, academia and, critically, the private sector to put children and young people at the centre of digital policies.
>
> *("Cyber Safety", 2019, para. 9)*

Beigbeder's statement connects us to the discussion on the need for a set of provisions and policies for children's digital media rights. As the digital environment is going to be crucial, in a report prepared for the Children's Commissioner for England in relation to UNCRC and digital media, Livingstone, Lansdown, and Third (2017) comment:

> At stake is identifying, anticipating and addressing the global relevance of the UNCRC in the "digital age", by and across geographic regions, and encompassing all dimensions of children's lives. If society can seize the opportunities, digital media will surely constitute a powerful tool for delivering on the promise of the Convention.
>
> *(p. 48)*

They caution that failure in this initiative would threaten to "undermine children's rights on a significant scale" (Livingstone, Lansdown, & Third, 2017, p. 48). In a roundtable jointly organised by United Nations Population Fund (UNFPA) Bangladesh and *The Daily Star*, discussants emphasised how youth could utilise digital spaces. They found potential for the robust engagement of young people in digital spaces. The discussants also think digital media is providing Bangladeshi young people with the freedom to express opinions and opportunities to interact virtually across borders ("Safe Spaces", 2018).

In the digital age, it is imperative that children's information and participation rights are respected and implemented. Therefore, "we need a *digital rights charter for children* based on the UN Convention" (Livingstone & Haddon, 2009, p. 189). The principles as outlined in CRC articles 12, 13, 16, and 17, for example, can be applied to children's digital media rights. In other words, as children's participation is still important for overcoming challenges that infringe upon their access to and participation in digital spaces, as well as to maximising opportunities offered by digital media, key provisions of UNCRC remain very much pertinent for the digital future. In addition to the CRC articles that encourage active children's participation in traditional broadcast media, other interrelated articles of the CRC, such as articles 2, 3, 6, 8, 28, 29, 30, and 31, can expedite children's safety and development in the digital age.

Conclusion and Recommendations

The study finds that the CRC 'media articles' are not yet used in legacy media to their full potential. In practice, there are very limited opportunities for children to participate in key stages of TV programming. Their access to the media is partial and indirect or secondary in nature. Media producers, initiators, and investors lack sufficient knowledge of the vitality of children's participation in the broadcasting process. Many of them do not seem to have enough knowledge of the Convention to which Bangladesh is a signatory. They have not mentioned their obligations to ensure child participation, although most of them referred to funding constraint as an outstanding challenge to the sustainability of child-focussed and child-led TV programmes. In this respect, one recommendation is that there should be mandatory policy provisions aimed at ensuring child participation in broadcasting media. In addition, in order to develop the skills to participate in the planning and production process, children should be able to receive training and supervisory guidance from the TV channels.

As a logical extension, the issue of children's participation in legacy media is linked to the concerns about and potential for their participation in the sphere of digital media. There are a few efforts to promote children's online safety and security but these do not recommend any charter to guarantee participation in the emerging digital media. However, there is an urgent need to develop a charter or convention for children's participation right in digital media. Deregulation and the liberalisation of communications along with a rise in economic growth in South Asia have triggered a sudden expansion of conventional broadcast media in the private sector. As a result, TV has once again become a powerful media-space for children to negotiate their rights. The parallel development of a digital media space and legacy media make it necessary to have a charter or convention in place to address new challenges to children's participation.

As participation has become a focus of increasing attention in safeguarding the rights of the child, it appears from this study that participation in terms of active media engagement needs to be revisited both for legacy and the burgeoning digital media. While it is now imperative to have a charter (or maybe a non-negotiable convention) for digital media, this raises further questions. Should there be a completely new convention for digital media? Should there be a new charter based on the UN Convention? Or should there be a modification of the UNCRC in line with digital communications? Bearing in mind the implications of this study and subsequently the scope of this chapter, until the State parties agree upon a new charter or convention (or propose to add new clauses to the existing Convention) for children's digital rights, in spirit, the fundamental principles that CRC outlines can still be applied to implement children's participation in the field of digital media.

References

BBC. (2011). *Understanding BTV's audiences*. London, UK: BBC World Service Trust.

Livingstone, S., & Haddon, L. (2009). Conclusion. In S. Livingstone & L. Haddon (Eds.), *Kids online: Opportunities and risks for children* (pp. 241–259). Bristol, UK: The Policy Press.

Livingstone, S., Lansdown, G., & Third, A. (2017). The case for a UNCRC general comment on children's rights and digital media. *LSE Consulting*. Retrieved from: www.childrenscommissioner.gov.uk/wp-content/uploads/2017/06/Case-for-general-comment-on-digital-media.pdf.

Nielson, R. K. (2013). The digital revolution remains unevenly distributed. *Digital News Report 2013*. Reuters Institute for the Study of Journalism. Retrieved from: www.digitalnewsreport.org/essays/2013/thedigital-revolution-remains-unevenlydistributed.

Staff Correspondent. (2011). 4 TVs to air one minute's free programme on child issues. *The Daily Star*, 4 November. Retrieved from: www.thedailystar.net/news-detail-209181.

Staff Correspondent. (2017). Five more TV stations to air children's content for a minute every day. *bdnews24*, July 18. Retrieved from: https://bdnews24.com/bangladesh/2017/07/18/five-more-tv-stations-to-air-childrens-content-for-a-minute-every-day.

Staff Correspondent. (2019). Cyber safety in Bangladesh: 32pc children bullied online. *The Daily Star*, 5 February. Retrieved from: www.thedailystar.net/country/safer-internet-day-2019-prevent-bullying-of-children-online-in-bangladesh-unicef-1697785.

Third, A., Bellerose, D., Dawkins, U., Keltie, E., & Pihl, K. (2014). *Children's rights in the digital age: A download from children around the world*. Melbourne, VIC: Young and Well Cooperative Research Centre and UNICEF. Retrieved from: http://aeema.net/WordPress/wp-content/uploads/2014/10/Childrens-Rights-in-the-Digital-Age.pdf.

The Daily Star. (2018, October 7). Safe spaces for youth. Retrieved from: www.thedailystar.net/round-tables/news/safe-spaces-youth-1643434.

Thorfinn, H. (2002). *Children ethics media*. Sweden: Save the Children.

UNICEF. (2017). *The state of the world's children 2017: Children in a digital world*. New York: UNICEF. Retrieved from: www.unicef.org/publications/files/SOWC_2017_ENG_WEB.pdf.

UNICEF. (2019). *Online safety of children in Bangladesh*. Bangladesh: UNICEF.

UNICEF. (n.d.). *A summary of the UN Convention on the Rights of the Child*. Retrieved from: www.unicef.org.uk/wp-content/uploads/2010/05/UNCRC_summary-1.pdf.

United Nations. (1989). *Convention on the rights of the children*. Retrieved from: www.cypcs.org.uk/rights/uncrc/full-uncrc.

51

CHINESE TEEN DIGITAL ENTERTAINMENT

Rethinking Censorship and Commercialisation in Short Video and Online Fiction

Xiang Ren

Introduction

The state censors in China use various reasons and rationales for content censorship in media and cultural industries and the protection of children from harmful content is a key one. However, China's restrictive censorship system has not fully protected children (including teenagers) from unsuitable content such as sex, violence, and profanity in practice. China has not established a content rating system to classify media content as to its suitability for children or teenagers, resulting in a censorship paradox of "restricted content and unrestricted access" (Tsui, 2017). As children and adults in China legally have the same access to all kinds of media content, censorship laws, including many specific guidelines, require most content to be suitable for children (Grealy et al., 2019). However, there is arbitrariness in practical implementation as the management of these censorship guidelines is sometimes open to interpretation. This provides certain space for media professionals to play the so-called 'edge ball game', producing the commercially appealing mature content without crossing the red lines of censorship, such as politics and nudity, to which children are exposed.

The internet further complicates censorship in China. While digital disruption has liberalised media in some ways since the 2000s, it brings new threats to children as both content viewers and participatory creators. As censorship normally lags behind technological innovation, many previously tightly controlled content areas turned into open markets for digital media industries, for example foreign novels, films, animations, and games that contain porn, violence, and politically sensitive or morally controversial content, which would otherwise hardly pass the official censorship. The rise of self-media (*zi mei ti*), or "social media entertainment" (Cunningham & Craig, 2017) in the platforms like Qidian for online fiction and Douyin (Tik Tok) for short video, led to a flood of uncensored digital content created by domestic amateur creators. Online writers, video bloggers, and live streamers often use mature and even controversial content to attract attention, increase popularity, and aggregate their fan communities.

Such content sometimes turns into a key selling point in many self-media outlets and digital entertainment platforms where no effective age restriction is in place. While Western scholars studying children and the internet pay much attention to online risks like online bullying, commercial exploitation of creative labour, and commodification of adolescence (Deutsch & Theodorou, 2010; Ko et al., 2007; McGuigan, 2010), it is a pressing problem in China that children and teenagers are exposed to a vast amount of harmful and unhealthy content online, as well as the competing values embedded in digital entertainment, which has been controlled and censored more effectively in the pre-digital age.

This chapter focusses on two popular areas of teen digital entertainment: short video and online fiction. These areas provide Chinese teenagers with opportunities to freely create and access digital content, and interact with social networks to express their identities, feelings, voices, and concerns. Many teenagers even become rich and popular by creating trendy content that attracts millions of fans. Digital teen entertainment has indeed achieved tremendous commercial success and formed strong influence over popular culture in China. However, it attracts wide public criticisms as well. Some parents, educators, and academics in China are concerned about the negative impact of unsuitable content on children, internet addiction, the poor cultural and aesthetic value of digital content, and the time spent (or wasted) on digital entertainment (Wang & Qi, 2017). These public discourses in both online and mainstream media tend to justify government censorship and regulation in digital entertainment in China, in the name of child protection.

Through two case studies of short video and online fiction, this chapter analyses Chinese teenagers' cultural participation in digital entertainment, the effectiveness, failure, and controversies of internet regulation in protecting teenagers from unsuitable content and other threats, and the role of censors, platforms, and publics in teens' online safety. It also discusses the evolving tension between censorship and commercialisation in the emergent context of China's teen digital entertainment, and concludes by commenting on the impact of a politically controlled but commercially (and sometimes morally) deregulated system on teenagers' cultural engagement and civic participation online.

Teen Digital Entertainment: Global Dynamics and Chinese Characteristics

New technologies allow teenagers to freely publish content, express themselves, share ideas, and interact with each other in social media, as well as collaborate massively for activism and social movements (Livingstone & Blum-Ross, 2017). However, the dynamic cultural participation does not exist in a vacuum or a tech-utopia. Henry Jenkins (2006) articulates 'participatory culture' as an emergent paradigm and believes that the bottom-up participatory cultures and creative fans/citizens are taking control of cultural production from corporate media. In contrast to optimistic views, scholars like Jim McGuigan (2009) and Srnicek (2017) understand digital innovation as a new 'cool' face of capitalism, in which platforms become a designed core architecture that mediates and governs human connections and interactions including cultural participation.

The tension between top-down corporate control and bottom-up participatory culture is more complicated in China's internet sphere due to its tight political restriction on the one hand, and relaxed regulations on platform monopoly on the other. This leads to a depoliticised internet sphere where platform-mediated entertainment becomes the most dynamic space for innovation and creativity. The commercialisation of participatory cultural production is one of the most noticeable trends. In 2011 the Chinese internet giant Tencent coined a concept, 'pan-entertainment', aiming to define digital entertainment and creative economy in the platform age. Huang Bin uses the Western idea of the Creator Economy to theorise China's digital entertainment industries, referring to a new-born digital model of cultural production that is totally dependent on internet intermediaries (platforms) to connect creators, producers, and users (Sohu.com, 2017). Huang and Xiang (2017) employ the term 'creators' network' to further explain the importance of internet giants' ecosystems in increasing the economic efficiency of participatory cultural production, in which platforms function as a combination of industrial operations, social communications, and governmental regulations. However, while the Chinese scholars cheer for platforms' powerful roles, they have not fully discussed the corresponding social responsibilities of platforms in the creator economy.

Censorship is evolving as well in platform-based digital entertainment. Since the rule of Xi Jinping in 2012, the interplay between commercial imperatives and Party control is becoming more complex (Tong, 2019). The space for cultural creation was extended for commercial exploitation based on entertainment platforms, though ideological control and news censorship are being tightened. As Curtin (2017, pp. 1390–1) observes, the government loosens the reins on content creators and distributors, and allows "trusted commercial enterprises to grow influence and achieve commercial ambitions, and passes out media control into their hands". Guo (2017, p. 487) further argues that the rise of digital publics and the increasingly central role of platforms in the internet led to "mutually reconfiguring relationships between official, commercial, and mainstream forces" in regulating digital entertainment. As a result, while political control is increasingly tight, emergent entertainment media such as short video and online fiction enjoy comparatively relaxed censorship. In the first years after launch, partially because technologies generally outpace regulation, these platforms even have a certain freedom in creating otherwise forbidden content types.

The platforms' power without responsibility and regulatory constraints in digital entertainment resulted in the problem that Chinese teenagers are exposed to the proliferation of controversial and vulgar content online. It is thus understandable that public discourses call for strong regulation aimed at reducing or removing the perceived threat. However, as Staksrud (2016, p. 1) argues, good intentions in internet regulations for child protection "might embed unintended consequences and hidden agendas". In China, child protection helps justify already tight internet censorship and could potentially be used to control and discourage youth online activism and protest.

Tao and Donald (2015, p. 40) believe that Asian young people's new media practices are "globally familiar but also fascinatingly uncommon due to the socio-cultural specificity". While Chinese teen digital entertainment is familiar in aspects like participatory culture and platform capitalism, it has unique cultural, economic, and political features largely resulting from the complex negotiation between commercialisation and censorship in China. Very few studies have been conducted to analyse the regulation of Chinese digital entertainment for protecting teenagers under such a special context. In the following sections, two case studies of short video and online fiction explore teenagers' cultural participation and the multidimensional regulatory issues in China's platform-mediated digital entertainment sphere.

Short Video and Chinese Teenagers

Online short video is one of the most rapidly growing digital entertainment industries in China and extremely popular among teenagers. In 2017 there were 240 million active users of short video apps in China and the total industry revenue reached a staggering RMB 5.73 billion ($ 913 million) (iiMedia Research, 2018). The report on Chinese teenagers' internet uses and online safety suggests that, among 13–18-year-olds, short video has bypassed online games and movies and become the most frequent online activity; about 20% of teenagers watch short video with all their play time (China National Radio, 2018). This case study examines one of the most popular short video apps, Douyin (Tik Tok), as an example to analyse the defining features of short video as a new form of digital entertainment, as well as its impact, controversy, and regulation relating to teens' safety and well-being.

Douyin was launched in 2016 and, within just one year, it became the most popular short video app in China, with 150 million daily active viewers (Clegg, 2018). Its international version, Tik Tok, also became the most downloaded app in the global Apple App Store in the first quarter of 2018. Douyin enables users to create and upload 15-second clips, offering them a series of editing tools, filters, and special visual effects. Starting with girl dancing, short-video content in Douyin soon became diverse, ranging from silly stunts to comedy skits and interesting snapshots of everyday life. Popular vloggers receive tips directly paid by users and commissions from online advertising. Some even run their own e-commerce business by adding online shopping links alongside video content. High economic rewards drive content creators in Douyin to do anything that could make them popular online.

To viewers, the design of Tik Tok is 'dangerously addictive' (Newby, 2018). The app shows viewers an endless feed of video automatically, which means, unlike YouTube, viewers do not need to hit a 'play' button to continue. If they are not interested in a video clip, viewers can easily move to the next with a quick flick of the screen. Douyin's interface design was very original and innovative in 2016, though it has been widely copied by competitors since launch. Furthermore, powered by its own patent-protected machine learning technology, the content-recommending algorithm in Douyin is very accurate based on viewing histories. All this makes Douyin so popular and addictive that its seven-day retention rate is as high as 73.8%, which means over 70% of users keep this app in their phones seven days after they initially installed it (JIguang Big Data, 2018).

Apart from technological innovation, Douyin's commercial success could also be attributed to its taking advantage of lagging censorship in the emergent short-video industry. Controversial, pornographic, and vulgar content prevails in Douyin, created and uploaded by individual vloggers with a thirst for popularity. The potential harmful impact on children captures public attention. In a widespread article titled "Douyin, please stay away from our children!", the author listed eight major types of unsuitable and unhealthy content for children, ranging from soft porn, to swear words, flaunting wealth, immoral or dangerous pranks, animal cruelty, and self-harm (Fast Microcourse, 2018).

Moreover, a large amount of controversial content is created or performed by teenagers themselves. The widespread videos of teen pregnancy and teen mothers could be a telling example, which even became a popular genre in short video. The popularity of such videos ceased after the closure of numerous vlogger accounts and a few platforms due to wide public criticism. Another controversial phenomenon is that some teachers inappropriately filmed students without parents' authorisation. In some short-video clips, students were filmed sleeping in the classroom, or embarrassed by learning difficulties; some teachers even played a prank on students or forced them to perform controversially.

Zhu Wei from China University of Political Science and Law points out in a media interview that some short-video creators love to do something immoral or unacceptable to please their fans, blurring the boundaries between ugliness and beauty, and between kindness and evil. "While content creators doing whatever to attract attention and become popular", he further argues, "watching such content is harmful for teenagers in many aspects ranging from mental health to moral/value systems" (Du & Chen, 2018). His view is representative in public criticisms of the out-of-control controversial content in short video, which usually concludes by calling for tight government control and censorship. According to a survey, 63.8% of respondents support the government to enhance regulation and censorship in short-video platforms; 61.9% urge short-video platforms to establish protective mechanisms for teenagers, restricting their registration, viewing time, and ability to watch unsuitable content (Du & Chen, 2018).

The Chinese government has issued some policies to protect children in digital entertainment, especially in online video. For instance, the National Internet Regulating Institute (*wang xin ban*) issued a regulatory note that banned child presenters and performers in the online video industry on 1 December 2016. The government also demands that short-video platforms like Douyin set age restrictions for users and send all users a notification after 90 minutes' continuous watching. The identity checks nowadays even involve advanced facial recognition, making it hard for the underage to take advantage of some loopholes. However, these regulations are poorly enforced in practice. For example, an investigation by *South China Morning Post* found that it is still easy to circumvent age restrictions in most platforms (Zhang, 2018).

Interestingly, Douyin was first banned by the Indonesian government because it "has a lot of negative and harmful content, especially for children" (Reuters Staff, 2018). Why does the Chinese censorship system respond to harmful content so slowly? Technically this could be attributed to the practical mechanism of digital censorship in China. The Chinese censor usually orders platforms to self-censor and delete their vulgar content before banning or closing down the apps. For instance, the Chinese government ordered a major short-video platform to self-check their content in 2017, partially because of the pressure from wide public criticism, and in part because of the growth of politically sensitive video spoofs that make fun of some heroes in Communist propaganda. In this censorship campaign, the major platforms closed over 40,000 accounts, banned 2,083 video presenters, and deleted over 13.5 million messages (Cheng, 2018).

However, the combination of platform self-censorship and top-down censorship campaigns has not 'cleaned' the online sphere, but turns digital censorship into "a tougher game of cat and mouse" (Mozur, 2017), an upgraded version of the edge-ball game in the platform age. It is crucial nowadays for the quick-fire, user-driven short-video apps like Douyin to "balance its exploding popularity with avoiding further interference from the censors" (Newby, 2018).

Online Fiction and Teen Readership

Online fiction started to boom in China in the mid-1990s. In the past 20 years or so it has evolved from amateur writing and fan-fiction into a digital entertainment industry with an economic scale of over RMB 9 billion yuan ($1.43 billion) in 2018. There are over 13 million registered online writers who publish 150 million words each day; among them, 600,000 become contracted authors who earn a stable income from platforms.[1]

Like short video, the online-fiction industry is based on commercialising armature creativity and participatory culture. Its commercial success largely results from a coincidence of the inability of China's print publishing sector to respond effectively to popular demand for entertaining works of fiction and the ability of the internet to enable every netizen to become an author. As online writers enjoy "a level of creative autonomy that could scarcely have been dreamed of before" (Ren and Montgomery, 2012, p. 121), it is unavoidable that many take advantage of censorship failure and attract readers by publishing vulgar content, pulp fiction, porn, and other traditionally unpublishable content, just like what happens in short video. This has certainly attracted similar public criticism since its very early age in the 1990s.

On the other hand, with over 20 years' development, online fiction as a digital entertainment industry has evolved and entered a mature stage with established genres, sustainable models, and a stable readership and fan-base. While self-publishing liberalises Chinese literature, it has also led to the prevalence of popular genre fiction and turned literature into an entertainment industry in China. Fantasy, romance, thrillers, crime stories, ghost stories, and Chinese martial arts fiction (*wuxia*), as well as some new-born digital genres like grave robbers' stories, time travel romance, and alternate history have become the mainstream in the online literary sphere, which, however, attracted very limited attention and interest from traditional writers and literary publishers in the print age.

The online fiction industry has been deeply integrated into the pan-entertainment ecosystem, characterised by IP franchising, fandom, and transmedia storytelling. Mainstream online authors nowadays intentionally avoid writing controversial content that challenges censorship lines (Ren, 2019) because they expect much more revenue from film/TV adaptations and franchising than from selling appealing content directly to readers. For this purpose, they self-censor to accommodate more restrictive censorship in the film and TV industries. In other words, the exposure to vulgar and unsuitable content remains a concern, but not a central issue, in teenagers' engagement in online fiction. Instead, the impact of online popular literature, and the benefits and harms of teens' writing and reading online fiction particularly, become the focus of public debates.

The freedom of online writing and publishing certainly encourages teenagers' participation in literature and this is important in the formation and self-expression of their cultural identities. For example, Jiu Yehui, a popular young novelist, described her motivation for writing as a wish to express herself on behalf of China's one-child generation who feel lonely and lost during their adolescence. Academics like Associate Professor Shao Yanjun from Beijing University also hold positive attitudes towards teen readers' reading of popular online fiction. She found those who grew up reading fantasy and online genre fiction were more imaginative and had higher emotional intelligence and better communication and writing skills (Du, 2017). Mr Jin Tao, a PhD student of Shao, examines middle-school students' participation in the social media discussions of online fiction and argues that social reading experience is beneficial for them in developing relevant skills and is valuable as a cultural memory of adolescence (Du, 2017).

On the other hand, the rise of online literature has divided China's literary realm, particularly between the so-called 'serious literature' and popular literature (Wang, 2015). It is thus understandable that some literary critics, scholars, and parents are resistant to children's participation in online fiction, either as writers or as participatory readers and fans. The time spent on digital entertainment especially concerns parents and educators given China's highly exam-oriented educational system, in which teens are expected to spend most of their time studying, while digital entertainment is regarded as nothing but a waste of time (Ren, 2017). Chinese parents and teachers expect teenagers to spend their precious spare time reading the books with approved cultural and intellectual value like classic literature and popular science, rather than self-published fantasy, time-travel romance, ghost stories, Chinese martial arts fiction, and other 'literary fast food'. Just as a parent criticises, there is nothing in this fiction but sexual and material demands and unrealistic imagination (Wang, 2013).

Deeper concerns and worries exist in the potential negative influences of online fiction on children's value systems, cultural tastes, and even mental health, as some works present controversial values against the mainstream, fake histories, low cultural and literary tastes, and money-worship, which is believed to be possibly imparted into teen readers' minds through entertaining and interesting storytelling (Todd, 1986). Public attention is also captured by some misleading industry narratives of creative entrepreneurship, illustrated by some school dropouts becoming quick-rich teen writers.[2]

The Chinese government has mixed but evolving attitudes towards online fiction. On the one hand, the control over digital content and online writing has become tighter and tighter, ranging from regular "Clean the Pornographic, Strike the Illegal" campaigns that close down numerous online fiction sites, to the requirement for real-name verification for registered online writers. On the other hand, the Chinese government increasingly recognises the economic value of online fiction as a digital creative industry and its value as an exemplar inspiring other media industries in digital innovation and upgrade, particularly relating to government-proposed themes like "Internet plus Arts and Literature", "Publishing/Culture Going Out", and "Mass Entrepreneurship, Mass Innovation" (Keane & Chen, 2019). In other words, due to its apolitical nature and huge economic scale, the Chinese government approves of and even encourages the commercialisation of online fiction and armature writing and the concentration of platforms' market power in digital entertainment. The policy agenda of protecting children from unsuitable and potentially harmful content is being discussed, but obviously has not been given a priority.

Discussion and Conclusion

In 2018 *The New York Times* published an article concerning a generation of Chinese young people who grow up without Google, Facebook, and Twitter. It argues that, "accustomed to the homegrown apps and online services", they are "uninterested in knowing what has been censored online, allowing Beijing to build an alternative value system that competes with Western liberal democracy" (Yuan, 2018). However, building such a value system is more complex and uncertain in reality. Authoritarian government and political censorship have led to de-politicisation of youth digital space in China, where entertainment, rather than politics, is the focus. However, digital entertainment is not totally under government control because platforms are able to circumvent regulation for commercial interests, even within a walled garden of internet. While censorship failure might grow the seeds for youth activism in digital entertainment, it also means big threats to teens' online safety and well-being.

Internet censorship in China is aimed at "preventing the spread of illegal information". In practice, censorship is implemented by pushing the burden of content monitoring and controls down to the lowest level possible, i.e., to platforms and individual content creators (Ruan, 2017). Unsurprisingly, priority is given to political control at all levels. Even for children's content, censorship of politically problematic content is extremely tight and effective. For example, the British animated children's programme Peppa Pig was banned because the main character became a 'subculture icon' on social media increasingly associated with cultural resistance and protests by grassroots young netizens (Walsh, 2018). Platforms are unwilling to challenge the political red line even for commercial interests.

Within apolitical entertainment areas, however, many platforms deliberately defy censorship rules and provide otherwise censored content like porn, controversial and vulgar content. Thus children are exposed to the flood of unsuitable and potentially harmful content due to censorship failure in practice, which has not attracted enough attention from Western researchers who study Chinese internet regulation.

Apart from unsuitable content, the threats to teenagers also include addiction and online bullying. For instance, an independent investigation found that many children use fake ID (over-18 identifications) in online entertainment platforms to avoid the protective measures against addition (Mozur, 2017). Over one third of Chinese teenagers experienced online bullying, scams, and sexual harassment in social media, online forums, and short video communities and only 10–15% told their parents (China National Radio, 2018).

The role of platforms in the less regulated digital entertainment areas is controversial. Though Facebook, Twitter, and Google cannot enter the Chinese market, China has its own internet giants like Tencent (owning the largest social media platforms WeChat and QQ), Baidu (the Chinese search engine), Alibaba (the e-commerce giant), and Toutiao (owning Douyin). There are similar communicative and social problems caused by the monopoly of platforms and digital capitalism in China, which deeply influence the regulation of teen digital entertainment.

Playbour, or the rapid commodification of informal creative labour, is one of the important issues in China's platform-mediated digital sphere for teens. In the field of short video, armature teen creators originally share videos for fun, but their creative labour has been commercially exploited by platforms and their creative practices are being shaped by the overall commercial atmosphere in entertainment platforms. As discussed earlier, some school teachers even forced their students to perform in short videos. In online fiction, internet platforms purposefully portray online creative writing as a fun and rewarding career through the appealing stories of quick-rich writers, sometimes school dropouts, who luckily made a fortune from an enjoyable and nice hobby. However, the commercialisation of online writing in practice is augmented precarity for most writers, including "risks of higher work intensity, diluted creative autonomy, dubious contract terms and less negotiation power against publishers" (Zhao, 2017, p. 1248). The issues around creative labour in China's teen digital entertainment sphere demands more attention from academics and policy makers, and more actions in platform governance and regulation for teenagers' rights as participatory creators.

Chinese scholars usually attribute the failure of regulation or censorship to the communicative model of participatory media, where no filters and gatekeepers stand in the way of the creation of content and children's access to content (*China News*, 2018). In the author's view, the fusion of state power and market power in China's internet industries is an important yet neglected perspective to understand the 'surprisingly' relaxed internet regulation in teen digital entertainment. In China, digital entertainment is valued as a pillar industry in the emergent digital economy because of its economic scale and potential. Such views dominate policy discourses and even academic publications in China. Chinese internet platforms thus operate with less pressure from government, academics, and even the general public than their Western counterparts. For these commercial platforms, implementing restrictive control for child protection would significantly increase operational cost and reduce commercial benefits. Therefore, it sounds like a mutually acceptable situation between state and capital that, while political control remains tight, platforms enjoy more relaxed regulations in terms of entertainment content, industrial monopoly, user privacy, and moral responsibilities, which enable them to explore more commercial opportunities and benefits. Despite some dynamics of teenagers' cultural participation, self-expression, and activism, children are largely unprotected in digital entertainment and the consequences could be serious.

In conclusion, while the Chinese internet regulations and censorship are effective in political control, they are much less effective in protecting children's safety and rights from the wide dissemination of unsuitable content and platforms' capitalising on teen creative labour. Further, the prevalence of digital entertainment reduces the space for youth activism and civic participation, and the less-regulated entertainment areas like online fiction and short video serve as a mechanism for strengthening the apolitical public sphere, spreading consumerism and capitalist values, and discouraging teen citizens' political interests in China.

Notes

1 These figures are from Mr Yijun Zhang, the head of the Digital Publishing Department of China's State Administration of Press, Publication, Radio, Film and Television, see relevant news report at www.xinhuanet.com/fortune/2017-8/14/c_1121481917.htm; there are other articles that provide similar statistics, for example, see www.xinhuanet.com/book/2018-01/31/c_129802946.htm; 333 million Chinese people are active readers in online fiction, accounting for 45.6% of total internet users. Several different sources of information estimate that the overall scale of online literature readership is over 300 million, between 300–400 million. See, for example, http://news.cctv.com/2017/03/29/ARTI4lmUyaPZPwEJ7B4m1C0f170329.shtml or http://tech.sina.com.cn/i/2018-01-31/doc-ifyqyuhy7671103.shtml .
2 See two examples: http://wemedia.ifeng.com/64927643/wemedia.shtml; www.sohu.com/a/121548997_132332.

References

Cheng, S. (2018, June 25). The regulation of short video shouldn't be "short". *People.cn*. Retrieved from: http://opinion.people.com.cn/n1/2018/0625/c1003-30081382.html.
China National Radio (2018, May 31). The launch of a report on Chinese teenagers' Internet uses. *China National Radio*. Retrieved from: http://tech.cnr.cn/techgd/20180531/t20180531_524253869.shtml.

China News (2018, June 1). Future Net and Douyin organise a symposium discussing children protection. *China News*. Retrieved from: www.chinanews.com/business/2018/06-01/8528158.shtml.

Clegg, W. (2018). Tik Tok viewers equal one fifth of China's Internet users. *Yicai Global*. Retrieved from: www.yicaiglobal.com/news/tik-tok-viewers-equal-one-fifth-of-china-internet-users.

Cunningham, S., & Craig, D. (2017). Being 'really real' on YouTube: Authenticity, community and brand culture in social media entertainment. *Media International Australia*, 164(1), 71–81. Retrieved from: https://journals.sagepub.com/doi/full/10.1177/1329878X17709098.

Curtin, M. (2017). Mediating Asia| between state and capital: Asia's media revolution in the age of neo-liberal globalization. *International Journal of Communication*, 11(2017), 1378–1396. Retrieved from: https://ijoc.org/index.php/ijoc/article/view/5156/1980.

Deutsch, N. L., & Theodorou, E. (2010). Aspiring, consuming, becoming: Youth identity in a culture of consumption. *Youth & Society*, 42(2), 229–254.

Du, L. (2017, October 23). Adolescence reading: When online fictions meet university entry exams. *China Youth Online*. Retrieved from: http://zqb.cyol.com/html/2017-10/23/nw.D110000zgqnb_20171023_1-09.htm.

Du, Y. (2017, August 11). Online literature: The age of lonely writing and reading is gone. *Guangming Daily*. Retrieved from: http://epaper.gmw.cn/gmrb/html/2017-08/11/nw.D110000gmrb_20170811_1-05.htm.

Du, Y., & Chen, Z. (2018, April 26). 88.1% respondents believe bad short videos have negative impact on teenagers. *China Youth Online*. Retrieved from: http://zqb.cyol.com/html/2018-04/26/nw.D110000zgqnb_20180426_2-07.htm.

Fast Microcourse. (2018). Douyins, please stay away from our children! Retrieved from: https://new.qq.com/omn/20180408/20180408A1G9BV.html.

Grealy, L., Driscoll, C., Wang, B., & Fu, Y. (2019). Resisting age-ratings in China: The ongoing prehistory of film classification. *Asian Cinema*, 30(1), 53–71. doi.org/10.1386/ac.30.1.53_1.

Guo, S. (2017). When dating shows encounter state censors: A case study of if you are the one. *Media, Culture & Society*, 39(4), 487–503. Retrieved from: https://journals.sagepub.com/doi/10.1177/0163443716648492.

Huang, B., & Xiang, Y. (2017). Creator network: On the evolution of creative class theory under the influence of Internet. *Journal of Shenzhen University (Humanities & Social Sciences)*, 34(2), 50–54.

iiMedia Research (2018). A report on the industrial trends and user behavior in China's short video industry in 2017–8. *iiMedia Research*. Retrieved from: http://iimedia.cn/60925.html.

Jenkins, H. (2006). *Convergence culture: Where old and new media collide*. New York: NYU press.

JIguang Big Data. (2018). Douyin in its rapid growth. *Sina*. Retrieved from: https://t.cj.sina.com.cn/articles/view/2975829210/b15f8cda001005bf7.

Keane, M., & Chen, Y. (2019). Entrepreneurial solutionism, characteristic cultural industries and the Chinese dream. *International Journal of Cultural Policy*, 25(6), 743–755. Retrieved from: doi:10.1080/10286632.2017.1374382.

Ko, C. H., Yen, J. Y., Yen, C. F., Lin, H. C., & Yang, M. J. (2007). Factors predictive for incidence and remission of Internet addiction in young adolescents: A prospective study. *CyberPsychology & Behavior*, 10(4), 545–551. Retrieved from: www.ncbi.nlm.nih.gov/pubmed/17711363.

Livingstone, S., & Blum-Ross, A. (2017). Researching children and childhood in the digital age. In P. Christensen & A. James (Eds.) *Research with children: Perspectives and practices* (pp. 66–82). Abingdon, UK: Routledge.

McGuigan, J. (2009). *Cool capitalism*. London: Pluto Press.

McGuigan, J. (2010). Creative labour, cultural work and individualisation. *International Journal of Cultural Policy*, 16(3), 323–335. Retrieved from: www.tandfonline.com/doi/full/10.1080/10286630903029658.

Mozur, P. (2017, August 3). China's Internet censors play a tougher game of cat and mouse. *New York Times*. Retrieved from: www.nytimes.com/2017/08/03/business/china-internet-censorship.html.

Newby, J. (2018). How Douyin became the most popular app in the world. *Technode*. Retrieved from: https://technode.com/2018/05/10/how-douyin-became-the-most-popular-app-in-the-world.

Ren, X. (2017). Electronic schoolbag and mobile learning in China: Design principles and educational innovations. In A. Murphy, H. Farley, L. E. Dyson, & H. Jones (Eds.) *Mobile learning in higher education in the Asia-Pacific region: Harnessing trends and challenging orthodoxies* (pp. 69–87). Singapore: Springer.

Ren, X. (2019). Publishing and innovation: Disruption in Chinese eBook industry. In D. J. Baker, D. L. Brien, & J. Webb (Eds.) *Publishing & culture* (pp. 199–219). Cambridge: Cambridge Scholars Press.

Ren, X. & Montgomery, L. (2012). Chinese online literature: creative consumers and evolving business models. *Arts Marketing: An International Journal*, 2(2), 118–130. doi.org/doi:10.1108/20442081211274002.

Reuters Staff. (2018). Indonesia bans Chinese video app Tik Tok for 'inappropriate content'. *Reuters*. Retrieved from: www.reuters.com/article/us-indonesia-bytedance-ban/indonesia-bans-chinese-video-app-tik-tok-for-inappropriate-content-idUSKBN1JU0K8.

Ruan, L. (2017). Internet censorship: How China does it. *The Strategist*. Retrieved from: www.aspistrategist.org.au/editors-picks-2017-forgetting-lessons-west.

Sohu.com. (2017, March 30). Chinese scholars conceptualised 'creator economy': A new era of cultural and creative industries? *Sohu.com*. Retrieved from: www.sohu.com/a/131064987_488901.

Srnicek, N. (2017). *Platform capitalism*. Cambridge: Polity.

Staksrud, E. (2016). *Children in the online world: Risk, regulation, rights*. New York: Routledge.

Tao, L., & Donald, S. H. (2015). Migrant youth and new media in Asia. In L. Hjorth & O. Khoo (Eds.) *Routledge handbook of new media in Asia* (pp. 40–50). New York: Routledge.

Todd, W. M. (1986). *Fiction and society in the age of Pushkin: Ideology, institutions, and narrative*. Cambridge, MA: Harvard University Press.

Tong, J. (2019). The taming of critical journalism in China. *Journalism Studies*, *20*(1), 79–96. doi:10.1080/1461670X.2017.1375386.

Tsui, C. (2017, March 8). China's film censorship paradox: Restricted content, unrestricted access. *South China Morning Post*. Retrieved from: www.scmp.com/magazines/post-magazine/arts-music/article/2076755/chinas-film-censorship-paradox-restricted-content.

Walsh, M. (2018, May 1). Peppa Pig blocked on Chinese video app after becoming a 'subculture icon'. *ABC*. Retrieved from: www.abc.net.au/news/2018-05-01/subculture-icon-peppa-pig-blocked-on-chinese-video-app/9713458.

Wang, F. (2013, December 4). Chinese parents' views on online literature: Reading online literature is nothing but wasting time. *China News*. Retrieved from: www.chinanews.com/cul/2013/12-04/5579709.shtml.

Wang, M., & Qi, W. (2017). Harsh parenting and problematic Internet use in Chinese adolescents: Child emotional dysregulation as mediator and child forgiveness as moderator. *Computers in Human Behavior*, *77*, 211–219. doi:10.1016/j.chb.2017.09.005.

Wang, X. (2015). 10 A realm divided in six: Chinese literature today. In K. Yu (Ed.) *On China's cultural transformation* (pp. 181–205). Leiden, The Netherlands: BRILL.

Yuan, L. (2018, August 6). A generation grows up in China without Google, Facebook or Twitter. *New York Times*. Retrieved from: www.nytimes.com/2018/08/06/technology/china-generation-blocked-internet.html.

Zhang, K. (2018, May 19). Hong Kong children expose their identities, thoughts and flesh to millions of strangers on popular iPhone app Tik Tok, post finds. *South China Morning Post*. Retrieved from: www.scmp.com/news/hong-kong/education/article/2146840/hong-kong-children-expose-their-identities-thoughts-and.

Zhao, E. J. (2017). Writing on the assembly line: Informal labour in the formalised online literature market in China. *New Media & Society*, *19*(8), 1236–1252. doi:10.1177/1461444816634675.

52

SEXUAL IMAGES, RISK, AND PERCEPTION AMONG YOUTH

A Nordic Example

Elisabeth Staksrud

Introduction

While it is possible to turn risk assessments into objective mathematical calculations of odds and probability, this is not how most people deal with risk. Instead, risk assessments and the psychological and behavioural consequences of these are based on subjective and often highly emotionally infused reasoning. Thus, risk can also be defined as "the possible effects of actions, which are assessed as unwelcome by the vast majority of human beings" (Renn & Klinke, 2001, p. 12). Two groups directly involved in daily risk management are parents and children/youth.

Looking at online risk in general and sexual risk in particular, this chapter seeks to explore some of the cultural contexts of risk management in one Nordic country. By first looking at the value-grounded roots of Nordic parental mediation strategies and then how children and youth define and experience sexual images online, the chapter aims to broaden the understanding of how sexual risk and, in particular, sexual images/pornography are defined and experienced by children.

Risk in Social Sciences and the Cultural Component of Risk Assessments

The theory underpinning this chapter originates from the 'psychometric paradigm' of risk research. It assumes that there are *several* factors influencing individuals' risk perceptions, including social, cultural, psychological, and institutional, and that it is possible to assess these and their influence on risk management and assessments through mapping and modelling using questionnaires (Wilkinson, 2006; Zinn & Taylor-Gooby, 2006, p. 29). The paradigm has facilitated theoretical frameworks, such as the 'social amplification of risk' framework (SARF) where one seeks to connect psychological, social, and cultural approaches (Pidgeon, Simmons, & Henwood, 2006), ranging from media research to issues of organisational response (see, for instance, Kasperson, Kasperson, Pidgeon, & Slovic, 2003; Kasperson & Kasperson, 2005a, 2005b; Leiss, 2003; Murdock, Petts, & Horlick-Jones, 2003; Pidgeon, Kasperson, & Slovic, 2003; Susarla, 2003). SARF describes and explains the various dynamic social processes that fuel risk perception and response (Kasperson et al., 2003). 'Signals' containing information about specific risks are by default fed through social 'amplification stations', such as experts, politicians, the media, interest groups, or governmental institutions, and their content is altered. Some aspects are intensified while others are suppressed, the result sometimes being unexpected public alarms (Pidgeon et al.,

2006, pp. 100–1). These amplification stations are, by definition, socially influenced (and influences), thereby rendering the final output culturally and contextually dependent. Consequently, it does provide a good tool for the understanding and the analysis of how risk perceptions are seldom context-free and isolated activities, but instead relationally created – and shared – with others (Pidgeon et al., 2006, p. 98).

One immediate benefit of using this analytical framework is its ability to explain otherwise peculiar differences between different national populations' perceptions of risk. For example, studies have found how, in the mobile-phone-saturated Scandinavian countries, there was little concern about health risks, while in (at the time of the sampling) poorly covered countries such as Australia and Italy, there were few phone masts, high levels of concern, and strict regulation (Alaszewski, 2006, p. 172; Burgess, 2002).

Parenting styles and approaches to balancing opportunities and risks are dependent on the type of risks one is concerned about. Risk is something infused with uncertainty but often instigated by a worry. Thus, when people deal with risks, they make decisions based on a potential future, transforming, altering, and reinterpreting risk messages through a variety of lenses. One of these is the cultural context. The hybrid approach is, therefore, at this stage, the one that provides the best insights.

Online Risk

Turning to the specifics of online risks for children, they arise in many varieties and definitions, and with different likelihoods of occurrence and various levels of potential harm. As the internet permeates most (if not all) aspects of society, including education and personal communication, separating online risk from all other risks becomes a complicated matter. In an attempt to systematise online risks as narrated in the public discourse the EU Kids Online networks proposed, and have in over a decade of research worked with, a typology of online risks considering the type of service and interaction facilitating the risk and the role of the child – being a recipient, a participant, or an actor in relation to the risk experienced or produced (see Table 52.1).

Table 52.1 EU Kids Online classification of online risks.

	Content – child as recipient	*Contact – child as participant*	*Conduct – child as actor*
Commercial	Advertising, spam, sponsorship	Tracking, harvesting personal info	Gambling, illegal downloads, hacking
Aggressive	Violent/gruesome/hateful content	Being bullied, harassed, or stalked.	Bullying or harassing one another
Sexual	Pornographic/harmful sexual material	Meeting strangers, being groomed	Creating/uploading pornographic material
Values	Racist, biased info/advice (e.g., drugs)	Self-harm, unwelcome persuasion	Providing advice, for example suicide/pro-anorexia

Source: adapted from Staksrud, E., Livingstone, S., Haddon, L., & Ólafsson, K. (2009). What do we know about children's use of online technologies? A report on data availability and research gaps in Europe (2nd Ed.), p. 18. The London School of Economics and Political Science: LSE Research Online: http://eprints.lse.ac.uk/24367.

Observing the risk of harm along three axes of risk types: encountering sexual images, meeting strangers, and bullying – and including the children (9–16-year-olds) in the 2010 EU Kids Online survey who had encountered risks online (N=5,722), Helsper, Kalmus, Hasebrink, Sagvari, and de Haan (2013) created a country classification model based on the distribution of children in different risk groups. Norway had the highest number of children in the sexual imagery risk group (20%), followed by the Netherlands, Finland, and Denmark, all belonging to a group characterised by a high risk of encountering sexual imagery (the other groups being Low Risk/Harm and Higher Risk/Harm). Interestingly, in this cluster of countries, most children mainly experience sexual risks, but do not encounter *other* risks or harm included in the study.

The same study also researched country-level differences in parental mediation strategies related to the internet. Previous research has looked into how European countries differ in patterns of parental mediation of children's online engagement, depending on the collectivistic versus individualistic orientation of the cultures in question (Kirwil, 2009; Kirwil, Garmendia, Garitaonadia, & Fernandez, 2009). By using cluster analysis, children were grouped together based on their parents' mediation styles, resulting in four groups of children: passive mediation preferred, restrictive mediation preferred, active mediation preferred, and all-rounders, using all the other three types of mediation (Helsper et al., 2013, pp. 27–8). As a result, almost mirroring the sexual imagery group, the Nordic countries and the Netherlands formed a separate group characterised by active mediation, having the highest proportion of parents preferring active mediation (47%), and less than average scores on parents preferring any of the other three mediation strategies. In addition, when looking at parental mediation, children's online opportunities, and children's online risk together, Denmark, Finland, the Netherlands, Norway, and Sweden formed a very clearly defined cluster, characterised by *low levels of restrictive mediation, high levels of sexual imagery risks*, and an advanced and experienced use of the internet, characterised by networking. The explanation for this is suggested to lie in the high internet diffusion and the generally high level of digital skills, also among parents.

Summing up, one of the main impressions and conclusions stemming from previous studies on European children and online risk was that Nordic children in general, and Norwegian children in particular, risk encountering more sexual imagery online, and that parents generally do not restrict their use of the internet – technically or otherwise – but rely considerably on active mediation strategies.

Research Questions

Against this background, seeing risks as potentially socially and culturally subjective constructs, this chapter seeks to further illuminate the *concept of sexual images as a risk for children* through five research questions (RQs).

In the 2010 EU Kids Online survey one in five (23%) of European children between 9 and 16 years said that they had seen obviously sexual images, such as naked people or people having sex. Fourteen per cent had seen such images on websites, while 12% had seen them on television, film, or video/DVD. The survey also revealed striking differences across Europe. In the Nordic countries the numbers were at the higher end of the scale. Forty-six per cent of Norwegian children (34% on websites), 37% in Finland (29% on the web), 41% in Sweden (26% on the web), and 42% in Denmark (28% on the web) had seen such images. This is in contrast to the other end of the scale with Italy (12%, 7% on the web) and Germany (10%, 4% on the web). While these numbers gave insights into the frequency of experiences, based on a single definition, it did not answer the question of what is *considered* sexual content by the children and youth themselves and *whether or not they perceive sexual content as a risk*. This is mirrored in a general challenge of definitions: when assessing sexual risks for children and youth online, it is not always clear what is being talked about and how to define it. In the survey, the measure used for online pornography and sexual content might have been a cultural caveat in itself. For instance, in attempts to operationalise 'pornography' in children's questionnaires into "picture of someone without clothes", this might in some cultures unequivocally connote sexual and pornographic content, but in other cultures it raises questions of context from the children (Was it on the beach? Do you mean breastfeeding? What if the pictures are just for laughs?), not necessarily triggering sexual alerts. Consequently, it is important to understand (RQ1): *what is considered sexual images among children and youth themselves?*

In research and in policy discourses, there is often an interest in frequencies of exposure as direct measurement of risk and harm. To assess the level of actual experience with online sexual content there was the question (RQ2): *how many children have seen sexual images, and from which sources?* Asking about the source of the images might provide further insights into the type of content in question.

However, seeing risk as a potentially subjective construct, *what happens after exposure* is of interest to assess risk perception; thus an important question is (RQ3): *how do children/youth feel after experiencing sexual content online?*

Several studies have linked parental mediation strategies to children's media use in general, as well as to actual online use and risk experiences (see, for instance, Austin, 1993; Haddon, 2015; Liau, Khoo, & Ang, 2008; Livingstone & Helsper, 2008; Livingstone, Mascheroni, Dreier, Chaudron, & Lagae, 2015; Livingstone et al., 2017; Lobe, Segers, & Tsaliki, 2009; Sarre, 2010; Shin & Huh, 2011; Van den Bulck & Van den Bergh, 2000). Assuming that parental mediation strategies influence children's potential risk behaviour online, it is of interest to ask (RQ4): *if and how are parents aware of their children's online viewing of sexual imagery?*

Research has also found how high-risk perception by parents does not mean more restrictive parental mediation. In a previous study on parental mediation of the internet in eight European countries, Livingstone et al. (2017) found that parents who judge risks to be higher are more likely to use enabling rather than restrictive mediation. Active parental mediation is a type of enabling mediation favoured by Norwegian and Nordic parents, which requires active communication with the child on the perceived risk in question. However, little is known about if, how, and to what degree Nordic parents perceive sexual content and interactions as a risk, or not, for children and youth. Thus, it is of interest to get a deeper understanding of (RQ5): *to what degree do Norwegian parents worry about sexual risk compared with other risks?*

Method

To answer the research questions, original analysis has been done using the EU Kids Online 2018 dataset from Norway. Norway is a particularly interesting case as it is the country with the highest score on the independence scale in the world value survey (World Values Survey, 2005–2009). Comparing the percentage of the general population in European countries that considers it to be especially important that a child learns independence at home, the Nordic countries all score high on the independence scale (NO 85%, SE 65%, IS 81%, DK 79%, and FI 51%). They are equally low on the obedience scale, only 21% of Norwegian parents feel it is very important that children learn to be obedient (SE 16%, IS 13%, DK 14%, and FI 20%). Norway is also the country with the highest risk of children seeing sexual images, according to the 2010 EU Kids Online survey (Livingstone, Haddon, Görzig, & Ólafsson, 2011, p. 51).

The data collection, part of a larger European study on opportunities and risks associated with children's use of the internet, was funded by the Norwegian Ministry of Justice and Public Security. The author was the principal investigator and responsible for the survey.

A representative sample of 1,001 children aged from 9 to 17 years and one of their parents was interviewed. The sampling frame was stratified by the economic statistics of municipalities and the number of children. The nationwide distribution of the parents' gender and education was taken into consideration during fieldwork. The data was collected by Ipsos and interviewers visited the recruited respondents at home, while the children and the parents filled out the survey using tablets. Written information about the survey was handed out to the parents and the children. Respondents were informed that they could stop the interview at any moment and that questions could be skipped on the wish of the respondent. Information was also given about national internet awareness centres and reporting hotlines that could be contacted if needed.

Analysis and Discussion

Sexual images, such as pornography, are a risk of the external kind; a concept, images, ideas, and influence that can pose potential psychological, cognitive, behavioural, and value-altering risk to a child if introduced. Against this backdrop, active mediation by talking to the child explicitly about pornography and other sexual risks is a mediation that in itself risks introducing these concepts where there were none before. At the same time, children and youths' own perception of risk – or of what actually constitutes sexual content – will also influence if and how they are able to absorb information, rules, and regulations. So, it is interesting to know what youth themselves consider sexual content (RQ1).

In the survey, a question was added to the Norwegian sample asking 15–17-year-olds what *they* considered to be sexual content (multiple answers possible). Table 52.2 shows the percentages of what is considered sexual content, based on all 15–17-year olds.

While there is a limitation in this particular study that all categories had to be pre-defined, it still provides some interesting insights. First of all, only 1% did not want to answer this question, and 5% said they did not know. This might indicate that most youths have a clear indication of what sexual content means to them. Table 52.2 also shows how, for the majority of youths, the content has to be *explicitly sexual* for them to consider it as 'sexual content'. Fewer than one in three (30%) think that images of half-naked people are sexual, and one in ten (12%) find

Table 52.2 Norwegian youth (15–17) definition of sexual content, in percentage (2018).

Movies or videos showing naked people participating in some form of sexual activity	79
One or more pictures of naked people	70
Sexual content in movies or videos showing naked people	64
Animations showing naked people	47
Images of one or more half-naked people (such as underwear or swimwear models, celebrities in private moments, celebrities in underwear)	30
Drawings of naked people	12
Something else	4
Do not know	5
Do not want to answer	1

Source: table generated from the 2018 EU Kids Online Norwegian dataset.
Notes: children born 2000 to 2002, n=246.

drawings of naked people sexual. This could be the reason why 'only' 42% say they have seen sexual images online during the past 12 months.

In the same way that definitions on what constitute sexual images can vary, so can the perception of risk. It could, for instance, be that Norwegian parents, or even Nordic cultures at large, perceive sexual images and interactions online as a lesser risk compared with others.

When it comes to actual experience with sexual content (RQ2), the data shows that 43% (9–17-year-olds) say they have seen sexual content. Television, movies, and online are the most common places to experience sexual content (Table 52.3). Relevantly, there is an almost complete overlap between seeing sexual images online, including on mobile phones (42%), and having seen sexual images at all (43%). Among the different online services available, 'pop-ups' on the internet and photo- and video-sharing platforms are most common. Interestingly, over half of those who have seen sexual content online (21% of all children) have done so at a pornographic website with adult or 'X-rated' content. Almost one in three (31%, 13% of all children) have experienced having sexual content sent directly to them via their mobile phone.

A way of looking at whether children perceive sexual content online as a risk (or perhaps an opportunity), is to look at how they felt after coming across such content (RQ4). Table 52.4 shows the distribution of children and whether or not they felt happy, upset, or neither happy nor upset.

What is striking is how the 'do not know' category is substantial, especially for the youngest children. One in three children (32%) and over half of the 9–11-year-olds *do not know how to interpret the feelings they have had about the sexual content that they have experienced online*. It also seems that the older you get, the more certain you are of your observation and how you feel about it. There are also gender differences. Most notably there are more boys (18%) than girls

Table 52.3 Where Norwegian children (9–17) have seen sexual content past 12 months (2018), by percentage.

Per cent of those who have seen sexual content . . .	
In a magazine or book	35
On television, film	80
Via a mobile phone, computer, tablet, or any other online device	90
On an online video-sharing platform or site (e.g., YouTube)	52
On an online photo-sharing platform (e.g., Instagram, Flickr)	59
On a social networking site (e.g., Facebook, Twitter)	40
In an online game	25
On a pornographic website (adult or X-rated website)	51
By pop-ups on the internet	68
By a message sent directly to me via my computer	12
By a message sent directly to me on my mobile phone	31
By e-mail	1
In an online advert	31
Some other way	28

Source: table generated from the 2018 EU Kids Online Norwegian dataset.

Table 52.4 How Norwegian children felt after being exposed to sexual content online, by age and gender (2018).

	Don't know	Happy	Neither happy nor upset	A little, fairly, or very upset
Boys	30	18	40	13
Girls	36	5	31	28
9–10 yrs	53	7	7	33
11–12 yrs	61	0	17	22
13–14 yrs	31	7	28	34
15–17 yrs	29	15	42	15
All	32	12	36	20

Source: table generated from the 2018 EU Kids Online Norwegian dataset.

(5%) who report being 'happy' after experiencing sexual content, while more girls (28%) than boys (13%) report having been upset. A logistic regression analysis (Figure 52.1) shows almost the same probability for girls being bothered when they're nine (0.33) as when they're 17 (0.31).

Exploring this further, a follow-up question was asked about other types of feelings. The largest group of children (42%) say that they did not feel anything special after being exposed to sexual content online. The list also shows further gender differences. Girls state embarrassment, anger, fear, and helplessness to a larger degree than boys, while boys to a larger degree express curiosity, excitement, and cheerfulness (Table 52.5).

An explanation for the gender differences might lie in the intentionality of the experience. Exposure to risk can come in many forms, and sexual content online can come as an unwelcome surprise or as an answer to an active request. A continuation question was therefore posed to those children and youths who had seen sexual images online, about whether this was intentional

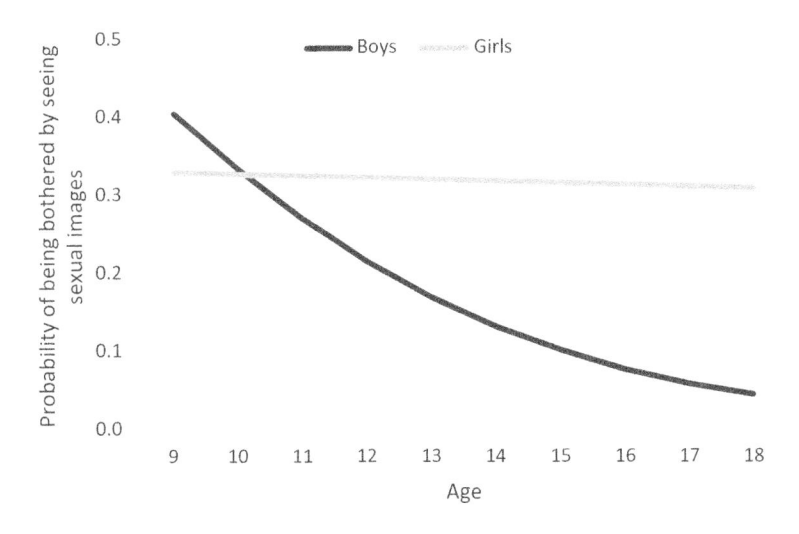

Figure 52.1 Logistic regression of probability for being bothered by seeing sexual images by age and gender (Norwegian Children, 2018).

Table 52.5 Stated feelings of Norwegian children after seeing sexual images (on- or offline), by gender 2018.

	Boys	Girls	All
I felt nothing special	39	46	42
Curiosity	25	13	20
Embarrassment	9	25	16
Excitement	16	6	12
Shame	9	8	8
Cheerfulness	10	1	6
Anger	2	9	5
Humiliation	5	4	5
Fear	2	6	4
Sadness	4	3	3
Helplessness	1	4	2
I don't know	14	6	11
Prefer not to say	8	3	6

Source: table generated from the 2018 EU Kids Online Norwegian dataset.

or not. The results (Table 52.6) show how boys to a larger degree than girls express that they *meant* to see the content in question.

Table 52.6 Intentionality of seeing sexual images online among Norwegian children, by gender (2018).

	Seen this type of content	Saw this material because it was their intention to see it	
		Boys	Girls
A sexual image or video of someone naked	78	74	28
A sexual image or video that shows someone's 'private parts'	69	75	28
An image or video that shows sexual acts or people having sex	67	83	37
An image or video that shows sexual acts in a violent way	17	47	38
Something else sexual	27	73	30

Source: table generated from the 2018 EU Kids Online Norwegian dataset.

Finally, the question of parental awareness of their children's experiences is assessed (RQ4). As Norwegian parents generally favour active mediation strategies, where co-use and dialogue are key factors, one could expect a high level of knowledge among parents regarding their children's online experiences.

Table 52.7 compares the parents' answer to the question "Has your child seen sexual images during the past year" with their child's answer to the question of having seen sexual images during the past year. Please note that both online and offline images are included.

Table 52.7 Parental awareness of children's experience with sexual images versus child's answer (Norwegian sample, 2018).

| | | Child's answer to whether they've seen sexual images (on- or offline) in the past year ||
		No	Yes
Parent's answer to whether their child has seen sexual images in the past year	Yes (22% of parents)	18	29
	No (35% of parents)	43	22
	Don't know (43% of parents)	39	49
	Total	100%*	100%**

Source: table generated from the 2018 EU Kids Online Norwegian dataset.
Note: *n = 526 **n = 377

The results show how the largest group of parents do not know if their child has seen sexual images, while 29% of the children have seen such images, and their parents know about this. Almost 1 in 5 parents think their child has seen sexual images when they have not.

In summary, the results show how some children, in particular younger children and girls, experience sexual images as unwelcome, while many parents are not aware of their experiences.

Sexual risk co-exists with other risks, both offline and online. In order to find out how parents perceive sexual risk compared with other risks (RQ5), two questions were asked about *worries* regarding 26 different (offline) risks and online risks: "thinking about your child, which of these things, if any, do you worry about a lot?" and "Still thinking about your child's internet use do you worry a lot that they may be ...". Following both questions, a list of alternatives was given with the options "yes/no/do not know/prefer not to say". Note that both questions asked about *substantial* worry ('a lot') only.

Table 52.8 ranks the risks according to descending level of worry. Out of the sexual risks (shaded options in the table), a large group of parents (40%) express substantial worry about their child being contacted by a stranger for sexual purposes, followed by exposure to pornography (36% of all parents, with parents of girls expressing more worry than parents with boys).

Generally, parents seem to have a stronger fear of and concern for risks that come as a threat from an external force. Parental awareness and fears related to the internet will typically lean towards content and *contact* risks, rather than *conduct* risks where the child itself plays an active role in creating or facilitating the risk in question. This means risks where something or someone else – a paedophile, a car, another child – initiates some sort of activity that harms your child.

Sexual images and online pornography is something that is made by others with the intent of creating sexual arousal within the recipient/onlooker (and sometimes also for the sender); access to online pornography does in most cases require some sort of action from the spectator. Very rarely, if ever, does one turn on the computer and experience porn that simply arrives on the

Table 52.8 Risks Norwegian parents worry about a lot, as a percentage, according to child's gender and age (2018).

No.	Norwegian parents with children 9–17 years old who answered the questions "Thinking about your child, which of these things, if any, do you worry about a lot?" and "Still thinking about 'your child's' internet use do you worry a lot that they may be ...", as a percentage (2018).	9–12 years Boys	Girls	13–17 years Boys	Girls	All
1	Your child receiving an injury on the roads	63	66	61	57	61
2	Experiencing something that makes my child feel bad about themselves	59	68	46	58	57
3	Using the mobile phone too much	53	57	53	61	56
4	Using the internet too much	56	52	49	53	52
5	A stranger contacting your child on the internet	54	65	42	48	51
6	Using computer games too much	76	36	69	21	51
7	Other children treating your child in a hurtful or nasty way	54	56	41	45	48
8	How your child is doing at school	45	37	45	36	41
9	Contacted by a stranger for sexual purposes	45	59	23	40	40
10	Your child becoming a victim of a crime	35	41	37	39	38
11	Exposed to pornography	40	54	25	32	36
12	Your child's health	38	37	33	34	35
13	Damaging their reputation either now or in the future	33	43	34	31	35
14	Your child revealing personal information online	36	42	33	30	34
15	Exposed to hateful or racist messages or activities	35	49	27	31	34
16	Your child seeing inappropriate material on the internet	44	47	29	21	34
17	Asked to send sexual images/nudes of themselves to someone	35	50	18	35	33
18	Your child treating other children in a hurtful or nasty way	38	38	28	19	30
19	Become socially isolated because of their technology use	33	20	33	18	26
20	Seeing content which encourages them to hurt or harm themselves	26	25	17	18	21
21	Learning to hack/drawn into cybercrime	23	12	14	6	14
22	Having enough money to care for your child	12	16	12	12	13
23	Your child getting into trouble with the police	13	8	16	10	12
24	Your child's sexual activities	8	10	10	13	10
25	Recruited by extremist or fundamentalist groups	9	11	6	9	9
26	Your child drinking too much alcohol/taking drugs	7	4	12	7	8

Source: table generated from the 2018 EU Kids Online Norwegian dataset.

screen. Usually there needs to be some sort of action, a search for something, or previous activities that result in cookies, spyware, or push-ads.

As seen in Table 52.8, sexual risks are risks that are high on the worry scale of Norwegian parents. Sexual conduct risks, such as the child itself creating, uploading, sending, or forwarding sexual images, texts, or other pornographic material, are something parents worry less about. This, in parallel to the general worry about children and youths' conduct – having sexual relations, along with taking drugs, having problems with the police, and drinking alcohol – is rather low.

Conclusion

The overall motivation for this study was to explore some of the cultural contexts of risk management and risk perceptions through one case.

If one accepts the notion of risks as being subjective and culturally dependent, then how risks are *perceived*, rather than a calculation of statistical risk of harm, is a factor to consider also when assessing the existence and quality of risk reduction strategies. Asking children and youth themselves about experiences with sexual images online gives information on this perception. This includes how children may – or may not – consider online activities labelled as 'risk' a problem and/or an opportunity. It also gives insights into how children have different experiences with sexual content online, pointing to the need for differentiated approaches in parental and public risk management strategies.

Sexual and pornographic content is often considered offensive, inappropriate, embarrassing, and sometimes harmful. It is also content that, regardless of how one feels towards the general concept of pornography, most adults will consider inappropriate for children and youth. This also goes for Nordic parents. The results show that Norwegian parents are worried about sexual risk in general and sexual content in particular. This is especially the case for parents with younger children and parents with daughters. The results also show that younger children and girls are those who are the most upset and have negative feelings after seeing sexual images online. Older boys seem to be the least affected by such content.

This study is based on one country alone. More research is needed before one can draw further conclusions on the relationship between cultural values, parental mediation, and online risk experiences among children and youth. It should also be emphasised that often the cultural variations within a country can be more substantial than the variations between countries, something that has not been considered for this present study. The results also point to a need for more research on the gender aspect of sexual risk assessment and experience among youth.

Linking the findings back to the SARF framework, where information about risks are seen to feed through social 'amplification stations', altering their content, culture, and the values embedded in them could be seen as such amplification stations. The output on how one perceives sexual risk – what it is, how big of a worry it is, and the impact it has, can be, at least in part, culturally and contextually dependent, and differ between parents and children.

The results on how children feel after seeing sexual content online show a differentiated pattern, where younger children and girls feel more upset than (older) boys. However, many children do not know how to feel about sexual images. This might pose a challenge and an opportunity for parents to aid children's coping.

Acknowledgements

The author would like to thank Kjartan Ólafsson for assistance in generating the figure for this chapter and Jørgen Kirksæther for valuable advice during the development of this chapter.

References

Alaszewski, A. (2006). Health and risk. In P. Taylor-Gooby & J. Zinn (Eds.), *Risk in social science* (pp. 160–179). Oxford and New York, NY: Oxford University Press.

Austin, E. W. (1993). Exploring the effects of active parental mediation of television content. *Journal of Broadcasting & Electronic Media, 37*(2), 147–158. doi:10.1080/08838159309364212.

Burgess, A. (2002). Comparing national responses to perceived health risks from mobile phone masts. *Health, Risk & Society, 4*(2), 175–188.

Haddon, L. (2015). Children's critical evaluation of parental mediation. *Cyberpsychology: Journal of Psychosocial Research on Cyberspace*, 9(1), Article 2. doi:10.5817/CP2015-1-2.

Helsper, E., Kalmus, V., Hasebrink, U., Sagvari, B., & de Haan, J. (2013). *Country classification: Opportunities, risks, harm and parental mediation*. Retrieved from: http://eprints.lse.ac.uk/52023.

Inglehart, R., Haerpfer, C., Moreno, A., Welzel, C., Kizilova, K., Diez-Medrano, J., ... & Puranen, B. (2014). *World values survey: Round five–country-pooled datafile 2005–2008*. Madrid: JD Systems Institute. Retrieved from: www.worldvaluessurvey.org/WVSDocumentationWV5.jsp.

Kasperson, J. X., & Kasperson, R. E. (2005a). *The social contours of risk: Publics, risk communication and the social amplification of risk (vol. 1)*. London and Sterling, VA: Earthscan.

Kasperson, J. X., & Kasperson, R. E. (2005b). *The social contours of risk: Vol II: Risk analysis, corporations and the globalization of risk*. London: Earthscan.

Kasperson, J. X., Kasperson, R. E., Pidgeon, N. F., & Slovic, P. (2003). The social amplification of risk: Assessing fifteen years of research and theory. In N. F. Pidgeon, R. E. Kasperson, & P. Slovic (Eds.), *The social amplification of risk* (pp. 13–46). Cambridge: Cambridge University Press.

Kirwil, L. (2009). Parental mediation of children's Internet use in different European countries. *Journal of Children and Media*, 3(4), 394–409. doi:10.1080/17482790903233440.

Kirwil, L., Garmendia, M., Garitaonadia, C., & Fernandez, G. M. (2009). Parental mediation. In S. Livingstone & L. Haddon (Eds.), *Kids online* (pp. 199–215). London: The Policy Press.

Leiss, W. (2003). Searching for the public policy relevance of the risk amplification framework. In N. F. Pidgeon, R. E. Kasperson, & P. Slovic (Eds.), *The social amplification of risk* (pp. 355–373). Cambridge: Cambridge University Press.

Liau, A., Khoo, A., & Ang, P. (2008). Parental awareness and monitoring of adolescent Internet use. *Current Psychology*, 27(4), 217–233. doi:10.1007/s12144-008-9038-6.

Livingstone, S., Haddon, L., Görzig, A., & Ólafsson, K. (2011). *Risk and safety on the internet. The perspective of European children. Full findings from the EU Kids Online survey of 9-16 year olds and their parents*. Retrieved from: http://eprints.lse.ac.uk/33731.

Livingstone, S., & Helsper, E. J. (2008). Parental mediation and children's Internet use. *Journal of Broadcasting & Electronic Media*, 52(4), 581–599.

Livingstone, S., Mascheroni, G., Dreier, M., Chaudron, S., & Lagae, K. (2015). *How parents of young children manage digital devices at home: The role of income, education and parental style*. Retrieved from: http://eprints.lse.ac.uk/63378.

Livingstone, S., Ólafsson, K., Helsper, E. J., Lupiáñez-Villanueva, F., Veltri, G. A., & Folkvord, F. (2017). Maximizing opportunities and minimizing risks for children online: The role of digital skills in emerging strategies of parental mediation. *Journal of Communication*, 67(1), 82–105. doi:10.1111/jcom.12277.

Lobe, B., Segers, K., & Tsaliki, L. (2009). The role of parental mediation in explaining cross-national experiences of risk. In S. Livingstone & L. Haddon (Eds.), *Kids online* (pp. 173–183). London: The Policy Press.

Murdock, G., Petts, J., & Horlick-Jones, T. (2003). After amplification: Rethinking the role of the media in risk communication. In N. F. Pidgeon, R. E. Kasperson, & P. Slovic (Eds.), *The social amplification of risk* (pp. 156–178). Cambridge: Cambridge University Press.

Pidgeon, N., Simmons, P., & Henwood, K. (2006). Risk, environment, and technology. In P. Taylor-Gooby & J. Zinn (Eds.), *Risk in social science* (pp. 94–116). Oxford and New York, NY: Oxford University Press.

Pidgeon, N. F., Kasperson, R. E., & Slovic, P. (2003). *The social amplification of risk*. Cambridge: Cambridge University Press.

Renn, O., & Klinke, A. (2001). Risk evaluation and risk management for institutional and regulatory policy. In A. Stirling (Ed.), *ESTO project report, on science and precaution in the management of technological risk. Volume II case studies* (pp. 11–37). Seville: European Commission – JRC Institute Prospective Technological Studies.

Sarre, S. (2010). Parental regulation of teenagers' time: Processes and meanings. *Childhood*, 17(1), 61–75. doi:10.1177/0907568209351551.

Shin, W., & Huh, J. (2011). Parental mediation of teenagers' video game playing: Antecedents and consequences. *New Media & Society*, 13(6), 945–962. doi:10.1177/1461444810388025.

Staksrud, E., Livingstone, S., Haddon, L., & Ólafsson, K. (2009). *What do we know about children's use of online technologies? A report on data availability and research gaps in Europe* (2nd ed.). Retrieved from LSE, London: www.eukidsonline.net.

Susarla, A. (2003). Plague and arsenic: Assignment of blame in the mass media and the social amplification and attenuation of risk. In N. F. Pidgeon, R. E. Kasperson, & P. Slovic (Eds.), *The social amplification of risk* (pp. 179–206). Cambridge: Cambridge University Press.

Van den Bulck, J., & Van den Bergh, B. (2000). The influence of perceived parental guidance patterns on children's media use: Gender differences and media displacement. *Journal of Broadcasting & Electronic Media, 44*(3), 329–348. doi:10.1207/s15506878jobem4403_1.

Wilkinson, I. (2006). Psychology and risk. In G. Mythen & S. Walklate (Eds.), *Beyond the risk society: Critical reflections on risk and human security* (pp. 25–42). Maidenhead and New York, NY: Open University Press.

Zinn, J., & Taylor-Gooby, P. (2006). Risk as an interdisciplinary research area. In P. Taylor-Gooby & J. Zinn (Eds.), *Risk in social science* (pp. 20–53). Oxford and New York, NY: Oxford University Press.

53

US-BASED TOY UNBOXING PRODUCTION IN CHILDREN'S CULTURE

Jarrod Walczer

Introduction

Are unboxing videos what they sound like? Media scholars Craig and Cunningham (2017, p. 78) note that despite its relative size and popularity that "unboxing is poorly defined and understood". To some, the popular internet genre is little more than one in which people mediate their opening up or otherwise unveiling of products followed shortly by their review, play, or other types of engagement with said product on-screen (for more general history, see Stoeber, 2018). Some toy unboxing content creators, however, have generated billions of video views and hundreds of millions of subscribers on the video-sharing platform YouTube and its child-centric subordinate YouTube Kids. These video views have generated substantial profit and notoriety for some, notably seven-year-old Ryan of *Ryan ToysReview*, who was YouTube's highest earner in 2018 at over $22,000,000 for his amassed 26 billion views and 17.3 million subscribers (Berg, 2018). Many of these views are assumed to be coming from children and their families, given the substantial number of videos focussed on the unpacking or unwrapping of toys, candy, surprise eggs, and other commercial products of interest to children varying in price and cultural capital depending on individual channel practices. Nevertheless, the toy unboxing phenomenon's commercial success is flavoured, if not tainted, by assertions that this segment of the children's media industry is manipulative and untoward in their content and that, by unveiling a product in a positive or celebratory light, these videos are necessarily commercial and possess explicit intentions to sell the product on the screen. Still, when pleasure is derived, as indicated by toy unboxing videos' popularity, one can challenge the basis for reductive assumptions and question the empirical grounding used to study this content, the creators who make this content, and the child viewers who engage with this content. This chapter draws from 25 in-depth semi-structured interviews with US-based toy unboxing content creators to position toy unboxing videos as having a rich and nuanced creator culture and as a disruptor to the children's media industry. This chapter seeks to brings balance to the more theoretical tensions of structure and agency in contemporary children's culture within which toy unboxing videos play an important role.

This research uses Jenkins' definition of children's culture and grounding "what it means to be a child, how adult institutions impact children's lives, and how children construct their cultural and social identities" (1998, p. 3) against the meanings currently constructed, defined, and circulated as being representative of toy unboxing videos as media. Doing so not only focusses the attention of this chapter on the diachronic cultural dynamics of children's media in a networked era but also considers children's culture theories within the broader circuit of culture that the researcher constructed and uses to examine toy unboxing. This chapter extends upon both Du Gay et al.'s (2013) updated circuit of culture framework and Buckingham's (2008) three-pronged circuit of culture. This chapter's circuit of culture, however, suggests that toy unboxing videos have their conventions, practices, and exchanges in which meanings are established, distributed, and negotiated within the networked interactions of content creators, content viewers, and YouTube as a platform, series of algorithms, and a corporation. This chapter, thus, frames the toy unboxing circuit of culture within a genre of content that is co-created, negotiated, and regulated by the actors above that also is indicative of and subject to contemporary children's culture debates. This research argues that it is the networked trust and tastes of the various channels and related personae that produce these texts, the audiences which consume and give their attention to these texts, and YouTube as the global firm and platform that houses and shape these texts which facilitate the political-economic conditions which have generated inquiry into the phenomenon itself.

Buckingham (2008) suggests that cultural studies theories and frameworks, like the circuit of culture, have long been concerned with "how cultural meanings and pleasures are produced and circulated within society and how individuals or social groups use and interpret cultural texts" (p. 2) and practices to construct social identities. As such, this research considers social negotiation over toy unboxing and the dynamics between adults and children who engage with them. It situates child viewers of unboxing videos as active viewers – not passive – with agency, though not wholly 'media-wise'. It does not take up the mantle that children's culture is de facto commercialised or commodified and instead looks to balance the 'power of the text' with the 'power of the audience' as "the relationship between children and the media can only be fully understood in the context of a wider analysis of the ways in which both are constructed and defined" (Buckingham, 2008, pp. 227–8). In this chapter, the practice of children's content creators (including those that are considered inimical to a child's well-being) are brought to light.

Making Sense of Toy Unboxing Videos

While academic research on unboxing videos, in general, has been scant in quantity, the interventions made thus far have been meaningful in laying the groundwork for this approach. Marsh, an academic researching young people's digital literacy practices, acknowledges that "[o]n the surface, the viewing of unboxing videos may appear to be a straightforward consumerist practice, which is focused on the desire of goods – a form of vicarious consumption" (Marsh, 2015, p. 375). However, she situates the viewing of unboxing videos within children's digital literacy practices in the home. Marsh acknowledges their value within the material culture of children and childhood as a "mode of cultural transmission [that] is a growing feature of online practices for this age group in the twenty-first century" (Marsh, 2015, p. 369). Other scholars, such as Nicoll and Nansen (2018), situate toy unboxing videos within children's affinity wherein children participate and co-create a space for unboxing videos to fit within children's culture by identifying and affiliating with them through informal literacies. Sharif Mowlabocus, a digital culture expert, has also published about unboxing videos, but has focussed on the unboxing of smartphones and discusses the pleasures of the broader unboxing genre. He writes that "communities of viewers are built up around [toy unboxing] channels and creators speak of how unboxing provides new ways to engage, share and interact with their children, as well as to generate an alternative revenue source" (Mowlabocus, 2018, p. 2).

These nuanced academic approaches, however, struggle for the spotlight as other concerns have been raised by popular press reporting on the same three toy unboxing channels – the hand-channel *FunToys Collector Disney Toys Review* (formerly known as *DisneyToyCollectorBR*) and child personality channels *EvanTubeHD* and *Ryan ToysReview*. It is not surprising nor undeserved that these channels receive such media attention when one considers their record-breaking view counts, subscriber bases, assumed monetary gains from AdSense revenues, and debated commercial ties (especially regarding sponsorship or branded content disclosures) despite their everyday relatability. It does, however, largely frame the broader toy unboxing phenomenon around these three individuals and pushes the thousands of other creators with less notoriety further out of the limelight.

Other concerns ranging from how YouTube videos are algorithmically suggested and made visible to audiences (Gillespie, 2014), to advertising disclosures (Campbell, 2017), to exposure to inappropriate or dangerous content (Bridle, 2017) have further compounded longstanding children's culture concerns and, through YouTube and YouTube Kids, created a perfect storm to frame toy unboxing videos as the new nadir of consumer capitalism and children's consumption in the digital age (Buckingham, 2011). However, moral panics around toy unboxing videos and their impact on children's culture are often bereft of the meaningful academic interventions listed above. Thus, the following sub-sections examine different facets of toy unboxing's circuit of culture intending to make sense of toy unboxing videos and open dialogues to discuss the impact they have on children's culture and the children's media industry.

Genre, Content, Texts, and Taste

As stated above, Mowlabocus (2018) focussed on smartphone unboxing to discuss the genre's propensity to touch and handle the objects, its cinematic perspective, and its audience orientation regardless of the products being unpackaged. He discusses the "affective intensities and tactile pleasures that structure these texts and which locate the genre within a broader landscape of consumer culture" (p. 3) – a chief concern of many children's culture critics. Mowlabocus writes that "it is possible to identify a set of common narrative tropes and visual conventions, some or all of which appear in the majority of unboxing videos" (p. 5). These techniques range from a narrative that documents a first engagement with the object being unboxed to a short discussion about how the product was acquired, whether for personal use or simple review, to the 'money shot' removal of the object before being temporarily set aside. The researcher deemed Mowlabocus's framework as applicable to toys, artifacts, and other products being unboxed that personify material children's culture, as Marsh suggests (2015; pp. 370–3). Many of these categories were also used in Nicoll and Nansen's (2018) content analysis of 100 toy unboxing videos, wherein they analysed varying levels of calibrated amateurism and professionalism (Abidin, 2017) and compared techniques of mimesis between professional and amateur channels and adult and child channels. By examining the practices and media rituals in these videos, they signpost a convergence of children's affinity spaces for different brands, products, and toys as well as newly developed affinity spaces around genre aesthetics, individual YouTubers, and broader internet genre content conventions. Here too, their invoking of mimesis suggests that amateur channels borrow techniques from and imitate professional channels and vice versa in the same way that adult-hosted channels and child-hosted channels imitate one another (pp. 9–11).

As both studies break down some of the conventions of unboxing videos, both allude to the inherently social and even participatory process that viewers – here, child viewers – engage in when constructing judgement about new genres of content (Jenkins, 1998). As such, understanding children's judgement of media and quality of children's media as a genre (both how adults and children construct and conceive of such judgements) is a matter of significant consideration in the digital age. Lauricella, Robb, and Wartella (2013) contend that making such determinations, however, is far from an easy task given the varied definitions of quality children's media.

This research contends that it is far more challenging to determine the quality of toy unboxing videos as opposed to other content of interest to children because of the particular political sensitivities and framing around under-aged children being on YouTube and platformised ambiguities of YouTube and YouTube Kids that shape the culture of toy unboxing videos (Hess, 2017; Rubin, 2018). Contemporary sentiments that position toy unboxing videos as far beyond the golden age of quality programming and as being too puerile or manipulative to be appropriate, let alone in good taste, are rampant in popular discourse. Drawing from Lauricella, Robb, and Wartella, however, one can look at "the age-appropriateness of material for the child, [the] characteristics of content, and the social experience of the context" to determine which toy unboxing videos and which toy unboxing channels are appropriate or quality by both children and adults and by both creators and viewers (2013, p. 5).

Channels and Personae

Where media and education scholar David Buckingham contends that "we need to pay careful attention to the ways in which those on all 'sides' of this debate construct and view children" (2011, p. 22), this research also suggests that careful attention is paid to how individual toy unboxing content creators are constructed and viewed given the networked co-construction of toy unboxing as a genre. Drawing from interviews with 24 different toy unboxing content creators in the United States, which represent 65 currently active channels on YouTube, this research acknowledges a wide variety of personalities, specialisations, and techniques that toy unboxing channels use to construct and calibrate their channels and online personae – many of which stand counter to channels like Evan's, Ryan's, and FunToyCollector's. Further, as both research on identity in children's culture and research on identity on social media platforms often discuss children's overall lack of agency, this research suggests that many toy unboxers are less agentic than popular discourse might lead readers to believe. Many creators, like Nat from the *Toys Unlimited* family of channels, expressed that they are, "left negotiating how [they] make [their] content between what [they] think a child viewer and their family might want or need and what will make [them] algorithmically visible" (Nathalie, personal communication, 2 December 2018).

This matter is further complicated as both adults and children, separately and jointly, have successfully established themselves as experts in the toy unboxing genre. Agentic concerns over whether or not parents are producing, co-producing, or sharenting their children's online identity have prompted concern over child labour laws for those younger YouTubers and questions about the blurred lines between playing in/on and working for social media (Blum-Ross & Livingstone, 2017; Leaver & Abidin, 2018). This research takes the position that the representation of adults in children's culture should not be restricted to the role of the adult but should also serve as an intersubjective 'voice' for children. To that end, many content creators described how their online identities and personae are modified or performed and sometimes turned into a series of digitally mediated and algorithmically determined tasks in order to pay their bills, let alone get close to their creative intentions.

The task of tailoring content to the algorithm, whether enacted by children or adults (with or without prompting or mimesis), has been identified as vital to toy unboxing channels' ability to further intimate connections with viewers and establish their expertise in various affinity networks. This tailoring does not diminish the tensions that have been raised between the social construction of a toy unboxer's presumed commerciality and their identity construction and personal practice on YouTube, however. With limited empirical scholarship on how much agency individual YouTube channels have to position their content within YouTube, let alone analysis for child-specific channels, one must consider how the global firm that YouTube has become will continue to impact children's culture with the content it privileges and the big data it generates from child viewers and creators alike.

YouTube as a Global Firm

Where digital media scholars Burgess and Green (2018) contend that one cannot look at YouTube as a platform without investigating its creators and users, so too does this research acknowledge that each toy unboxing video's success is shaped by the YouTube platform and the networked data it generates. Media scholar and COPPA architect Kathryn Montgomery explained that "the imperatives and practices of the Big Data era are also having a transformative impact on children's media culture, fostering new data-driven business models, ushering in a new generation of digital platforms, and influencing social, personal, and cultural practices" (Montgomery, 2015, p. 267). Montgomery, in turn, prompting researchers to reconsider how they study children's content on YouTube by citing the significance that big data could have in datafying and subsequently commercialising children's culture. Montgomery contends that "data-driven media for children and teens may also encourage and reward certain tendencies and behavior patterns ... that could, in turn, become internalised and normalised" (Montgomery, 2015, p. 270).

A recent Pew Research Center study found that YouTube is a key content provider for children's culture with 10% of all YouTube views in 2016 coming from kids entertainment, in some cases representing more than half of a given country's entire view count (Smith, Toor, & van Kessel, 2018). The study goes on to note that 81% of parents with children under the age of 11 allow their children to watch content on YouTube, with 34% allowing this to become a regular activity, despite 61% having found at least some content that was deemed unfit for child consumption. Further still, the study found that "videos suggested by the site's recommendation engine finds that users are directed to progressively longer and more popular content". This research contends, therefore, that YouTube's recommendation system uses the data generated by child and parent users of the platform to suggest content that the algorithm determines will keep users engaged longer, thus pulling users in for longer viewing sessions by pushing targeted and individualised content towards them. Further, in the interviews conducted for this research, many creators indicated that they were wholly dependent upon YouTube and that, despite having reservations about some of their practices, they would not survive without the platform (see Nieborg & Poell, 2018 for discussion on platform dependency).

Pairing YouTube's use culture and media rituals together with these figures about YouTube's platform and algorithmic design directives highlight how YouTube's prominence as a media and data firm spans not only across the globe but across the networked era in which contemporary children's culture resides. It is here that one can look at YouTube as a global firm and question what roles it may have in prompting consumer enculturation or what Cook describes as "the variety of ways in which children come to 'know' and participate in commercial life" and what the implications of this are (Cook in Buckingham & Tingstad, 2010, p. 70). Here too, one can look at how the political-economic dimensions of YouTube as a platform have incentivised individuals to join the platform while concurrently shaping the production culture of some genres, like toy unboxing, and allowing them to be framed as the root cause of consumerist concerns in contemporary children's culture despite having little to no agency over platformised decisions.

The Production Culture and Political Economy

Using Mowlabocus's notion that "[u]nboxing is integral to the broader YouTube economy", (2018, p. 5), it is unsurprising that creating like Ryan and Evan won the war for eyeball attention among children. However, toy unboxing is also shaped by the YouTube recommendation system and the content creators making or optimising their content to be algorithmically privileged. Thus, participants in and critics of children's culture should question how to untangle the economic and corporate dimensions of YouTube, toy companies, and intermediaries from the more social, creative, conceptual, and interpersonal dynamics of these creators and their production culture. Drawing from Caldwell's (2009) point that content creators "seldom systematically elaborate on [questions of production] in lengthy spoken or written forms" (p. 7), this chapter recognises how the existing framing of toy unboxers has not yet prompted the recording of personal reflections.

Toy unboxing videos' place in children's culture has primarily been one where objectors to the genre or critics of the culture have read into a varied ensemble of media texts but have been unsuccessful or have not attempted to look over the shoulder of those whom they belong to or who place value in them. While meaningful ground setting has been done by Craig and Cunningham (2017) in their initial conjecture that toy unboxing embodies a form of creator labour within their political-economic framework of social media entertainment as a media industry, this research seeks to extend their notion. This research sees the political-economic dimensions of toy unboxing entwined with the production culture that is informed by those dimensions. This research, therefore, positions the rituals, production practices, and working methods of toy unboxing creators as being even more precarious than Craig and Cunningham proposed in 2017. This research also sees toy unboxing as wildly misunderstood and understudied – particularly regarding how it has been framed as positioning child audiences and their data as commodities to be exchanged for advertising revenue or toy company cash.

As this scholarship has developed, nuances have surfaced even amongst some toy unboxing sceptics and critics. Common Sense Media, a non-profit focussed on promoting safe media and technology for children and their families, wrote that

> Companies don't usually pay [a toy unboxer] directly for featuring their product in a video. When an unboxer becomes super popular (with tens of millions of views and subscribers), companies may send them products for free, but not always. Sometimes hosts disclose this, sometimes not.
>
> *(Common Sense Media, 2018)*

This acknowledgement alone brings the political-economic question of whether children are commodified by the toy unboxing community or not to a head by challenging presumptions about toy companies holding puppet strings over creators in producing toy unboxing videos. While Common Sense Media does acknowledge that "extremely popular and influential YouTubers [are monetarily compensated] in other areas [like making] a personal appearance at a toy store or a toy convention", this has no measurable direct effect on how much algorithmic visibility is given to that channel's video or even if a given toy company will send free product to that channel. Despite this clash between the political-economic frameworks and the production culture which shape the contextual dynamics of toy unboxing, it *is* the desire of both YouTube and the toy unboxer to obtain the audience's attention and have them consume the videos being made.

Audience Attention and Consumption

In examining the relationships between the object being unboxed, the creator unboxing and mediating the unboxing of the object, the viewer of the video, and the YouTube platform itself, this portion of the circuit of culture induces a multidimensional sociality of emotion which can prompt or foster audience attention and channel video, platform, or product consumption. This demonstrates a noteworthy change in children's culture by exploring how intimate communications can be mediated, structured, and utilised through the conditions of its existence by all actors involved. At the apex of this attention and consumption is the contentious blurring of play and work, material and immaterial, and online and offline, which parents struggle to navigate alongside their children as viewers and content creators (Sefton-Green, 2018). Such context collapses are complicated when family entertainment channels on YouTube have had an average of roughly 200% year-over-year growth.

Such figures beg the question about whether it is the platform, the videos, the YouTuber, the affinity networks, or a confluence of them all, which creates a desire for children to give their attention to YouTube, YouTubers, and toy unboxing videos. Jackie Marsh explained that the attention children pay to toy unboxing videos is primarily based on pre-existing interests in the brands or toys being unboxed (Craig & Cunningham, 2017, p. 82). Marsh also noted that little research has been conducted around how the videos prompt buying or further consumption beyond the videos themselves. An additional consideration regarding consumption comes from a consensus between academics like Seiter (2005) and industry practitioners like Rosenberg (2004) that kids are interested in learning about or playing with other kids and that they trust other kids to a higher degree than adults. Where some might suggest that toy unboxing creators bilk off this and blend advertising and children's content conventions to foster and nurture child viewer attention and prompt consumption (Ramos-Serrano & Herrero-Diz, 2016; Campbell, 2017), this research suggests that more pertinent matters obfuscate the severity of any supposed commodification of children's culture with other issues of trust and regulation that children's culture faces through digital media.

Trust and Regulation

In 2017, author James Bridle wrote a viral article detailing what is now called the 'ElsaGate' scandal on YouTube and YouTube Kids. This scandal, in which dubious and satirical content featuring popular branded characters like Spiderman impregnating Disney princess Elsa or Peppa Pig drinking bleach made it onto YouTube and, to a lesser degree, onto YouTube Kids, rocked the children's media industry and children's culture experts and critics alike. While journalist Ben Popper explained that, "YouTube announced that it would no longer allow creators to monetise videos which 'made inappropriate use of family-friendly characters'", and that it was "in the process of implementing a new policy that age restricts this content in the YouTube main app when flagged", stating that "age-restricted content is automatically not allowed in YouTube Kids", fears were already rampant (Popper, 2017).

The difficulty for the toy unboxing community, whose largest concern or critique is the commercialisation of childhood argument rehearsed above, was that Bridle wrote about their content (as well as children's nursery rhymes) in the same article – framing their content and the concerns held about their content alongside more egregious and devious content. In doing so, the toy unboxing genre suffered by Bridle's association, ranging from losing algorithmic visibility, to loss of advertising revenue, to having a more staunchly negative connotation being associated with them than before. This article brought to light that YouTube and YouTube Kids have both algorithmic filters and employees and volunteers working across different time zones to review content. However, it also brought about additional questions ranging from how children may or may not be an algorithm's or a creator's unwitting target to why YouTube is not prepared to "ban the use of family-friendly characters by creators who are not the original copyright holders" (Popper, 2017). These have both positive and negative connotations for toy unboxing creators, viewers, and content as a whole. As screens continue to be used for a blend of "entertainment, learning, discovery, communication, play, creation, and more", each of which is prompted by an algorithmic suggestion, it is not surprising that parents and lobbyist groups are concerned about digital media's impact on children's culture (Kleeman, 2017). However, as parents and children tread the uncharted territories and increasingly porous boundaries between algorithms, platforms, tablets and mobile technologies, commercial brands, native YouTube channels, advertising, and content, this research argues that there is still room for, and indeed a need for, toy unboxing videos to be seen as pleasurable texts. One might even consider toy unboxing videos to be positive and important to children's culture on the whole – notwithstanding those channels that subversively push the purchase of commodities or commercial goods of poor quality and value without disclosing as much.

Looking Forward

Today's children are dually framed as being empowered through their having a digital childhood – or one that has never known content that was not mostly accessible anywhere and anytime, interactive, and customisable – and being in the direct line of fire for the risks of big data culture, niche algorithmic targeting, and covert advertising. Today's adults, as shapers of children's culture, examine these risks and will inevitably create appropriate parental controls, policies, and regulatory efforts to mitigate them and protect children's rights (Livingstone & Third, 2017). It is this research's conjecture, however, that they should also look at the content in question and ask if a toy unboxing video, an interaction with a given YouTuber, or even the toy being unboxed will provide a benefit to the child in question. Drawing from industry strategist David Kleeman, this research would like adults overseeing YouTube and content like toy unboxing videos, parents, and toy unboxing creators alike to ruminate on the idea that "child development doesn't change, but the context in which children grow and learn does" (Kleeman, 2017).

As children's culture changes with and through digital media, toy unboxing videos have brought to a head both longstanding cultural anxieties and new concerns as parenting transcends the physical into the digital and everyday children experience elevated access to and participation in social media attention economies. Children's culture, therefore, should not view children's digital practices as wholly separate from those in the 'real world' or even from the platforms and content that are deemed for adults. Furthermore, before regulatory efforts are made by state governments, YouTube, lobbyists, parents and guardians, and toy companies, this research entreats such parties to consider the entire circuit of culture surrounding toy unboxing videos and the agency that children's culture theories may have in shaping active engagements on YouTube. By acknowledging that the production of toy unboxing videos stems primarily from individuals who are not necessarily beholden to the commercial toy companies but are dependent upon the algorithmic pressures of YouTube, the uses of these videos and the intentions behind them may be better understood and may find a place in children's culture beyond being kindling for commodification and commercialisation discussions.

References

Abidin, C. (2017). #familygoals: Family influencers, calibrated amateurism, and justifying young digital labor. *Social Media + Society*, *3*(2), April–June 2017, 1–15.
Berg, M. (2018). How this 7-year-old made $22 million playing with toys. *Forbes*. 3 December 2018. Retrieved from: www.forbes.com/sites/maddieberg/2018/12/03/how-this-seven-year-old-made-22-million-playing-with-toys-2/#235819154459.
Blum-Ross, A., & Livingstone, S. (2017). 'Sharenting', parent blogging, and the boundaries of the digital self. *Popular Communication*, *15*(2), 110–125.
Bridle, J. (2017). Something is wrong on the Internet. *Medium*. 06 November 2017. Retrieved from: https://medium.com/@jamesbridle/something-is-wrong-on-the-internet-c39c471271d2.

Buckingham, D. (2008). Children and media: A cultural studies approach. In K. Drotner & S. Livingstone (Eds.), *Handbook of children, media, and culture* (pp. 219–236). London, UK: Sage.

Buckingham, D. (2011). *The material child: Growing up in consumer culture*. Cambridge, MA: Polity.

Burgess, J., & Green, J. (2018). *YouTube: Online videos and participatory culture* (2nd Edition). Cambridge, MA: Polity.

Caldwell, J. (2009). Cultures of production: Studying industry's deep texts, reflexive rituals, and managed self-disclosures. In J. Holt & A. Perren (Eds.), *Media industries: History, theory, and methods* (pp. 199–212). Malden, MA: Blackwell.

Campbell, A. J. (2017). Rethinking children's advertising policies for the digital age. *Georgetown University Law Center*. 01–55. Retrieved from: http://scholarship.law.georgetown.edu/facpub/1945.

Common Sense Media. (2018). What are YouTube unboxing videos? *Common Sense Media*. Retrieved from: www.commonsensemedia.org/youtube/what-are-youtube-unboxing-videos.

Cook, D. T. (2010). Commercial enculturation: Moving beyond consumer socialization. In D. Buckingham & V. Tingstad (Eds.), *Childhood and consumer culture* (p. 70). London, UK: Palgrave Macmillan.

Craig, D., & Cunningham, S. (2017). Toy unboxing: Living in a(n unregulated) material world. *Media International Australia*. Online First. Retrieved from: http://journals.sagepub.com/doi/abs/10.1177/1329878X17693700.

Du Gay, P., Hall, S., Janes, L., Madsen, A. K., MacKay, H., & Negus, K. (2013). *Doing cultural studies: The story of the Sony Walkman* (2nd Edition). London, UK: The Open University Press.

Gillespie, T. (2014). The relevance of algorithms. In T. Gillespie, P. J. Boczkowski, & K. A. Foot (Eds.), *Media technologies* (pp. 167–193). Cambridge, MA: MIT Press.

Hess, A. (2017). How unboxing videos soothe our consumerist brains. *The New York Times*. Retrieved from: www.nytimes.com/video/arts/100000005777067/unboxing-videos-internet.html.

Jenkins, H. (1998). *The children's culture reader*. New York, NY: New York University (NYU) Press.

Kleeman, D. (2017). The genius of play is in the child, not the toy. *KidScreen*. 23 February 2017. Retrieved from: http://kidscreen.com/2017/02/23/the-genius-of-play-is-in-the-child-not-the-toy.

Lauricella, A., Robb, M., & Wartella, E. (2013). Challenges and suggestions for determining quality in children's media. In D. Lemish (Ed.), *The Routledge international handbook of children, adolescents, and media* (pp. 425–432). New York, NY: Routledge.

Leaver, T., & Abidin, C. (2018). From YouTube to TV, and back again: Viral video child stars and media flows in the era of social media. Internet Research 2018, Selected Papers of #AoIR2018, Montreal, Canada, 10–13 October.

Livingstone, S., & Third, A. (2017). Children and young people's rights in the digital age: An emerging agenda. *New Media & Society*, *19*(5), 657–670.

Marsh, J. (2015). 'Unboxing' videos: Co-construction of the child as cyberflaneur. *Discourse: Studies in the Cultural Politics of Education*, *37*(3), 369–380.

Montgomery, K. C. (2015). Children's media culture in a big data world. *Journal of Children and Media*, *9*(2), 266–271.

Mowlabocus, S. (2018). "Let's get this thing open": The pleasures of unboxing videos. *The European Journal of Cultural Studies*. Retrieved from: http://sro.sussex.ac.uk/id/eprint/78712.

Nicoll, B., & Nansen, B. (2018). Mimetic production in YouTube toy unboxing videos. *Social Media + Society*, *4*(3), 1–12.

Nieborg, D. B., & Poell, T. (2018). The platformization of cultural production: Theorizing the contingent cultural commodity. *New Media & Society*, *20*(11), 4275–4292.

Popper, B. (2017). YouTube says it will crack down on bizarre videos targeting children. *The Verge*. 9 November 2017. Retrieved from: www.theverge.com/2017/11/9/16629788/youtube-kids-distrubing-inappropriate-flag-age-restrict.

Ramos-Serrano, M., & Herrero-Diz, P. (2016). Unboxing and brands: YouTubers phenomenon through the case study of EvanTubeHD. *Prisma Social: Revista de ciencias sociales*, May 2016, 90–120.

Rosenberg, M. B. (2004). *Getting past the pain between us: Healing and reconciliation without compromise*. Encinitas, CA: PuddleDancer Press.

Rubin, M. (2018). The world of kids on YouTube is wild, weird, and almost entirely unregulated. *Quartz News*. Retrieved from: https://qz.com/1500662/the-world-of-kids-on-youtube-is-wild-weird-and-almost-entirely-unregulated.

Sefton-Green, J. (2018). Changing family cultures: The politics of learning with digital media, mapping a provocation. *The YCC Network*. 01 October 2018. Retrieved from: https://yccnetwork.net/wp-content/uploads/2018/09/Provocation-paper-v3.1.pdf.

Seiter, E. (2005). *The internet playground: Children's access, entertainment, and mis-education*. New York, NY: Peter Lang.

Smith, A., Toor, S., & van Kessel, P. (2018). Many turn to YouTube for children's content, news, how-to lessons. *Pew Research Centre*. 7 November 2018. Retrieved from: www.pewinternet.org/2018/11/07/many-turn-to-youtube-for-childrens-content-news-how-to-lessons.

Stoeber, J. (2018). A brief history of unboxing videos. *Polygon*. 25 May 2018. Retrieved from: www.polygon.com/2018/5/25/17393882/unboxing-video-history.

54
THE ROLE OF DIGITAL MEDIA IN THE LIVES OF SOME AMERICAN MUSLIM CHILDREN, 2010–2019

Nahid Afrose Kabir

Introduction

Many Muslim children in America are growing up within the realm of two worlds, their parents' country of origin and their place of birth or residence, America. They acquaint themselves with their parental culture in their home and when they visit their parents' home country. For example, a US-born child of Bangladeshi heritage would learn about his ethnic culture from family and extended family living in Bangladesh or America. At the same time, the child would become familiar with his American surroundings from his Day Care Centre, then from his school, teachers, and American friends. He is also growing up in a digital age, finding the use of internet, social media, Snapchat, etc., useful and entertaining. Being a digital child can help him negotiate his hybrid cultures. This chapter explores the role of digital media in the lives of some Muslim American children, 18 in 2010 and 4 in 2016–2019. Within the framework of social constructivism (Charmaz, 2006), the research question informing this chapter is whether digital media is helping some young Muslims in the negotiation of their identity/identities and assisting them in their communication skills.

Earlier research on Muslim children growing up in America has found that many are living in extremely challenging times (Garrod & Kilkenny, 2014). The challenges are multi-layered, with Kabir (2014, 2017) finding that many second-generation Muslim youth face tremendous challenges in both cultures – cultural restrictions in their family environment and Islamophobia (fear of Muslims) within wider society. Most of their parents are first-generation immigrants who arrived in the US under either the skilled or humanitarian categories. Initially, many first-generation immigrants experience culture shock (Ahmed, 2013; Kibria, 2011; Mir, 2014). In this new cultural environment, many Muslim parents living in a diaspora become overprotective of their children (Haddad, Smith, & Moore, 2006, pp. 14, 84–5).

Brubaker (2006) observed that a diaspora is an immigrant population that lives as a minority and envisions a real and imagined homeland (Anderson, 1983) by maintaining a collective memory and myth about their birthplace. But Muslim youth are able to manoeuvre between both their ethnic/religious culture and mainstream American culture by using their bicultural skills (Bhabha, 2004). That is, they retain their ethnic culture (language and traditional culture) and Islamic culture (religion) while also adopting American culture (English language, music, and sports).

Islamophobia

Following the Twin Towers attacks by the Al Qaeda Muslim terrorists in New York on 11 September 2001, Islamophobia became more evident in American society, manifesting in the physical and verbal abuse of people with a Muslim appearance, particularly women wearing a *hijab* (headscarf); and including resistance from the wider society to Muslim initiatives such as new mosques, and racial profiling at airports (Bayoumi, 2015; Kabir, 2018; Sirin & Fine, 2008).

Following the election of the Trump administration in 2016, Islamophobia has become exacerbated. Early in his term of office, the President ordered a ban on immigration from some Muslim countries (Thrush, 2017), increasing the anxiety of many Muslims in America. This has helped create conditions where young American Muslims may feel excluded from broader American society, potentially increasing their risk of disaffection. According to the United States Pew Survey report (July 2017), 48% of Muslims reported that they experienced at least one incident of discrimination in the past 12 months. The Council of American-Islamic Relations (Bharath & Gazzar, 2018) report found that President Trump's 'anti-Muslim rhetoric' has been a contributor to the increased hate crimes against Muslims. Negative Islamophobic influences have impacted upon the lives of the research participants, for example Samiha (16 years) said:

> I had an experience in a park where my friend and I were walking. I didn't wear the *hijab* but my friend did at the time. And we were waiting for the slide when two girls said, "why don't you fix your faces?" They then followed us when we left, pulled my hair and my friend's scarf off.
>
> *(Interview, New York, 2016)*

Another participant, Suraiya (16 years), said:

> I am a hijabi and I had a headphone in my ear listening to music when I was in an elevator. Within a crowd in the elevator, one man asked me to press the button on the elevator for him. I did not hear at first hand … what he said. He repeated, and I finally did what he asked. Then within the ride, he started yelling at me. He said I am a retard. That if I don't understand the language I should go back to my country. "You and your people not the type to be here". There were seven other people in the elevator and no one said anything. It all happened so fast, yet the moment felt so long.
>
> *(Interview, New York, 2019)*

Research (Iner & Esposito, 2019; Kabir, 2019) indicates that experience of Islamophobia can be very challenging for young people and may occasionally lead to the radicalisation of young Muslims. In such circumstances, one or more of the "seven other people in the elevator" might helpfully have intervened and Suraiya may have felt less exposed.

Research Methodology

This chapter draws upon interviews with 22 young people. Eighteen interviews were conducted in 2010 in Massachusetts and New York, with a further four between 2016 and 2019 in Michigan, New York, and Virginia. The participants were 15 to 18 years old. The participants attended public and Islamic schools (Table 54.1). Under the United States immigration law, a child refers to anyone who is under the age of 21. This research uses a qualitative method, namely in-depth interviews, which were recorded either digitally or by note-taking. The first project (Kabir, 2014) focussed on young American Muslims' identity and sense of belonging.

Table 54.1 Participants, with pseudonyms, from Massachusetts, Michigan, New York, and Virginia, USA, aged 15–18 years. Interviews conducted in 2010* and 2016–2019^.

No	Pseudonym & gender	Age	Nationality	Identity, as stated by participant	Use of digital media
1*	Mateen Male	16	US-born of Sudanese origin	Sudanese American Muslim	Uses iPod. Part-time job. Assisted youth in job search through the use of computer.
2*	Faisal Male	16	US-born of Lebanese origin	Arab American	Computer business, fixes people's computers and gets paid.
3*	Aida Female	16	US-born of Indian origin	Just Muslim	I did a computer job in the wider community during the summer break.
4*	Muzna Female	16	Overseas-born of Pakistani origin	I am proud to say that I am from Pakistan	I have computer class that's Excel. I watch some religious programmes, I also listen to songs.
5*	Fahima Female	16	US-born of Pakistani origin	Pakistani Muslim American	Computer games are more of a boy thing. I use computer for my emails and chat with my friends. I hang around with my *Desi* community.
6*	Nargis Female	16	Overseas-born of Pakistani origin	I am a Pakistani American	We watch new movies on the internet. My older sister has a laptop from school. We have a house computer so we just use that to watch cricket.
7*	Hanif Male	16	US-born of Pakistani origin	100% American	I watch sports through internet. My favourite team is New York Giants. I never went to the stadium to watch the game.
8*	Yasmeen Female	15	US-born of Pakistani and American origin	Muslim American	I read Quran through the internet. I like to read the translation in English and read the actual word in Arabic.
9*	Sultana Female	16	US-born of Pakistani origin	Pakistani	I sometimes play computer games with my brothers.
10*	Farzana Female	17	Overseas-born of Bangladeshi origin	I am a pure Bengali	I listen to Bengali songs through computer. I like songs of the Renaissance band. I hear it through YouTube.
11*	Lokman Male	16	Overseas-born of Pakistani origin	Pakistani American	I have Computer Science as a school subject.
12*	Nusrat Female	15	US-born of Palestinian origin	Muslim Palestinian	No computer. Father does not allow it.
13*	Fatima Female	16	US-born of Egyptian origin	Arab American	I have the Google phone. I play games that come with it. Google phone, it's expensive, it's like $300. My dad got it for my birthday.

(Continued)

Table 54.1 (Cont.)

No	Pseudonym & gender	Age	Nationality	Identity, as stated by participant	Use of digital media
14*	Afrosa Female	15	US-born of Pakistani origin	Muslim Pakistani American	I am not allowed to use a mobile phone or computer.
15*	Sulaiman Male	15	Overseas-born of Egyptian origin	Muslim Egyptian	I have an iPod. I listen to Islamic artists. Like Native Deen, like Naeem, Joshua. Their latest song is "Not Afraid to Stand Alone". In TV Iqraa Channel, I watch Islamic programmes with my grandmother. Also, I watch English programmes, *The Simpsons*, Forensic Science, etc.
16*	Ahmed Male	15	US-born of Egyptian origin	Egyptian	On my phone I have Egyptian and American music. I use computer for emails. I don't have much time for computer. I attend school, do my homework, and memorising the Quran. My mother is my Quran teacher.
17*	Habib Male	16	Overseas-born of Egyptian origin	Egyptian	Yes, computer, email, and listen to music on phone. I always call my cousins in Egypt. I am in touch with them every week on the email.
18*	Salma Female	15	US-born of Sudanese origin	African American	I have iPod. I listen to music, Hip Hop, Rhythm and Blue.
19^	Samiha Female	16	Overseas-born of Bangladeshi origin	Muslim American	I have Facebook account. I use Instagram, Snapchat, Facebook messenger. Digital media carried stories of Omran Daqneesh. Digital media can provide ISIL's counter-narratives.
20^	Nasreen Female	16	US-born of Bangladeshi origin	Muslim American Bangladeshi	I use Instagram for my photographs. I am connected with my cousins in Bangladesh through Snapchat. Digital media can be powered by gossips.
21^	Mahmud Male	17	Overseas-born of Yemeni origin	Sunni Muslim	Digital media can dispel stereotypes.
22^	Suraiya Female	16	US-born of Bangladeshi origin	Muslim American	I listen to music through my iPhone. I have Facebook account. I have experienced Islamophobia for my *hijab*.

This data is used as a background and counterpoint to the more recent interviews, which were conducted from 2016 to 2019 as part of a project investigating the possible association of digital media with the radicalisation of young American Muslims. The researcher collected four interviews (one digitally recorded and three by note-taking).

This chapter employs grounded theory (Glaser & Strauss, 1967). Its goal is to gain a better understanding of participants' identity formation and negotiation as American Muslims, as supported by or manifested in their use of digital media. The analysis applies a constructivist method of interpretation (Charmaz, 2006) and emphasises the participants' capacity to create meaning in their lives and social contexts. All recorded interviews were transcribed and the transcriptions and the contemporaneous notes were coded and analysed.

Muslim Children's Identity and Their Use of Digital Media

The 22 participants identified themselves as having a single identity, a dual identity, or multiple identities. As Kabir (2012, 2014) argues, identity represents a process and is in a constant state of flux: negotiable, contextual, situational, and circumstantial. Emotion plays an important role in the formation of a person's identity, reflecting dynamics of 'us' and 'them'. This section examines how participants constructed their identity/identities and how digital media plays a vital part in that construction. It also reflects upon how some Muslim American children negotiate their identity, moving between being an American child and a Muslim child while being part of a cultural/ethnic diaspora (see Table 54.1).

The first 18 interviews, consisting of 7 males and 11 females, were conducted in 2010. All 18 interviewees used digital media except two 15-year-old female participants, Nusrat and Afrosa, whose parents did not allow them to do so. A common theme across the participants at that time was their familiarity with digital media, including the use of emails, internet chatting, entertainment (music, movies, and sports), and access to cultural and Islamic websites. Two 16-year-old male participants, Mateen and Faisal, and one 16-year-old female participant, Aida, did part-time computer-related jobs.

The most recent interviews consisted of one male and three female participants, and they were immersed in social media, discussing their use of Facebook, Instagram, Snapchat, and Twitter. The four interviewees, Samiha, Nasreen, Mahmud, and Suraiya, kept abreast of current news via the internet.

The Role of Digital Media in Young Migrants' Diasporic Lives

Hossain and Veenstra (2017, pp. 6–7) argue that digital media allow diasporic peoples to maintain their family and friendship ties. Young migrants learn how to use emails and social networks to feel closer to their family members in their parents' country of origin and this helps them to use their native language with their fellow country folk, strengthening their sense of identity. Immigrants use communication technologies for a range of different purposes including mitigating the trauma of separation and handling life in their new communities. These technologies can also aid in the adaption process of integrating within their host society (Fortunati, Pertierra, & Vincent, 2012, p. 10).

Alba and Nee (2005) have argued that second-generation migrants are unlikely to engage with their parents' country of origin with the same intensity and frequency as their parents. Green and Kabir (2012) observed, for example, that information and communication technologies (ICTs) assist second-generation Australian migrant children to negotiate their cultural difference by engaging with the majority culture, establishing friendships with their mainstream Australian counterparts, and also exercising their rights as global citizens by expressing opinions on political activity at home and abroad. Yet Green and Kabir (2012, pp. 96–7) also found that a few conservative immigrant parents imposed restrictions relating to ICTs because they feared digital media would lead to cultural erosion (see also Table 54.1).

Digital Media in American Muslim Children's Lives, 2010

In 2010, two of the 18 participants said they were not allowed to use computers. In some families, the decision not to have a computer may indicate a religious or cultural concern about external influences (Green & Kabir, 2012, p. 94). The remaining 16 participants said they generally used digital media for entertainment, online games, music (hip hop, etc.), movies, sport (football, cricket), email, and internet chat. Although these may seem like ephemeral pastimes, important themes emerged from the interviews.

Integration within the Muslim Community

Fahima (female, 16 years, Pakistani heritage) identified as Pakistani Muslim American (Table 54.1). She thought that computer games were "more of a boy thing", so she focussed her computer use on emails and chatting with her friends. Fahima said, "I have friends from any culture. But I hang around with people from different backgrounds. It's like a whole, a *desi* [South Asian diasporic] community". Sometimes she had differences of opinion and arguments with her friends, but she resolved them through internet chatting. Fahima commented:

> You know how Bengalis and Pakis (Pakistanis) don't get along, right? Yeah, history influences people but I have Bengali friends. When some Bengali girls find out that I'm Paki, right? They started saying things about me. I don't say anything back to them. I was like, "you think of me that way", but after they got to know me they wanted to become my friend. I said "you shouldn't judge a person by if they come from a certain country, and I don't like it when somebody says something bad about my country".
> *(Interview, New York, 2010)*

Before the partition of India in 1947, there was one Bengal that included East and West Bengal. With the partition of India, East Bengal became East Pakistan (1947–1971) and, from 1971, East Pakistan became an independent country, Bangladesh. Throughout this time, West Bengal remained part of India. People from these two regions are called Bengalis because they speak the same language, Bangla/Bengali. However, for Fahima, her use of Bengali referred to Bangladeshis because of the previous political conflict between East Pakistan (now Bangladesh) and West Pakistan (now Pakistan). Fahima's views reflect upon the old enmities that exist in South Asian diasporic communities. Apart from political issues, there are cultural differences between Bangladeshi and Pakistani Muslims including language and dress. So sometimes diasporic communities bring their cultural differences with them to their host country, and it can impact on their children. In her interview, however, Fahima demonstrates her willingness to forge "a whole, a *desi* community" (interview, New York, 2010).

This perspective is further reinforced in Fahima's construction of her faith. There are two major denominations of Islam, Sunni and Shia Islam. Globally, Sunni Muslims form a majority (about 85%) and Shia Muslims a minority (about 15%) (Nasr, 2002). But there can be tensions between these two communities and ISIL (Islamic State of Iraq and the Levant), for example, has waged "a genocidal anti-Shia campaign conducted under the guise of resurrecting the caliphate" (Gerges, 2017, p. 24). Fahima commented:

> Sunni, Shias yeah, it's like Bengalis and Pakistanis, they don't get along. But I don't have a problem because we're all Muslim, we all pray to one God. We all believe in one thing. It's like fighting with your own self.
> *(Interview, New York, 2010)*

Digital media proved useful for Fahima to negotiate her *desi* Pakistani Muslim identity. Through emails and chatting she has negotiated differences with her friends from diverse backgrounds, building a sense of what they have in common as they make their way within American society.

Teens Mateen and Faisal were sufficiently digitally skilled to have part-time computer repair jobs. Mateen (male, 16 years, Sudanese heritage) attended an Islamic school and identified himself as Sudanese American Muslim. He had already performed *Umrah Hajj* (a pilgrimage to Mecca that can be performed anytime in the year except the *Hajj* period) and through his part-time job Mateen assisted young people to navigate digital media. Mateen stated:

> I worked with children, mostly Americans and Hispanic community, who have disabilities or come from low-income families. I would help them find jobs [by navigating the internet] in the summer to pretty much get them out of trouble. I felt like that was the job that suited me perfectly, because I gave back to the community in a certain way by helping those young adults.
>
> *(Interview, Massachusetts, 2010)*

In 'othering' Americans and the Hispanic community, Mateen implicitly identifies himself as 'not-them', yet his American pride in having given 'back to the community' identifies Mateen's perception that he and the young people he worked with are all part of the same broader community within the USA. Mateen is grateful to digital media because his technical skills allow him to help the broader community.

Faisal (male, 16 years, Lebanese heritage), like Mateen, attended an Islamic school, but he identified as 'just Muslim'. He considered listening to music as *haram* (forbidden in Islam) and only listened to *nasheeds* (devotional Islamic songs). However, Faisal did not restrict himself only to his Muslim community: "I have a small business that I run. I manage IT, computers, phones, computer management, and software unlocking. I advertise online. I've recently finished building a website". Faisal also helped his school with IT. "It's a [religious] requirement to do certain volunteer work in the community. I've worked as an aide to the school in terms of technological help as well as advertising" (interview, Massachusetts, 2010). Faisal's voluntary work with local non-Muslim community organisations helping the poor and homeless gave him an insight into the many different groups and communities disadvantaged within American society. This led Faisal to believe that Muslim Americans are not always particularly marginalised.

Digital Media in American Muslim Children's Lives, 2016–2019

By 2016, participants' focus on digital media had become more diversified, reflecting the rise in social networking and app use. In the 2016–2019 interview cohort, all four participants mentioned their use of Facebook and Twitter, and two specifically discussed Islamophobia (see also Table 54.1). These four participants attended public schools.

Samiha (female, 16 years, Bangladeshi heritage) said that she offered prayers, but in a way that integrated her religious identity within her school context: "I try to pray three times out of the five mandatory prayers. I try to pray *Asr*, *Maghrib* and *Isha*. I miss the rest of it because of school and other activities" (interview, New York, 2016). Samiha identified as Muslim American and became especially passionate when discussing her concern about how ISIL was exploiting USA foreign policy as a strategy for recruiting disaffected young American Muslims. She referred to an August 2016 media story about five-year-old Syrian boy Omran Daqneesh from the war zone in Aleppo, Syria (see CNN, 2016). Samiha commented:

> Most young Muslims noticed that America is going into war with many Islamic countries and, between these wars, these young American Muslims notice the violence that is occurring, e.g., a bomb blast in Syria killed a family and left a little boy [Omran Daqneesh] alive

with long-lasting mental and physical injuries. Now these young Muslims are questioning what was the fault of [the] innocent Syrian child [to provoke this attack]?

(Interview, New York, 2016)

Samiha went on to share her views on how to counter ISIL's narratives of radicalisation through digital media by, "circulating the aftermath of the choices of these ISIL fighters and so-called jihadi brides in news and digital media so these people [audiences] can understand the reality of this matter, which is violence and hatred" (interview, New York, 2016). Having rejected ISIL's purported religious identity, Samiha suggested that young American Muslims could be protected against radicalisation by "posting on digital media, e.g. Instagram, Twitter, Facebook, we can make aware to other people of these horrendous outcomes of the militants and what happens to the ISIL fighters, as well as their violent actions" (interview, New York, 2016). In this way, Samiha identifies digital media as enabling users to challenge dominant narratives (USA foreign policy) and the potential radicalisation of audiences.

Projecting a Public Image

In her 2018 interview, Nasreen (female, 16 years, Bangladeshi heritage) identified herself as being Muslim American Bangladeshi. Nasreen said, "I am connected with my cousins in Bangladesh through Snapchat. You take pictures and send it to your friends – texting with the picture but picture disappears" (interview, Virginia, 2018). Nasreen's Muslim identity was revealed when she spoke of her digital media activities with her friends:

> I wear *hijab* and I use Instagram for my photographs. My other *hijabi* friends are very much into fashion. They use [follow] bloggers and Instagram. They gain support through positive feedback or may get discouraged with negative feedback. But it should not affect them because, Islamically, it is important for individuals to find peace within oneself. Once they find peace in themselves and have a strong bond with God, so negative comments would not affect them.
>
> (Interview, Virginia, 2018)

Nasreen noted as a negative that digital media is often powered by gossip, and that people make assumptions about others rather than hearing from the person themselves. Although she hoped faith would help young people feel strong enough to be unaffected, Nasreen said, "it can hurt another person if their [other people's] comments are consistently rude. For example, if they post something without the other person's permission" (interview, Virginia, 2018). Nasreen also noted the role of digital media in challenging popular stereotypes, however, "Muslim girls are usually misunderstood as shy, quiet, composed women. But through the digital media they can express themselves as outgoing despite what society says about them" (interview, Virginia, 2018).

Nasreen went on to discuss how digital media has provided a platform for different social and political movements such as the Women's March (responding to President Trump's inauguration and now an annual and global movement #WomensWave), Black Lives Matter, lesbian, gay, bisexual and transgender matters, and gun control. These media create an outlet for ideas to be spread. She also discussed how digital media can mobilise a community, for example after the horrendous rape and murder of 17-year-old Muslim girl Nabra Hassanen in July 2017. About 5,000 mourners attended Nabra's funeral (Barakat, 2017). Nasreen said, "The community came together … There is a website called 'GoFundMe' so that people can donate for Nabra" (interview, Virginia, 2018).

An Outlet for Muslim and Non-Muslim Understanding

Echchaibi (2013) observes that American Muslims have created a range of alternative digital media sites such as the blog site *AltMuslims*, which was developed immediately after 9/11 to counter anti-Muslim sentiment. The site offers Muslims an opportunity to discuss cultural issues and connect with non-Muslims. *Muslimah Media Watch* allows feminist Muslims to critique the representation of Muslim women in popular culture and advocate for more diverse voices in discussions of Islam in America and beyond. It addresses the topics of misogyny, sexism, patriarchy, Islamophobia, and racism (Echchaibi, 2013, pp. 129–30).

In 2016 some American Muslims in Fremont, California, started a #MeetAMuslim Campaign with a sign, "I am a Muslim, Ask Me Anything". They also opened up a Facebook account, "Meet A Muslim", to dispel misconceptions about the faith (www.facebook.com/MeetAMuslim Community), and the campaign has since spread throughout America.

The last 2016–2019 interviewee, Mahmud (male, 18 years, Yemeni heritage), did not specifically mention his ethnic or civic identity but said that he was a Sunni Muslim. His views on digital media reflected his Muslim American identity, however, while his interests demonstrate his engagement in the local community politics of his area, as represented on Facebook:

> The other day I was on Facebook, so it's a lot of non-Muslims in this group, so it's like to revitalise the city. And someone commented about infidels [non-believers]. There's some debates politically happening right now, the Muslim voting block on the council has a view on one thing and then coincidentally the non-Muslims voting block have a view on another thing. It's not a religious issue, it's more of a city management issue. But that's how the coalitions have been split [constructed, it] is the Muslims and then the non-Muslims. So that amplifies this whole [… division]. From time to time you'll hear someone spewed out something, "Oh, this is *Sharia* law", or, "I'm an infidel", and they don't really understand. It's like, "No, you're not an infidel". I spoke to someone and he knows I'm Muslim and he knows I'm Yemeni and I asked him, "Why aren't you running for office?" because he's involved in politics and he says, "Because I'm an infidel". And although I'm sure he meant it [as] a joke it's kind of concerning that this is how some people [are] thinking.
>
> *(Interview, Michigan, 2017)*

These comments reveal Mahmud's view that the ongoing anti-Muslim rhetoric that Muslims want to introduce *Sharia* law is not helpful or accurate; nor is the perception of some non-Muslims that they could not be elected as representatives of a predominantly Muslim area because they are 'infidels'.

Islamophobia and Its Consequences

Lean (2017, p. 105) offers a range of examples to demonstrate that digital media can serve as a platform for Islamophobia. This can be counterproductive when it comes to supporting the social integration of Muslims in the USA, and the development of integrated American Muslim identities. Lean (2017, p. 64) noted that some bloggers such as Robert Spencer and Pamela Geller, identified by Islamic community leaders as anti-Islam, publish around 300 blog posts every month by simply re-blogging or copying chunks of previously written news stories with new titles and new images to portray Islam in a negative light. Phrases such as "jihad mass murder", "jihad suicide bombing" and "jihad martyrdom" frequently appear on Robert Spencer's blog *Jihad Watch*. Teen interviewee Nasreen said that the "media such as CNN, Fox News often stereotype Muslims as terrorists. Teenagers are easily susceptible and influenced by what they hear" (interview, Virginia, 2018). Although young Muslims like Nasreen might try to counter negative perceptions, she finds that, "It is tough to have decent conversation through the digital media. Things may be taken out of context" (interview, Virginia, 2018).

Mahmud noted how Islamophobia can help create the conditions for the radicalisation of American Muslim children:

> If I'm a 13-year-old boy who lives in a suburb that's predominantly white but I live there because my dad's a wealthy doctor or whatever the case may be, and I'm the only person of colour there or the only Muslim person there and they mock me and tease me, and Trump says this [Muslim ban], and then I discover an ISIL [Islamic State of Iraq and the Levant] website. I may have an interest now because the government hates me, my friends hate me, this group of people [ISIL] send message through their Twitter accounts, saying, "Hey, we're willing to help you", the children may fall into ISIL trap.
>
> *(Interview, Michigan, 2017)*

Perhaps partly in response to President Trump's Muslim ban (Thrush, 2017) and a perceived permission to be more openly Islamophobic, the Council on Islamic-American Relations identified a significant increase in the number of anti-Muslim hate groups in America during 2017 (Bharath & Gazzar, 2018). Thirteen states in the USA also introduced anti-*Sharia* bills, with Texas and Arkansas going as far as enacting legislation. In addition to this negative fear-mongering, there were anti-Muslim hate rallies in 28 cities on 10 June 2017, indicating that Islamophobia was on the rise (Beirich & Buchanan, 2018).

Arguably, digital media is implicated in these dynamics. Ott argues (2017, p. 64) that Trump's use of Twitter in particular and digital media in general constitutes a "politics of debasement", stating that his "simple, impulsive, and uncivil Tweets do more than merely reflect sexism, racism, homophobia, and xenophobia; they spread those ideologies like social cancer". Kharakh and Primack (2016) argue that these divisive ideologies resonate with white supremacist rhetoric.

This is the digital environment in which young American Muslims are being socialised, constructing personal identities and assuming their role as the next generation of American Muslim citizens.

Conclusion

This research shows young American Muslims using digital media to negotiate community relations and explore differences, developing friendships through emails and internet chatting as Fatima did in 2010; with Mateen and Faisal using digital media to assist the wider non-Muslim community. Samiha, Nasreen, and Mahmud continued these practices in 2016–2019. Throughout the past decade, digital media have helped participants negotiate their identity/identities through their communication skills and through connecting with family and friends locally, nationally, and globally.

With the growing popularity of Twitter, Instagram, and Snapchat, the more recent participants had adopted apps and specialised digital platforms, for example Nasreen mentioned the fun of Instagram. But three participants, Samiha, Nasreen, and Mahmud (2016–2019), were also wary of the power of digital media in alienating their peers and providing possible opportunities for ISIL and others to radicalise vulnerable youngsters. Some Muslim Americans try to effect social cohesion with initiatives such as the #MeetAMuslim campaign.

References

Ahmed, S. (2013). Adolescents and emerging adults. In S. Ahmed & M. Amer (Eds.), *Counselling Muslims: Handbook of mental health issues and interventions* (pp. 251–280). New York, NY: Routledge.

Alba, R., & Nee, V. (2005). *Remaking the American mainstream: Assimilation and contemporary immigration.* Cambridge, MA: Harvard University Press.

Anderson, B. (1983). *Imagined communities: Reflection on the origin and spread of Nationalism* (revised ed.). London: Verso.

Barakat, M. (2017, June 21). Thousands attend slain Muslim teen's funeral in Virginia. *USA Today.* Retrieved from: www.usatoday.com.

Bayoumi, M. (2015). *This Muslim American life: Dispatches from the war on terror.* New York, NY: New York University Press.

Beirich, H., & Buchanan, S. (2018, February 11). 2017: The year in hate and extremism. *Southern Poverty Law Centre Intelligence Report.* Retrieved from: www.splcenter.org.

Bhabha, H. K. (2004). *The location of culture.* London: Routledge.

Bharath, D., & Gazzar, B. (2018, 23 April). Hate crime against Muslims up 15%, say CAIR. Retrieved from: https://ca.cair.com/losangeles/news/hate-crimes-against-muslim-up-15-says-cair.

Brubaker, R. (2006). The 'diaspora' diaspora. *Ethnic and Racial Studies, 28*(1), 1–19.

Charmaz, K. (2006). *Constructing grounded theory: A practical guide through qualitative analysis.* London: Sage.

CNN. (2016, August 18). Story of Syrian boy moves CNN anchor to tears [Video file]. Retrieved from: www.youtube.com/watch?v=PJOzBRy7dWs.

Echchaibi, N. (2013). American Muslims and the media. In J. Hammer & O. Safi (Eds.), *The Cambridge companion to American Islam* (pp. 119–138). Cambridge: Cambridge University Press.

Fortunati, L., Pertierra, R., & Vincent, J. (2012). Introduction. In L. Fortunati, R. Pertierra, & J. Vincent (Eds.), *Migration, diaspora and information technology in global societies* (pp. 1–17). New York, NY: Routledge.

Garrod, A., & Kilkenny, R. (Eds.). (2014). *Growing up Muslim: Muslim college students in America tell their stories.* Ithaca, NY: Cornell University Press.

Gerges, F. A. (2017). *ISIS: A history.* Princeton, NJ: Princeton University Press.

Glaser, B. G., & Strauss, A. L. (1967). *The discovery of grounded theory: Strategies for qualitative research.* London: Weidenfeld and Nicholson.

Green, L., & Kabir, N. A. (2012). Australian migrant children: ICT use and the construction of future lives. In L. Fortunati, R. Pertierra, & J. Vincent (Eds.), *Migration, diaspora and information technology in global societies* (pp. 91–103). New York, NY: Routledge.

Haddad, Y. Y., Smith, J. I., & Moore, K. M. (2006). *Muslim women in America: The challenges of Islamic identity today.* New York, NY: Oxford University Press.

Hossain, M. D., & Veenstra, A. S. (2017). Social capital and relationship maintenance: Uses of social media among the South Asian diaspora in the U.S. *Asian Journal of Communication, 27*(1), 1–17.

Iner, D., & Esposito, J. L. (Eds.). (2019). *Islamophobia and radicalization: Breeding intolerance and violence.* Cham, Switzerland: Palgrave Macmillan.

Kabir, N. A. (2012). *Young British Muslims: Identity, culture, politics and the media.* Edinburgh: Edinburgh University Press.

Kabir, N. A. (2014). *Young American Muslims: Dynamics of identity.* Edinburgh: Edinburgh University Press.

Kabir, N. A. (2017). *Muslim Americans: Debating the notions of American and un-American.* London: Routledge.

Kabir, N. A. (2018). Young Muslims identity in Australia and the US: The focus on the 'Muslim question'. In A. W. Ata & J. A. Ali (Eds.), *Islam in the west: Perceptions and reactions* (pp. 129–155). New Delhi, India: Oxford University Press.

Kabir, N. A. (2019). Can Islamophobia in the media serve Islamic state propaganda? The Australian case, 2014–2015. In D. Iner & J. L. Esposito (Eds.), *Islamophobia and radicalization: Breeding intolerance and violence* (pp. 97–116). Cham, Switzerland: Palgrave Macmillan.

Kharakh, B., & Primack, D. (2016, March 22). Donald Trump's social media ties to White Supremacists. *Fortune.* Retrieved from: http://fortune.com/donald-trump-white-supremacist-genocide.

Kibria, N. (2011). *Muslims in motion: Islam and national identity in the Bangladeshi diaspora.* New Brunswick, NJ: Rutgers University Press.

Lean, N. (2017). *The Islamophobia industry: How the right manufactures hatred of Muslims.* London: Pluto Press.

Mir, S. (2014). *Muslim American women on campus: Undergraduate social life and identity.* Chapel Hill, NC: University of North Carolina Press.

Nasr, S. H. (2002). *The heart of Islam: Enduring values for humanity.* New York, NY: HarperOne.

Ott, B. L. (2017). The age of Twitter: Donald J. Trump and the politics of debasement. *Critical Studies in Media Communication, 34*(1), 59–68.

Sirin, S. R., & Fine, M. (2008). *Muslim American youth: Understanding hyphenated identities through multiple methods*. New York, NY: New York University Press.

Thrush, G. (2017, March 6). Trumps new travel ban blocks migrants from six nations, sparing Iraq. *The New York Times*. Retrieved from: www.nytimes.com/2017/03/06/us/politics/travel-ban-muslim-trump.html.

INDEX

AAC *see* augmentative and alternative communication
AAP *see* American Academy of Pediatrics
Abiala, K. 265
Abidin, Crystal 6, 21, 221, 226–234, 236
Abueva, Amihan 384, 385, 387
abuse 379, 382, 427
access 43, 379; Africa 503–504; barriers to connectivity 500; Brazil 419, 515; Global South 535; inequalities 435, 436, 437–439, 443, 514; right to 510, 536; television in Bangladesh 527–528
action research 493, 498
active mediation 338, 346, 551, 552, 556
activism 1, 535, 540, 579; cancer survivors 416, 419, 421; China 545, 546; climate 374; disability 363, 365; education 67; rights 219
Adams, D. 502
Adams, R. E. 464–465
addiction 19, 21, 261, 351, 407; China 540, 542, 545; sexuality 425
adolescence: autism 349; commodification of 539–540; cyberbullying 462–463, 466; death and bereavement 485–486; digital media use 510–511; friends 157, 158; identity development 173–175, 182; parental tools 195–203; participation in television 534–535; self-exploration 173; sharenting 238; sleep 405, 406; social and cultural conditions 20; *see also* teenagers
advertising 8, 221, 286, 291, 568–569; child micro-celebrities 231, 232; consumer culture 207, 208, 210, 211–212, 214; digital literacy 495; games 208; retargeting 287, 290; social media 287–288, 290, 291–292; tweens in Brazil 271; UGC games 279; YouTube 212–213, 227–228; *see also* marketing
affordability 152
affordances: creativity 75; digital game making in school 149; digital storytelling 469; expectations regarding technology 509; grandparents 97; *Minecraft* 147; mobile devices 114; moral agency 368, 374; parental tools 195, 197–200, 201; street children 452–453, 457
Africa 12, 500–507
age: access to ICT 500; cyberbullying 462; digital divide 106; girls' video performances 54; inequalities 43, 421, 438–443, 444; moral agency 374; nineteenth-century discourses 430; research ethics 32; understanding of marketing 291
age restrictions 288, 298–299, 380, 543, 568
agency 2, 21, 261; children as active agents 62, 201, 265, 290; children as architects 146; digital citizenship 343, 346; law 8–9, 318; little c creativity 76; makerspaces 83; media socialisation 9, 327, 328, 330–334; moral 9, 368–377; participatory research 54; possibility thinking 78; research ethics 31; sexual 427, 428, 430; sick children 416; social media 220–221; sociology of childhood 53; structures and 48; surveillance 187, 192; tastes and identities 24; touchscreen technologies 90, 94; toy unboxing 563, 565; UGC games 282
aggression 464, 465
Ågren, Ylva 6, 207–216
Aitken, K. J. 124
Akanle, O. 502
Akiwowo, A. A. 501
Alba, R. 576
Albury, K. 428, 430, 523–524
Alckmin, Geraldo 508
alertness 404, 405
algorithms 565, 566, 568–569
Alibaba 545
Allan, Alicia 10, 403–413
Allen, L. 429
Alper, Meryl 9, 348–357, 358–359, 363, 420–421
AltSchool 246

Index

Amazon 218, 246
American Academy of Pediatrics (AAP) 58, 239, 409
American Civil Liberties Union 322–323
American Psychological Association 286
Anderson, A. 34
Anderson, H. 238
Andrade, N. 175
Andrejevic, Mark 22
anonymous communication 5, 173–184, 416
Anti-Defamation League 339
anti-sociality 351–352, 354
anxiety: autistic children 348, 350, 351; cyberbullying 463, 464–465, 466; pre-sleep arousal 406; pregnancy and parenting apps 398, 399–400; sick children 418
Anyanwu, Chika 12, 500–507
Apart of Me 481–482
Appadurai, A. 48, 470
Apperley, T. 338, 340
Apple 111, 115, 117, 247; *see also* iPad
apps: autistic children 353–354; child micro-celebrities 230; children's learning apps 7, 245–255; coding 73; communication 38; consumer culture 207; digital play 59; domestication of touchscreen technologies 90, 91, 92, 93; Douyin (Tik Tok) 539, 541–542, 545; engagement with 57–58; grandparents 99, 101, 105; haptic interface design 115; hook-up 519; i-Cut 505; in-app purchases 289–290, 291; mobile marketing 289, 291; moral agency 369; parental influence 60–61, 63; possibility spaces 82; pregnancy and motherhood 393–402; privacy issues 239–240, 241–242; research ethics 34; sibling influence 61; sleep 10, 408; social narrative 350; YouTube Kids 218, 481
Archard, David 314–315
architects, children as 144–151
Ariès, Phillipe 20
Arminen, I. 130
Arnett, J. J. 329, 331, 333
Arnott, L. 62
Arnstein, S. R. 302
arousal 404, 406–407, 410
artificial intelligence 262, 380
Ash, J. 78, 81, 83
Ask.fm 173, 174, 175–178
aspirational labour 218, 222, 227
assemblages: consumer culture 214; feminist new materialism 10, 395; makerspaces 83; posthumanism 3, 23, 78, 80, 81, 82, 84; pregnancy and parenting apps 399, 400
assent 32
assistance 130, 131–142
Asuwada 501, 502
asylum seekers 381
ATN Bangla 531–532, 533, 534
Attwood, F. 429

audiences 302–303, 451, 457, 458, 472, 477
augmentative and alternative communication (AAC) 353, 360
Australia: child influencers 236; children as architects 144; children as consumers 285; children with disabilities 361–362; dataveillance 394; e-Safety Commissioner 314, 318; Early Years Learning Framework 246; Games of Being Mobile project 186–187; haptic interfaces 113; inequalities 43–44; law 311, 313–314; migrant children 576; mobile technologies 550; parental surveillance 188–192; pregnancy and parenting apps 393, 395; screen time 287; sexting 371, 425, 518–526; sexuality 425, 426; sibling interactions 132; social media 39, 287; Steam 41; Toddlers and Tablets project 3, 79, 82, 89–93
Autcraft 352
autism 9, 348–357, 363
auto-play features 408, 410
autonomy 24, 339; digital citizenship 342; parental tools 6, 195, 197, 199–200, 201; rights 308, 318, 321–322; sexual 424; street children 452; surveillance 187; tweens 266; two-year olds 121
avatars 210

Baidu 545
Bak, M. 276
Bale, C. 429
Ballestrini, F. 457
Balmford, William 5, 185–194
Bandura, A. 330
Bangladesh 13, 527–538, 572, 577, 579
Bar Lev, Y. 123
Barad, K. 79–80, 81, 83
Barbie Girls 208
Barbosa, M. 513
Barnes, B. 330
Barnes, R. F. 44
Bauman, Z. 207, 214
Bauwens, Joke 9, 368–377
Bazalgette, Cary 4, 120–129
BBC 218
becoming 2, 21, 26, 48; moral 370, 372; peer culture 370; posthuman entanglements 79, 83
Beer, D. 162
Beghetto, Ronald 75
behavioural control 196, 197, 201
Beigbeder, Edouard 536
being 2, 21, 48, 79, 370
Belgium 437
Bellerose, D. 500
belonging 32, 370, 371–372, 442; consumer culture 211; digital culture 267; social media 182, 271, 363
bereavement 11–12, 480–488
Beresin, Anna 50
Berg, L. 429
Berger, Guy 386, 387

best interests 8–9, 311–312, 316, 319–322, 324, 380–381
Bickel, B. 471
big C creativity 75–76
Big Data 185, 238, 242, 380, 565, 566, 569
Biggs, S. N. 406
Bitaña, Hazel 386
Blackman, S. 430
blogs 236, 416, 580
Bloustien, G. 54
Blum-Ross, Alicia 21, 191, 192, 221, 227
body 431
body image 269–270, 272
Boerman, S. C. 292
Bolivia 11, 449–459
Bolsonaro, Jair Messias 266
Bond, E. 373, 430
Bourdieu, Pierre 112
boyd, d. 40, 165–166, 421, 510–511
Boyden, J. 23
Bragg, S. 429
Braidotti, R. 79
brands 285–286, 288
Braun, V. 176
Brazil: *CarecaTV* 417–420; schools 12, 508–517; sick children 416; tweens 7, 265, 266–272
Brewer, Holly 310
Bridle, James 227, 568
Briggs, M. 122
Brites, Maria José 12, 491–499
Britt, C. 29
Brochado, S. 462
Brooker, E. 62
Brown, P. 248–250
Brubaker, R. 572
Bryer, T. 260
BTV 527, 529, 531, 533
Buckingham, David: agency 330; childhood identities 213–214; circuit of culture 563; class 214; consumption 208, 212; 'digital generation' 510; meanings and uses of technology 511–512; media socialisation 333; parental responsibilisation 245; sexuality 429, 430; toy unboxing 565; under-use of technology 42
Buckleitner, W. 115–116
bugs 71–72, 73
Bulger, Monica 378
bullying 11, 418, 466, 550, 551; definition of 461; prevalence 461–462, 464; teacher training 495; traditional/cyberbullying relationship 463–465; *see also* cyberbullying
Burgess, J. 227, 566
Burnard, Pamela 77, 78, 82, 83
Burroughs, Benjamin 6, 217–225
Burton, P. 491
business sector 385
Byrne, J. 43, 504
Byron, P. 428

Cabello, P. 491
Caldeira, J. 509, 511, 514, 515
Caldwell, J. T. 58, 567
Canada: children as architects 144; dataveillance 394; media literacy education 258; refugees 471–478; sexting 523
cancer 415, 416, 417–420
capitalism 22, 25–26, 208, 222, 540, 546, 564
care 35–36
CarecaTV 10, 417–420, 421
career planning 73
caring dataveillance 394, 399, 400
Carrington, V. 144, 493
Carter, Michelle 322–324, 325
Carvalho, Raiana de 10, 414–423
Castells, Manuel 44
censorship 13, 385, 427, 539–546
Center for Digital Democracy (CDD) 338
Centofanti, S. A. 406
Central African Republic 505
Chakraborty, K. 223
Chalklen, C. 238
Chambers, D. 167
Chan, Philip 535
Channel *i* 531, 532, 533
Chappell, K. 78–79
Chaudron, S. 59, 61, 492
Chester, K. L. 462
Child Bereavement UK 481
child-centred policy 297–307
child-created content 6, 24, 217–225, 228, 236, 261; *see also* user-generated content
child labour 6, 218–220, 226, 233, 266
child, notion of the 2, 19, 20–21, 25, 201, 320
child pornography 12–13, 371, 425, 518–525
child sexual abuse 379, 382, 427
childhood 2, 19; conceptualising children 28–29; emergence as a category 430; law 309–310, 316, 319, 321–322; paradigms of scholarship 21–25; romantic notions of 219, 309, 313; sexuality 429, 430; social construction of 20–21, 22, 23, 25, 48; understandings of 358; *see also* sociology of childhood
childhood studies 369–370
Children's Online Privacy Protection Act (COPPA, 1998) 228, 288
Chile 513
China 13, 393, 539–548
Chronaki, Despina 10, 424–434
circadian rhythms 405
Circle 199
circuit of culture 563, 569
citizenship 364, 431; Brazil 266; consumption 42; digital 9, 299, 301, 304, 337–347, 381, 492, 496–497; intimate 431; research ethics 33; sexual 429, 430
civic engagement 162, 163, 166, 338, 436

Clark, Lynne Schofield 185, 187, 190, 191, 339, 358–359, 420–421
Clarke, V. 176
Claro, M. 491
class 214, 428; Brazil 511, 512; children with disabilities 362; Global Kids Online 513; nineteenth-century discourses 430; *see also* socio-economic status
ClassDojo 246
Club Panfu 210–211
Club Penguin 208–209, 210–211
co-location 191–192
co-use 195–196, 197
co-viewing 97, 102–104, 125–126, 127
coding 3, 67–74, 145–146, 149, 382, 506
cognition 125, 470–471
cognitive development 80, 87, 403; touchscreen technologies 88, 93; understanding of advertising 286, 291; Wonder Weeks app 397
Coleman, S. 301
Collin, P. 301
Collins, W. A. 121
Colvert, A. 493
commercialism 6, 8, 22, 38, 246–247, 286
commodification 207, 208–209, 210, 381, 539–540; children's culture 568; data 22; exclusion of children 214; 'playbour' 13; toy unboxing 567, 569
Common Sense Media 48, 222, 339, 567
communication: anonymous 5, 173–184; augmentative and alternative 353, 360; children with disabilities 361–362; 'communication risk' approach 424; death and bereavement 480–481; digital images 519; inequalities 436; interactive 301; media messages 493; 'normal' 359, 361; parental mediation 195–196; research ethics 34; sexual 425–426; teens' sociability 152, 156, 157, 158; tweens in Brazil 269; use of technology 42
competence 131
computer science (CS) 67–68, 69
connections 77, 82, 125
connectivity 153; Africa 503–504; barriers to 500; Brazil 269, 272, 515, 516
consent 32, 310, 311–312, 318–319, 338; age of sexual consent 520; sexting 425; sick children 416; street children 452
Constant Comparative Analysis (CCA) 340
constructionism 428, 429; *see also* social constructionism
consumer culture 6, 207–216, 426
consumer socialisation 286
consumption 6, 42, 48, 207–208, 214, 221; child-created content 223–224; children as consumers 285–286; as cultural practice 49; parents' roles 212; toy unboxing 563, 564, 567–568
content creation 38, 42; child-created content 6, 24, 217–225, 228, 236, 261; inequalities 435–436, 440; tweens in Brazil 269; *see also* user-generated content
context collapse 241, 455, 568
convergence 40, 81
conversation analysis 131, 132, 133–141
Cook, Daniel T. 22, 208, 566
copyright 7, 276, 281–282, 372
Coronovirus (COVID-19) 7, 14
Costa, Daniela 12, 508–517
Costa, E. 454
Couldry, N. 519
Coulter, Natalie 2, 19–27
Council of Europe 300
Craft, Anna 75–76, 77–78, 82, 84
Craig, D. 220, 562, 567
Cramer, F. 115
Crawford, K. 428, 523–524
CRC *see* United Nations Committee on the Rights of the Child
creativity 3, 75–86; African children 506; benefits of digital media 414; cognitive development 93; UGC games 276, 277, 279; vernacular 227
creators network 540–541
criminalisation 521, 522
crip theory 350
critical consciousness 35
critical discourse analysis (CDA) 247
critical engagement 337, 344–345
critical perspective 63–64
Crofts, T. 519, 520
Cross, Gary 219
CRPD *see* United Nations Convention on the Rights of Persons with Disabilities
Csikszentmihalyi, M. 76
cultural capital 156–157, 362
cultural-historical perspective 57, 60, 64
cultural knowledge 57, 64
cultural perspective 63–64
cultural phenomenology 113, 116
cultural studies 113, 426, 429–430, 563
cultural tools 57, 62, 63, 64, 80
culture 20, 24, 48–49, 562–563; African 500, 502; Brazil 266; global 23; habitus 112; methodological issues 49, 54–55; Muslim American children 572, 577; participatory research 54; toy unboxing 569
Cumiskey, Kathleen M. 11–12, 480–488
Cummins, J. 470, 472
Cunningham, S. 220, 562, 567
curation 261, 262, 270
Curbi 199
Curran, Tillie 360
curriculum 144, 148, 246, 257, 258, 506
Curtin, M. 541
Curtis, Pixie 236
customisation 69, 73, 276
cyberbullying 11, 19, 299, 379, 460–468, 539–540; African children 501–502; anonymous communication 5, 174, 176, 182; autistic children

352; Bangladesh 536; China 545; definition of 461; extreme cases 368; gender differences 43; increase in 42; inequalities 436; law 313, 319, 324; moral agency 9, 374; parental tools 200; prevalence 461, 462–463, 464

da Silva, Luís Inácio 266
DaddyOFive 228
Danby, Susan 4, 130–143
dances 261
dangers 19, 261
Dash 229, 231–232, 233
data 22–23, 261; Big Data 185, 238, 242, 380, 565, 566, 569; coding 67; educational 256–257; GDPR 318–319; location-based marketing 289; privacy issues 238–240, 241, 242, 325; rights-respecting treatment 386; smart toys 379; social media advertising 287–288; unlawful collection of 228
data protection 298–299
datafication 394
dataveillance 10, 223, 252–253, 394–395, 399, 400; *see also* surveillance
Davidson, C. 131, 140
Davis, L. 362
Davis, Natalie Zemon 20
de Bono, Christopher 378
de Haan, J. 551
De Lange, N. 451
de Luca, F. 152
De Ridder, S. 428, 430
death 11–12, 480–488
debugging 71–72, 73
deception 288
decision-making 302–303, 304, 333, 384
deficit approaches 361, 363, 421
Dehaene, S. 126
democratic participation 310, 516
Denmark 437, 551
deontology 368
depression: autistic children 348; cyberbullying 463, 464–465, 466; parental tools 200
Dessie, Betelhem 505
Deuze, M. 214
diakresis 126
dick pics 519, 520, 523
DigiLitEY 83, 258–259
digital affective cultures 481
digital citizenship 9, 299, 301, 304, 337–347, 381, 492, 496–497
digital divide 302, 491; Africa 504; age-related 106; Brazil 512, 515; street children 452; *see also* inequalities
digital environment 380–386, 420, 491
Digital Kids Asia-Pacific 337, 338
digital literacy 4, 7, 42, 144–145, 256–264; Africa 505; child micro-celebrities 226, 229, 232; digital play 144; education 385; family practices 142; grandparents 99, 105; legal issues and copyright 281, 282; makerspaces 83; marketing 291; privacy 242; rights 300, 301, 379, 387; social media 452; technical skills 430; young children 491–499

digital natives 24, 44, 62; Brazil 267; critique of concept 30, 435; haptic media habitus 116; inequalities 11, 435, 436, 443–444
digital policy 298–299
digital storytelling 11, 469–479
dignity 312, 373, 452
Diniz de Oliveira, J. 500
disability 9, 349, 354, 358–367, 381, 382, 462
discourse 20, 79, 361
discrimination 270, 271–272, 381, 384, 509
Disney 218, 222
Disney Infinity 276
displacement of sleep 404, 407–408
DiSTO see From Digital Skills to Tangible Outcomes
distraction 91, 93, 114
diversity 33, 358, 374
Dobson, Amy Shields 12–13, 518–526
Dobson, Madeleine 2, 28–37
Doe, Kelvin 505
domestication 3, 87–95
Donald, S. H. 541
Donkin, Ashley 7, 245–255
Donnison, David 324
Donovan, Sheila 386–387
Dooley, K. T. 470
Doretto, Juliana 12, 508–517
Dorrian, J. 406
Doshi, M. J. 399
Dota 2 game 338, 339, 340–346
Douyin 539, 541–543, 545
Döveling, K. 482
Drew, P. 130, 131
Drotner, Kirsten 358
Drouin, M. 520
Du Gay, P. 563
due process 315–316
Duffy, B. E. 218
Duronto TV 531, 532, 533
dynamic literacies 7, 258, 262–263

Early Childhood Australia (ECA) 31, 32, 33
Early, M. 472
Early Years Foundation Stage (EYFS) 246
Early Years Learning Framework (EYLF) 246
Easy Solar 505
Echchaibi, N. 580
education 256–257; Africa 505, 506; Brazil 12, 508–517; children with disabilities 363; digital game making in school 148–150; digital literacy 385; grandparents 101, 105; inequalities 438–443; learning apps 245, 247–253; media literacy 258; *Minecraft* 147–148; moving-image media 122; parental responsibilisation 7, 245, 252–253; refugees 469–470; right to 381, 382;

588

Index

schoolification 246; Sustainable Development Goals 384; *see also* pedagogy; teachers
educational software 99, 100–101
edutainment 131, 248, 250, 251–252
Edwards, S. 58, 59, 63, 81, 82, 494
EECERA *see* European Early Childhood Education Research Association
Eekelaar, John 320
'effects' paradigm 420
Egan, D. 429, 430
Eichhorn, K. 240–241
Eklund, L. 339
El Emam, K. 415
Eliana 229, 230–231, 232, 233
Elias, Nelly 3, 96–107, 123
Ellis, Katie 9, 358–367
Ellison, N. 40
Elmer, Greg 22
'ElsaGate' Scandal 568
eMarketer 288
embodied cognition 122, 124–125, 127
embodiment 112, 113, 114, 115, 117
Emert, T. 471
emotion 125
emotional problems 439–440, 441–442, 443
empathy 125, 351
empowerment 325, 535, 569; African children 506; digital literacy 492; digital storytelling 470, 471; girls 381; grandparents 97; information 301; parental tools 200, 201; participation 300; participatory research 54; research ethics 33, 35; sick children 415; street children 453, 457; surveillance 192; YouTube 223
encounters 113, 114, 115, 117
enculturation 113, 114, 115, 116, 117
engagement 57–58, 163, 165
Ennew, Judith 314, 325
entanglements 78–79, 80, 83
entrepreneurship 504–505
Epson 231
equality 358, 381
equity 32, 43
Erickson, I. 492
Erstad, O. 471
Ess, C. 154
ethics 2, 6, 28–37, 50; child-created content 223; digital socialisation 353; sexual 428; street children 451–452
Ethiopia 505
ethnicity: Brazil 266; coding study 68; inequalities 436; influence on everyday experience 60; *see also* race
ethnography 25, 49, 364; fan communities 164; Games of Being Mobile project 186; online harassment 339; participatory research 54; visual 50
ethnomethodology 131
EU Kids Online 265, 267, 426, 491; anonymous communication 5, 175, 176, 177; inequalities 436; media socialisation 327; research ethics 34; risks 427, 550–551, 552; siblings 131
Europe: inequalities 437; internet use 503; makerspaces 83; media literacy education 258
European Early Childhood Education Research Association (EECERA) 31–32, 33
European Union: Audiovisual Media Services Directive 298; digital citizenship 337–338; GDPR 298–299, 318–319, 338; *see also* EU Kids Online
EvanTube HD 220, 222, 563–564, 565
Event Handling Guide for iOS 113, 115
exclusion 214, 266, 272, 372, 381, 384
expertise 41; health information 415; learning apps 248, 249, 251, 253
exploitation 21, 42, 381; Brazil 266; child-created content 228; protection from 31; sharenting 227; *see also* sexual exploitation
EYFS *see* Early Years Foundation Stage
EYLF *see* Early Years Learning Framework

Facebook 44, 262; age requirement 288; China 545; death and bereavement 486; digital storytelling 473, 477; Meet A Muslim campaign 580; Muslim American children 576, 578, 579, 580; parental surveillance 189; popularity of 460; retargeting 290; sharenting 237, 238; sibling influence 61; sick children 416, 418; street children 11, 449–459; teens' sociability 155, 156; tweens in Brazil 268, 270
Facetime 58, 90
facework 211
Fairclough, N. 247
'fake news' 258, 301, 379
family 60–62, 130–131; child-created content 217; digital literacy skills 142; influencers 221, 226, 228, 233; media socialisation 333; sleep 408; *see also* parents
fan communities 5, 161–172
fanarts 163
fanfiction 163, 165, 166, 168–169, 170
Farman, J. 190
Farrell, A. D. 463–464
Farrugia, Lorleen 5, 173–184
fast food 289
fear of missing out (FOMO) 407
Featherstone, M. 210
Federal Trade Commission (FTC) 289
feedback 158, 175–176, 182, 303
Feller, Gavin 6, 217–225
feminism 10, 29, 371; feminist new materialism 395; moral agency 374; Muslims 580; political/relational model of disability 350; sexuality 426, 428; sharenting 227; youthful bodies 522; *see also* gender; women
femtech 393
Fernandes, N. 513
Ferreira, M. 268
fiction 539, 540, 541, 543–546

field notes 51
Fillol, Joana 4–5, 152–160
filmmaking 260
filter bubbles 157, 301
filters 345
Finkelhor, D. 425, 520
Finland 551
Fischel, J. 428, 431
Fiske, J. 451
flawed consumers 214
Flick, U. 31
Flood, M. 425
Flores, A. 373
Floridi, Luciano 5, 153–154, 157
flow 408
FOMO *see* fear of missing out
Fortunati, L. 152
Foucault, Michel 187, 430
4Ps 78
Fraga, S. 462
Fredstrom, B. K. 464–465
free speech 322–323, 324
freedom of association 381, 382
freedom of expression 31, 299, 300, 321, 381, 382, 530
Freeman, Michael 321
frexting 519
friendships 157, 158, 163, 166, 167–168
Frith, H. 52
From Digital Skills to Tangible Outcomes (DiSTO) 437–443
FTC *see* Federal Trade Commission
Fuchs, Christian 22, 325
Fuente, Julián de la 5, 161–172
Fuller, M. 115
functional qualities 198, 199, 200, 201
FunToys Collector Disney Toys Review 563–564, 565

Gallacher, Leslie 53
Gallagher, Michael 53
Gallese, V. 125
gambling 227–228
game jams 277, 278–279, 282n1
GameMaker 148
games 38, 39, 42; advertising 212; Apart of Me 481–482; autistic children 351, 352; children with disabilities 361; coding 71, 72, 73; concerns about 339; consumer culture 207, 208–209; content creation 24; data 22; digital citizenship 338, 340–346; digital game making in school 148–150; engagement with 57–58; grandparents 99, 100–101, 105; in-app purchases 289–290; learning 59; Muslim American children 577; parental influence 61; parental surveillance 5, 188–189, 191–192; pre-sleep arousal 406; sibling interactions 61, 131, 132–138, 140; sleep interference 407–408; Steam 41; teaching practices 494; tweens in Brazil 269; user-generated content 7, 275–284; virtual worlds 147–148; young children 494
Games of Being Mobile (GoBM) project 186–187, 190, 191, 192
gamification 250, 251–252
Gardner, H. 75–76
Garland-Thomson, Rosemarie 362
gaspard, luke 2, 38–47
Gasser, U. 44
Gauntlett, D. 277
GDPR *see* General Data Protection Regulation
Gee, J. P. 157
geeking out 41
Geller, Pamela 580
gender: access to ICT 500; *CarecaTV* 419; child-created content 217; digital culture 267; digital gender gaps 43; identities 431; inequalities 43, 421, 436, 438–443, 444; influence on everyday experience 60; intersectionality 23; learning apps 248, 249, 252, 253; moral agency 374; online harassment 339; pornography 429; sexting 371, 523; sexual content 13, 425–426, 427, 428, 554–556, 559; tweens in Brazil 270, 272; *see also* feminism; women
General Data Protection Regulation (GDPR) 298–299, 318–319, 338
geolocation 22–23
Gerber, H. R. 276
Germany 303, 393, 551
gestures 4, 113, 114–117, 118
Ghana 502, 504, 505
Gibbs, L. 223
Gibson, James 197
Giddens, A. 330
Giddings, S. 81
Gidget 68, 72, 73
Gillen, J. 492
Gillespie, T. 281
Gillick competence 319, 320–321
Gilman, R. 464–465
Giumetti, G. W. 464
Gleeson, K. 52
global culture 23
Global Kids Online 265, 378–379, 382, 436, 491, 512–513
Global South 23, 272, 378; access 535; barriers to connectivity 500; inequalities 45, 379, 436; lack of research 445
Goggin, Gerard 9, 358–367
Goodyear, V. A. 415
Google 6, 212–213; China 545; digital storytelling 473–474, 478; right to be forgotten 240–241
Google Glass 351
Google Play 245, 247, 248
Görzig, A. 338
Grace, Sophia 23
Grainger, Teresa 77, 82
grandparents 3, 96–107

Index

Green, B. 150, 493
Green, J. 227, 566
Green, Lelia 1–14, 337–347, 576
Green, Maxine 78
grief 11–12, 481–482, 486
Grimes, Sara M. 7, 22, 275–284
Grindr 519
grounded theory 122, 575
Grusec, J. 328
GSM Association (GSMA) 503
Guerra, N. G. 466
Gunderson, L. 469
Guo, S. 541

habitus 111, 112–113, 114–118
Hacker, K. 512, 514, 516
hacking 22–23, 72
Haddon, Leslie 1–14, 24, 87–95, 152, 157, 269, 338
Hamilton, Alexander 218–219
Hand, M. 519
Hansson, K. 361
haptic interfaces 4, 111–119
Haque, Ashfara 13, 527–538
harassment 339, 427, 521, 524, 550; autistic children 352; Bangladesh 536; China 545; inequalities 436
Harbaugh, A. G. 466
Hargittai, E. 512
harm 8, 9, 312–313, 325, 368, 382, 524, 550–551
Hart, R. A. 53, 302
Hasebrink, U. 551
Hasinoff, A. A. 428, 519, 521
Hassanen, Nabra 579
hate speech 270, 272, 299, 301–302
hauls 213, 215n2
Hawkes, G. L. 429, 430
Hazer, O. 98
HBO 218
HCI *see* human-computer interaction
health: access to information 382; benefits of digital media 414; health media literacy 420; right to 381; self-tracking 398; sick children and social media 414–423; sleep 10, 403, 408–409; UNCRC 530; women and digital health 395
Heath, Shirley Brice 50
Hecht, Albie 222
Heigl, Katherine 239
Helmersson Bergmark, K. 339
Helsper, Ellen J. 11, 97, 265, 435–448, 551
Henderson, M. 494
Henry, Nzekwe 505
Hernwall, P. 265
Hess, M. 502
heteronormativity 371, 428, 523
Highfield, T. 237
Hillman, A. 53
Hjorth, Larissa 5, 185–194
Hodge, B. 126
Hodkinson, P. 54, 340

Holland, S. 53
Holloway, Donell 1–14, 82, 245–255
home life 59, 62, 256
homophobia 270, 430, 581
Horst, Heather 2, 38–47, 188
Horvath, M. A. H. 425
Hossain, M. D. 576
Houen, Sandy 4, 130–143
Hour of Code 67
HTML *see* HyperText Markup Language
Huang, B. 540–541
Hull, G. A. 471, 472
human-computer interaction (HCI) 113, 116, 360
Humphreys, Lee 187
Hunt, P. 429
HyperText Markup Language (HTML) 68, 69–70, 73

i-Cut 505
Iannotti, R. J. 462
ICT in Education survey 514–515
ICT Kids Online Brazil 267–272, 511, 512, 514
identity: adolescent development 173–175, 182; anonymous communication 173, 177; digital storytelling 11, 469, 472, 478; fan communities 5, 162; gender 431; intersectionality 420–421; learner 262; moral agency 369, 371; Muslim American children 13–14, 572, 573, 576, 577, 579, 580; plurality of identities 78; research ethics 32; research on 565; right to an 325; self-socialisation 329; sexual 371; sick children 415, 417, 418–419, 420; social distinctiveness 358; social media 40; social networks 24, 163; street children 453, 455–456, 457, 458; teens' sociability 158; toy unboxing 565; tweens 265, 269–270; video research 54
ideology 250–251, 257, 309, 319, 360
IELS *see* International Early Learning and Child Well-being Study
ignorance 314–315
Ihde, Don 113
illegal downloading 372
illness 10, 414–423
imagination 77, 81–82, 83
immaturity 310–311, 313, 316, 323
immersion 77, 82
in-app purchases 289–290, 291
In re Gault (1967) 315–316
In Re Kelvin 320
inappropriate content 42, 177, 290, 313–314, 542, 546, 559
inclusion 303, 360, 364, 516
India 43
inequalities 11, 43–44, 45, 156, 379, 435–448; Brazil 7, 266, 271–272, 515, 516; children with disabilities 360; intersectionality 420–421; networked illness 421; reducing 514; social media 416; structural 512, 513; *see also* digital divide
influence 302–303

influencers 207, 213, 220; child 25–26, 217, 218, 221–222, 226–234, 236; family 221, 226, 228, 233; marketing 8, 288; parent 235, 236–237, 241; social media 221, 227
informal learning 44, 256, 380
information: empowerment 301; health 414–415, 420; right to 299, 300, 380, 381, 382, 530
INGOs *see* international non-governmental organisations
innocence 21, 312–315, 316; romanticisation of childhood 219; sexuality 426, 427, 428, 430–431
insider research 50, 54
Instagram 262; age requirement 288; dances 261; data collection 289; fan communities 169; influencers 221, 235, 236; marketing 8, 287; Muslim American children 576, 579, 581; parental surveillance 189–190; popularity of 460; sharenting 237; sick children 416, 418; teens' sociability 155, 156; tweens in Brazil 270
instant messaging 269, 462, 463
intellectual disability 311–312
intellectual property 7, 277, 281–282
inter-connectedness 40
interaction 81
interactivity 70–71, 285, 301
interfaces 4, 111–119
International Early Learning and Child Well-being Study (IELS) 246
international non-governmental organisations (INGOs) 528, 529, 535
internet 39, 265, 378–379; Africa 503–504; Bangladesh 535; barriers to connectivity 500; Brazil 267–272, 510, 511–512, 513–515, 516; child-centred policy 297, 301; China 539, 540–546; commercial interests 44–45; concerns about 58; fan communities 161–172; gender differences 43; identity development 173–174; increase in children's use 207; inequalities 43–44, 438–440, 442–443; informal learning 380; mediation 97; Muslim American children 577; parental tools 199–200; safety 313–314; teens' sociability 155; time spent on the 287; as transnational technology 387; young children 491, 493–494; *see also* social media; websites
Internet Governance Forum 297
internet of things 22–23, 58, 379, 380
Internet of Toys 82–83
interpretive paradigm 164
intersectionality 23, 354, 358, 359, 365, 420–421
intersubjectivity 368
intertextuality 257
intimate surveillance 188, 189, 190, 227, 239
intra-action 81–82, 83
iPad 79, 145, 351; haptic media habitus 111, 115, 117; Minimum User Competency 116; parental surveillance 189–190; robots 146; sibling interactions 134–135, 138
iPhone 34, 111

iPod 38, 145, 574, 575
Ireland 174, 393, 437
Irons, Madison 9, 348–357
Islamophobia 572, 573, 578, 580–581
Israel 98
Italy 437, 462, 550, 551
Ito, Mizuko 41, 163, 166, 191

Jacenko, Roxy 236
Jackson, S. 429
James, Allison 21–25, 26
James, C. 373
James Playz 482–484
Jansz, J. 339
Japan 185
Javascript 71, 72
Jenkins, Henry 20, 540, 562
Jenks, C. 19, 20, 21, 277
JillianTube HD 222
Jiming, W. 502
Jin Tao 544
Jiow, H. J. 338
Jiu Yehui 544
Jobim, Tom 266
John-Steiner, V. 76, 80
Johnson, Lauren 11, 469–479
Jones, B. L. 419
Jor, Jorge Ben 266
Jordan, Amy 121, 359
Jorge, Ana 10, 414–423
journeys 90–91
Joyce-Gibbons, A. 504
Juan, L. 502
Jurassic World 290
juvenile justice 315–316, 318, 319, 323–324

Kabir, Nahid Afrose 14, 572–583
Kagan, J. 126
Kaji, Ryan *see* Ryan Toys Review
Kalmus, V. 551
Kanchev, P. 491
Kapp, K. M. 252
Kardefelt Winther, D. 491
Katz, M. 471, 472
Katz, Vikki S. 62, 358–359, 420–421
Kaufman, James 75
Kendrick, K. H. 130, 131
Kendrick, Maureen 11, 469–479
Kennelly, J. 25
Kent, Mike 9, 358–367
Kenya 505
Kervin, L. 61
Kharakh, B. 581
Kibby, M. D. 162
KidGuard 200
Kidron, Beeban 387
Kim, Jung Soo 3, 67–74
Kincaid, James 314

Index

King, D. 252
Kirby, A. V. 352
Kirby, P. 302
Kitzinger, Jenny 314
Kleeman, David 569
Klinke, A. 549
knowledge: cultural 57, 64; expert knowledge discourse 251, 253; media socialisation 333; participatory research 53–54; persuasion 292; teacher training 496
Kolko, B. 458
Kowalski, Robin M. 11, 460–468
Krämer, B. 328, 332–333
Krcmar, M. 96–97
Kress, Gunther 48–49, 169, 470–471
Kuby, C. 78
Kudos 200
Kulju, P. 495
Kumar, P. 237
Kumpulainen, K. 492

La Rue, Frank 387
Lacasa, Pilar 5, 161–172
ladder of participation 53, 302, 491
Laidlaw, Linda 4, 144–151
Lala, G. 500
Lambert, J. 471
Lancaster, L. 125, 127
Lange, Patricia 24
language 34, 35, 144, 247, 470
Lankshear, C. 150
Lansdown, Gerison 9–10, 368, 378–389, 535, 536
laptops 39
Laroche, M. 504
Lauder, H. 248–250
Lauri, Mary Anne 5, 173–184
Lauricella, A. 564–565
law 8–9, 308–317, 318–326; child-created content 219–220; child labour 226; sexting 518, 520–525; user-generated content 276, 281–282; Youth Law Australia 518; *see also* policy
Law, J. 50
Le, A. H. 463–464
Lealand, G. 121
Lean, N. 580
learned qualities 198
learning 59–60, 64; benefits of digital media 408, 414; business of 246–247; children's learning apps 7, 245–255; digital 146; informal 256; lifelong 333; moving-image media 122; parental influence 61; participatory 276; refugees 477–478; sleep 403; young children 121, 492
Leaver, Tama 1–14, 188, 190, 235–244
Lee, Michael J. 3, 67–74
Leeson, C. 34
legacy media 13, 527–528, 537; *see also* television
Lemineur, Marie-Laure 386
Lemish, Dafna 3, 23, 96–107, 121–122

Lenhart, A. 371
Let's Play videos 213, 215n1, 281
Levesque, R. J. R. 330
Levy, S. T. 123
Lewis, J. B. 180
LGBTQI children 382, 428
Liddiard, K. 365
life, right to 381
lifelong learning 333
light exposure 404, 405–406, 409–410
Lim, Sun Sun 153, 338
Limber, S. P. 465
Lin, J. 338
Lindgren, S. 212
Lindgren, Therese 213, 214
Ling, R. 157
Linville, H. A. 471
Linzer, D. A. 180
listening 33, 35
literacy 144, 257, 262; access to ICT 500; apps 247, 248; attainment gaps 469; cognitive development 93; learning and teaching 145; moving-image media 122; parental responsibilisation 245, 253; right to 381, 382; schoolification 246; young children 492; *see also* digital literacy
Lithuania 462
Little Big Planet 276, 277–278
little c creativity 75–76, 77, 79–80, 81–82, 83, 84
Livingstone, Sonia: access 510; audiences 451; autonomy 24; children with disabilities 359; data harvesting 22; debates over children and media 358; differences 420; ethnography 25; expectations regarding technology 509; family practices 61; global networks 518; the home 130; intersubjectivity 368; ladder of opportunities 265, 491; mediation 97, 338; parental mediation 552; privacy 452; protection 337; rights 9–10, 378–389, 535, 536; risky media engagement 187; screen time 191, 192; sharenting 221, 227; social networks 157; stimulation hypothesis 153; 'The Class' project 332
Ljung-Djärf, A. 62
location data 289
Lomax, H. 53
Loomis, C. P. 502
Lüders, M. 153
Lundy, L. 302–303, 304
Lupton, Deborah 10, 223, 393–402

Mabovula, N. N. 501
Mac Operating System 199
Macbeth, Jamie C. 3, 67–74
MacDougall, C. 223
Mackay, R. W. 131
maker movement 4, 145
Maker Studios 222–223
makerspaces 79, 83
MakEY project 83, 259

Malaguzzi, L. 29
Malta 175–182
Mantilla, A. 494
Marcon, A. 457
marginality 421
Marji, M. 149
marketing 8, 42, 112, 212, 285–294; influencers 213; mobile phones 217; responsibilisation discourse 245, 251; tweens in Brazil 271, 272; YouTube 227–228; *see also* advertising
Marôpo, Lidia 10, 414–423
Marseille, N. M. 96–97
Marsh, Jackie A. 92, 94; family schedules 61; online/offline practices 146; parental influence 60–61; play 78, 81, 82–83; playground games 53–54; toy unboxing 563, 564, 568; virtual worlds 208–209, 210
Martínez, C. 208, 209
Marwick, Alice 187, 192
Masanet, M.-J. 430
Mascheroni, Giovanna 7, 245–255
massively multiplayer online games (MMOs) 338, 407
materialism 286, 290, 428
materiality 113
mathematics 77, 147
Matsuda, M. 185
Mauss, Marcel 112
Máximo, Thinayna 7, 265–274
Maxwell, C. 247
Mayer-Schonberger, V. 240
McCord, Annie 11, 460–468
McDonald's 286
McDougall, J. 258
McGuigan, Jim 540
McLachlan, J. 29, 33
Mead, Margaret 20, 334
meaning-making 24, 29, 55; death and bereavement 486; digital storytelling 471, 472; literacy 257, 258, 259, 263; moving-image media 4, 121; multimodal 492; parental tools 198
media: childhood 21; Islamophobia 580–581; media socialisation 332; research 48; street children 450; *see also* internet; social media; television
'media articles' 535, 537
media literacy 258, 420
media socialisation 9, 327–336
mediascapes 48
mediation: active 338, 346, 551, 552, 556; grandparents 3, 96–97, 101–104, 105–106; moving-image media 125–126; parental 195–197, 199, 201, 338–339, 492, 494, 551, 552, 556; visual 519
medical model of disability 349, 362
Meet A Muslim campaign 580, 581
Mehari, K. R. 463–464, 465
melatonin 404, 405, 409
Meltzer, L. J. 406

memes 163
Menesini, E. 464
mental health 321, 398, 486, 530, 544
Merleau-Ponty, M. 112–113, 115
Merriman, Vincent 7, 275–284
Mesch, Gustavo 153, 156
Messenger 155
metagaming 41
methodological issues 2, 25, 33, 48–56, 409; child-centred policy 302–304; ICT Kids Online Brazil 267; media socialisation 332; Transmedia Literacy project 154
Meyers, E. M. 492
Mick, D. 248
micro-celebrities 21, 25–26, 207, 220; commodification 209; consumer culture 213, 214; hauls 215n2; micro-microcelebrities 226, 228, 233, 236; pre-schoolers 226–234; rise of 221
Microsoft 279, 280, 281
Miller, Pernilla 4, 130–143
mimesis 564
Minchin, J. 466
Minecraft 7, 70, 147–148, 276, 277–281, 289, 352
Minimum User Competency (MUC) 112, 116, 117
mirror neurons 125
Misslissibell 209, 213
Mitchell, C. 451
Mitchell, K. 425
MMOs *see* massively multiplayer online games
mobile technologies 5, 39–40, 144, 287, 568–569; Africa 503, 504; autistic children 352; Bangladesh 535; Brazil 7, 508–509, 511, 512, 514, 515, 516; death and bereavement 480, 485–486; engagement with 57–58; gender differences 43; haptic interfaces 111, 112; haptic media habitus 117; health risks 550; inequalities 438–440; Israel 98; marketing 217; media socialisation 327; mobile marketing 289–290, 291; parental surveillance 185–194; refugees 384; sexual content 554; teens' sociability 153, 155; *see also* smartphones; tablets
modality judgements 126–127
Modecki, K. L. 466
Mojang 279, 280
Moletsane, R. 451
monitoring: mediation 97; parental mediation 195–197, 199; sexual content 424; touchscreen technologies 92–93; *see also* surveillance
Monteiro, M. C. 268, 271–272
Montgomery, Kathryn 566
Montgomery, L. 543
Montreuil, M. 370
Moonves, Jon 222
Moore, D. C. 281–282
moral agency 9, 368–377
moral horizons 369, 370, 374
moral panics 58, 88, 207, 241, 363, 564
Moran, S. 76, 80
Morduchowicz, R. 457

Moreno, M. A. 465
Mosia, Nthabiseng 505
Mostmans, Lien 9, 11, 368–377, 449–459
Mother Pukka 236
mothers 10, 393–402
Moura, Pedro 4–5, 152–160
movie-watching 124–125, 126–127
moving images 4, 120–129; *see also* video
Mowlabocus, Sharif 114, 563, 564, 566
Mozur, P. 543
MUC *see* Minimum User Competency
Mulholland, Monique 429
multiliteracies 259, 472
multimodality: digital storytelling 470, 471, 478; fan communities 161, 163, 165, 168–170; learning 477–478; meaning-making 257; modality judgements 126–127; moving-image media 121, 124–125; multiliteracies 259; young children 492
Murris, K. 80–81
music 54, 121, 577, 578
Muslims 13–14, 572–583
Mutsvairo, B. 504
MySkool Portal 505
MySpace 41

Nadchatram, Indra Kumari 384, 385
Nadesan, M. H. 251
Nakamura, L. 458
Nandagiri, R. 452
Nansel, T. R. 462
Nansen, Bjørn 4, 111–119, 220, 223, 563, 564
narratives: moral agency 370, 373–374; moving-image media 120, 125, 127; situated child consumption 214
National Alliance for Grieving Children 481
native advertising 288
natural user interfaces (NUIs) 116
Nee, V. 576
NEETs *see* Not in Employment, Education, or Training
Nelissen, S. 329
neoliberalism 245, 248, 252, 253, 369, 372, 373
Neopets 22, 208
Net Children Go Mobile 265, 268, 437–443, 510
Netflix 218
Netherlands 339, 551
netnography 41
networked publics 165–166, 368, 415
Neumann, D. L. 92
Neumann, M. M. 92
neurodiversity 350, 363
new literacy studies 257, 259
New London Group 259, 472
new materialism 10, 23
Newby, J. 543
newsfeed ads 288, 292
newspaper project 496–498
Nicoll, B. 220, 563, 564

Niemeyer, D. J. 276
Nigeria 500, 502, 505
Nikken, P. 339
Nimrod, Galit 3, 96–107
Nolan, A. 494
non-discrimination 380–381
non-verbal communication 34
Norman, Donald 116
norms: autistic children 349; gender 371, 374; law 308, 309, 324, 325; media socialisation 328, 329, 331, 333, 334; moral 370; sexual 429
Norway 13, 551, 552–559
Not in Employment, Education, or Training (NEETs) 437, 439–440, 441, 443, 444
Nouwen, Marije 5–6, 195–203
nudes 519
NUIs *see* natural user interfaces
numeracy 245, 246, 248, 253

obesity 408–409, 462
observations 49–50, 51, 122, 186
Ochs, Elinor 350
Odom, S. L. 363
Ogusemo, Temitope 505
O'Kane, C. 53
Ólafsson, K. 338
Olson, K. R. 277, 282
Olsson, T. 209
Olweus, D. 464, 465
O'Mara, Joanne 4, 144–151
Omobowale, A. O. 502
One Direction 5, 164, 165–170
O'Neill, Brian 8, 297–307
onlife concept 153–154, 157, 158
online fandom 5, 161–172
online fiction 539, 540, 541, 543–546
online/offline distinction 5, 144, 146, 153–154, 157, 162, 370
online viewing 99, 100, 105
ontology 368
Opie, Iona 50, 260, 261
Opie, Peter 260, 261
Ott, B. L. 581
OurPact 200
outcome inequalities 437, 442–443, 444
Ovia 396
Owlet 239, 241
ownership 7, 277, 279–280, 282
Oyedemi, T. 503
Öztürk, M. S. 98

pace of research 34, 35
Pakistan 577
Palaiologou, I. 495, 498
Palfrey, J. 44
pan-entertainment 540, 543

Panksepp, J. 125
Papacharissi, Z. 158
parenting 196, 250, 569; 'good' and 'bad' 320; learning apps 251, 253; nineteenth-century discourses 430; opportunities and risks 550; parental tools 5–6, 201; permissive 286; pregnancy and parenting apps 10, 393–402
parents: African 502, 506; best interests of children 311–312; child bereavement 481; child micro-celebrities 232–233; children's consumption 212; children's 'pestering power' 286; China 544; cyberbullying 466; digital citizenship 9, 339, 341–346; domestication of touchscreen technologies 3, 88, 89–94; educational use of *Minecraft* 148; haptic media habits 114, 117; ICTs used as babysitters 88; influence of 42, 60–61, 94; influencers 226, 235, 236–237, 241; media socialisation 332, 333, 334; mediation 195–197, 199, 201, 338–339, 492, 494, 551, 552, 556; parental tools 5–6, 195–203; possibility spaces 82; privacy issues 6–7, 235–242; response to the digital age 63–64; responsibilisation discourse 7, 245, 247, 248–251, 252–253; responsibilities 384; sexual risk 552, 556–558, 559; sharenting 6–7, 21, 221, 227, 235, 237–238, 241–242; surveillance by 5, 185–194; tweens in Brazil 268; UGC games 279; young children 493–495
Parisi, D. 117
Park, H. W. 503
participation 2, 12, 24, 38, 40–42, 44, 308; African children 505; children with disabilities 360; creativity 78; democratic 310, 516; digital citizenship 337, 346; fan communities 163, 165, 166; inequalities 437; ladder of 53, 302, 491; law 311, 321; moral agency 369; participatory culture 540, 543; participatory research methods 53–54, 277; policy 298–304; right to 343, 379, 381, 420, 527, 529–530, 535–537; sick children 416; street children 457; Sustainable Development Goals 384; television in Bangladesh 13, 527–528, 529, 530–535, 537; UGC games 282
partnership 33–34
passing-back 114
Pasupathi, M. 373–374
paternalism 316, 318, 319–320, 321
Paterson, Mark 190
Paul, Jake 227–228
PBS Kids 218
pedagogy: digital literacy 257; digital storytelling 470, 471; dynamic literacies 258; multiliteracies 472; parental responsibilisation 250–251; possibility thinking 77, 82; teacher training 496; 'third space' 259–260
Peekaboo Moments 239–240, 241
peer culture 370
peer-pressure 181, 182
Peeters, A. L. 96–97
Peppa Pig 59, 138–139, 545, 568

Pereira, Sara 4–5, 152–160
Peres-Cajías, Guadalupe 11, 449–459
performativity 262, 370
Perkel, Dan 41
personalisation: coding 68, 69; devices 378; marketing 287–288, 290, 291–292
persuasion knowledge 292
'pestering power' 286
Peter, J. 153, 157, 158, 175, 425
phatic communication 188
phenomenology 25, 112–113, 116
photo voice 25
photographs 51, 473, 474–476, 478, 518–519, 579; *see also* sexting
Phyfer, J. 491
Piaget, J. 286
Pink, Sarah 188
place 2, 38–39, 43–44, 152
platforms 2, 38, 39–40, 44, 568–569
play: child-created content 223–224; cognitive development 80, 93; collaborative 62, 191–192; digital 59, 60, 75, 80–83, 114, 144, 275; Games of Being Mobile project 186; methodological issues 49; possibility thinking 77, 79, 82; postdigital 83; right to 325, 381; toy industry 219
'playbour' 13, 545
playfulness 78, 192, 261
playground research 49–54, 260–261
Plowman, L. 59, 60, 62, 88, 142, 494
Plummer, K. 431
Pocket Watch 222–223
Podlas, K. 220
Pokémon Go 6, 209, 211–212, 213
police 353–354
policy 297–307, 337, 379, 380, 386–387, 542–543; *see also* law
political/relational model of disability 350
politics 309, 354, 419, 539, 545
Ponte, Cristina 7, 265–274
Popper, Ben 568
popular culture 53, 260, 275, 279
pornification 424, 429
pornography 19, 227, 298, 379, 425; anonymous communication 176; China 539, 545; gendered performance 429; online risks 550, 551–552, 553–554, 557–558, 559; tweens in Brazil 268; *see also* child pornography; sexual content
Portugal 12, 154–157, 158, 437, 492–498
possibility spaces 75–80, 82–83, 84
Post, D. G. 174
post-natal anxiety 398
postcolonialism 25
postdigital play 83
postfeminism 428
posthumanism 3, 23, 75, 78–82, 83, 84
poststructuralism 29, 429
Potter, John 7, 256–264
poverty 271, 381, 438, 439–440, 441, 443

power: bullying 464, 465; children with disabilities 360; digital storytelling 470; law 309; research ethics 30, 35; surveillance 187, 192
powerlessness 21
Poyntz, S. R. 25
pre-schoolers: digital literacy 491–499; grandparents 97; haptic interfaces 113; learning apps 7, 247–253; moving-image media 120–129; schoolification of education 246; touchscreen technologies 87–95; YouTube stars 6, 226–234
pre-sleep arousal 404, 406–407, 410
pregnancy 10, 237–238, 393–402
Prendella, Kate 359
Prensky, M. 44, 62, 435
pride 477
Primack, D. 581
privacy 6–7, 22–23, 235–244, 325, 370, 452; autistic children 353; digital citizenship 343; health information 414; learning apps 248, 250, 252–253; location-based marketing 289; marketing 288, 290, 291; moral agency 369, 371–372, 373; parental surveillance 6, 185, 190, 197, 199–200; right to 219, 381, 383, 420; self-disclosure 175; sick children 415, 416, 420; smart toys 379; social media 415; teens' sociability 157; tweens in Brazil 268, 270, 272
problem-solving 64, 72, 145, 437, 439–440, 443, 444
programming 67–74
Project Spark 278
prosumers 40
protection 310–311, 312–315, 316, 319, 529; China 540, 541, 546; digital citizenship 337; focus on 384; international cooperation 386; rights 309, 321, 325, 379, 420, 535
Prout, Alan 21–25, 26
provision rights 379, 420, 529, 535
Pruulmann-Vengerfeldt, P. 265–266
pseudonyms 174, 182
psychological control 196, 197, 201
psychometric paradigm 549
Pugh, A. J. 211

Qidian 539
Qun, W. 502

race: attainment gaps 469; discrimination 270, 272; inequalities 421; intersectionality 23; nineteenth-century discourses 430; online harassment 339; police brutality 354; sexualisation 521; sexuality 428; *see also* ethnicity
racism 430, 580, 581
radicalisation 301–302, 573, 575, 579, 581
Ragnedda, M. 504
Raskauskas, J. 173
reading 59, 61, 257, 405, 407, 494
reality television 219
Reddit 235
reflection 33–34

reflexivity 55, 262
refugees 11, 381, 384, 469–479
Reggio Emilia 29
Reginato, Lorena 10, 417–420
relational materialism 81
relational qualities 198
relationships: autistic children 349; fan communities 162–163, 165, 167–168, 170; siblings 142; sociability 152; young children 62
religion 267, 339, 577
remix 163, 165, 169–170, 277
Ren, Xiang 13, 539–548
Renn, O. 549
Renold, E. 53
reputation 19, 240, 371, 372, 373, 524
research: children with disabilities 360–361, 365; ethics 2, 28–37, 50; ethnographic 25; EU Kids Online 426; inequalities 436, 444–445; media socialisation 330–334; methodological issues 2, 48–56; sleep 410; young children and media 121–122
resilience 187, 314, 501
Resnick, M. 149
respect 35–36
respectful connectedness 185
responsibilisation 7, 198, 201, 245, 247, 248–251, 252–253
responsibilities 337, 343–344, 431
responsibility 372–373
restrictions 195–196, 197, 199, 494, 551; age 288, 298–299, 380, 543, 568; grandparental mediation 97, 102–104; parental surveillance 191–192
retargeting 287, 290
reverse socialisation 334
reward processing 407, 410
Reynolds, A. C. 406
Reza, S. M. Shameem 13, 527–538
Rezende, A. S. B. 268
Ribble, M. 492
Richards, Chris 2, 48–56
Richardson, Ingrid 5, 112, 113, 114, 116, 185–194, 394, 399
Riesmayer, Claudia 9, 327–336
right to be forgotten 240–241, 338, 420
right to be heard 298, 299, 300, 321, 381
rights 6, 8–9, 219, 358–359, 378–389; autonomy 308, 318, 321–322; children with disabilities 363–364, 365; children's capacity 314; claiming 324–325, 338–339; cultural 275, 282; dataveillance 223; digital citizenship 337, 342–343; due process 315–316; 'effects' paradigm 420; intellectual property 281–282; law 308–317, 319–322; meaning of the child 25; ownership 280; parental tools 201; participation in television 13, 527–528, 535; policy 299–301; privacy 240–241, 242, 369; protection 309, 321, 325, 379, 420, 535; research ethics 31, 35–36; school newspaper project 496, 497; sexual 10, 12–13, 428, 429, 431, 525; social

inequality 272; street children 457; Ubuntu 501; Youth Law Australia 518; *see also* United Nations Convention on the Rights of the Child
Rinaldi, C. 35
Ringland, K. E. 352
Ringrose, J. 520
risk 42, 261, 382–383; anonymous communication 177, 181, 182; children with disabilities 363; 'communication risk' approach 424; creativity 76; inequalities 43, 440; learning apps 249–250; moral agency 372–373; moving-image media 121; parental tools 201; responsibilisation discourse 252–253; sexual 13, 426–427, 549–561; street children 451, 452, 457; teens' sociability 158; tweens in Brazil 269
risk taking: parental tools 199–200; possibility thinking 77, 79, 82; self-disclosure 175
Robb, M. 564–565
Robinson, M. 122
Roblox 276, 278
robots 71, 145–147, 351, 352, 380
Rodman, G. 458
Roedder-John, D. 286
Romania 437
Rose, G. 451, 472
Rosenberg, M. B. 568
Ross, J. 520
Ross, N. J. 53
Rowe, D. 121
Rucker, T. 78
Runions, K. C. 466
Runnel, P. 265–266
Runswick-Cole, Katherine 360, 361
rural areas: Brazil 511, 512, 513, 514–515; inequalities 43, 436; teens' sociability 156–157
Ryan Toys Review (Ryan's World) 23, 218, 221–222, 223–224, 228, 236, 562, 563–564, 565

Safer Internet Programme 198
SafeToNet 199–200
safety 182, 383, 537; African children 501; Australian law 313–314; autistic children 353; China 545, 546; parental concerns 384; parental tools 199–200; responsibilisation discourse 252
Sagvari, B. 551
Saleh, A. 470
Sampaio, Inês Vitorino 7, 265–274
Samsung 117
Sandin, B. 208
Sandland, Ralph 364
Sarandos, Ted 218
SARF *see* social amplification of risk
scaffolding 82, 93
Scanlon, M. 245
Scarcelli, M. 429
Scarman, Lord 320
schedules 61

Schoenebeck, S. 237
Scholz, Trebor 22
schoolification 246
Schor, Juliet 22
Schouten, A. P. 158
Schroeder, Ralph 153, 158
Scott, H. 406
Scratch 68, 71, 73, 149
screen time: AAP guidelines 409; children with disabilities 363; grandparental mediation 98; measurement issues 409; moral panics 241, 363; physical activity 408–409; responsibilisation discourse 252; restriction of 191–192, 341; sleep 403, 405, 407, 408; surveys on 287; teens' sociability 156; UGC games 278
security 72, 240, 248, 253; *see also* safety
Sefton-Green, Julian 24, 25, 332, 491–492, 493, 495
Seiter, Ellen 22, 568
self-advocacy movement 350
self-awareness 182, 226, 232
self-care 400
self-determination 76, 77, 82, 192, 332
self-disclosure 158, 175, 182, 285, 291, 371–372, 452
self-esteem: adolescent identity development 174; cyberbullying 464–465; inequalities 437, 438, 439–440, 441–442, 443, 444; teens' sociability 158
self-expression 173, 324, 416, 469, 544, 546
self-harm 550
self-media 539
self-presentation 175, 270, 272, 414
self-regulation 369, 408
self-responsibility 373
self-socialisation 327, 328–329, 330–334
self-stimulation 352
self-tracking 398, 400
selfies 230, 519
Selman, R. L. 286
Selwyn, N. 58, 59, 62
sensory experience 117–118, 352
Sesame Street 122, 218, 251
sexism 430, 580, 581
sexting 12–13, 425–426, 427, 428, 518–526; moral agency 9, 371, 372, 373, 374
sexual abuse 379, 382, 427
sexual consent, age of 520
sexual content 314, 424–427, 431; anonymous communication 176; critical approaches 428–429; inequalities 440; online risks 13, 550, 551–559; *see also* pornography
sexual exploitation 314, 379, 382; Brazil 266; sexting 12–13, 519–525
sexual identity 371
sexualisation 227, 424, 426, 428, 430, 520, 521
sexuality 10, 314, 424–434; criminalisation of 522; critical approaches 428–429; discrimination 270; girls' video performances 54; inequalities 421; intersectionality 23; online harassment 339; right to 380

Index

Shade, Leslie Regan 22, 187
Shantanu, Fahmidul 528
Shao Yanjun 544
sharenting 6–7, 21, 221, 227, 235, 237–238, 241–242
Shaw, A. 277, 282
Shepherd, T. 519
Shin, Wonsun 8, 285–294
short video 539, 541–543, 545
siblings 4, 130–143, 192; child bereavement 481; consumer culture 210, 211; influence of 61; UGC games 279
sick children 414–423
Sieghart, Paul 325
Sierra Leone 505
sign making 49
Silseth, K. 471
Simmel, G. 152
Simões, J. A. 510
Simon, J. 154
Simpson, Brian 8–9, 308–317, 318–326, 425
Simun, M. 44
Singapore 226, 229
Singh, R. 187
Siraj-Blatchford, J. 62
situated child consumption 208, 214
skill inequalities 435–436, 437, 438–440, 444
Skouteris, H. 494
Skype 58, 90, 97, 131
sleep 10, 398, 403–413
Small, R. V. 492
'Smart Sock' 239, 241
smartphones 38, 39–40, 58, 87, 287; African children 504; Bangladesh 535; child-created content 217; child micro-celebrities 230; concerns about 351; domestication of touchscreen technologies 88–89, 90–91; grandparents 101, 105; haptic media habitus 111, 114; home life 59; inequalities 43, 45, 438–440, 442; moving-image media 123; parental surveillance 188, 189–190; parents 494; photography 518–519; pre-sleep arousal 406; prevalence 460; sexuality 430; street children 449–450; teens' sociability 157; tweens in Brazil 268, 272; YouTube 261; *see also* mobile technologies
Smith, Hannah 173
Smith, P. K. 98, 461
Smith, Simon 10, 403–413
Snapchat: age requirement 288; Muslim American children 576, 579, 581; popularity of 460; sick children 418; teens' sociability 155
sneaky-hat images 519
Snowden, Edward 394
Snyder, I. 150
Soares, S. 462
sociability 4–5, 152–160, 163, 414, 450
social amplification of risk (SARF) 549–550
social capital 502–503
social construction of childhood 20–21, 22, 23, 25, 48

social constructionism 80, 424, 429
social development 88
social justice 510
social learning 162, 163
social media 5, 19, 39–40, 261, 287, 308; adolescent identity development 174, 175; advertising 287–288, 290, 291–292; agency 220–221; anonymous platforms 182; autistic children 349; child micro-celebrities 226, 236; China 539; coding 68, 69–70, 73; concerns about 58; cyberbullying 460, 462; data 22; death and bereavement 485, 486; digital citizenship 381; fan communities 167; inequalities 44; 'infinite scroll' 408; influencers 221, 227, 236; legal discourse 325; marketing 8; media socialisation 333; moral agency 369; Muslim American children 576, 578; parental consent 318–319; place 38; play 261; policy 298–299; pre-sleep arousal 406; pregnancy and parenting 399; privacy 415; reward processing 407; right to be forgotten 240; sharenting 237–238; sick children 10, 414–423; street children 11, 449–459; surveillance 187, 189–191; teens' sociability 155, 158; tweens in Brazil 269, 270–271; *see also* Facebook; Instagram; Twitter; WhatsApp
social model of disability 349–350, 364
social narrative apps 350
social networking sites (SNS) 40, 41; anonymous communication 5, 173–174; mobile phones 287; teens' sociability 155, 157; *see also* social media
social networks 41–42, 509; companionship of 486; diasporic peoples 576; fan communities 161, 162, 163, 165, 166, 170; inequalities 512; street children 453, 458; tweens in Brazil 271
social skills 351, 414
social surveillance 187, 189
socialisation: autistic children 349, 350–351, 352–353, 354; consumer 286; definition of 328; media 9, 327–336; research as 53
sociality 348, 350, 352, 354, 374
socio-culturalism 29
socio-digital ecologies 444–445
socio-economic status: access to ICT 500; Africa 504; Brazil 266, 268, 269, 272; digital culture 267; Global Kids Online 513; inequalities 11, 43, 436, 437, 438–443, 444; influence on everyday experience 60; intersectionality 23; *see also* class
socio-emotional development 349, 350
socio-emotional skills 246, 337, 341–342, 345–346
sociology of childhood 21–25, 26, 48, 53, 265, 277, 426
software 100–101, 105
Solomon, Olga 350
sound recording 51
South Africa 501–502, 505
South African Kids Online 500, 501
South Korea 228–229, 393
space 302–303
Sparrman, A. 208

Spencer, Robert 580
Spigel, Lynn 223
Spotify 155, 353
Spyzie 199
Srnicek, N. 540
Stage, C. 420
Staksrud, Elisabeth 13, 541, 549–561
status 211
Steam 41
Steemers, J. 124
Stephen, Christine 2–3, 57–66, 88, 92
stereotypes 252, 523, 579, 580–581
sterilisation 311–312
Stevenson, Kylie J. 1–14, 75–86
stimulation hypothesis 152–153
Stoilova, M. 452
Stoltz, A. D. 173
Stone, Lawrence 20
storytelling: digital 11, 469–479; research ethics 33, 35
StoryVisit 97
strangers 550, 551
Street, Brian 257
street children 11, 449–459
stress 416, 418, 464–465
Styles, Harry 5, 164, 165, 166, 167, 169–170
subjectivity 23
substantive approach 63
suicide 173, 174, 182, 227, 322–324, 550
Super Mario Maker 276, 277–278, 281
supervision 97, 102, 103–104, 105; *see also* mediation
support, parental 196–197, 201
surveillance 5, 22, 185–194, 261, 343; children's rights 385; data 22–23; intimate 239; sexuality 522; *see also* dataveillance
Süss, D. 329
Sustainable Development Goals 384
Sweden 6, 207, 209–214, 339, 551
swiping 114–115, 140
Swist, T. 80, 420
Sylvestre, V. 457

tablets 38, 39, 87, 568–569; autistic children 353; children with disabilities 362; domestication of touchscreen technologies 89–94; engagement with 57–58; grandparents 101; haptic interfaces 111; home life 59; impact on sleep 405; mobility of 114; moving-image media 123; young children 494; YouTube 261; *see also* iPad; mobile technologies
Taddicken, Monika 452
Taipale, S. 152
Tanzania 504
Tao, L. 541
Target 222
Taylor, C. 369, 372, 373, 374
teachers 63–64, 493–495; Africa 506; Brazil 509–511, 515; digital game making in school 148–150; *Minecraft* 147–148; moving-image media 122; newspaper project 496–498; training 495–496, 498; *see also* education
technological determinism 19, 63, 64, 509
technology 39, 44, 386; affordances 197; dystopian view of 313; engagement with 57–58; home and school spaces 256; material culture 262; sociability 152
Technology and Play project 82
teenagers: Brazil 265; China 13, 539, 540–546; conceptualisation of children 310; digital media use 460; grandparents 97; illness 415; online fan communities 5, 161–172; parental surveillance 185, 188–190, 192; personal identity 371; sleep 403; sociability 4–5, 152–160; social media 287; *see also* adolescence
Teichert, L. 34
teleology 368
teleplasty 78, 81
television 39, 48, 121; autistic children 351–352; Bangladesh 13, 527–535, 537; children's programming 218; consumer culture 207; on demand 58; grandparents 98, 99, 100, 101, 102–103, 104, 105; mediation 96–97; reality 219; sexual content 554; social context of viewing 122–123; street children 450; teens' sociability 155; young children 121–124, 125–127, 493–494
Temer, Michel 266
Tencent 540, 545
Terranova, Tatiana 22
texting 1, 369, 485; *see also* sexting
texts 144, 145, 168–170, 247, 248, 492
Thangaperumal, P. 470
Theakstone, G. 500
thing-power 10, 395, 399, 400
Third, Amanda: African children 501, 503; barriers to connectivity 500; children with disabilities 359; cultural phenomenology 113, 116; differences 420; digital citizenship 301; global networks 518; haptic interfaces 116; intersubjectivity 368; protection 337; rights 9–10, 378–389, 535, 536
'third space' 259–260
Thomas, G. M. 399
Thomas, Jenny 387
Thompson, J. 50–51
Thorfinn, H. 529, 530
Tiilikainen, S. 130
Tik Tok 539, 541–543
time 152
Tinder 519
Tisdall, K. 302
Tobin, E. 520
Toddlers and Tablets project 3, 79, 82, 89–93
tokenism 302
Tomé, Vítor 12, 491–499
Tönnies, F. 502

touchscreen technologies: children's haptic media use 4, 111–112, 113, 114–118; domestication 3, 87–95; literacy activities 260; *see also* smartphones; tablets
Toutiao 545
Toyota 286
toys: child-created content 218, 221–223; children as consumers 285; converged play 81; data 22, 241; home life 59; Internet of Toys 82–83; smart 22, 379; toy industry 219; unboxing 13, 220–221, 562–571
tracking 22–23, 289, 290
trafficking 384, 452
transferable skills 72–73
transmedia learning 44
Transmedia Literacy project 154–157
transparency 6, 32, 301, 303
Treseder, P. 302
Trevarthen, C. 124
Tripp, D. 126
Trump, Donald 573, 579, 581
trust 199–200, 201
Tsaliki, Liza 10, 424–434
Turkey 393
Turkle, Sherry 40, 158
Turnbull, B. 122
tweens 5, 7, 265–274
Twitter 262; age requirement 288; China 545; fan communities 168, 169; Muslim American children 576, 578, 579, 581; sick children 418; teens' sociability 155; Trump 581

Ubuntu 501, 502
UGC *see* user-generated content
ultrasound images 237–238
unboxing 145–146, 209, 215n2, 220–221, 228, 236, 562–571
UNCRC *see* United Nations Convention on the Rights of the Child
UNESCO *see* United Nations Educational, Scientific and Cultural Organization
UNICEF *see* United Nations Children's Fund
United Kingdom: assessment-driven curriculum 258; Child Bereavement UK 481; children's viewing habits 123; dataveillance 394; digital resilience 314; Early Years Foundation Stage 246; *Gillick* competence 319, 320–321; inequalities 437–444; informal learning 256; internet use 287; parents 60; pornography 298; sexting 523, 524; sexualisation 426; suicides 174; Technology and Play project 82; television 39; Toddlers and Tablets project 3, 79, 82, 89–93
United Nations Children's Fund (UNICEF) 297, 379; Africa 500–501, 502, 504; Bangladesh 529, 536; Brazil 271; inequalities 43; rights 530
United Nations Committee on the Rights of the Child (CRC) 299–300, 337, 379–380, 385, 387
United Nations Convention on the Rights of Persons with Disabilities (CRPD) 363–364
United Nations Convention on the Rights of the Child (UNCRC) 1, 8, 9–10, 299, 316, 378–388, 420; children's capacity 321; discursive bias 23; General Comment 10, 299–300, 337, 379–380, 384–386, 387–388; implementation 383–386; Lundy's work 302–303; participation 13, 298, 527, 529–530, 535–537; privacy 240; research ethics 2, 31, 33; sexual exploitation 519; US non-ratification 6
United Nations Educational, Scientific and Cultural Organization (UNESCO) 337, 338
United States: bullying 461–462; Center for Digital Democracy 338; child labour 218–220, 226; child micro-celebrities 229; children as consumers 285; children's media consumption 48; coding study 68–69; cyberbullying 462, 465; dataveillance 394; digital media use 510–511; internet use 287; juvenile justice 315; makerspaces 83; media literacy education 258; Muslim children 13–14, 572–583; National Alliance for Grieving Children 481; participation 41; pregnancy and parenting apps 393; reading 59; sexting 371, 425, 521, 523; sexuality 425, 426; smartphone use 39, 287; social media surveillance 187; social media use 39; suicides 174; toy unboxing 562, 565
universal child 23
urban areas 43, 156–157, 511, 512, 514–515
Uruguay 512–513
user experience (UX) design 112, 115–116, 117
user-generated content (UGC) 7, 275–284; *see also* content creation

Vaala, S. 247
Valkenburg, Patti M. 42, 96–97, 153, 157, 158, 175, 425
values 20, 63, 64; China 545; media socialisation 331, 333, 334; moral agency 374; online risks 550; social ties 502
Van Bauwel, S. 428, 430
van den Bulck, J. 329
Van der Velden, M. 415
van Dijk, J. 512, 514, 516
van Kruistum, C. 64
Van Leeuwen, Karla 5–6, 195–203
van Leeuwen, T. 470
van Steensel, R. 64
Vanden Abeele, M. M. P. 153
Vanobbergen, B. 250
Vásquez, C. 175
Veenstra, A. S. 576
Velasco, Marcela Losantos 11, 449–459
Verenikina, I. 61
Verizon Wireless 40
Vetere, F. 223
Viacom 223

video: data collection 49–50, 51–52; on demand 58; filmmaking 260; moving-image media 122; participatory research 54; school newspaper project 497–498; sexual content 554; short video in China 539, 541–543, 545; teaching practices 494; Toddlers and Tablets project 89; toy unboxing 562–571; tweens in Brazil 269, 271; *see also* moving images; YouTube
Vimeo 40
Vincent, C. 247
Vincent, J. 269
Vinogradova, P. 471
violence 227, 339, 381, 522, 536, 539
virtual goods 289–290
virtual reality (VR) 350–351
virtual worlds 79, 147–148, 208–209, 210–211
visibility 363, 364, 373
visual ethnography 50
visual meaning-making 472
visual resources 35
vlogging 218, 219, 221, 230, 542
voice 31, 35, 297, 302–303, 457, 516
VR *see* virtual reality
Vromen, A. 301, 304
Vygotsky, L. S. 3, 75, 76, 80

Wainryb, C. 373–374
Walczer, Jarrod 13, 562–571
Wall, J. 369, 374
Walmart 222
Wang, J. 462
Wang, W. 289
Wartella, E. 564–565
Wasko, J. 208
Wästerfors, D. 361
Wattpad 168–169
wearable devices 239, 351, 353, 393
Webkinz 208
websites: coding 70, 71, 73; commercial imperatives 42; grandparents 100–101; parental tools 196, 199; retargeting 287; *see also* internet
WeChat 262
Weinshenker, Daniel 478
Weiss, G. 222
well-being: benefits of digital media 414; China 541, 545; collective 502; death and bereavement 485; digital socialisation 352; inequalities 443, 444; International Early Learning and Child Well-being Study 246; marketing impact on 286, 291; moving-image media 120; pregnancy and parenting apps 393, 398, 399–400; responsibilisation discourse 252; sexting 524; sick children 417, 421; sleep 403, 408, 409; social 370; UNCRC 530
Western perspective 23

What to Expect When You're Expecting 396
WhatsApp 262, 382; Brazil 509; fan communities 168; street children 449; teens' sociability 155; tweens in Brazil 269–270
Whitehouse, Anna 236–237
wi-fi: Brazilian schools 508, 510, 511, 514, 516; inequalities 438; tweens in Brazil 268, 272
Wilken, R. 112
Willett, Rebekah 2, 48–56, 208, 213–214, 276, 338
Williams, Chris M. 222
Williams, R. A. 309
Williamson, B. 223
Willson, Michele 346, 362
Wing, J. M. 67–68
Wohlwend, K. 81
Wojciechowski, H. C. 126
Wojdynski, B. W. 292
Wolak, J. 425, 520
women: apps for pregnancy and motherhood 10, 393–402; internet use 43; learning apps 248, 252, 253; Muslim 580; sexting 425, 523, 524; social model of disability 349–350; *see also* feminism; gender
Wonder Weeks 396, 397
Wong, Suzanna So Har 4, 144–151
Woods, H. C. 406
Woolley, J. D. 127
WordPress 262
Words With Friends 188–189

Xi Jinping 541
Xiang, Y. 540–541
Xiaxue 229, 231–232

Yang, L. 289
Yang, Z. 504
Ye Bin 228, 229–230, 232, 233
Youngswood, Steve 218
Youth Law Australia 518
YouTube: adult concerns 23; autistic children 352, 353, 354; *CarecaTV* 10, 417–420; child-created content 6, 217, 218, 219–220, 221–224, 236; children's use of touchscreen interfaces 115; coding 382; consumer culture 209, 212–214; death and bereavement 481, 482–484; digital play 59; digital storytelling 473–474; 'ElsaGate' Scandal 568; as a global firm 566; HTML 70; inequalities 44; Israel 98; marketing 8; playground games 260–261; *Pokémon Go* 211; popularity of 460; pre-school stars 6, 226–234; prosumers 40; sibling interactions 138–139; sick children 416; social networks 24; Steam platform 41; Sweden 207; teens' sociability 155; toy unboxing 13, 562, 563, 564–565, 566–569; tweens in Brazil 7, 271–272; UGC games 278, 281; young children

123, 493–494; YouTube Kids 218, 481, 562, 564–565, 568
Yuan, L. 545

Zaman, Bieke 5–6, 195–203, 495
Zarouali, B. 290
Zehle, S. 117

Zelizer, Vivian 20–21, 219
Zhang, Q. 289
Zhang, Tony Boming 3, 67–74
Zhao, E. J. 546
Zhu Wei 542
Zinnecker, J. 329

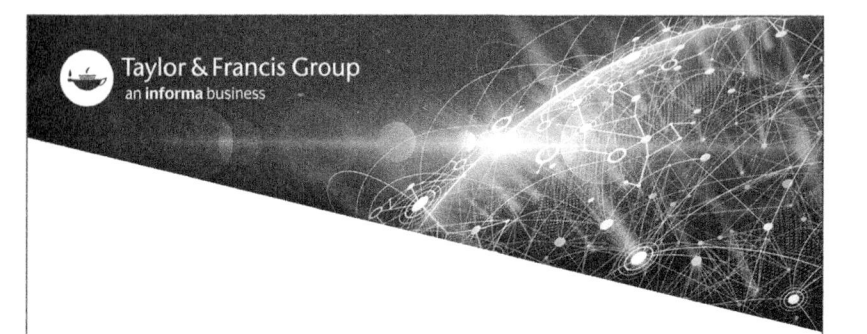

Printed in Great Britain
by Amazon